MULTIDISCIPLINARY MANAGEMENT OF FEMALE PELVIC FLOOR DISORDERS

Commissioning Editor: Rebecca Gaertner
Development Editors: Hilary Hewitt and Claire Bonnett
Project Manager: Rory MacDonald
Designer: Andy Chapman
Illustrators: Sandie Hill, Gillian Lee and Richard Morris
Marketing Managers (UK/USA): Brant Emery/Lisa Damico

MULTIDISCIPLINARY MANAGEMENT OF FEMALE PELVIC FLOOR DISORDERS

Edited by

Christopher R Chapple BSc MD FRCS(Urol)
Professor of Urology, The Royal Hallamshire Hospital & Sheffield Hallam University, Sheffield, UK

Philippe E Zimmern MD FACS
Professor of Urology, Director, Bladder and Incontinence Treatment Center,
Department of Urology, University of Texas Southwestern Medical School, Dallas, TX, USA

Linda Brubaker MD MS
Assistant Dean for Clinical and Translational Research, Professor, Department of Obstetrics and Gynecology
Director and Fellowship Director, Division of Female Pelvic Medicine and Reconstructive Surgery,
Loyola University Medical Center, Maywood, IL, USA

Anthony R B Smith MD FRCOG
Consultant Gynaecologist, Department of Urological Gynaecology, Saint Mary's Hospital for Women and Children,
Manchester, UK

Kari Bø PT PhD
Professor of Exercise Science, Norwegian School of Sport Sciences, Oslo, Norway

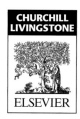

CHURCHILL LIVINGSTONE

ELSEVIER

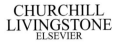

CHURCHILL
LIVINGSTONE
ELSEVIER

An imprint of Elsevier Inc.

ISBN-13: 978–0–443–07272–7
ISBN-10: 0–443–07272–8
   Reprinted 2007

British Library Cataloguing in Publication Data
A catalogue record for this book is available from the British Library

Library of Congress Cataloging in Publication Data
A catalog record for this book is available from the Library of Congress

Notice
Medical knowledge is constantly changing. Standard safety precautions must be followed but as new research and clinical experience broaden our knowledge, changes in treatment and drug therapy may become necessary or appropriate. Readers are advised to check the most current product information provided by the manufacturer of each drug to be administered to verify the recommended dose, the method and duration of administration, and contraindications. It is the responsibility of the practitioner, relying on experience and knowledge of the patient, to determine dosages and the best treatment for each individual patient. Neither the Publisher nor the author assumes any liability for any injury and/or damage to persons or property arising from this publication.

The Publisher

Printed in China
Last digit is the print number: 9   8   7   6   5   4   3   2

Contents

Section 8: Fistula

Section 9: Intraoperative Injury

Section 10: Congenital Abnormalities of the Female Genital Tract

Section 11: Irritative Conditions of the Genitourinary Tract

Section 12: Neurogenic Bladder

Section 13: Statistics

List of Contributors

Cindy L Amundsen MD
Associate Professor of Obstetrics and
Gynecology
Division of Urogynecology
Duke University Medical Center
Durham, NC, USA

Karl-Erik Andersson MD PhD
Professor of Clinical Pharmacology
Lund University Hospital
Lund, Sweden

Kari Bø PT PhD
Professor of Exercise Science
Norwegian School of Sport Sciences
Oslo, Norway

Timothy B Boone MD PhD
Russell and Mary Hugh Scott Professor and
Chairman
Scott Department of Urology
Baylor College of Medicine
Houston, TX, USA

Muriel K Boreham MD
Assistant Professor of Obstetrics and
Gynecology
University of Texas Southwestern Medical
Center
Dallas, TX, USA

Linda Brubaker MD MS
Assistant Dean for Clinical and Translational
Research
Professor, Department of Obstetrics and
Gynecology
Director and Fellowship Director, Division of
Female Pelvic Medicine and Reconstructive
Surgery,
Loyola University Medical Center
Maywood, IL, USA

**Christopher R Chapple BSc MD
FRCS(Urol)**
Professor of Urology
The Royal Hallamshire Hospital & Sheffield
Hallam University
Sheffield, UK

C Sage Claydon MD
Assistant Professor of Obstetrics and
Gynecology
Division of Female Pelvic Medicine and
Reconstruction
Brody School of Medicine
East Carolina University
Greensville, NC, USA

Firouz Daneshgari MD
Director
Center for Female Pelvic Medicine and
Reconstructive Surgery
Cleveland, OH, USA

Donna Deng MD
Clinical Instructor
Reconstructive and Female Urology
David Geffen School of Medicine at UCLA
Los Angeles, CA, USA

Naresh V Desireddi MD
Department of Urology
Feinberg School of Medicine
Northwestern University
Chicago, IL, USA

Roger R Dmochowski MD FACS
Professor of Urologic Surgery
Vanderbilt University Medical Center
Nashville, TN, USA

Catherine E DuBeau MD
Associate Professor of Medicine
Section of Geriatrics
Department of Medicine
University of Chicago
Chicago, IL, USA

Michael K Flynn MD MHS
Assistant Professor of Obstetrics and
Gynecology
University of Rochester
Rochester, NY, USA

Jason P Gilleran MD
University of Texas at Southwestern Medical
Center at Dallas
Urology, Dallas, TX, USA

Noelani M Guaderrama MD
Department of OBGYN, Female Pelvic
Medicine and Reconstructive Surgery
Southern California Permante Medical
Group
Irvine, CA, USA

Adam P Klausner MD
Assistant Professor of Urology Research
Department of Urology
University of Virginia Health Science Center
Charlottesville, VA, USA

Gary E Lemack MD
Associate Professor of Urology
Residency Program Director
University of Texas Southwestern Medical
Center
Dallas, TX, USA

Malcolm Lucas MD
Consultant Urological Surgeon
Swansea NHS Trust
Morriston Hospital
Swansea, UK

Courtenay Moore MD
Fellow
Glickman Urological Institute
Cleveland, OH, USA

Charles W Nager MD
Professor
Department of Reproductive Medicine
Division of Female Pelvic Medicine and
Reconstructive Surgery
University of California, San Diego
La Jolla, CA, USA

Christine Norton PhD MA RN
Professor of Gastrointestinal Nursing,
King's College London
Nurse Consultant,
St Mark's Hospital,
Harrow, Middlesex, UK

Andrew Pickersgill MD
Consultant Obstetrician and Gynaecologist
Stepping Hill Hospital
Stockport, UK

Christina J Poon MD
Clinical Instructor
Lions' Gate Hospital
Vancouver, BC, Canada

Shlomo Raz MD
Professor of Urology
Co-Director, Division of Female Urology,
Reconstructive Surgery and Urodynamics
University of California Los Angeles
Los Angeles, CA, USA

Larissa Rodriguez MD
Assistant Professor of Urology
Reconstructive and Female Urology
David Geffen School of Medicine at UCLA
Los Angeles, CA, USA

Matthew P Rutman MD
Assistant Director of Urology
Co-Director of Incontinence, Voiding
Dysfunction and Urodynamics
Department of Urology
Columbia University
New York, NY, USA

Harriette M Scarpero MD
Assistant Professor of Urologic Surgery
Vanderbilt University Medical Center
Nashville, TN, USA

Anthony J Schaeffer MD
Department of Urology
Feinberg School of Medicine
Northwestern University Medical School
Chicago, IL, USA

Joseph I Schaffer MD
Associate Professor of Obstetrics and
Gynecology
Chief of Gynecology
Director, Division of Urogynecology and
Reconstructive Pelvic Surgery
University of Texas Southwestern Medical
Center
Dallas, TX, USA

Anthony R B Smith MD FRCOG
Consultant Gynaecologist
Department of Urological Gynaecology
Saint Mary's Hospital for Women and
Children
Manchester, UK

William D Steers MD
Hovey Dabney Professor and Chair
Department of Urology
University of Virginia
Charlottesville, VA, USA

**Richard Turner-Warwick CBE FRCP
FRCS FRCOG**
Emeritus Consultant
The Middlesex Hospital & Institute of
Urology
London, UK

Clifford Y Wai MD
Assistant Professor of Obstetrics and
Gynecology
University of Texas Southwestern Medical
Center
Dallas, TX, USA

Kristene E Whitmore MD
Professor of Surgery, Urology and OBGYN
Drexel University
Philadelphia, PA, USA

Philippe E Zimmern MD FACS
Professor of Urology
Director, Bladder and Incontinence
Treatment Center
Department of Urology
University of Texas Southwestern Medical
School
Dallas, TX, USA

Preface

Three years ago Philippe Zimmern and I asked ourselves the question is there a role for yet another book looking at female urology and disorders of the female pelvic floor? We carefully reviewed existing publications and decided that there was a potential role for just such a book targeted at clinicians of all disciplines interested in this sub-specialty area. With this in mind we felt it was important to critically review all of the important areas within the sub-specialty using a multi-disciplinary approach. Thereby making this an internationally applicable book, which will be useful to clinicians with all levels of interest, experience and expertise. As you will see the sections on both urinary and fecal incontinence are written by experts from many disciplines, covering these topics in detail in what we hope to be a very readable and interesting style.

We hope that you will agree with the fundamental ethos of this book that the multi-disciplinary approach to management is not only preferable but also essential to achieve the best results for our patients.

Christopher R Chapple
Philippe E Zimmern
2006

Foreword

In the past decade there has been a long overdue recognition that collaboration between urologists, obstetrician-gynecologists, colon and rectal surgeons, physiotherapists, physiologists, pharmacologists, and nurse practitioners is essential if we are to enhance our care of women with disorders of the pelvic floor. The editors of *Multidisciplinary Management of Female Pelvic Floor Disorders* have assembled an experienced, well balanced group of authors from various disciplines as well as geographically diverse institutions to share their own knowledge of these frequently inter-related disorders.

The format of the book is logical, beginning with the recognition that we must understand normal anatomy and physiology of the pelvic floor before dealing with the abnormal and progressing from diagnosis and management eventually to a review of statistics for the clinician.

The readers will appreciate the balanced approach to treatment options. Women with disorders of the pelvic floor can not all be managed in a standardized fashion. Some complaints are best managed non-surgically and others, such as fistulas, may always require surgical intervention for ultimate cure. The editors have purposefully provided a comprehensive approach to patient care, recognizing that only the patient and her personal doctor should make the ultimate decision regarding management.

One of the hidden treasures in such a comprehensive text authored by a diverse group of people is the set of bibliographies following all chapters. The truly curious reader will find an endless source of references not only to classic but also to current literature.

Personally, I have had a long interest in caring for women with disorders of the pelvic floor. My patients and I have regularly benefited from the on-going work of the men and women who have edited and contributed to this text. The women of the world owe a debt of gratitude to the editors and contributors not only for their past work but to their commitment to providing us this comprehensive, up to date resource.

Bob L Shull MD
Professor of Obstetrics and Gynecology
Texas A&M University Health Science Centers
Scott & White Clinic and Hospital
Temple, TX, USA

At first glance this text might seem to be just another addition to the ever increasing library of texts dealing with portions of what is termed "female urology" or "urogynecology," depending on ones specialty. It is, however, considerably more than that. The well respected editorial board, consisting of 2 urologists, 2 urogynecologists and an expert in pelvic floor physiotherapy, has put together a veritable handbook for a fellowship in female pelvic medicine and reconstructive surgery. Each subject encompassed in this area, with the possible exception of female sexual dysfunction, is covered in a succinct but authoritative manner by a carefully chosen roster of authors. The result, in my opinion, is a comprehensive text which will give the reader a working knowledge of the pertinent concepts and current data in each area and provide a basis on which to build an individual library or reference file in those areas. Fellows and residents will find the text extremely useful, as will those urologists and gynecologists whose practices are concentrated in this area. If one took each of the 30 chapters and constructed 2 teaching conferences around each, one would have a very impressive and nearly complete curriculum for female pelvic medicine and reconstructive surgery.

Alan J Wein MD PhD(Hon)
Professor and Chair of the Division of Urology
University of Pennsylvania Health System
Philadelphia, PA, USA

SECTION 1

Anatomy

Pelvic Anatomy for the Surgeon

Harriette M Scarpero and Roger R Dmochowski

INTRODUCTION

Significant advancements in computer and imaging technology in recent years have enabled more realistic rendering of human pelvic anatomy. Magnetic resonance imaging (MRI) has provided unsurpassed soft tissue visualization and the ability to see structures in several spatial planes. Dynamic MRI offers the opportunity to see anatomic structures altered by intraabdominal pressure and provides clarification of the contents of the prolapse in unclear cases (Fig. 1.1). Using interactive rotation of the three-dimensional (3D) model of the human pelvis, as well as cine films of the pelvic floor and portions of the lower urinary tract (LUT) during straining and relaxation, we may also improve our understanding of the pathophysiologic mechanisms of stress incontinence.[1] Computed tomography (CT) images can be reconstructed in three dimensions, creating images of greater definition and realism. Just as simulators have become standard in the fields of aviation and aerospace, virtual reality models of the human may replace cadavers in the gross anatomy laboratory.

This chapter will highlight some of these new areas of anatomic research as well as review pelvic anatomy and the surgical relevance of key anatomic structures. For the purpose of this chapter, pelvic anatomy is divided into three main areas: pelvic musculature, ligaments and fascia, and neurovascular supply to the pelvic organs.

THE PELVIC FLOOR

The term "pelvic floor" refers to more than just the muscles that support the pelvic viscera. The viscera are actually a component of it. The entity of the "pelvic floor" includes the pelvic viscera, the peritoneum overlying it, endopelvic fascia, levator ani muscles, coccygeus, obturator internus, piriformis, and perineal membrane.[2] The muscles, associated fascia and ligaments and the fascial attachments of the viscera work in concert to support the contents of the abdominopelvic cavity. The load carried by the pelvic floor is shared by all its components. Damage to the pelvic muscles by injury, disease or surgery increases the load on the fascia and vice versa.

Points of origin and insertion of pelvic muscles are on the bony pelvis which can therefore be considered the foundation on which the pelvic floor is built. Areas of interest to the pelvic surgeon on the bony pelvis include the pubic symphysis, pubic rami, ischial spines, ischial tuberosities, and coccyx. The sacrospinous ligaments attach to the ischial spines. Extending laterally from the spines is the arcus tendineus that attaches anteriorly to the lower pubic bone. Near its pubic end, the arcus tendineus splits into two portions: the tendinous arch of the pelvic fascia from which the pubocervical fascia arises, and the tendinous arch of the

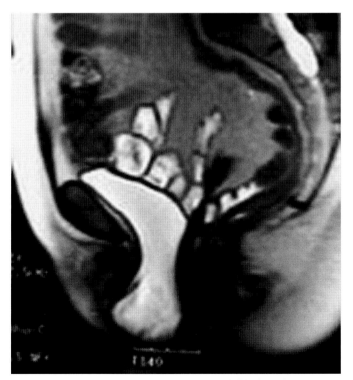

Figure 1.1 A sagittal image from a dynamic MRI of the female pelvis during Valsalva maneuver. A prominent cystocele is identified as the contents of the anterior compartment prolapse.

levator ani from which the levator ani muscles arise. These areas are pertinent landmarks for many of our common transvaginal and transabdominal procedures. Being familiar with the location of these bony structures will direct the surgeon toward other structures of importance such as ligaments and help prevent inadvertent injury to structures in close proximity such as the ureter or neurovascular bundles.

PELVIC MUSCULATURE

The muscles of the pelvic floor consist of a group collectively known as the levator ani and the coccygeus. The levator ani muscles are known separately as the pubococcygeus (PC), iliococcygeus, and puborectalis. These muscles take their names from their points of origin on the pelvis. They extend together as an expansive sheet from the inner surface of the pubic bone, just lateral to the symphysis, to the pelvic surface of the ischial spines (Fig. 1.2). At the pelvic side wall, the levator ani are attached to the arcus tendineus. Posteriorly, they extend from their origin on both sides and travel medially to a midline raphe between the rectum and coccyx. Physiologic studies have demonstrated that the levator ani exhibit constant activity which allows them to work as a functional shelf in support of the pelvic viscera.[3]

The pubococcygeus is the most medial of the group. From its origin at the pubis, it surrounds the vagina medial to it and may have attachments to the urethra. In the posterior pelvis it surrounds the anus between the internal and external sphincters. Histochemical analysis of the PC muscles has identified both slow-twitch and fast-twitch fibers indicating that the muscle works to provide static visceral support as well as maintaining tone and active closure of urethra, vagina, and rectum.[4] These muscles are the ones contracted during a Kegel exercise, so their strength can be assessed at least subjectively by palpation while the patient contracts the muscle. The PC muscles have a role in sexual function as well. Tension or spasm in these muscles has been implicated in the painful disorder of vaginismus as well as the pleasurable rhythmic contractions during orgasm.

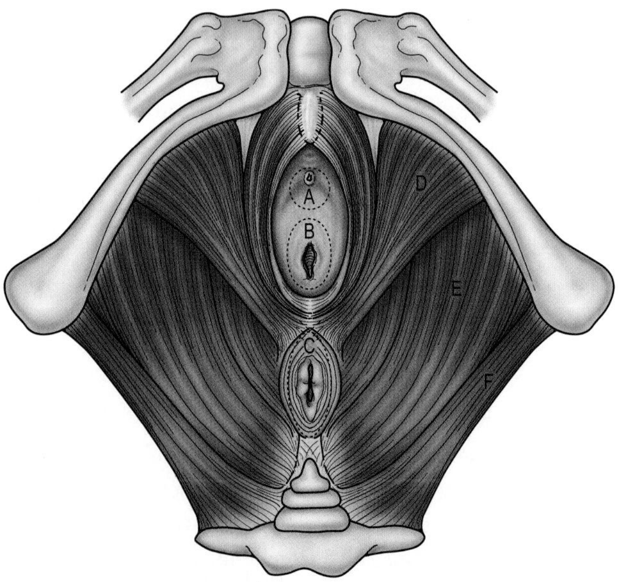

The origin of the iliococcygeus is the posterior portion of the tendinous arch and ischial spine. From either side of the pelvis, they join into a midline raphe just above the anal–coccygeal body. The puborectalis is more medial than the iliococcygeus, originates at the posterior surface of the pubis and inserts at the midline to the rectum. On contraction, this muscle is pulled toward its pubic attachment, effectively closing the proximal anal canal. It further aids anal continence by maintaining the anorectal angle. There are two areas of discontinuity within the levator ani known as the urogenital hiatus anteriorly and the anorectal hiatus posteriorly. The vagina and urethra traverse the more anterior hiatus and the rectum passes through the posterior hiatus.

The levator ani muscles share in the mechanisms of defecation and urination as well as visceral support. Levator dysfunction as a result of vaginal delivery may lead to loss of pelvic organ support, as well as constipation or fecal and urinary incontinence. A test of levator ani muscle response to stimulation measured by EMG found diminished response at rest and on contraction in multiparous women with a prolonged second stage of labor.[5]

The coccygeus muscle, which is continuous with the iliococcygeus anteriorly, originates at the ischial spines and sacrospinous ligament and then inserts on the lateral sacrum and coccyx. These attachments give it a triangular configuration. The coccygeus is more posterior than the levator ani and overlies the sacrospinous ligaments.

The obturator muscles, typically considered as muscles of the lower extremity, are nonetheless intimately connected to the muscles of the pelvic floor. They compose the lateral pelvis or pelvic side walls. Their origin is the internal surface of the obturator membrane, posterior bony margins of the obturator foramen, the pubic rami, and ramus of the ischium. They insert into the medial surface of the greater trochanter of the femur. The arcus tendineus fascia pelvis or "white line" that has been previously described is a condensation of obturator fascia and endopelvic fascia. This pelvic landmark may be attenuated or torn, contributing to a defect in anterior compartment support. The obturator foramen within the bony pelvis and the associated obturator canal within the muscle are other important landmarks. The obturator neurovascular bundle runs through these openings and is of particular concern in a newer variant of the midurethral polypropylene sling known as the transobturator tape.

Figure 1.2 The levator ani muscles and levator hiatuses. **A,** urethra; **B,** urogenital hiatus; **C,** rectal hiatus; **D,** pubococcygeus; **E,** iliococcygeus; **F,** coccygeus (adapted from Wahle GR, Young GPH, Raz S. Anatomy and pathophysiology of pelvic support. In: Raz S, ed. Female urology. Philadelphia: WB Saunders; 1996).

The piriformis, which lies in the same plane as the coccygeus, arises from the sacrum and inserts on the greater trochanter. It has special significance because the sacral plexus lies on top of it on its course beneath the coccygeus.

Perineal membrane. Below the levator ani is the perineal membrane which is a dense triangular area of fascia in the anterior half of the pelvic outlet. It arises from the inferior ischiopubic rami and attaches medially to the urethra, vagina, and perineal body. Like the levators above, it is pierced by the vagina and urethra. Some authors refer to the perineal membrane as the urogenital diaphragm but this term is incorrect. As classically described, a true urogenital diaphragm, consisting of two layers of fascia enclosing the deep transverse perineal muscle and sphincter urethrae and creating a closed compartment, does not exist.[6]

Perineum. The anatomy of the perineum is important to any discussion of the pelvic floor because these muscles lie beneath the muscles of the pelvic floor, and reconstruction of the perineum may be undertaken along with pelvic prolapse surgery. Commonly, the anatomy of the perineum is described as being divided into an upper urogenital triangle and a lower anal triangle. The points of the triangle are the pubic symphysis, ischial tuberosity, and tip of coccyx. A line through the anterior ischial tuberosities forms the shared base of the two triangles.

The perineal body is a tendinous structure located midline between the anus and vagina. It is the central fixation point of the perineum. The muscles of the urogenital triangle include the median bulbocavernosus, right and left ischiocavernosus, and superficial transverse perineal muscle (Fig. 1.3). The bulbospongiosus muscle surrounds the vaginal introitus and covers the lateral part of the vestibular bulbs. It also attaches to the corpora of the clitoris

and the perineal body. The ischiocavernosus muscle covers the crura of the clitoris. The superficial transverse perineal muscle extends from the ischial tuberosity to the perineal body. It can be poorly developed or absent. A deep transverse perineal muscle originates at the ramus of the ischium and joins the urethral and anal sphincters as well as the perineal body. The ischiorectal fossa is a wedge-shaped space in the anal triangle between the levator ani and obturator internus. This anatomic space is important because of its relationship to the pudendal neurovascular bundle. The internal pudendal vessels and nerve are within the lateral wall of the ischiorectal fossa and the obturator internus muscle. The fascial sheath covering this space creates the pudendal or Alcock's canal.

PELVIC FASCIA AND LIGAMENTS

There is often confusion regarding the divisions and naming of various portions of the pelvic fascia known as endopelvic fascia. The fascia investing the levator ani may be referred to separately as the levator fascia. The levator–endopelvic fascia can be subdivided further into the pubourethral ligaments, urethropelvic ligaments, pubocervical fascia, and uterosacral ligament complex (Fig. 1.4). These subdivisions help to distinguish the importance of the fascia for specific support roles.

Many structures commonly referred to as ligaments are really condensations of levator fascia, so they differ from the tough connective tissue composing ligament elsewhere in the body. As visceral ligaments, these condensations are just loosely organized connective tissue, containing considerable amounts of smooth muscle.[7] The fibers of visceral ligaments are far less regular than the fibers of true ligaments. The pubourethral ligaments are the fascial support of the midurethra to the inner surface of the inferior pubis. They

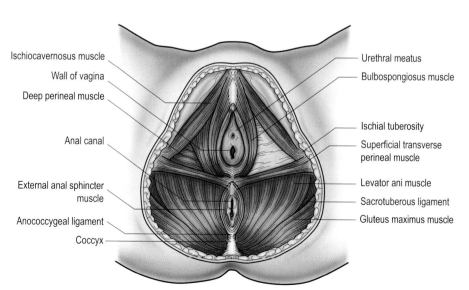

Ischiocavernosus muscle
Wall of vagina
Deep perineal muscle
Anal canal
External anal sphincter muscle
Anococcygeal ligament
Coccyx

Urethral meatus
Bulbospongiosus muscle
Ischial tuberosity
Superficial transverse perineal muscle
Levator ani muscle
Sacrotuberous ligament
Gluteus maximus muscle

Figure 1.3 Muscles of the perineum (from DeLancey JO, Richardson AC. Anatomy of genital support. In: Benson JT, ed. Female pelvic floor disorders. New York: WW Norton; 1992).

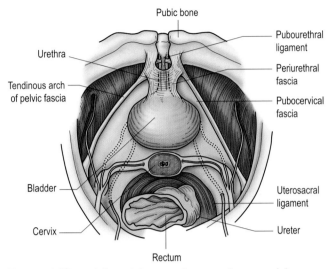

Pubic bone

Urethra

Tendinous arch
of pelvic fascia

Bladder

Cervix

Rectum

Pubourethral
ligament

Periurethral
fascia

Pubocervical
fascia

Uterosacral
ligament

Ureter

Figure 1.4 View of the pelvic musculature and some pelvic organs in relation to the fascial layers of the pelvic floor.

support and stabilize the urethra and anterior vaginal wall. The external sphincter is located just distal to these ligaments. They have been examined grossly and histologically and found to be very consistent structures that demonstrate dense collagen fibers.[8] Laxity or failure of these ligaments is partially responsible for stress urinary incontinence (SUI) as described by the integral theory.[9] The midurethral sling reconstitutes these structures to restore continence. The urethra is also supported on both sides by levator fascia. Proximally this lateral urethral support is termed the urethropelvic ligaments which are the endopelvic fascia that fuses the periurethral fascia to the arcus tendineus. It is the major support for the bladder neck and proximal urethra. Again, these areas are contiguous and not truly distant structures. They are specialized areas of the endopelvic fascia.

Urethral support is not determined by fascia alone. The pelvic muscles are also responsible. The fascial attachments responsible for urethral support are those of the pubourethral ligaments, periurethral tissue, and anterior vaginal wall to arcus tendineus fascia pelvis (paravaginal fascial attachment) (see Fig. 1.4). The muscular component is the connection of periurethral tissues to the levator ani muscles. When these attachments are intact, continence is maintained. During increased abdominal pressure, the urethra is compressed against this firm supportive layer as explained by the "hammock theory" of continence.[10] Weakening of these supports can lead to anterior wall relaxation and diminishment of the occlusive action of the vaginal support.

Connective tissue disorders have been implicated as a cause and/or contributor to significant pelvic organ prolapse.[11] It may also be possible that aging and hormonal changes associated with menopause may alter the composition and strength of connective tissue.[12-14] Immunohistochemical staining of periurethral fascia from continent and incontinent postmenopausal women with pelvic organ prolapse demonstrated differences and reductions of the types of collagen found in incontinent women compared to continent. The investigators theorize that these alterations indicate an alteration in metabolism of connective tissue in the periurethral region leading to a significant decrease in collagen in postmenopausal women.[15] In a study to assess whether menopause was associated with connective tissue weakening, the uterosacral ligament resilience was assessed in hysterectomy specimens. It was significantly reduced with vaginal delivery, menopause, and older age.[16]

The genital tract (ovary, uterus, cervix, and vagina) is attached on each side to the pelvic side walls by endopelvic fascia. In relation to a specific organ, the fascia is often referred to as the mesentery of the organ. The mesenteries not only support the organs but also carry their blood supply. The mesentery of the ovary containing its vascular pedicle is found at its craniolateral aspect and is known as the infundibulopelvic ligament. Other mesenteries referred to as ligaments include the broad ligament which, as the name implies, is a wide expansive ligament on either side of the uterus that attaches to the pelvic side wall. The broad ligament contains the fallopian tubes, ligament of the ovaries and uterus, and the uterine vasculature. The round ligament is an additional uterine support found within the broad ligament. The mesenteries blend into fibrous sheets that become the cardinal and uterosacral ligaments. The cardinal ligament is found at the base of the broad ligament. It contains veins and the uterine artery and supports the uterus along with the round ligament, ovarian ligament, and uterosacral ligament. In all, there are six ligamentous supports of the pelvic viscera: the broad, round, uterosacral, cardinal, ovarian and infundibulopelvic. The origin of the cardinal ligament is the greater sciatic foramen. The uterosacral ligament arises from the second through fourth sacral vertebrae. Both surround the cervix and suspend it to the pelvic sidewall. They extend downward from the cervix to suspend the upper vagina as well.

There is no real separation between the cardinal and uterosacral ligaments. The entire support apparatus is continuous from the uppermost cardinal–uterosacral complex to the pubocervical fascia. The cellular make-up of these ligaments is a mixture of smooth muscle and connective tissue. There has been histologic examination of some of these tissues. The cardinal ligament, for instance, has been shown to be primarily perivascular connective tissue running parallel to the uterine vessels.[17] In a small histopathologic evaluation of the uterosacral ligament, investigators could not consistently identify normal ligamentous tissue, particularly in the posthysterectomy pelves.[18] The lack of solid ligamentous tissue suggests that this structure may not be a reliable fixed structure for prolapse repair but this remains to be determined by larger studies.

Continuous with the cardinal–uterosacral complex but having its own anatomic distinction is the pubocervical fascia. It is the endopelvic fascia lower in the pelvis where the vagina meets the pelvic wall. The pubocervical fascia attaches the vagina laterally to the arcus tendineus of the fascia pelvis and supports the bladder to the same. Posteriorly it blends with the cardinal ligaments and is encountered when dissecting laterally beneath the vaginal wall at the level of the bladder during anterior vaginal wall surgery. Defects in this fascia produce anterior compartment prolapse. In description of anterior compartment prolapse, the term "paravaginal defects" refers specifically to detachment of the pubocervical fascia from the arcus tendineus. The arcus tendineus may itself detach from the pubis or ischial spine. In 71 retropubic operations, the arcus tendineus fascia pelvis was noted to be detached from the ischial spine over the pubis in a significant majority of cases (97.6% versus 2.8%).[19]

The anatomy of vaginal support has been described in terms of levels of support, a concept which helps conceptualize the role of each ligament (Fig. 1.5).[20] Level I support at the vaginal apex is provided by the upper divisions of endopelvic fascia, collectively known as paracolpium. These fibers extend vertically and posteriorly toward the sacrum. In level II the midportion of the vagina is connected laterally to the pelvic walls by the paracolpium. This structural layer is intimately related to the anterior vaginal wall and stretches the vagina transversely between bladder and rectum. At level III, the distal vagina is attached directly to the surrounding organs and muscle without any intervening fascia.

Just beneath and adjacent to the vagina in the posterior compartment is a layer of fibromuscular tissue known as the rectovaginal septum (Denonvillier's fascia). It is a fascial continuation of the peritoneal cavity between the apex of the vagina and anterior rectum. More distinctly, it is the fusion of the posterior vaginal fascia and the prerectal fascia. It too blends with the cardinal–uterosacral complex superiorly and fuses with the perineal body inferiorly. Laterally the fused layers are known as pararectal fascia. Monoclonal and polyclonal antibody tissue analysis of fetal and newborn pelvic specimens has revealed that the rectogenital septum is formed by mesenchyme in the early fetal period. There is apparent coinnervation of the rectal muscle layers and adjacent longitudinal muscle fibers of the septum. These tissue findings support a functional correlation between rectum and rectogenital septum; therefore, careful dissection in this area during pelvic surgery could limit neural damage and defecatory disturbance.[21]

VASCULAR AND NEUROLOGIC SUPPLY TO ALL PELVIC ORGANS

The blood supply of the levator ani, coccygeus, and piriformis is the inferior gluteal artery. The innervation of the levator muscles is a bit controversial. In a recent study, detailed pelvic dissections of female cadavers were undertaken to elucidate the peripheral innervation of the female levator ani muscles. Nerve biopsy specimens were obtained to confirm the gross findings. The authors point out that despite "specific and exhaustive attempts to locate pudendal nerve branches to the levators, none could be demonstrated in any cadaver."[22] Instead the levator ani were found to be innervated by a nerve that originates from the third to fifth sacral foramina which they termed the "levator ani nerve." These findings contradict the belief that the pelvic floor muscles are innervated by branches of the pudendal nerve.[22-25] The authors found that the pudendal nerve innervated the external anal sphincter, external urethral sphincter, perineal muscle, clitoris, and perineal skin.[22]

Another important finding from these dissections was that the levator ani nerve crosses the coccygeal muscle precisely at the point traditionally considered safe for sacrospinous ligament fixation sutures, namely two fingerbreadths medial to the ischial spine. Therefore, sacrospinous ligament fixation (SSLF) would have a high potential for nerve injury or entrapment. The authors postulate that injury to the levator ani nerve and subsequent pelvic floor denervation and atrophy could be another explanation for the high occurrence of anterior vaginal wall prolapse reported after SSLF.[22]

The autonomic inferior hypogastric plexus (IHP) (left and right pelvic plexuses) is the major nerve supply to pelvic organs.[26,27] It is located on pelvic side walls bilaterally beneath the fascia and medial to the vasculature and extends from the sacrum to the genital organs at the level of the lower sacral vertebrae.[28] It is composed of parasympathetic fibers from sacral nerve roots S3–4 (nervi erigentes or pelvic splanchnic) and occasionally S2 (sacral splanchnic nerves) as

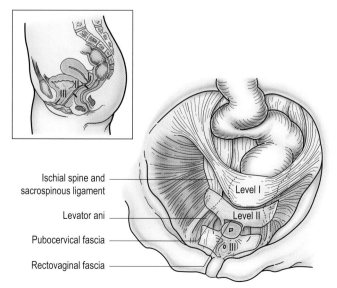

Figure 1.5 Levels of vaginal support (from reference 2).

Ischial spine and sacrospinous ligament

Levator ani

Pubocervical fascia

Rectovaginal fascia

Level I

Level II

well as some sympathetic fibers from T11–12/L1–2 from the lumbosacral trunk (hypogastric nerve). The IHP is believed to supply all the pelvic viscera. The posterior portion supplies the rectum to the level of the internal anal sphincter via the inferior mesenteric plexus branches, the bladder and urethral sphincter via vesical branch and the uterus and upper third of the vagina. It may also be supplemented by autonomic supply from the ureter and arteries. In one study of female cadavers, sacral splanchnic nerves were derived from either S1 or S2 sympathetic ganglia, in contrast to males in which all sacral sympathetic ganglia were involved.[28]

The location of the IHP within the pelvis may vary between gender and between individuals of the same gender. In females, the IHP nerve fibers were identified in four locations and a total of 60 locations were observed in 49 female hemipelves. In 57% of cases, the IHP was found in the uterosacral ligament. It was found parametrially in 30% of cases. It was found pararectally and in the fold between the bladder and uterus in 2% and 11% of cases respectively.[28]

The medial position of the IHP has important implications for surgical procedures. More detailed knowledge of IHP location can predict areas of concern for iatrogenic injury during pelvic surgery. The sacral promontory is the most superior region where operative injury may occur. Operations such as aortocaval lymph node dissections, colorectal surgery, and abdominosacral colpopexies may injure the superior hypogastric plexus.[28] Dissection of the mesorectum or retrorectal space risks the superior hypogastric plexus and pelvic and sacral splanchnic nerves. Pelvic lymph node dissections around the internal iliac artery can injure the IHP itself as well as dissection along the middle rectal artery. Injury to the anterior IHP may occur during intervention near the distal ureter, uterine or inferior vesical arteries, and Denonvillier's fascia.

Pelvic nerve damage is a well-known complication of radical hysterectomy that may lead to bladder, anorectal, and sexual dysfunction. Delineation of the anatomic distribution of important pelvic plexuses can help prevent inadvertent injury and resultant neurogenic dysfunction. From dissection of nerve branding and distribution of the pelvic plexus of 12 female cadavers, the pelvic plexus and subsidiary plexuses are laid closely to the lateral walls of the pelvic organs. The pelvic plexus and the uterosacral–cardinal ligaments are closely related.[29]

In radical hysterectomy as it is classically described, branches of the pelvic plexus may be divided. Modifications such as preservation of the lateral 1–2 cm of the cardinal ligament has been shown to reduce the incidence of postoperative urinary dysfunction compared to hysterectomy requiring transection of the cardinal ligament flush with the pelvic side wall and uterosacral ligament flush with the

rectum.[30,31] The cardinal ligament and uterosacral ligament contain considerable nerve tissue, including major nerve trunks, ganglia, and free nerve fibers.[32] The nerve content is higher at the origin on the pelvic sidewalls than at their insertion into the uterus. In a follow-up study by the same investigators, different nerve types within the uterosacral ligament and cardinal ligament were identified and quantified with neuropeptide markers.[33] The content of nerve fibers is different between the ligaments, and total nerve content is higher in the uterosacral ligament. The uterosacral ligament had a greater amount of sympathetic nerve compared with cardinal ligament. Sympathetic and parasympathetic nerve content was similar in the cardinal ligament. The sensory and sensorimotor components of the cardinal ligament were less than those of the uterosacral ligament. Larger diameter trunks were found in greater numbers in the uterosacral ligament and likely represent nerve supply to more distant pelvic organs supplied by the IHP (bladder, large bowel, and uterine body). Radical hysterectomy modifications that focus on less radical transection of the uterosacral ligament may reduce surgical morbidity.[33] Surgical technique may continue to evolve as our knowledge of the autonomic nervous system in the pelvis grows.

The genital organs within the female pelvis (ovaries, fallopian tubes, uterus, and vagina) do not all have common embryology; therefore, their blood supply and innervation differ. Despite their differences, the internal iliac artery or hypogastric artery is the main blood supply to the pelvis and pelvic viscera. The ovary receives parasympathetic fibers from the vagus nerve and sympathetics from T10, the lesser splanchnics, via the inferior hypogastric plexus. Ovarian arteries are direct branches from the ventral aorta. There is anastomotic connection to the uterine artery. Venous drainage is accomplished by a pampiniform plexus that coalesces into a single ovarian vein. Ovarian venous drainage is not symmetric. The right ovarian vein drains directly into the vena cava and the left into the left renal vein. The fallopian tubes receive a dual blood supply from the ovarian artery which supplies the lateral third and uterine artery which supplies the medial two-thirds. The fallopian tubes receive parasympathetic and sympathetic innervation along the ovarian and uterine arteries.

The uterus receives vascular supply from the uterine artery, a branch of the anterior trunk of the internal iliac artery. There are contributions as well from the ovarian artery and vaginal artery. The uterine artery also supplies the cervix and gives contributions to the vagina. These vessels run in a circuitous path within the broad ligament. The pelvic ureter is in close proximity to the uterus and its vasculature. Attention to its location is necessary during many pelvic procedures to avoid ureteral injury. Near the infundibulopelvic ligament, the ureter is crossed by the gonadal vein. The ureter crosses the cardinal ligament at its lowest portion and travels caudally. In this area it is surrounded by the uterine venous plexus and uterine artery. It then passes the supravaginal portion of the cervix approximately 1.5 cm from it on either side to reach the bladder. The venous drainage of the uterus is a plexus with several levels converging into a main vein within the myometrium. This uterine plexus communicates with ovarian and vaginal plexuses as well. Innervation to the uterus arises from the inferior hypogastric plexus. The vaginal blood supply travels laterally within the cardinal ligaments and through the paravaginal suspensory ligaments to the vagina. The main artery is the vaginal branch of the internal iliac artery but there may be vaginal arteries that arise from the uterine artery or inferior vesical artery. Additionally there is a vaginal arterial plexus that extends to a midline vaginal artery, sometimes referred to as the azygous artery of the vagina. A vaginal venous plexus communicates through the cardinal ligament with the venous system of the bladder, rectum, and paravaginal tissues.

The nerve supply to the vagina is extensive. Of greatest importance are the pudendal nerve (S2–4) and the inferior hypogastric plexus. Sensory afferents to the skin and subcutaneous tissues of the lower two-thirds of the vagina are via the pudendal nerve. Efferent motor somatic supply is not significant to the vaginal wall since there is no striated muscle. Visceral nerve supply for the upper vagina, musculature, and glands arises from the inferior hypogastric plexus. Afferent fibers transmit noxious stimuli from the peritoneum and pouch of Douglas, cervix and upper third of the vagina to the nerve roots S2–4. Efferent fibers supply the smooth muscle and glands of the vagina. Sympathetic nerves accompany sacral nerves of the hypogastric plexus. Parasympathetic fibers are carried by the pudendal nerve in the inferior hypogastric plexus to the lower portion of the vagina.

The arterial supply to the bladder includes a variety of vessels. Superior vesical arteries (1–4) arise from the umbilical artery to supply the upper bladder. The middle vesical artery may arise from the umbilical artery or as a branch of the superior vesicle artery and supplies the bladder body. The vaginal artery may supply the inferior bladder neck. Additional supply may be given by the obturator or inferior gluteal arteries. Most arteries to the bladder arise from the umbilical artery trunk of the internal iliac artery, except the inferior vesical artery which is its own branch off the internal iliac. Venous return is by a vesical plexus. Innervation of the bladder can be divided into that to the bladder itself and that to the bladder outlet. The bladder is innervated by the pelvic plexus found just lateral to the rectum. The plexus has input from S2–4 spinal segments by the pelvic splanchnic nerve and input from T10–L2 segments by the presacral nerve. The detrusor receives parasympathetic input from the pelvic nerve. Sympathetic input is carried on the hypo-gastric nerve. The female urethra receives arterial supply from branches of the vaginal artery. Venous drainage is via the pelvic venous plexus.

According to recent studies of the lower urinary tract in fetuses, the anatomy of the urethral sphincter differs by gender. The continence mechanism is composed of detrusor, trigone, and urethral sphincter muscle with distinctive histologic features in both sexes.[34] In females, the external urethral sphincter covers the ventral surface of the urethra in a horseshoe shape. Inferiorly, the size of the external sphincter increases and envelops the distal vagina. The levator ani muscles do not support the proximal urethra and may not actively control continence.[34]

The blood supply to the anorectum is provided by the inferior hemorrhoidal artery and a perineal artery, both branches of the pudendal artery. The superior hemorrhoidal, a continuation of the inferior mesenteric artery, supplies the rectum above the anorectal junction. The middle rectal artery, which may arise from the internal iliac artery or internal pudendal artery, is also a contributor. The venous drainage follows arterial supply. The sympathetic innervation to the anorectum is the superior and inferior hypogastric plexuses. Parasympathetic innervation is carried on the second, third and fourth sacral spinal nerves. Sensory and motor innervation are distributed on several peripheral nerves.

RESEARCH IN ANATOMY

Several MRI studies of the pelvic floor have been undertaken to describe both normal and abnormal pelvic floor anatomy.[35-40] The levator ani anatomy and endopelvic fascia and urethra have been examined with MRI to detect anatomic variations in nulliparous women. Certainly, the establishment of normal variation in healthy women is important prior to description of differences related to trauma, injury or aging. Even in 20 healthy continent nulliparous women with normal pelvic examinations and normal urodynamic results, there was considerable difference in MRI findings that were not attributable only to technical limitations in measuring technique. There was an absence of visible insertion of the levator ani inside the pubic bone bilaterally in 10% of all women, which contradicts the classic description of normal anatomy in textbooks. The variations observed clearly point out the need for further studies before standardizing an imaging technique for assessment of the pelvic floor.[35]

Since vaginal delivery is considered a major risk factor for levator ani damage and the development of SUI, an interesting study utilizing MRI from nulliparous women and vaginally primiparous women was undertaken. The authors proposed that the comparison of images would describe the appearance and occurrence of abnormality in levator muscles in nulliparous women and in women after their first vaginal birth.[39] Additionally, images of continent and incontinent women were compared. Abnormality in levator muscles was found in both continent and incontinent women but was demonstrated only in women who had delivered vaginally and not nulliparous women. Within the primiparous group, 28% of incontinent women demonstrated a defect in the levator ani, compared to 11% of continent women, making stress incontinent primiparous women twice as likely to have a muscle abnormality. The authors conclude that these findings are the first scientific evidence in support of vaginal birth as a source of levator ani muscle damage. Furthermore, the MRI images have provided visualization of the type of pelvic floor injury that occurs during vaginal birth. They suggest that further research with a population-based study is needed, as well as additional research to identify induced CT rupture in the vaginal supports that play a role in pelvic floor dysfunction. Another interesting concept put forth in this study is using MRI and electromyography as complementary techniques in order to also assess pelvic nerve injury. This may help define the relationship between nerve injury and MRI-visible abnormalities.[39]

Three-dimensional MRI has been used to assess levator ani morphologic features among different grades of prolapse and comparison was made with nulliparous asymptomatic women as controls.[36] The authors were able to identify patterns of change in the levator ani but alterations in levator ani morphology were not dependent on the grade of prolapse. Additionally, not all women with pelvic organ prolapse (POP) had abnormal levator morphology. What did seem to change with increasing grade of prolapse was the gap between levator and pubic symphysis and the levator hiatus. Further study of MRI in POP may find it a useful predictor as to which patients might develop recurrent prolapse after surgery.[36]

One limitation of current MRI technique is that, at present, studies are all performed in the supine position which may or may not introduce distortion. Technical advances in MRI are needed before images of satisfactory detail can be obtained in standing subjects. The choice of slice thickness for images on MRI is a compromise. Thinner slices offer higher spatial but poorer image resolution whereas thicker slices offer the converse. There is also the possibility of subjective bias in reading the scans.[36]

MRI has been employed to examine the structural regions of the urethra in nulliparous women and was determined to be successful at showing the normal appearance and location in continent, nulliparous women.[37] This may help with future investigations to describe structural abnormalities that might be associated with urinary incontinence.

Three-dimensional reconstruction from serial histologic sections allows for precise description of morphometry and appreciation of spatial relationships of one structure to another. Such an investigation has been undertaken of the hypogastric plexus of a human fetus.[40] Serial pelvic histologic sections were digitized from slides directly. Using a reconstruction program, the image treatment and reconstruction were performed manually. Results allowed the HP to be visualized and studied in three dimensions. Although the technique is time consuming, advancing technology may simplify and streamline the technique. Studying anatomy and embryology may be dramatically changed by these revolutionary imaging/computer technologies.[40]

Another intriguing modern investigation in human anatomy is the Visible Human Project through the National Library of Medicine.[41] Established in 1989, this undertaking sought to build a digital image library of volumetric data representing the complete adult anatomy of both sexes. It defines the anatomy of the adult human in three dimensions and at high resolution (Fig. 1.6). The visible human female data set was released in 1995 and contains 5189 anatomic

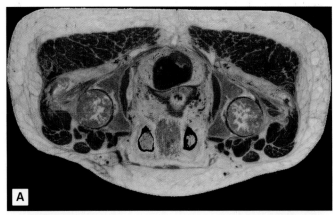

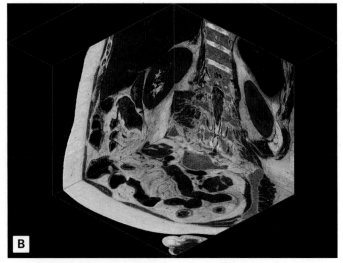

Figure 1.6 Transverse and three-dimensional images created from the female human database project.[41]

images.[41] It is currently used as a tool to teach anatomy and in the future it may be combined with surgical and anesthesiology simulators to create a virtual operating room.[42] It could then be used to teach surgical skills to physicians in training or to allow practicing physicians to gain skill in new techniques, to give researchers clinical insight into the diseases they investigate or perhaps as a tool to educate a patient about a disease state or possible treatment.

REFERENCES

1. Stenzl A, Kolle D, Eder R, et al. Virtual reality of the lower urinary tract in women. Int Urogynecol J 1999;10:248–253.
2. Wei JT, DeLancey JOL. Functional anatomy of the pelvic floor and lower urinary tract. Clin Obstet Gynecol 2004;47(1):3–17.
3. Parks AG, Porter NH, Melzak J. Experimental study of the reflex mechanism controlling muscles of the pelvic floor. Dis Colon Rectum 1962;5:407–414.
4. Koelbl H, Strassegger H, Riss PA, et al. Morphologic and functional aspects of pelvic floor muscles in patients with pelvic relaxation and genuine stress incontinence. Obstet Gynecol 1989;74:789–793.
5. Shafik A, El-Sibi O. Study of the levator ani muscle in the multipara: role of levator dysfunction in defecation disorders. J Obstet Gynecol 2002;22(2):187–192.
6. Mirilas P, Skandalakis JE Urogenital diaphragm: an erroneous concept casting its shadow over the sphincter urethrae and deep perineal space. J Am Coll Surg 2004;198(2): 279–290.
7. Walters M, Weber AM. Anatomy of the lower urinary tract, rectum and pelvic floor. In: Walters MD, Karram MM, eds. Urogynecology and reconstructive pelvic surgery. St Louis: Mosby; 1999.
8. Vazzoler N, Soulie M, Escourrou G, et al. Pubourethral ligaments in women: anatomic and clinical aspects. Surg Radiol Anat 2002;24(1):33–37.
9. Petros PE, Ulmsten U. An integral theory and its method for the diagnosis and management of female urinary incontinence. Scand J Urol Nephrol Suppl 1993;153:1–93.
10. DeLancey JO. Structural support of the urethra as it relates to stress urinary incontinence: the hammock hypothesis. Am J Obstet Gynecol 1994;170(6):1713–1720.
11. Carley ME, Schaffer J. Urinary incontinence and pelvic organ prolapse in women with Marfan or Ehlers Danlos syndrome. Am J Obstet Gynecol 2000;182(5):1021–1023.
12. Ulmsten U. Connective tissue factors in the aetiology of female pelvic disorders. Ann Med 1990;22(6):403.
13. Falconer C, Ekman-Ordeberg G, Blomgren B, et al. Paraurethral connective tissue in stress-incontinent women after menopause. Acta Obstet Gynecol Scand 1998;77(1):95–100.
14. Falconer C, Ekman-Ordeberg G, Ulmsten U, et al. Changes in paraurethral connective tissue at menopause are counteracted by estrogen. Maturitas 1996;24(3):197–204.
15. Goepel C, Hefler L, Methfessel HD, et al. Periurethral connective tissue status of postmenopausal women with genital prolapse with and without stress incontinence. Acta Obstet Gynecol Scand 2003;82:659–664.
16. Reay Jones NH, Healy JC, King LJ, et al. Pelvic connective tissue resilience decreases with vaginal delivery, menopause and uterine prolapse. Br J Surg 2003;90(4):466–472.
17. Range RL, Woodburne RT. The gross and microscopic anatomy of the transverse cervical ligaments. Am J Obstet Gynecol 1964;90:460–467.
18. Cole E, Leu PB, Gomelsky A, et al. Histopathological evaluation of the uterosacral ligament: is this a dependable structure for pelvic reconstruction? J Urol Abstract 2004; 171(4):304–305.
19. DeLancey JO. Fascial and muscular abnormalities in women with urethral hypermobility and anterior vaginal wall prolapse. Am J Obstet Gynecol 2002;187(1):93–98.
20. DeLancey JO. Anatomic aspects of vaginal eversion after hysterectomy. Am J Obstet Gynecol 1992;166:1717–1724.
21. Aigner F, Zbar AP, Ludwikowski B, et al. The rectogenital septum: morphology, function, and clinical relevance. Dis Colon Rectum 2004;47(2):131–140.
22. Barber MD, Bremer RE, Thor KB, et al. Innervation of the female levator ani muscles. Am J Obstet Gynecol 2002;187:64–71.
23. Wall LL. The muscles of the pelvic floor. Clin Obstet Gynecol 193;36:910–925.
24. Retzky SS, Rogers RM, Richardson AC. Anatomy of female pelvic support. In: Brubaker L, Saclarides T, eds. The female pelvic floor: disorders of function and support. Philadelphia: FA Davis; 1996.
25. DeLancey JO. Surgical anatomy of the female pelvis. In: Rock JA, Thompson JP, eds. TeLinde's operative gynecology. Philadelphia: Lippincott-Raven; 1997.
26. Mundy AR. An anatomic explanation for bladder dysfunction following rectal and uterine surgery. Br J Urol 1982;54:501–504.
27. Hockel M, Konerding MA, Heussel CP. Liposuction-assisted nerve-sparing extended radical hysterectomy: oncologic rationale, surgical anatomy, and feasibility study. Am J Obstet Gynecol 1988;178:971–976.
28. Baader B, Herrmann M. Topography of the pelvic autonomic nervous system and its potential impact on surgical intervention in the pelvis. Clin Anat 2003;16:119–139.
29. Tong XK, Huo RJ. The anatomic basis and prevention of neurogenic voiding dysfunction following radical hysterectomy. Surg Radiol Anat 1991;13(2):145–148.
30. Forney P. The effects of radical hysterectomy on bladder physiology. Am J Obstet Gynecol 1980;138:374–382.
31. Piver SM, Rutledge F, Smith JP. Five classes of extended hysterectomy for women with cervical cancer. Obstet Gynecol 1974;44:623–644.
32. Butler-Manuel SA, Buttery LDK, A'Hern RP, et al. Pelvic nerve plexus trauma at radical hysterectomy and simple hysterectomy: the nerve content of the uterine supporting ligaments. Cancer 2000;89:834–841.
33. Butler-Manuel SA, Buttery LDK, A'Hern RP, et al. Pelvic nerve plexus trauma at radical hysterectomy and simple hysterectomy: quantitative study of nerve types in the uterine supporting ligaments. J Soc Gynecol Investig 2002;9(1):47–56.
34. Yucel S, Baskin LS. An anatomic description of the male and female urethral sphincter complex. J Urol 2004;171(5):1890–1897.
35. Tunn R, DeLancey JO, Howard D, et al. Anatomic variations in the levator ani muscle, endopelvic fascia and urethra in nulliparas evaluated by magnetic resonance imaging. Am J Obstet Gynecol 2003;188:116–121.
36. Singh K, Jakab M, Reid WM, et al. Three-dimensional magnetic resonance imaging assessment of levator ani morphologic features in different grades of prolapse. Am J Obstet Gynecol 2003;188(4):910–915.
37. Umek WH, Kearney R, Morgan DM, et al. The axial location of structural regions in the urethra: a magnetic resonance study in nulliparous women. Obstet Gynecol 2003;102(5 Pt 1): 1039–1045.
38. Parikh M, Rasmusssen M, Brubaker L, et al. Three dimensional virtual reality model of the normal female pelvic floor. Ann Biomed Eng 2004;32(2):292–296.

39. DeLancey JOL, Kearney R, Chou Q, et al. The appearance of levator ani muscle abnormalities in magnetic resonance images after vaginal delivery. Obstet Gynecol 2003;101:46–53.

40. Hounnou GM, Uhl JF, Plaisant O, et al. Morphometry by computerized three-dimensional reconstruction of the hypogastric plexus of a human fetus. Surg Radiol Anat 2003;25:21–31.

41. United States National Library of Medicine. National Institutes of Health. Available online at: www.nlm.nih.gov/research/visible/visible_human.html

42. Center for Human Simulation, University of Colorado. Available online at: www.uchsc.edu

SECTION 2

Physiology

The Physiology of Micturition and Urine Storage

William D Steers and Adam P Klausner

INTRODUCTION

The lower urinary tract is composed of the bladder and an outlet that includes the bladder neck, urethra, and external urethral sphincter. These structures form a functional unit that switches between urine storage and release depending on the status of the nervous system. Urine storage requires a low bladder pressure that does not exceed outlet resistance. Urine release requires intact innervation, adequate detrusor contractility, and coordinated relaxation of the bladder outlet and pelvic floor. Failure to meet these basic requirements can produce residual urine, urinary incontinence, hydronephrosis, urinary tract infections, calculi or deterioration of bladder and renal function. Both passive and active mechanisms participate in the maintenance of continence. Urinary continence relies on an active relaxation of the bladder body and maintenance of tone by the bladder neck and urethra. Continence also relies on the passive, viscoelastic properties of these tissues and their pelvic supports.

The nervous system, the muscular and connective tissue components of the detrusor, urethra, and pelvic floor, as well as the urothelium itself all play significant roles in bladder function. The role of the nervous system in the lower urinary tract is unique. Central neural input is crucial for bladder function in contrast to its modulatory role in other viscera. This neural input is the result of integration and coordination of autonomic and somatic pathways, and these neural networks can rapidly reorganize following injury or disease. Such unique neurophysiologic properties accentuate the importance of understanding how reflex pathways control bladder and urethral function. Apart from the nervous system, the bladder, urethra, and supporting tissues have unique, intrinsic properties which contribute to the continence mechanism. In addition, there is a growing body of evidence which demonstrates that the urothelium functions as a mechano- and chemosensor and that intraluminal contents can influence urine storage and release. By gaining a comprehensive understanding of voiding and storage mechanisms, the clinician can formulate a rational plan for the treatment and prevention of urinary incontinence.

ANATOMY

Bladder. The urinary bladder is a hollow viscus composed of coarse bundles of smooth muscle fascicles. Connective tissue and extracellular matrix consisting of collagen and elastin are interspersed between the muscle fascicles. In addition, intramural ganglia and interstitial cells may control discrete bladder regions and form functional modules.[1] There is not a one-to-one relationship between free nerve endings and smooth muscle cells. Rather, excitation spreads throughout an interconnected syncytium of cells. Gap junctions composed of connexin 43 may enhance coupling and facilitate the initiation, maintenance, and modulation of detrusor contractions. Indeed, this arrangement may explain how the bladder sustains a contraction even with progressive shortening of fiber length. With overactive states, it has been postulated that increased coupling between cells produces involuntary contractions.[2] Furthermore, the electrochemical excitability of smooth muscle cells increases with some overactive conditions.

Urethra. The urethra is composed of epithelium surrounded by lamina propria and a thin layer of circular smooth muscle. Beneath this, a thick longitudinal layer of smooth muscle runs along the entire urethral length. More distally, the urethra is surrounded by a horseshoe-shaped mass of striated muscle termed the external urethral sphincter (EUS). Resting tone is myogenic since nerve-blocking agents such as tetrodotoxin, guanethidine, and atropine fail to abolish contractile activity of urethral smooth muscle strips. Figure 2.1 depicts a sagittal section of the human female urethra.

External urethral sphincter. Striated muscle extends over the distal two-thirds of the female urethra. This muscle has been termed the EUS and is derived from the puborectalis muscle; 87% of the muscle fibers are Type I which produce slow, nonfatigable contractions. However, significant racial differences may exist in the types of fibers which make up the EUS. The EUS receives somatic innervation

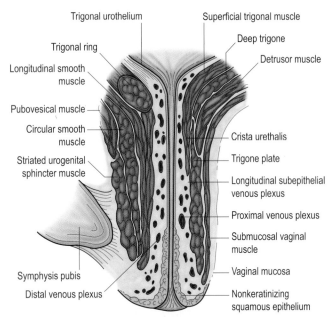

Figure 2.1 Sagittal section through the human female urethra. The diagram depicts the layers of circular and horizontal smooth muscle as well as the supporting structures that comprise the urethra.

from the pudendal nerve and previous investigators have found that pudendal nerve block reduces maximal urethral pressure in female volunteers.[3]

Urethral support system. The pubourethral ligaments fix the midurethra and suburethral vaginal wall to the pubic symphysis. The suburethral vaginal wall serves as the floor for the urethra and, in women with bladder descent, facilitates bladder neck closure by mechanical compression. A rise in urethral pressure occurs prior to a rise in intra-abdominal pressure, indicating an active role for this support system. In addition to active urethral tone, the passive tissue properties of the bladder and outlet participate in this process. The endopelvic fascia and levator ani, by providing pelvic support, also facilitate urine storage in women. However, recent work has revealed that the levator ani muscles are not innervated by the pudendal nerve as previously believed. Rather, sacral roots S3–5 give rise to a separate levator ani nerve.[4] Therefore, demonstration of pudendal neuropathy on electrophysiologic studies may approximate, but not define, neurologic damage to the levators since this nerve does not provide their neural input. Structural damage to these tissues or their innervation allows less resistance to deformation during abdominal straining. Thus, urethral closure would not be assured.

LOWER URINARY TRACT INNERVATION

Reflex pathways to the lower urinary tract consist of an afferent limb, that relays information to the central nervous system, and an efferent limb, which provides motor outflow to the bladder and urethra. By definition, afferent refers to input *to* a dendrite or soma of a neuron. Efferent refers to axonal transmission *from* a neuron. The lower urinary tract receives afferent and efferent innervation from the pelvic, hypogastric, and pudendal nerves as well from the sympathetic chain (Fig. 2.2). Direct nerve pathways to the lower urinary tract derive from both the spinal cord and the brain. Spinal pathways can be classified as parasympathetic, sympathetic or somatic. Brain pathways originate mainly from the pons; however, the cerebral cortex and diencephalon also influence micturition.

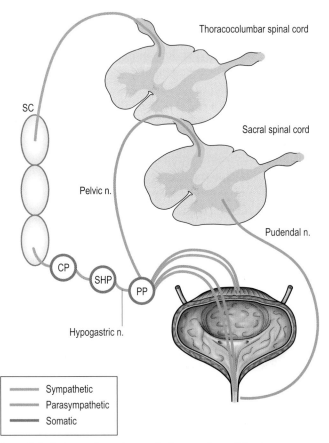

Figure 2.2 Autonomic and somatic innervation of the lower urinary tract. Sympathetic (yellow) preglionic outflow emerges from the thoracolumbar spinal cord, enters the sympathetic chain (SC) and then travels via the lumbar splanchnic nerve to the celiac plexus (CP) and superior hypogastric plexus (SHP). The hypogastric nerve then conveys these preganglionic and postganglionic fibers to the pelvic plexus (PP) or the bladder and urethra. Parasympathetic (green) preganglionic outflow to the lower urinary tract arises in the sacral spinal cord S2–4 and runs in the pelvic nerve to the pelvic plexus or to bladder wall ganglionic cells. Somatic (brown) neural output to the external urethral sphincter and the pelvic floor originates from the sacral cord segment S2–4 and runs in the pudendal nerve.

Spinal pathways to the lower urinary tract

Parasympathetics

AFFERENT PATHWAYS. Parasympathetic sensory neurons reside in the S2–4 dorsal root ganglia. These bipolar cells send long processes to the urinary smooth muscle and epithelium. Low-threshold myelinated (Aδ) and unmyelinated (C) afferent fibers convey mechanical or noxious (nociceptive) stimuli to the dorsal horn of the spinal cord.[5,6] The mechanoceptive afferents responsible for initiation of micturition travel in the pelvic nerve.[7] The presence of urine in the urethra probably activates additional afferents that reinforce the micturition reflex.[8] This reflex may explain the common coexistence of detrusor overactivity and stress incontinence, also called "stress hyperreflexia" (Fig. 2.3).

Bladder and urethral afferents enter the dorsal horn of the spinal cord and project laterally toward the sacral parasympathetic nucleus (SPN).[9] Overlap of bladder and urethral afferents suggests that these regions coordinate vesicosphincteric reflexes.[38] Second-order neurons relay afferent input to supraspinal sites including the hypothalamus and pons.[10] The hypothalamus coordinates autonomic activity between multiple organ systems.[10] The pons controls visceral functions, including micturition and defecation.

In addition to providing information to the central nervous system on the status of the lower urinary tract, afferents can directly influence bladder and urethral function. Electrical, chemical, and mechanical stimulation of bladder afferents results in an alteration of smooth muscle contractility, blood flow, and immune response. These alterations are mediated through the release of neuropeptides from peripheral nerve terminals.[11]

EFFERENT PATHWAYS. Parasympathetic outflow to the bladder and urethra originates in the sacral parasympathetic nucleus (SPN). The SPN is located in the intermediolateral cell column of the S2–4 sacral spinal cord. This nucleus contains the cholinergic preganglionic neurons responsible for micturition, defecation, vaginal relaxation, and clitoral engorgement. Injuries to these regions can result in the triad of bladder, bowel, and sexual dysfunction. Preganglionics exit the spinal cord in the ventral spinal nerves to form the pelvic nerve and then synapse on postganglionic neurons in pelvic ganglia. The pelvic ganglia reside on either side of the rectum and vagina and in the walls of the bladder and urethra.

PHARMACOLOGY AND THERAPEUTIC TARGETS. Nerves in the human bladder contain an assortment of neurotransmitters including acetylcholine, noradrenaline, and neuropeptides.[12] Preganglionic parasympathetic efferents contain acetylcholine as well as enkephalins (ENK), galanin, cholecystokinin (CCK), and nitric oxide (NO).[13-16] Cholinergic efferents activate nicotinic receptors on postganglionic neurons in the pelvic plexus. These postganglionic nerves release acetylcholine which excites muscarinic receptors (M3/M2) expressed by bladder and urethral smooth muscles as well as by the urothelium itself. Thus, antimuscarinic drugs provide useful therapy for detrusor overactivity and increase bladder compliance.[17] The muscarinic receptor responsible for human bladder contraction is the M3 subtype.[18] Although this subtype predominates, the M2 receptor is mainly responsible for turning off cAMP-mediated relaxation mechanisms of the detrusor.[19] Oxybutynin, tolterodine, and trospium are nonselective antimuscarinics. Newer antimuscarinics darifenacin and solafenacin act predominantly on M3 receptors. Unfortunately, M3 receptors are also expressed by the gut and salivary glands. Thus, side effects of dry mouth and constipation still occur with M3 antagonists (Ikeda, Kobayashi et al. 2002).

Nonadrenergic noncholinergic (NANC) transmitters, most notably adenosine triphosphate (ATP), act in conjunction with acetylcholine to contract detrusor smooth muscle. Antimuscarinics often fail to abolish bladder overactivity because of their inability to block noncholinergic excitatory transmission to the bladder.[21] Purinergic transmission (ATP) provides a greater share of excitatory input to the bladder with aging or after pelvic surgery with presumed partial denervation.[22]

In the urethra, cholinergic transmission appears to play only a modulatory role in smooth muscle relaxation. Cholinergic innervation of the urethra is not completely understood. However, electrical stimulation of the ventral

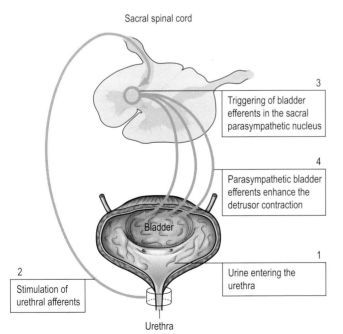

Sacral spinal cord

3 — Triggering of bladder efferents in the sacral parasympathetic nucleus

4 — Parasympathetic bladder efferents enhance the detrusor contraction

Bladder

1 — Urine entering the urethra

2 — Stimulation of urethral afferents

Urethra

Figure 2.3 Stress hyperreflexia. In this diagram, the presence of urine in the urethra (voluntary or involuntary) triggers afferents which reinforce the micturition reflex.

sacral nerve roots reduces urethral pressure, implying that there is a parasympathetic-induced urethral relaxation. Activation of muscarinic receptors on adrenergic nerve terminals in the lower urinary tract inhibits noradrenaline release.[23] Therefore, presynaptic inhibition of noradrenaline release may be regulated by cholinergic nerves in the urethra. This mechanism may contribute in part to parasympathetic-induced urethral relaxation (Fig. 2.4). On the other hand, direct, noncholinergic reflex relaxation of the urethra has been attributed to the inhibitory transmitter nitric oxide (NO).[24] Nitric oxide synthase (NOS) is an enzyme which catalyzes the production of NO from L-arginine. Nerve terminals in the bladder and urethra are immunoreactive for this enzyme[25] and inhibition of NOS reduces urethral relaxation.[24] Considering these data, it is tempting to speculate that NO is responsible for neurogenic relaxation of urethral smooth muscle.

Sensation of bladder fullness and pain is mediated by afferent nerves which relay information to the sacral dorsal root ganglia. Afferents in the sacral dorsal root ganglia contain VIP, substance P (SP), calcitonin gene-related peptide (CGRP), ENK, CCK, glutamate, ATP, and NO.[10] Therefore, it is not surprising that anticholinergic drugs have less effect on sensory than motor disorders of the lower urinary tract. Depletion of SP and related peptides with the vanilloid receptor agonists capsaicin or resiniferatoxin depresses the micturition reflex.[10,11] In humans, intravesical administration of capsaicin/resiniferatoxin transiently reduces bladder sensation and irritable voiding.[26] These agents reduce incontinent episodes in some patients.[27] This implies that SP or a related peptide is involved in the micturition reflex. SP and related neurokinins act via NK-1 and NK-2 receptors. Selective NK-2 receptor antagonists inhibit bladder contraction.[28] In the dorsal horn, NK-1 receptor antagonists inhibit micturition. These findings indicate that neurokinins play an important role in afferent transmission from the bladder.[29]

More recently, ATP has been shown to play a prominent role in afferent transmission from the bladder. P2X3 receptors reside on bladder afferents.[30] Mice with homozygous deletion of the gene for this receptor demonstrate enlarged bladders and reduced intravesical sensation.[31] Clinically, changes in expression of this receptor have been shown in patients with detrusor overactivity.

Sympathetics

EFFERENT PATHWAYS. Sympathetic preganglionics in the lower urinary tract arise from the intermediolateral cell column, and possibly the nucleus intercalatus, in the T11–L2 segments of the spinal cord. Preganglionics leave the spinal cord in the ventral roots and enter the sympathetic chain. Axons coursing through the sympathetic chain without synapsing form the lumbar splanchnic nerves which then project to the superior hypogastric plexus. Some preganglionics may synapse in the superior hypogastric plexus, while other axons travel in the hypogastric nerve toward the pelvic plexus (see Fig. 2.2). It is important to note that pelvic surgery often injures some of these nerves. Preganglionics in the hypogastric nerve then synapse within the pelvic plexus or on bladder or urethral ganglion cells. Postganglionic nerves from the sympathetic chain ganglia travel toward the bladder and urethra in the pelvic nerve.

PHARMACOLOGY AND THERAPEUTIC TARGETS. Sympathetic preganglionics release acetylcholine which excites nicotinic receptors on postganglionic neurons. These postganglionic cells contain noradrenaline. Noradrenaline released from postganglionics contracts smooth muscle in the urethra and bladder base. This contraction is due to stimulation of α_1-adrenoceptors.[32] The α_{1d} receptor subtype is found in the bladder neck while the α_{1a}-receptor predominates in the urethra.[33] In contrast, β_3-adrenoceptors inhibit smooth muscle activity in the bladder body, base, and urethra.[34] Moreover, stimulation of α_1 and β receptors facilitates transmission in pelvic ganglia whereas α_2 stimulation inhibits transmission (see Storage Reflexes, below).

The noradrenergic innervation of the human urethra is sparse relative to other species. However, an increase in noradrenergic innervation and response to adrenergic drugs occurs in several pathologic conditions including obstruction of the bladder outlet and denervation.[35] These pharmacologic changes explain the clinical efficacy of α_1-adrenergic blockers in obstructive and hyperactive voiding

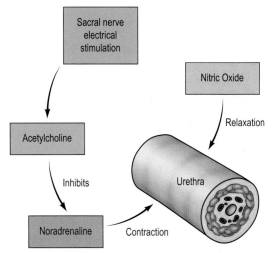

Figure 2.4 Parasympathetic-induced urethral relaxation. Electrical stimulation of pelvic efferents may contribute to urethral relaxation *indirectly*. In this diagram, electrical stimulation triggers parasympathetic efferents which then synapse on adrenergic terminals in the urethra. This inhibits adrenergic tone and allows nitric oxide-mediated relaxation to predominate. In this manner, parasympathetic tone induces urethral relaxation.

disorders, yet the minimal effect of these drugs in normal individuals.[36]

Somatics

EFFERENT PATHWAYS. The neurons innervating the striated muscle of the EUS and pelvic floor emerge from the anterior horn of the second to fourth sacral spinal cord segments, from an area termed Onuf's nucleus. Efferents to the EUS and the periurethral striated muscle travel in the pudendal nerve (see Fig. 2.2).[37,38] However, efferents to the levator ani do not travel in the pudendal nerve as previously believed. Rather, these nerves originate in the lower portion of the sacral spinal cord and travel in a nerve variously termed the coccygeal nerve or nerve to the levator ani.[4] Importantly, branching sacral preganglionic axons project to Onuf's nucleus, providing the substrate for inhibition of these neurons during voiding.[39]

AFFERENT PATHWAYS. Afferents from the EUS travel in the pudendal nerve. The termination of pudendal nerve afferents in the spinal cord overlaps with afferents in the pelvic nerve from the bladder.[37] However, afferents in the pudendal nerve demonstrate a more diffuse and central termination in the dorsal horn than those from the pelvic nerve.[37,38] Stimulation of these afferents as well as those of the posterior tibial nerve inhibits detrusor contraction. Clinically, sacral neuromodulation using InterStim (Medtronic, Minneapolis, MN) as well as pelvic floor muscle exercise have been shown to be useful for treating bladder overactivity and urge urinary incontinence[40] and may rely on activation of these and other somatic afferents from pelvic muscles such as the levator ani.[41]

PHARMACOLOGY AND THERAPEUTIC TARGETS. Striated muscles of the lower urinary tract and pelvis are innervated by cholinergic fibers in the pudendal nerve.[42] Acetylcholine acts on nicotinic receptors located at the motor endplate. Activation of nicotinic receptors on striated muscle elicits contraction. Overactivity of the EUS is reduced by botulinum toxin, which prevents neurotransmitter release.[43] Similarly, pancuronium paralyzes the EUS.[44] After treatment of the EUS with botulium toxin or pancuronium, incontinence at rest does not occur, a finding which is seen after blockade or transaction of the pudendal nerve. This implies that incomplete EUS inhibition is occurring with these pharmacologic agents.

Muscle fibers of the EUS contain noradrenergic varicosities and blockade of α_1-receptors is another pharmacologic mechanism through which EUS relaxation can be produced.[45] However, α_1-blockers may also work directly in the spinal cord to reduce EUS activity.[46] Onuf's nucleus is surrounded by noradrenergic and serotoninergic (5-HT) fibers originating from the brainstem. NA and 5-HT activate α and 5-HT-1 receptors that influence pudendal nerve activity. The selective NA/5-HT reuptake inhibitor duloxetine enhances pudendal nerve activity and reduces stress incontinent episodes.[47]

Brain pathways to the lower urinary tract

AFFERENT PATHWAYS. Ascending tracts arising in the dorsal horn of the spinal cord transmit sensory information from the lower urinary tract to the pons.[48] These dorsal horn neurons are located in areas that receive dense projections from bladder afferents including lateral lamina I and lamina V–VII.[9]

EFFERENT PATHWAYS. There does not appear to be a distinct pontine micturition center; rather, several regions of the pons initiate, coordinate, and integrate lower urinary tract function. Anatomic, pharmacologic, and electrophysiologic evidence implicates several pontine sites in the control of bladder function, including the locus ceruleous alpha, dorsolateral tegmentum, and periaqueductal gray.[49,50] Stimulation of the dorsomedial pons duplicates events that occur during micturition such as bladder contraction and synchronous inhibition of the EUS.[50] Conversely, stimulation of the dorsolateral pons imitates functions necessary for urine storage including increased activity of the EUS and inhibition of the bladder.[49] Together these observations provide compelling evidence for pontine regulation of urine storage and release.

There is substantial anatomic overlap in the brain sites involved in both the stress response and the control of micturition. Foot shock stress produces significant increases in corticotropin-releasing factor (CRF) mRNA in Barrington's nucleus, the region that controls micturition in rodent brains.[51] Likewise, injection of pseudorabies virus into the bladder labels neurons in the amygdala, bed nucleus stria terminalis, hippocampus, and prefrontal cortex, areas which are important in the central stress response.[52] Interestingly, these areas are also activated after chemical cystitis[53] and electrical stimulation of these areas affects bladder activity.[54] Therefore, it appears that the areas critically important in the central stress response also participate in bladder activity. CRF given within the spinal cord reduces the threshold for micturition, an action blocked by CRF antagonist astressin.[55] Thus it is not surprising that stressful conditions can elicit bladder overactivity, possibly via CRF modulation.

PHARMACOLOGY AND THERAPEUTIC TARGETS. A variety of excitatory and inhibitory inputs regulate pontine function. Enkephalinergic varicosities have been demonstrated in the pons, SPN, and Onuf's nucleus[14] and a group of pontine neurons is under tonic inhibition by enkephalinergic neurons. Intrathecal administration of μ- and δ-opiate agonists inhibits the micturition reflex, whereas κ-receptor agonists inhibit sphincter reflexes.[56,57] In humans, systemic and intrathecal naloxone, an opioid antagonist, decreases bladder compliance, supporting the concept of an endogenous opiate mechanism in the regulation of urine storage.[58] Postoperative urinary retention has been attributed to the action of either endogenous opiates or narcotic analgesics in the CNS. Furthermore, opiate agonists are being investigated as possible treatments for overactive bladder.

Nonopiate transmitters also influence lower urinary tract function. Glycine, GABA, and 5-hydroxytryptamine (i.e. serotonin or 5-HT) inhibit bladder activity by interaction with afferent terminals or parasympathetic preganglionics in the sacral spinal cord.[59] Intrathecal baclofen, a GABA-B agonist, raises the threshold for micturition in patients with spinal pathology, probably by inhibiting afferent input.[60,61] Similarly, administration of 5-HT to thoracolumbar preganglionic neurons facilitates vesicosympathetic storage reflexes. Many 5-HT agonists when administered systemically inhibit micturition.[62] Consistent with these observations, drugs that inhibit 5-HT uptake such as tricyclic antidepressants are useful for treating urge urinary incontinence and enuresis.[63]

The primary neurotransmitter contained within ascending and descending pathways involved in micturition and storage is glutamate, which acts at several types of receptors. Activation of NMDA/AMPA/kianate receptors facilitates neurotransmission in the pons and spinal cord, thereby lowering the micturition threshold.[50,64] Dopamine influences micturition and storage through activation of excitatory D1 receptors and inhibition of D2 receptors in the brain.[65] Oxytocin and NO inhibit voiding.[66]

It is easy to envision how any disruption of central inhibitory pathways with tumor, stroke, inflammation or trauma may shift the balance of positive and negative inputs on micturition pathways. Bladder overactivity and urge incontinence could develop by facilitation of a voiding reflex or inhibition of a storage reflex.

NEUROPHYSIOLOGY
Voiding reflexes

The sensory reflex limb. Mechanoreceptive and possibly chemoreceptive suburothelial nerve endings coursing between muscle fascicles in the bladder wall are responsible for initiation of the voiding reflex.[67,68] Bladder afferents are quiescent at low bladder volumes but fire at threshold intravesical pressures of 15–20 cmH$_2$O.[5] Their conduction velocities range from 1.2 to 30 m/s which is consistent with activation of Aδ, lightly myelinated fibers.[69] Bladder afferents in the pelvic nerve synapse on neurons in the sacral spinal cord. Some of these second-order neurons, in turn, project rostrally to the pons. In humans, bilateral lesions of the spinothalamic tracts abolish bladder sensation

and disturb normal voiding, a finding which indicates that ascending inputs from the bladder travel in or in proximity to these pathways[70] (Fig. 2.5).

Afferent inputs from the urethra also influence micturition. As urine flows through the bladder outlet, afferent fibers send sensory information to the spinal cord and higher centers. In turn, these fibers synapse onto pathways which facilitate a more forceful and complete bladder contraction.[8] With stress urinary incontinence, urine entering the urethra may activate this urethrovesical reflex and trigger involuntary detrusor contractions. This mechanism could explain the relatively common association of stress and urge (due to involuntary detrusor contractions) urinary incontinence, sometimes termed "stress hyperreflexia" (see Fig. 2.3).

Central coordination of voiding reflexes. A substantial body of evidence suggests that the pons serves as the command and control center for micturition. Lesioning experiments offered the earliest evidence that the pons was important for voiding.[71] Subsequently, it was shown that injection of viral retrograde tracers into the bladder labeled pontine neurons.[72] More recently, positron emission transmission (PET) and functional blood oxygen level depletion (fBOLD) magnetic resonance imaging (MRI) have demonstrated activation of a pontine micturition center during

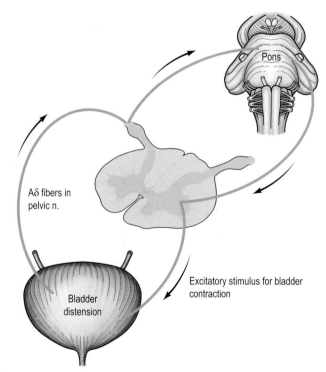

Pons

Aδ fibers in pelvic n.

Bladder distension

Excitatory stimulus for bladder contraction

Figure 2.5 Distension of the bladder triggers firing in Aδ afferents conveyed by the pelvic nerve. These afferents synapse in the spinal cord and second-order neurons relay the input to neurons in the pons. Excitatory descending pontine input to sacral preganglionics initiates a detrusor contraction.

voiding.[73] Furthermore, electrical and chemical activation of discrete areas of the pons induce bladder contraction and coordinated relaxation of the EUS.[49,50]

The motor reflex limb. A voiding reflex directly stimulates bladder contraction mainly by activation of M3 muscarinic receptors on bladder smooth muscle. However, other reflexes promote emptying by reducing outlet resistance. Pudendal efferents originating from Onuf's nucleus become quiescent during voiding.[50] During micturition, descending input from the pons inhibits these somatic motoneurons. Additionally, axon collaterals from sacral preganglionic neurons project to Onuf's nucleus.[9] Thus, with firing of bladder preganglionics, inhibition of sphincter motoneurons occurs, possibly by hyperpolarizing these cells.[74] In addition, efferent parasympathetic pathways in the pelvic nerve appear to be involved in relaxation of the bladder outlet. This is inferred because electrical stimulation of sacral nerve roots lowers urethral pressure[75] (see Fig. 2.4). In this regard, it is possible that afferents in the bladder trigger a pelvic nerve-mediated urethral relaxation reflex mediated by a substance such as NO.

Storage reflexes

Detrusor-sphincter reflex. To promote bladder accommodation and urethral sphincter contraction during urine storage, the parasympathetic pathway is inhibited while sympathetic and somatic pathways are activated. A detrusor-sphincter reflex exists in which bladder distension produces afferent firing in the pelvic nerve. An intersegmental pathway from the sacral to thoracolumbar cord stimulates preganglionics in the hypogastric nerve. This provides excitatory outflow to the bladder base and urethra, resulting in increased outlet resistance. Overactivity of sympathetic efferents supplying the bladder outlet may contribute to functional obstructive disorders found in anxious young women.

Guarding reflex. Bladder afferents in the pelvic nerve also trigger motoneurons in Onuf's nucleus, causing somatic outflow to the EUS manifested as the guarding reflex. EUS motoneurons exhibit a tonic discharge that increases during bladder filling. Overactivity of the guarding reflex may contribute to urinary retention after pelvic surgery.

Central coordination of storage reflexes. The urine storage center resides in a lateral pontine area. This supraspinal site inhibits sympathetic and somatic nerves during voiding. The cerebral cortex must also project to the EUS neurons since voluntary interruption of micturition or an enhanced guarding reflex is possible. This pathway forms the anatomic substrate for the nonneurogenic, voluntary dyssynergia syndrome observed in some children.

Reflex control of bladder compliance. During bladder filling, the intravesical pressure remains low and constant (5–10 cmH$_2$O). Viscoelastic properties of the bladder wall and the electromechanical properties of smooth muscle contribute to bladder compliance during filling.[76] However, bladder compliance must also be influenced by sacral neural input because intrathecal drugs can dramatically alter this value.[56,60,61] In addition, stretch-induced production of local factors such as prostaglandins, NO or parathyroid hormone-related protein could theoretically influence bladder compliance through urothelial reflexes. In animals, the hypogastric pathway inhibits the detrusor smooth muscle.[77] However, in humans, the importance of sympathetic innervation on bladder during filling is controversial.[78]

Reflex inhibition of efferent pathways. In addition to activation of sympathetic and somatic pathways, urine storage relies on inhibition of central and peripheral parasympathetic efferent pathways. Descending supraspinal input restricts sacral preganglionic outflow to the bladder. This inhibition may be due to the release of transmitters that depress neural activity at several key sites, including afferent receiving areas and preganglionic neurons. Peripheral mechanisms can also turn off excitatory parasympathetic pathways. Adrenergic sympathetic fibers synapse on parasympathetic postganglionic neurons or interneurons in the pelvic plexus. Heightened sympathetic activity stimulates α_2-adrenoceptors on parasympathetic ganglion cells that block cholinergic ganglionic transmission.[79] Purinergic (ATP), enkephalinergic, tachykinin, GABAminergic, and serotonergic mechanisms also inhibit cholinergic transmission in bladder ganglia. These mechanisms allow the pelvic ganglia to function as high-pass filters. Prejunctional M2 receptors reduce the release of acetylcholine. Conversely, prejunctional nicotinic receptors facilitate its release.[80] Finally, local factors such as endothelin can depress ganglionic transmission in pelvic ganglia.[81]

Other storage reflexes. A profound degree of integration and coordination exists in central autonomic pathways. Therefore it is not unexpected that neural activity from a variety of somatic and visceral tissues affects voiding and storage reflexes. For example, distension of the rectum, probing the cervix and stimulation of the perineum transiently inhibit voiding.[82] These reflexes probably prevent urination during defecation or sexual activity. They also provide the neurophysiologic basis for cutaneous, anal or vaginal stimulators used in the treatment of urinary incontinence.

Although the physiologic basis for neuromodulation is unclear, sacral nerve root stimulation (Interstim) may activate pelvic afferents that reflexively inhibit micturition. The mechanism must rely on supraspinal centers since Interstim is rarely effective for OAB in the setting of complete spinal cord transection.

SUMMARY

Voiding and continence require switching from activation of a micturition reflex, with inhibition of storage reflexes, to inhibition of the micturition reflex, with activation of storage reflexes. The association of many neurologic dis-orders with disturbances in voiding reflects the extensive integration and coordination between neural networks. Complex excitatory and inhibitory mechanisms through-out the neuraxis regulate this switching network. Drugs used to treat voiding disorders work by affecting these pathways or by acting directly on the bladder and its outlet. Precise delineation of these networks will produce refinements in the treatment of many types of bladder dysfunction.

REFERENCES

1. Drake MJ, Mills IW, et al. Model of peripheral autonomous modules and a myovesical plexus in normal and overactive bladder function. Lancet 2001;358(9279):401–403.
2. Turner WH, Brading AF Smooth muscle of the bladder in the normal and the diseased state: pathophysiology, diagnosis and treatment. Pharmacol Ther 1997;75(2):77–110.
3. Thind P, Lose G The effect of bilateral pudendal blockade on the static urethral closure function in healthy females. Obstet Gynecol 1992;80(6):906–911.
4. Barber MD, Bremer RE, et al. Innervation of the female levator ani muscles. Am J Obstet Gynecol 2002;187(1):64–71.
5. Bahns E, Halsband U, et al. Responses of sacral visceral afferents from the lower urinary tract, colon and anus to mechanical stimulation. Pflugers Arch 1987;410(3): 296–303.
6. Habler HJ, Janig W, et al. Activation of unmyelinated afferent fibres by mechanical stimuli and inflammation of the urinary bladder in the cat. J Physiol 1990;425:545–562.
7. Mallory B, Steers WD, et al. Electrophysiological study of micturition reflexes in rats. Am J Physiol 1989;257(2 Pt 2):R410–421.
8. Jung SY, Fraser MO, et al. Urethral afferent nerve activity affects the micturition reflex; implication for the relationship between stress incontinence and detrusor instability. J Urol 1999;162(1):204–212.
9. Morgan C, Nadelhaft I, et al. The distribution of visceral primary afferents from the pelvic nerve to Lissauer's tract and the spinal gray matter and its relationship to the sacral parasympathetic nucleus. J Comp Neurol 1981;201(3):415–440.
10. De Groat WC, Downie JW, et al. Basic neurophysiology and neuropharmacology. In: Wein AJ, ed. Incontinence. Plymouth, UK: Health Publications; 1999.
11. Maggi CA, Meli A. The role of neuropeptides in the regulation of the micturition reflex. J Auton Pharmacol 1986;6(2):133–162.
12. Gu J, Blank MA, et al. Peptide-containing nerves in human urinary bladder. Urology 1984;24(4):353–357.
13. Batra S, Biorklund A, et al. Identification and characterization of muscarinic cholinergic receptors in the human urinary bladder and parotid gland. J Auton Nerv Syst 1987;20(2):129–135.
14. de Groat WC, Kawatani M. Enkephalinergic inhibition in parasympathetic ganglia of the urinary bladder of the cat. J Physiol 1989;413:13–29.
15. Morris JL, Gibbins IL, et al. Galanin-like immunoreactivity in sympathetic and parasympathetic neurons of the toad Bufo marinus. Neurosci Lett 1989;102(2-3): 142–148.
16. Dun NJ, Dun SL, et al. Nitric oxide synthase immunoreactivity in the rat, mouse, cat and squirrel monkey spinal cord. Neuroscience 1993;54(4):845–857.
17. Yoshimura N, Chancellor MB. Current and future pharmacological treatment for overactive bladder. J Urol 2002;168(5):1897–1913.
18. Chess-Williams R, Chapple CR, et al. The minor population of M3-receptors mediate contraction of human detrusor muscle in vitro. J Auton Pharmacol 2001;21(5-6):243–248.
19. Wang P, Luthin GR, et al. Muscarinic acetylcholine receptor subtypes mediating urinary bladder contractility and coupling to GTP binding proteins. J Pharmacol Exp Ther 1995;273(2):959–966.
20. Ikeda K, Kobayashi S, et al. M(3) receptor antagonism by the novel antimuscarinic agent solifenacin in the urinary bladder and salivary gland. Naunyn Schmiedebergs Arch Pharmacol 2002;366(2):97–103.
21. Burnstock G, Dumsday B, et al. Atropine resistant excitation of the urinary bladder: the possibility of transmission via nerves releasing a purine nucleotide. Br J Pharmacol 1972;44(3):451–461.
22. Yoshida M, Miyamae K, et al. Management of detrusor dysfunction in the elderly: changes in acetylcholine and adenosine triphosphate release during aging. Urology 2004;63(3 Suppl 1):17–23.
23. Mattiasson A, Andersson KE, et al. Interaction between adrenergic and cholinergic nerve terminals in the urinary bladder of rabbit, cat and man. J Urol 1987;137(5):1017–1019.
24. Bennett BC, Kruse MN, et al. Neural control of urethral outlet activity in vivo: role of nitric oxide. J Urol 1995;153(6):2004–2009.
25. Persson K Alm P, et al. Nitric oxide synthase in pig lower urinary tract: immunohistochemistry, NADPH diaphorase histochemistry and functional effects. Br J Pharmacol 1993;110(2):521–530.
26. Fowler CJ, Jewkes D, et al. Intravesical capsaicin for neurogenic bladder dysfunction. Lancet 1992;339(8803):1239.
27. Lazzeri M, Spinelli M, et al. Intravesical vanilloids and neurogenic incontinence: ten years experience. Urol Int 2004;72(2):145–149.
28. Giuliani S, Patacchini R, et al. Characterization of the tachykinin neurokinin-2 receptor in the human urinary bladder by means of selective receptor antagonists and peptidase inhibitors. J Pharmacol Exp Ther 1993;267(2):590–595.
29. Lecci A, Giuliani S, et al. Effect of the NK-1 receptor antagonist GR 82,334 on reflexly-induced bladder contractions. Life Sci 1992;51(26):PL277–280.
30. Birder LA, Ruan HZ, Chopra B, et al. Alterations in P2X and P2Y purinergic receptor expression in urinary bladder from normal cats and cats with interstitial cystitis. Am J Physiol Renal Physiol 2004; 287(5):F1084–1091.
31. Vlaskovska M, Kasakov L, et al. P2X3 knock-out mice reveal a major sensory role for urothelially released ATP. J Neurosci 2001;21(15):5670–5677.
32. Nordling J. Influence of sympathetic nervous system on lower urinary tract in man. Neurourol Urodyn 1983;2:3.
33. Kirby R, Andersson KE, et al. Alpha(1)-adrenoceptor selectivity and the treatment of benign prostatic hyperplasia and lower urinary tract symptoms. Prostate Cancer Prostatic Dis 2000;3(2):76–83.
34. Morita T, Iizuka H, et al. Function and distribution of beta3-adrenoceptors in rat, rabbit and human urinary bladder and external urethral sphincter. J Smooth Muscle Res 2000;36(1):21–32.
35. Rohner TJ, Hannigan JD, et al. Altered in vitro adrenergic responses of dog detrusor muscle after chronic bladder outlet obstruction. Urology 1978;11(4):357–361.
36. Christmas T, Kirby R Alpha-adrenoceptor blockers in the treatment of benign prostatic hyperplasia. World J Urol 1991;9:36–40.

SECTION 2 Physiology

37. Roppolo JR, Nadelhaft I, et al. The organization of pudendal motoneurons and primary afferent projections in the spinal cord of the rhesus monkey revealed by horseradish peroxidase. J Comp Neurol 1985;234(4):475–488.

38. McKenna KE, Nadelhaft I. The organization of the pudendal nerve in the male and female rat. J Comp Neurol 1986;248(4):532–549.

39. Morgan CW, de Groat WC, et al. Axon collaterals indicate broad intraspinal role for sacral preganglionic neurons. Proc Natl Acad Sci USA 1991;88(15):6888–6892.

40. Siegel SW, Catanzaro F, et al. Long-term results of a multicenter study on sacral nerve stimulation for treatment of urinary urge incontinence, urgency-frequency, and retention. Urology 2000;56(6 Suppl 1):87–91.

41. Dattilo J. A long-term study of patient outcomes with pelvic muscle re-education for urinary incontinence. J Wound Ostomy Continence Nurs 2002;28(4):199–205.

42. Morita T, Nishizawa O, et al. Pelvic nerve innervation of the external sphincter of urethra as suggested by urodynamic and horse-radish peroxidase studies. J Urol 1984;131(3):591–595.

43. Dykstra DD, Sidi AA, et al. Effects of botulinum A toxin on detrusor-sphincter dyssynergia in spinal cord injury patients. J Urol 1988;139(5):919–922.

44. Lapides J. Function of striated muscle in control of urination II. Effect of complete skeletal muscle paralyis. Surg Forum 1955;6:613–615.

45. Gosling JA, Dixon JS, et al. The autonomic innervation of the human male and female bladder neck and proximal urethra. J Urol 1977;118(2):302–305.

46. Gajewski J, Downie JW, et al. Experimental evidence for a central nervous system site of action in the effect of alpha-adrenergic blockers on the external urinary sphincter. J Urol 1984;132(2):403–409.

47. Dmochowski RR, Miklos JR, et al. Duloxetine versus placebo for the treatment of North American women with stress urinary incontinence. J Urol 2003;170(4 Pt 1): 1259–1263.

48. De Groat WC, Steers WD. Autonomic regulation of the urinary bladder and sexual organs. In: Spyer M, ed. Central regulation of the autonomic functions. Oxford: Oxford University Press; 1990.

49. Holstege G, Griffiths D, et al. Anatomical and physiological observations on supraspinal control of bladder and urethral sphincter muscles in the cat. J Comp Neurol 1986;250(4):449–461.

50. Kruse MN, Noto H, et al. Pontine control of the urinary bladder and external urethral sphincter in the rat. Brain Res 1990;532(1-2):182–190.

51. Imaki T, Nahan JL, et al. Differential regulation of corticotropin-releasing factor mRNA in rat brain regions by glucocorticoids and stress. J Neurosci 1991;11(3):585–599.

52. Grill WM, Erokwu BO, et al. Extended survival time following pseudorabies virus injection labels the suprapontine neural network controlling the bladder and urethra in the rat. Neurosci Lett 1999;270(2):63–66.

53. Kergozien S, Menetrey D. Environmental influences on viscero(noci)ceptive brain activities: the effects of sheltering. Brain Res Cogn Brain Res 2000;10(1-2):111–117.

54. Koyama K. Effects of amygdaloid and olfactory tubercle stimulation on efferent activities of the vesical branch of the pelvic nerve and the urethral branch of the pudendal nerve in dogs. Urol Int 1991;47(Suppl 1):23–30.

55. Klausner A, Na YG, Tuttle JB, Steers WD. Corticotropin releasing factor (CRF) lowers micturition threshold through sites in the brainstem and spinal cord. Auton Neurosci: Basic Clinical 2005; in press.

56. Roppolo JR, Booth AM, et al. The effects of naloxone on the neural control of the urinary bladder of the cat. Brain Res 1983;264(2):355–358.

57. Herman RM, Wainberg MC, et al. The effect of a low dose of intrathecal morphine on impaired micturition reflexes in human subjects with spinal cord lesions. Anesthesiology 1988;69(3):313–318.

58. Booth AM, Hisamitsu T, et al. Regulation of urinary bladder capacity by endogenous opioid peptides. J Urol 1985;133(2):339–342.

59. DeGroat WC. The effects of glycine, GABA and strychnine on sacral parasympathetic preganglionic neurones. Brain Res 1970;18(3):542–544.

60. Nanninga JB, Frost F, et al. Effect of intrathecal baclofen on bladder and sphincter function. J Urol 1989;142(1):101–105.

61. Steers WD, Meythaler JM, et al. Effects of acute bolus and chronic continuous intrathecal baclofen on genitourinary dysfunction due to spinal cord pathology. J Urol 1992;148(6):1849–1855.

62. Lee KS, Na YG, et al. Alterations in voiding frequency and cystometry in the clomipramine induced model of endogenous depression and reversal with fluoxetine. J Urol 2003;170(5):2067–2071.

63. Hunsballe JM, Djurhuus JC. Clinical options for imipramine in the management of urinary incontinence. Urol Res 2001;29(2):118–125.

64. Yoshiyama M, Roppolo JR, et al. Effects of MK-801 on the micturition reflex in the rat—possible sites of action. J Pharmacol Exp Ther 1993;265(2):844–850.

65. Seki S, Igawa Y, et al. Role of dopamine D1 and D2 receptors in the micturition reflex in conscious rats. Neurourol Urodyn 2001;20(1):105–113.

66. Pandita RK, Nylen A, et al. Oxytocin-induced stimulation and inhibition of bladder activity in normal, conscious rats—influence of nitric oxide synthase inhibition. Neuroscience 1998;85(4):1113–1119.

67. Uemura E, Fletcher TF, et al. Distribution of sacral afferent axons in cat urinary bladder. Am J Anat 1973;136(3):305–313.

68. Jensen D Jr. Pharmacological studies of the uninhibited neurogenic bladder. III. The influence of adrenergic excitatory and inhibitory drugs on the cystometrogram of neurological patients with normal and uninhibited neurogenic bladder. Acta Neurol Scand 1981;64(6):401–426.

69. Vera PL, Nadelhaft I. Conduction velocity distribution of afferent fibers innervating the rat urinary bladder. Brain Res 1990;520(1-2):83–89.

70. Nathan PW, Smith MC. The centrifugal pathway for micturition within the spinal cord. J Neurol Neurosurg Psychiat 1958;21:177–189.

71. Tang PC, Ruch TC. Localization of brainstem and diencephalic area controlling the micturitio reflex. J Comp Neurol 1956;20:213–245.

72. Nadelhaft I, Vera PL, et al. Central nervous system neurons labelled following the injection of pseudorabies virus into the rat urinary bladder. Neurosci Lett 1992;143(1-2):271–274.

73. Kershen RT, Kalisvaart J, et al. Functional brain imaging and the bladder: new insights into cerebral control over micturition. Curr Urol Rep 2003;4(5):344–349.

74. Shimoda N, Takakusaki K, et al. The changes in the activity of pudendal motoneurons in relation to reflex micturition evoked in decerebrate cats. Neurosci Lett 1992;135(2):175–178.

75. McGuire EJ, Herlihy E. Bladder and urethral responses to isolated sacral motor root stimulation. Invest Urol 1978;16(3):219–223.

76. De Groat WC, Lalley PM. Reflex firing in the lumbar sympathetic outflow to activation of vesical afferent fibres. J Physiol 1972;226(2):289–309.

77. Nergardh A, Boreus LO. Autonomic receptor function in the lower urinary tract of man and cat. Scand J Urol Nephrol 1972;6(1):32–36.

78. Steers WD. Physiology of the urinary bladder. In: Vaughan ED, ed. Campbell's urology. Philadelphia: WB Saunders; 1992.

79. De Groat WC, Booth AM. Inhibition and facilitation in parasympathetic ganglia of the urinary bladder. Fed Proc 1980;39(12):2990–2996.

80. Somogyi GT, de Groat WC. Evidence for inhibitory nicotinic and facilitatory muscarinic receptors in cholinergic nerve terminals of the rat urinary bladder. J Auton Nerv Syst 1992;37(2):89–97.

81. Nishimura T, Krier J, et al. Endothelin causes prolonged inhibition of nicotinic transmission in feline colonic parasympathetic ganglia. Am J Physiol 1991;261(4 Pt 1):G628–633.

82. Sato A, Schmidt RF. The modulation of visceral functions by somatic afferent activity. Jpn J Physiol 1987;37(1):1–17.

SECTION 2 Physiology

Anatomy and Physiology of Anorectal Function

Christine Norton

INTRODUCTION

Fecal continence is achieved via the integrated neuro-muscular functioning of the bowel and its sphincters.

COLONIC MOTILITY

The colon is composed of an inner mucosa and an outer serosa with two muscle layers in between: an inner layer of circular smooth muscle and an outer layer of longitudinal smooth muscle. Together, the activity of these muscles achieves mixing and movement of colonic contents, mediated by the local enteric nervous system, with some influence from the central nervous system. The presence of the rich enteric nervous system within the gut wall means that colonic motility is largely maintained after spinal transsection. The colon has frequent forward and retrograde churning activity, mostly via contractions of the circular muscle layer, which ensures exposure of the contents to the colonic mucosa for fluid reabsorption. About 1500 ml of ileal contents is delivered to the cecum via the ileocecal valve each day. About 150–200 ml of stool is passed daily, the balance being mostly accounted for by water reabsorption. The faster contents move through the colon, the less opportunity there is for this absorption, intestinal hurry thus leading to loose stool.

Periodically, high-amplitude propagated contractions (HAPCs) move stool along the colon in the direction of the rectum, primarily by contraction of the longitudinal layer of muscle. These pressure waves can be of great amplitude, especially in people with irritable bowel syndrome, in whom they can be up to 500 cmH$_2$O.[1] These mass movements occur regularly and are most pronounced after eating or drinking—the "gastrocolic response," mediated hormonally. In health the bowel is relatively inactive while asleep and most active in the first few hours after waking, with additional stimulation to motility coming from mobility and eating. This is the reason why the most usual time for a bowel action is after eating breakfast.

The right side of the colon acts to store stool and absorb fluid. By the time stool reaches the left colon, it is relatively solid and the major activity is propulsion and storage. Average transit time through the colon is 36–72 hours and this does not change with healthy aging.[2]

RECTUM

The rectum is approximately 15 cm long and has a reservoir function. It is composed of the same two layers of smooth muscle as the colon, as well as a mucosa and submucosa and an outer serosa. There is no somatic nerve supply and the rectum is thus not under voluntary control. It has both sympathetic (via lumbar nerve roots) and parasympathetic (via sacral nerve roots) autonomic innervation, as well as enteric (intrinsic) nerves. The anterior and posterior walls are somewhat shorter than the lateral walls, giving the classic three-section appearance of the rectum (sometimes referred to as the valves of Houston). The rectum is a compliant organ, gradually relaxing and accommodating stool and flatus.

The first sensation of rectal filling seems to be a mucosal sensation responding to stretch. Sensation can be perceived at volumes as low as 10 ml. Pressure receptors in the pelvic floor detect rectal distension,[3] although the feeling described is often a rather vague notion of "fullness." Rectal sensation is an important determinant of continence.[4,5] Pain receptors in the serosa mediate the sensation of maximal filling, although the rectum is relatively insensitive to pain.

A normal rectum has considerable ability to expand, often accommodating stool volumes of up to 300 ml without discomfort. Rectal filling is achieved with minimal or no increase in intrarectal pressure.[3] Resting pressure in the rectum is low, at approximately 5–20 cmH$_2$O and this increases little with rectal filling except at very large volumes.[6] Gradual rectal filling seems to produce less sensation of urgency than the sudden arrival of a bolus, especially of loose stool, which will usually result in urgency.

Inflammation can increase sensitivity and lessen compliance of the rectum. Advancing age is associated with both a blunted rectal sensation and reduced tone and increased compliance,[7] sometimes termed "rectal dyschezia."[2]

The anterior rectal wall is adjacent to the posterior vaginal wall, with a thin rectovaginal fascial septum dividing them. Some herniation of the rectum into the vagina (rectocele) may be normal as it is found in up to 80% of asymptomatic women.[8,9]

ANAL SPHINCTERS

There are two anal sphincters responsible for maintaining continence. They appear as two concentric sleeves surrounding the anal canal (Fig. 3.1).

Internal anal sphincter. The internal anal sphincter (IAS) is a smooth muscle in continuity with the circular muscular layer of the rectum, but about three times thicker. It is approximately 2–3 mm thick and 3 cm long, terminating about 1 cm above the anal verge, with men having a longer IAS than women. It normally becomes thicker with age. Like the rectum, it has both sympathetic (via lumbar nerve roots) and parasympathetic (via sacral nerve roots) autonomic innervation. Its normal state is contracted and it is able to generate a constant tension over long periods of time, thus maintaining anal closure at rest. It contributes about 75–85% of resting anal pressure,[10,11] with the balance contributed by the external anal sphincter and the anal mucosa and anal cushions. Normal anal resting pressure is 60–100 cmH$_2$O, which is increased during physical activity, with a decrease with advancing age.[12] Phasic slow-wave pressure variations are normal and more pronounced distally, which

may protect against incontinence during sampling (see below). As patients with a damaged IAS most often report symptoms of passive soiling, it may be deduced that the IAS is largely responsible for passive stool retention at rest in the absence of an urge to defecate.

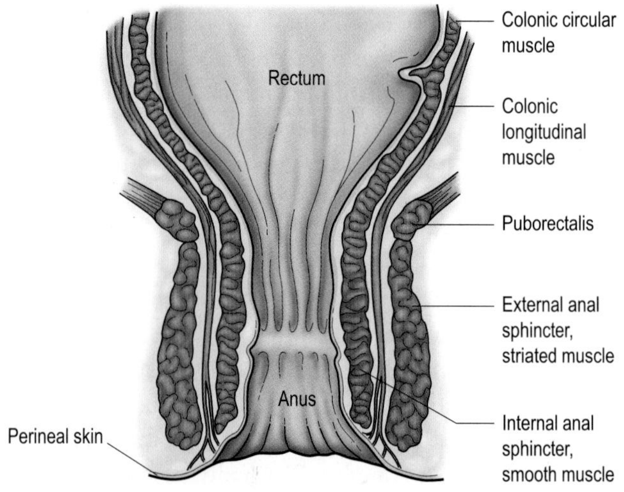

External anal sphincter. Between the internal and external anal sphincters there is a layer of longitudinal muscle continuous with that in the bowel wall. This muscle does not seem to contribute to the continence mechanism but probably has a role in "splinting" the anal canal during defecation.

The external anal sphincter (EAS) is a striated muscle, 6–10 mm thick, in continuity with the muscles of the pelvic floor and extending the length of the anal canal, terminating immediately beneath the perianal skin. It is innervated by branches of the pudendal nerve. Some authors have identified three sections to the sphincter, although functionally they act as a unit. High in the anal canal, the puborectalis can be seen inserting into the EAS. Anteriorly, the sphincter does not usually form a continuous ring caudally in women and this U-shape appearance of the puborectalis merging into the EAS may be misinterpreted as an anterior sphincter defect by inexperienced endosonographers.[13] The normal appearance is for the anterior EAS to be present much lower down the anal canal anteriorly than posteriorly in women;[14,15] this is less pronounced in men.

The EAS contracts reflexly in response to sudden rises in intraabdominal pressure such as coughing or lifting heavy weights. Voluntary squeeze increment over resting pressure is usually 50–100% higher pressure but may reach pressures as high as 300 cmH$_2$O or more, with lower pressures in women than in men and an age-dependent decrease.[12,16] The EAS has a higher proportion of fast-twitch fibers than the pelvic floor and is observed to fatigue rapidly. It is thought that excessive fatigability of the EAS may be associated with fecal incontinence.[17]

With an empty rectum, EAS tone is low. The tone increases with rectal filling and this compensates for the falling IAS pressure with increasing stool volume in the rectum. However, at rectal volumes greater than about 200 ml there is reflex relaxation of the EAS. When the urge to defecate is felt, a voluntary contraction of the EAS is needed to counteract this urge. Once thought to be a reflex, this contraction is found to be voluntary.[18] Patients with damage to the EAS complain primarily of urge fecal incontinence as this ability to squeeze hard enough or long enough to resist the urge to defecate is impaired.

Figure 3.1 Anal sphincters.

Labels:
- Colonic circular muscle
- Rectum
- Colonic longitudinal muscle
- Puborectalis
- External anal sphincter, striated muscle
- Anus
- Perineal skin
- Internal anal sphincter, smooth muscle

PELVIC FLOOR MUSCLES

The muscles of the levator ani, the puborectalis in particular, act as a sling to help create an angle between the rectum

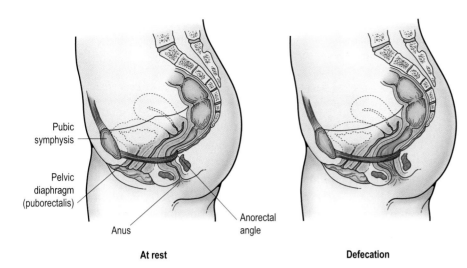

At rest

Defecation

Pubic symphysis

Pelvic diaphragm (puborectalis)

Anus

Anorectal angle

Figure 3.2 Representation of the pelvic floor at rest and during defecation. Note that, at rest, the puborectalis and the rest of the pelvic diaphragm are in tonic contraction to maintain an acute anorectal angle, contributing to continence. During defecation, relaxation of the puborectalis results in straightening out of the angle to ease rectal evacuation.

and the anus by pulling the lower rectum forward towards the pubic bone[19] (Fig. 3.2). The normal angle at rest is approximately 90°.[20] The muscle fibers are a combination of approximately 70% slow-twitch and 30% fast-twitch fibers, as in the anterior pelvic floor. However, the fibers in the perianal levator ani tend to be slightly smaller in diameter than those more anteriorly.[21] The levator ani muscles are innervated by the pudendal nerve arising from S2–4 and maintain a constant resting tone via the slow-twitch fibers.

In health, the position of the pelvic floor maintains the anorectal junction within 4 cm below the level of the coccyx; positions lower than this are considered as abnormal perineal descent.[22] The anorectal angle can be made more acute by voluntary or reflex contraction of the fast-twitch fibers. It is possible that this reflex helps to maintain continence during increases in abdominal pressure. There is also a flap valve effect: when intraabdominal pressure is raised, that rise in pressure acts to close the angle more tightly with rectal mucosa occluding the upper anal canal (Fig. 3.3). There is also a reflex contraction of the pelvic floor as well as the anal sphincter itself.[20]

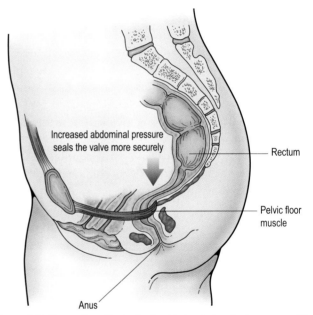

Increased abdominal pressure seals the valve more securely

Rectum

Pelvic floor muscle

Anus

Figure 3.3 Flap valve effect of raised intraabdominal pressure. The arrangement at the anorectal junction results in the formation of a flap valve. The anterior wall of the lower rectum impinges upon the closed anal canal, and any increase in abdominal pressure appears to seal the valve more securely.

STOOL

The content of stool is 70–80% water. The lower the water content, the firmer the stool and the longer stool remains in the gut, the more water will be reabsorbed; hence the observation that constipated people produce lower stool volumes than the nonconstipated. On an average western diet, adults produce about 150–200 ml of stool per day. The balance of the solid matter is some indigestible residue from food. However, colonic bacteria are very effective in utilizing the majority of digestive waste. The flora of the colon have been considered as separate "organ" in their own right, with numerous symbiotic roles for their host. The average colon contains 1–2 kg of bacteria, with as yet poor understanding of the full range of their activity in maintaining health. The majority of solid content of stool is dead (and some live) bacteria.

Stool consistency varies a lot between individuals and with diet: in women only 56% of stools are what is usually considered the "normal" soft formed stool.[23]

ANAL CANAL

The anal canal is 3–5 cm in length, with women having a shorter canal than men. The proximal anal canal is lined with mucosa continuous with the rectal mucosa. At the dentate line there is a "transition zone" to squamous epithelium of the perianal skin, and also a rich sensory innervation with the ability to distinguish between gas, liquid or solid matter. Anal glands at this level may become infected, creating an abscess or even a perianal fistula. Anal sensation is mediated via the pudendal nerve arising from S2–4.[16] This rich innervation means that some anal conditions such as fissure can be extremely painful. There are three anal cushions at the 3, 7, and 11 o'clock positions in the anal canal, contributing 10–20% to resting anal pressure and augmenting the ability of the anus to maintain a mucosal airtight and watertight seal.[24,25] If these cushions become dilated, they are termed hemorrhoids. The mechanism for the ability to selectively release gas while retaining liquid and solid is not yet fully understood.

When the rectum contains stool or flatus, periodic rectal contractions trigger the rectoanal inhibitory reflex, with reflex relaxation of the upper IAS and a consequent fall in anal pressure. This allows stool to enter the upper anal canal where it is "sampled" by the sensory nerves of the anal epithelium at the dentate line.[20,26] Sampling takes place for about 10 seconds approximately every 8–10 minutes throughout rectal filling[6] but seldom reaches conscious appreciation unless a decision is needed as to the social appropriateness of passing stool or flatus. Incontinent people appear to sample less often than continent subjects.[26] The anal canal is also highly sensitive to temperature changes and as the anal temperature is lower than rectal temperature, this may also form part of the sampling mechanism.[27] Resting pressure in the IAS falls progressively as the rectum fills.

NEUROLOGY OF DEFECATION

The neurologic control of the bowel is the result of an intricate balance between the extrinsic nervous system, the enteric nervous system, and the intestinal smooth muscle cells.

The extrinsic nervous system.

The extrinsic nervous system of the bowel is the nervous system which is external to the bowel itself. It consists of autonomic, sensory, and motor nerves (Fig. 3.4).

The **autonomic (smooth muscle, involuntary)** nervous system of the bowel comprises an integrated complex system of parasympathetic (predominantly stimulating motility) and sympathetic (predominantly inhibiting motility) fibers. The parasympathetic vagal nerves originate from the medulla within the brain and supply motor and sensory input to the proximal (upper) colon. The parasympathetic sacral nerves originate from the spinal level S2–4 and contain both motor and sensory fibers to distal (lower) colon.

The sympathetic nerve supply arises from between the 10th thoracic and third lumbar segments. It is composed of fibers that synapse with enteric ganglionic plexuses within the colon wall.

Somatic (voluntary) nerves provide both sensory and motor supply to the pelvic floor and external anal sphincter, via the nervi erigentes (from S2 to S4), direct sacral root branches (from S1 to S5) and the pudendal nerve.

The enteric nervous system.

The enteric nervous system is the internal nervous system of the gut itself. It has an essential role in the control of motility, blood flow, water and electrolyte transport, and acid secretion in the digestive

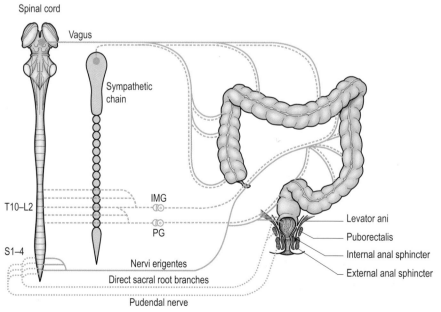

Figure 3.4 Extrinsic nerve supply to gut. The extrinsic nervous system of the bowel and pelvic floor consists of the parasympathetic vagal and sacral innervation (*solid lines*) and the sympathetic outflow from the intermediolateral column of the spinal cord (*dashed lines*). The parasympathetic system is composed of preganglionic fibers that synapse the pre-programmed circuits in the ganglionated enteric plexuses within the colon wall. The sympathetic nerves synapse in the prevertebral celiac (PG), superior and inferior mesenteric (IMG) ganglia. Sensory and motor innervation of the bowel and pelvic floor occurs through the vagus, the nervi erigentes, direct sacral root branches, and the pudendal nerve. Mixed nerves supply the somatic voluntary musculature of the pelvic floor and the external anal sphincter (*dotted lines*).

Spinal cord
Vagus
Sympathetic chain
T10–L2
IMG
PG
S1–4
Nervi erigentes
Direct sacral root branches
Pudendal nerve
Levator ani
Puborectalis
Internal anal sphincter
External anal sphincter

tract. This system is organized in ganglionated plexuses within the bowel wall itself and is separated from the autonomic nervous system. The enteric nervous system has several components: sensory receptors (mechano- and chemoreceptors), interneurons (processing input and controlling effector units, motor and secretory) and effector motor neurons involved in motility of the gut. Enteric nervous control of the bowel is modulated through connections from the autonomic nervous system to the brain. The enteric nervous system has the unique capacity to mediate reflex activity independently of input from the central nervous system. This is why even people with complete destruction of central neurologic input to the bowel maintain some gut motility, as the intrinsic nervous system keeps the bowel working to at least some extent (unlike the bladder which can become totally atonic).

Delaying defecation. At a critical level of rectal filling, sensation is relayed centrally to the cerebral cortex. This volume is dependent upon stool consistency and rectal capacity and compliance. If conditions are not right when the urge to defecate is felt, it is possible to defer defecation. A voluntary contraction of the EAS will counteract the drop in anal pressure from IAS relaxation during the rectoanal inhibitory reflex. This reflex lasts 5–20 seconds, with increasing duration as rectal volume increases,[20] and then resting pressure in the anus is restored as the IAS recovers its normal state of contraction. This EAS contraction is often performed at a subconscious, yet still voluntary, level, without the individual necessarily being aware of the action. The anal contraction returns stool to the rectum, the urge to defecate subsides, and this may initiate retrograde peristalsis in the rectum, with stool pushed back up into the sigmoid colon in some cases. This leads to the experience that if defecation is delayed, sometimes if it is attempted later there is no stool in the rectum to pass. In normal individuals, repeatedly ignoring the call to stool can result in self-induced constipation.[28] The longer stool remains in the rectum, the greater the opportunity for water absorption and the likelihood of hard stool.

DEFECATION

Once conditions are right, a sitting or squatting posture is adopted and a brief push, raising intraabdominal pressure, with coincidental pelvic floor relaxation is usually sufficient to augment rectal wall contractions and propel stool into the anus. The anorectal angle should become more obtuse as the puborectalis relaxes, aligning the rectum and anus. Squatting is a more physiologic position than sitting as it achieves a better alignment of the anus and rectum. If the pelvic floor fails to relax, this can lead to incomplete or ineffective evacuation, sometimes termed rectoanal dyssyn-

ergia or "anismus."[29] The EAS relaxes, reducing intraanal pressure. Rectal contraction means rectal pressure is above anal pressure. Evacuation is normally rapid and completely empties the rectum within a few seconds via a relaxed anus. Sensation from the anus seems to maintain rectal propulsive contraction until evacuation is complete.[6] Reflex defecation is maintained even in complete spinal cord transsection providing that spinal reflexes at the sacral level are intact.

After defecation is completed, there is a reflex after-contraction of the external anal sphincter which should "snap shut" with a higher than resting pressure.[6] This high pressure serves to clear the anal canal of any residual stool, which is either returned upwards to the rectum or expelled. Thus the anal canal should not normally contain stool in the resting state.

Normal frequency of defecation in western populations varies between three times per day and three times per week,[30] with only a minority (approximately 40% of men and 33% of women) having a single bowel action on a daily basis.[23] There are many influences on stool frequency including diet, mobility, emotional state, lifestyle and even personality, with extraverts producing larger and more frequent stools than introverts.[31] Young women in particular are likely to have an irregular bowel habit. Very hard or soft stool and low-volume pellet stool may be more difficult to evacuate completely than soft formed stool.

Toilet training. Continence is a learned social and physiologic skill. The newborn infant does not have the neuromuscular maturity to allow control, nor the social realization that continence is a desirable achievement. The complex coordination needed to delay defecation cannot be "taught" but when the child has the physical maturity (about the age of 2 years), most will acquire continence fairly readily via a combination of imitation and positive reinforcement for the desired behavior. Cognitive impairment or emotional problems may delay or even preclude acquisition of continence skills.

Once continent, the body "knows" how to do it but that knowledge is often not accessible consciously, meaning that many people struggle to describe what actions they take to defer defecation.[32] Once the skill has been acquired, control usually operates at a subconscious but still voluntary level. Overemphasis on the importance of clean pants or punishment for "accidents" can lead to deliberate retention of stool and may be the basis for retentive encopresis in some children, where the rectum becomes overloaded and then soiling occurs as an "overflow."[33]

FECAL AND ANAL INCONTINENCE

Fecal incontinence (FI) has been defined in different ways. The colorectal literature distinguishes loss of solid, liquid or gas.[34] The Royal College of Physicians has proposed "the involuntary or inappropriate passage of faeces."[35] An international panel of experts has defined "functional fecal incontinence" as "recurrent uncontrolled passage of fecal material for at least one month, in an individual with a developmental age of at least four years...."[36] Some authors also include inability to control passage of flatus or an arbitrary frequency with which symptoms must occur to be included.

The term "anal incontinence" (AI) is usually used to denote any involuntary leakage, whether of solid, liquid or gas. The International Consultation on Incontinence has proposed: "Anal incontinence is the involuntary loss of flatus, liquid or solid stool that is a social or hygienic problem," with FI defined identically except for the omission of flatus incontinence.[37] This definition recognizes the fact that people react very differently to the same objective situation. For example, involuntary loss of flatus which is hardly noticed by one person is experienced as socially incapacitating by another.

Prevalence of fecal incontinence. Fecal incontinence is much more common in the general population than is often realized. Although the problem does increase with advancing age and disability, there are also large numbers of young, otherwise healthy adults with this distressing symptom. Studies have found widely varying prevalence rates of fecal incontinence, depending upon the definition of incontinence used and the population studied. The largest community study in the UK was a postal survey with over 15,000 respondents,[38] in which 5.7% of women and 6.2% of men over 40 years old living in their own homes reported some degree of fecal incontinence, with prevalence increasing with age. Overall, 1.4% of adults reported major fecal incontinence (at least several times per month) and 0.7% had disabling fecal incontinence (major incontinence with major impact on their life). Two-thirds of those with disabling fecal incontinence said that they wanted help with symptoms.

Different methods have yielded different results. In the USA a telephone survey found that 2.2% of the population reported some anal incontinence (0.8% were incontinent of solid stool, 1.2% to liquid stool, and 1.3% to flatus). Two-thirds of those reported as anally incontinent were under 65 years old, and 63% were female. These results are in response to the question "In the last year, have you or anyone in your household experienced unwanted or unexpected or embarrassing loss of control of bowels or gas?."[39]

This study excluded people who live in nursing homes but separate data enabled a calculation that 1.1% of the total population are incontinent of solid stool and 2.6%

have some form of anal incontinence. Ten percent of those reporting incontinence had more than one episode per week, one-third had restricted their activities as a result of their incontinence, and only 36% had consulted a doctor about it.[39]

Overall, between 2% and 24% of the population have been found to report AI and 0.4–18% FI, depending on the methodology of prevalence studies.[40]

At present, the majority of people with fecal incontinence do not present for, or receive, professional help.[41,42] There is a dual problem of reluctance to face the embarrassment of admitting to the problem and a lack of knowledgeable health professionals with an interest in the subject, with few specialist facilities to manage those who do present for help.

Johanson & Lafferty studied 881 people consulting a general practitioner (GP) or gastroenterologist. Overall, 18.4% admitted to at least one episode of stool leakage. As might be expected, the rate amongst those consulting a gastroenterologist was double that in the GP attenders, with 2.7% reporting daily incontinence and 4.5% weekly. Except in the under-30 year olds, more men than women were incontinent in all age groups. Of those with incontinence, only 20% of those attending the GP had mentioned their incontinence and under half had told their gastroenterologist, while 10% avoided leaving their home for fear of an accident.[42] Drossman similarly found more men than women over 45 years with some symptoms, 7.9% versus 7.7%, but the men were more likely to have minor soiling while more women were grossly incontinent (0.9% women versus 0.5% of men).[43]

In people over 65 living at home, 3.7% report fecal incontinence at least once a week and 6.1% need to wear pads in case of bowel leakage.[44] Kok et al found that 16.9% of Dutch women over 85 years reported occasional involuntary loss of feces but that only 4.2% of 60–85 year olds have a problem.[45] Twenty-one percent of elderly people living in a home or hospital are fecally incontinent at least weekly[46] and for most people in institutional care, fecal incontinence is compounded by urinary incontinence. Among the frail elderly in nursing homes, prevalence of over 20% is common but rates of over 90% are also reported,[47] suggesting that variation may be due to factors other than the aging bowel (such as institutional regimes and policies).

Although childbirth is commonly cited as the most widespread causative factor for fecal incontinence, many studies have shown an equal prevalence in men and women. The reasons for this are at present unclear. There is also a large overlap between symptoms of urinary and fecal incontinence,[48] and especially an association between overactive bladder and overactive bowel.[49]

REFERENCES

1. Herbst F, Kamm MA, Morris GP, Britton K, Woloszko J, Nicholls RJ. Gastrointestinal transit and prolonged ambulatory colonic motility in health and fecal incontinence. Gut 1997;41:381–389.

2. Harari D. Bowel care in old age. In: Norton C, Chelvanayagam S, eds. Bowel continence nursing. Beaconsfield: Beaconsfield Publishers; 2004: 132–149.

3. Williamson ME. Pathophysiological correlations in anorectal conditions. In: Duthie GS, Gardiner A, eds. Physiology of the gastrointestinal tract. London: Whurr Publishers; 2004: 73–86.

4. Read M, Read NW. Role of anorectal sensation in preserving continence. Gut 1982;23:345–347.

5. Wald A. Biofeedback for neurogenic fecal incontinence: rectal sensation is a determinant of outcome. J Ped Gastroenterol Nutrition 1983;2:302–306.

6. Emmanuel AV. The physiology of defecation and continence. In: Norton C, Chelvanayagam S, eds. Bowel continence nursing. Beaconsfield: Beaconsfield Publishers; 2004: 8–13.

7. Read NW, Abouzekry L, Read M, Howell P, Ottewell D, Donnelly TC. Anorectal function in elderly patients with fecal impaction. Gastroenterology 1985;89:959–966.

8. Shorren P, McHugh S, Diamant NE. Defecography in normal volunteers: results and implications. Gut 1989;30:1737–1749.

9. Ikenberry S, Lappas JC, Hana MP. Defecography in healthy subjects: comparison of three contrast media. Radiology 1996;201:233–238.

10. Frenckner B, Euler CV. Influence of pudendal block on the function of the anal sphincters. Gut 1975;16:482–489.

11. Schweiger M. Method for determining individual contributions of voluntary and involuntary anal sphincters to resting tone. Dis Colon Rectum 1979;22:415–416.

12. McHugh S, Diamant NE. Effect of age, gender and parity on anal canal pressures. Dig Dis Sci 1987;32(7):726–736.

13. Bollard RC, Gardiner A, Lindow S, Phillips K, Duthie GS. Normal women have natural sphincter defects. Dis Colon Rectum 2003;46(8):1083–1088.

14. Aronson MP, Lee RA, Berquist TH. Anatomy of anal sphincters and related structures in continent women studied with magnetic resonance imaging. Obstet Gynecol 1990;76:846–851.

15. Bartram CI, DeLancey JO. Imaging pelvic floor disorders. Berlin: Springer-Verlag; 2003.

16. Farouk R. Anorectal physiology. In: Duthie GS, Gardiner A, eds. Physiology of the gatrointestinal tract. London: Whurr Publishers; 2004: 87–105.

17. Marcello PW, Barrett RC, Coller JA, et al. Fatigue rate index as a new measure of external sphincter function. Dis Colon Rectum 1998;41:336–343.

18. Whitehead WE, Orr WC, Engel BT, Schuster MM. External anal sphincter response to rectal distension: learned response or reflex. Psychophysiology 1982;19(1):57–62.

19. DeLancey JO. Functional anatomy of the pelvic floor and urinary continence mechanism. In: Schussler B, Laycock J, Norton P, Stanton SL, eds. Pelvic floor re-education. London: Springer-Verlag; 1994: 9–21.

20. Rao SS. Pathophysiology of adult fecal incontinence. Gastroenterology 2004;126(suppl)(1):S14–S22.

21. Dixon J, Gosling J. Histomorphology of the pelvic floor muscle. In: Schussler B, Laycock J, Norton P, Stanton SL, eds. Pelvic floor re-education. London: Springer-Verlag; 1994: 28–33.

22. Goei R, Van Engelshoven J, Schouten H. Anorectal function: defecographic measurement in asymptomatic subjects. Radiology 1989;173:137–141.

23. Heaton KW, Radvan J, Cripps H, Mountford RA, Braddon FEM, Hughes AO. Defecation frequency and timing, and stool form in the general population: a prospective study. Gut 1992;33:818–824.

24. Lestar B, Penninckx F, Rigauts H, Kerremans R. The internal anal sphincter cannot close the anal canal completely. Int J Colorectal Dis 1992;7:159–161.

25. Lestar B, Penninckx F, Rigauts H, Kerremans R. The composition of anal basal pressure. An in vivo and in vitro study in man. Int J Colorectal Dis 1989;4:118–122.

26. Miller R, Bartolo DCC, Cervero F, Mortensen NJ. Anorectal sampling: a comparison of normal and incontinent patients. Br J Surg 1988;75:44–47.

27. Miller R, Bartolo DC, Cervero C. Anorectal temperature sensation: a comparison of normal and incontinence patients. Br J Surg 1987;74:511–515.

28. Klauser AG, Voderholzer WA, Heinrich CA, Schindlbeck NE, Mueller-Lissner SA. Behavioural modification of colonic function—can constipation be learned? Dig Dis Sci 1990;35:1271–1275.

29. Preston DM, Lennard-Jones JE. Anismus in chronic constipation. Dig Dis Sci 1985;30(5):413–418.

30. Connell AM, Hilton C, Irvine G, Lennard-Jones JE, Misiewicz JJ. Variation in bowel habit in two population samples. BMJ 1965;ii:1095–1099.

31. Tucker DM, Sandstead HH, Logan GM, et al. Dietary fiber and personality factors as determinants of stool output. Gastroenterology 1981;81:879–883.

32. Norton C. Nurses, bowel continence, stigma and taboos. J Wound Ostomy Cont Nurs 2004;31(2):85–94.

33. Clayden GS, Hollins G. Constipation and fecal incontinence in childhood. In: Norton C, Chelvanayagam S, eds. Bowel continence nursing. Beaconsfield: Beaconsfield Publishers; 2004: 217–228.

34. Jorge JM, Wexner SD. Etiology and management of fecal incontinence. Dis Colon Rectum 1993;36(1):77–97.

35. Royal College of Physicians. Incontinence. Causes, management and provision of services. A Working Party of the Royal College of Physicians. J Roy Coll Phys London 1995;29(4):272–274.

36. Whitehead WE, Wald A, Diamant NE, Enck P, Pemberton JH, Rao SSC. Functional disorders of the anus and rectum. Gut 1999;45(Suppl 11):1155–1159.

37. Norton C, Whitehead WE, Bliss DZ, Metsola P, Tries J. Conservative and pharmacological management of fecal incontinence in adults. In: Abrams P, Khoury S, Wein A, Cardozo L, eds. Incontinence (Proceedings of the Third International Consultation on Incontinence). Plymouth, UK: Health Books; 2005.

38. Perry S, Shaw C, McGrother C, et al. The prevalence of fecal incontinence in adults aged 40 years or more living in the community. Gut 2002;50:480–484.

39. Nelson R, Norton N, Cautley E, Furner S. Community-based prevalence of anal incontinence. JAMA 1995;274(7):559–561.

40. Macmillan AK, Merrie AEH, Marshall RJ, Parry BR. The prevalence of fecal incontinence in community-dwelling adults: a systematic review of the literature. Dis Colon Rectum 2004;47:1341–1349.

41. Leigh RJ, Turnberg LA. Fecal incontinence: the unvoiced symptom. Lancet 1982;1:1349–1351.

42. Johanson JF, Lafferty J. Epidemiology of fecal incontinence: the silent affliction. Am J Gastroenterol 1996;91(1):33–36.

43. Drossman DA, Li Z, Andruzzi E, Temple RD, Talley NJ, Thompson WG. U.S. householder survey of functional gastrointestinal disorders. Dig Dis Sci 1993;38(9):1569–1580.

44. Talley NJ, O'Keefe EA, Zinsmeister AR, Melton LJ. Prevalence of gastrointestinal symptoms in the elderly: a population-based study. Gastroenterology 1992;102:895–901.

45. Kok ALM, Voorhorst FJ, Burger CW, Van Houten P, Kenemans P, Janssens J. Urinary and fecal incontinence in community-residing elderly women. Age Ageing 1992;21:211–215.

46. Peet SM, Castleden CM, McGrother CW. Prevalence of urinary and fecal incontinence in hospitals and residential and nursing homes for older people [see comments]. BMJ 1995; 311(7012):1063–1064.

47. Brocklehurst JC, Dickinson E, Windsor J. Laxatives and fecal incontinence in long term care. Nurs Standard 1999;13:32–36.

48. Khullar V, Damiano R, Toozs-Hobson P, Cardozo L. Prevalence of fecal incontinence among women with urinary incontinence. Br J Obstet Gynaecol 1998;105:1211–1213.

49. Monga AK, Marrero JM, Stanton SL, Lemieux M-C, Maxwell JD. Is there an irritable bladder in the irritable bowel syndrome? Br J Obstet Gynaecol 1997;104:1409–1412.

Physiology of the Vagina

Linda Brubaker

INTRODUCTION

Clinicians who provide pelvic care for women benefit from a thorough understanding of vaginal anatomy, function, and physiology. Although this is an understudied area, a solid basis in our current knowledge is helpful. This chapter will review the normal anatomic and physiologic features of the adult vagina. Clinically relevant topics related to vaginal health are also discussed.

ANATOMIC FEATURES THAT RELATE TO VAGINAL FUNCTION

The embryologic development of the vagina is controversial. The two most popular theories of vaginal development propose:

- formation entirely by the lower end of the fused paramesonephric ducts
- dual origin, with the upper vagina forming from the fused paramesonephric ducts while the lower portion forms from the sinovaginal bulbs which in turn arise from the epithelium of the urogenital sinus.

Abnormalities of development may occur, including complete absence of vaginal development or partial malformations, including various forms of septate vaginae. Rarely, portions of the mesonephric duct persist and may cause symptoms or abnormal findings on physical examination. The typical appearance is a lateral vaginal cyst, often called Gartner's duct cysts. Very rarely, these malformations are associated with ectopic ureters that may enter the vagina at this point, leading to unusual forms of urinary incontinence.

The hymen separates the vaginal canal from the vulva. The adult vagina is not cylindric but has an H-shaped configuration in cross-section and a sigmoid curve in sagittal section. Reconstructive surgeons may occasionally overlook these normal characteristics; however, much literature supports the strong relationship between successful repairs and re-creation of the normal anatomic features. Specifi-cally, repairs that shorten or straighten the vagina, distort the normal vaginal axis or significantly narrow the vaginal caliber are associated with undesirable anatomic and functional consequences.

The normal length of the vagina is approximately 10–12 centimeters with the posterior wall typically being somewhat longer than the anterior wall. The upper vagina normally has a greater diameter than the lower third. Given its close proximity to the lower urinary and bowel systems, disorders of these neighboring systems can affect vaginal anatomy and/or function. Likewise vaginal disorders or treatments can affect the neighboring systems. The levator support of the vagina appears to be an important factor in determining shape, topography, and some aspects of function.[1,2]

The blood supply is rich and variable and has many collaterals and a vigorous anastomotic vascular network, sometimes called the "azygous artery." This rich vasculature is clinically important during both medical and surgical treatments. Many medications are rapidly and easily absorbed transvaginally (including estrogens and progesterones).

A branch of the uterine artery and the superior vesical branch of the internal iliac artery typically supply the upper vagina. Branches from the inferior vesical and middle rectal (of the internal iliac) supply the middle vagina, while the distal vaginal blood supply originates from the pudendal and inferior rectal branches of the internal pudendal. The venous drainage flows into the internal iliac veins.

Vaginal innervation originates from the perineal branches of the internal pudendal nerve and the pelvic autonomic plexus, supplying the thin outer layer of vaginal smooth muscle. Although much work has been done to delineate vaginal innervation, there is still a limited understanding of neural injury and repair in the vagina. Distension of the vagina in experimental conditions results in altered visceral function.[3] The human pudendal nerve has been monitored in experimental situations and is known to undergo adverse changes during vaginal delivery.[4] The long-term conse-quences of these changes remain under study. However, it is

33

clinically apparent that the neural pathways of the vagina may allow central sensitization, similar to establishment of chronic pain elsewhere in the body.[5,6]

The lining of the vagina is stratified, nonkeratinizing squamous epithelium without glands. This allows the vagina to expand without rupture (for example, during childbirth) and return to a near-normal configuration. Lubrication of the vagina is actually a transudate from the vascular vaginal plexus, rather than secretions from vaginal glands, as there are no glands in the vaginal skin.

NORMAL FUNCTION OF THE VAGINA

The vagina plays important anatomic and functional roles throughout the reproductive and postreproductive years. Physiologically, there are many highly interconnected neural and endocrine systems that contribute to proper vaginal function. Following puberty, the vagina lengthens, widens, and thickens. Coitus prior to puberty is associated with high rates of anatomic and psychologic injury.

Reproductive years. During the reproductive years, the principal estrogen is estradiol, which is made almost entirely by the ovary. The vagina is moist, rugous, and pliable and has abundant hormone receptors. A normal thin secretion is observed as a normal vaginal discharge with a normal musty scent. Physicians play an important role in educating women regarding their normal anatomy and physiology. Familial and cultural habits of regular douching should be discussed with the goal of discouraging these practices, as they confer no benefit and may disrupt the normal vaginal flora.

Menopause transition. As menopause approaches, the ovaries become less responsive to pituitary gonadotropins. Ovulation becomes irregular and infrequent, finally stopping entirely. Typically this transition begins in the late 40s for American women. The serum pituitary gonadotropin levels are high, although the levels of gonadotropin-releasing hormone (GnRH) remain unchanged.

The onset of clinical symptoms (and bother from those symptoms) is highly variable. Common symptoms include the hot flush that affects up to 85% of postmenopausal women. This symptom typically decreases after 2 years, although in a minority of women it may continue for many years. Physiologically there is a pulsatile release of LH with the onset of each hot flush, apparently accompanying a central hypothalamic mechanism that triggers the clinical event.

Other clinical symptoms include alterations in sleep, mood, and memory. A full discussion of the care of these symptoms is beyond the scope of this text.

Postmenopausal years. Following menopause, there is a marked decline in ovarian follicle stimulation. Circu-lating estradiol levels fall significantly. The principal circulating estrogen is estrone, more of which is derived from extraovarian sources or produced in extraglandular tissues, such as adipose tissues. The clinical impact of this is that slender women convert less androstenedione to estrone in peripheral tissues and therefore have less circulating estrone than obese women. Testosterone production is slightly lower than during the premenopausal years. However, because of the marked decrease in estrogen production, there is a relative androgen excess in post-menopausal women.

The vagina changes significantly in this altered hormonal milieu. The vaginal epithelium is much thinner, the normal rugae are decreased and may become absent, and lubrication decreases. Clinicians often prescribe adjunctive estrogen for postmenopausal women.[7] Sexual dysfunction may occur secondary to hormonal deficiencies.

THE ROLE OF THE VAGINA IN SEXUAL FUNCTION

As with most voluntary human functions, the brain plays a central role in female sexual function. As physicians, our role in assessing and treating sexual dysfunction requires an awareness of the many illnesses, drugs, and surgical treatments that affect normal function. Although patients may present to a pelvic clinician with a perception that sexual problems are centered in the vagina, it is the clinician's responsibility to screen more broadly for causes.

Most heterosexual physicians assume their patient is heterosexual as well. This assumption may limit the ability to obtain an optimal history. Many lesbian women have had relationships with men (including marriage) and nearly half of lesbian women may bear or raise a child. Therefore, these are not reliable proxy measures for determining sexual orientation. Questionnaires (even demographic questionnaires) should be carefully assessed to determine whether an inadvertent heterosexual bias may limit the quality and quantity of information that women provide regarding sexual function. For example, for a lesbian woman, repeated questions about how often intercourse occurs are inappropriate. Not all patients wish to share their sexual orientation with their healthcare team but it is useful to have some knowledge about the sexual health of all patients presenting for pelvic care. Survey data suggest that approximately 4% of US women are lesbians.[8]

In the US, women are more likely to be assaulted, injured, raped or killed by a male partner than by any other type of assailant.[9] Domestic violence is often underreported and frequently not recognized by healthcare teams. Therefore it is important that every pelvic physician is alert to signs and symptoms of domestic violence and includes screening questions during routine history taking. Questions may include whether the patient has ever been physically hurt by someone close to her. If your index of suspicion is high, this topic should be initiated again even if the patient defers the question or denies violence. Clinical presentations that should heighten screening efforts include women with frequent physician visits for nonspecific pelvic complaints such as pelvic pain or vaginal irritation. Suspicion should be heightened when a male partner insists on staying unusually close to the woman, answering questions for her or being verbally abusive to healthcare staff.

Normal sexual function. Sexual practices vary widely. The preponderance of sexual activity in heterosexual women includes vaginal intercourse and, less commonly, oral sex. The preponderance of lesbian sexual activity consists of direct manual, digital, and mostly oral stimulation of the clitoris.

The classic description of the female sexual response cycle includes excitement, plateau, orgasm, and resolution. These changes are determined by physiologic events, predominantly vasocongestion and increased muscle tension. Interested readers are referred to classic texts for more details regarding the entire sexual cycle.[10] Desire is also a clinically relevant portion of this cycle. Loss of desire (low libido) may obviate the sexual response cycle.

During the excitement phase, the vagina responds to effective sexual stimulation with a clear secretion that effectively lubricates the vagina. This transudate has an important reproductive function as it buffers the normal acidic pH of the vagina to improve sperm survival. Certain contraceptive agents may alter this action.[11] Anatomically, the vagina lengthens (up to 3 cm) and increases in diameter up to 4 cm. The normal pink-red color of the vagina darkens secondary to the vasocongestion.

Once the plateau is reached, vaginal secretions slow and the anatomic changes of the vagina are more pronounced. The distal vagina is relatively small compared to the upper vagina. It is believed that this enhances sperm collection in the upper vagina.

During the orgasmic phase, the vagina remains essentially unchanged, although a woman may perceive vaginal and/or uterine contractions. It is believed that these contractions actually originate from the pelvic and perineal muscles underlying the labia minora.

The resolution phase is a physiologic return to baseline. The vasocongestion reverses, the vagina returns to its preexcitement size and the secretions return to their low normal levels.

Sexual function after childbirth. It is well known that the physiologic and emotional demands of childbirth and the early parenting experience affect sexual functioning for many women. Although more than half resume sexual activity by 6 weeks postpartum, nearly half of new mothers desire intercourse less or much less. Klein et al surveyed 484 women using a postal questionnaire.[12] Nearly 70% reported less frequency, and up to one-quarter of women have not resumed sexual activities by 6 months postpartum. Perineal injury at the time of delivery is associated with postpartum dyspareunia.

Changes in menopause. Although most clinicians assume that sexual function decreases in the menopausal years, some postmenopausal women report improved sexual function. There is no longer a fear of undesired pregnancy and typically the family and work demands of younger years have abated somewhat. Although rates of sexual activity decline with age, nearly half of married women aged 66–71 and one-third of women over 78 years of age continue sexual activity.[13-15]

In coitally active women, there are changes to the normal sexual response. All the normal events occur but may happen more slowly. Excitation, elevation of the clitoral hood, and vaginal lubrication may take longer. Also, skin flush, muscle tension, vaginal lengthening, and vascular congestion may be decreased in menopause. Orgasmic function occurs but may have a decreased duration and more rapid resolution.

ASSESSMENT OF SEXUAL FUNCTION

When pelvic physicians do not assess sexual function, it is most commonly because the provider is uncomfortable. Physicians can enhance their skills in this area by improving their knowledge base, setting aside personal judgments and preferences, and being less worried about offending patients. The sensitive and mindful physician may initiate a discussion but find it appropriate to revisit the topic at subsequent visits. Sexual function should be routinely assessed prior to pelvic intervention such as surgery.[16] Several validated questionnaires are helpful in gathering this information.[17-19]

Sexual dysfunction. Sexual dysfunction is common, affecting 20–50% of women. Clinicians may not feel proficient at evaluating sexual dysfunction. Loss of libido appears to be the most common form of sexual dysfunction, followed by anorgasmia (25%), lack of lubrication (20%), and lack of pleasure.[20,21] These disorders can be cataloged clinically as shown in Box 4.1. Anorgasmia is reported by approximately 12% of heterosexual women and 3% of lesbian women.[22]

A common presenting symptom is dyspareunia. Painful intercourse may be due to problems within the vagina itself or external to the vaginal lumen. Painful intercourse may also occur when there is a lack of vulvovaginal lubrication or the presence of infectious or inflammatory vulvovaginal

---

BOX 4.1   Sexual dysfunction[40]

Sexual desire disorders
Hypoactive sexual desire disorder
Sexual aversion disorder

Sexual arousal disorder

Orgasmic disorder

Sexual pain disorders
Dyspareunia
Vaginismus
Noncoital sexual pain disorder

---

conditions. New-onset postoperative dyspareunia may be related to alterations in vaginal caliber or length, foreign body problems or scar formation. Sexual function may be altered following prolapse or incontinence surgery.[23] Certain procedures are associated with higher rates of dyspareunia, including episiotomy,[24,25] posterior vaginal prolapse repairs,[26,27] radiation,[28,29] perineorrhaphies and levator plications for any purpose.[30] Women who undergo sacrocolpopexy tend to have a longer vagina than women who are treated with transvaginal suspensions.[31]

Problems external to the vaginal lumen may also cause painful intercourse. A variety of pelvic conditions, including pelvic masses, bowel or bladder disorders and painful pelvic muscles, may be detected.[32]

Following childbirth, many women experience at least a transient decrease in sexual functioning.[33] This may be due to a combination of psychosocial, anatomic, and functional causes. Fortunately, this resolves without residual problems for most women.

Medical illnesses or their treatments may contribute to sexual dysfunction. Drugs that decrease estrogen availability are commonly associated with decreased sexual function as well as causing visible changes to the vagina.[34] Many psychotropic and hypertension agents affect sexual function. Close collaboration with the prescribing physician may promote appropriate medication substitutions.

Women with incontinence may have other specific impacts on their sexual function. Although rare, incontinence during sexual activities is a very disturbing symptom for affected women. Hilton reported that loss of urine during penetration or orgasm was relatively common but rarely volunteered to clinicians providing incontinence care.[35] Two community surveys report that this symptom is experienced by approximately 13% of women.[36,37] Women with prolapse and/or incontinence generally have less frequent sexual activity.[19] While sexual satisfaction in women with pelvic floor disorders is similar to unaffected groups, women with detrusor overactivity suffer more adverse sexual impact than women with stress incontinence.

Effects of pelvic floor disorder treatments on sexual function.
Stress incontinence surgery variably affects sexual function. Haase et al reported that the majority (67%) of women reported unchanged sexual function following surgery, whereas 24% found improvement and 9% experienced deterioration.[38] Berglund et al prospectively evaluated women undergoing stress incontinence as well as their partners. Male partners reported an increase in desire following surgery, whereas only a third of women experienced increased desire.[41]

Three hundred and sixty women who participated in a multicenter study of stress incontinence surgery were assessed for sexual functioning at baseline and postoperatively at 3, 6, and 12 months. The majority reported no change in sexual function, whereas nearly one-quarter (22%) experienced deterioration and 13% reported improvement.[39] The effect of continence surgery on coital urine loss is summarized in Table 4.1.

Table 4.1   The effects of incontinence surgery on coital urine loss and sexual function

Author	N	Improvement	No change	Deterioration
Berglund et al[41]	45	1/3 increased desire	Frequency unchanged	Increased
Black et al[39]	239	13%	65%	22%
Weber et al[23]	81		Frequency unchanged	8–19% dyspareunia 22–26% coital UI
Lemack et al[42]	22		No change	
Barber et al[17]	21	Less worried about coital UI		

Women with pelvic organ prolapse may withdraw from sexual activities due to fears of themselves or their partner. However, the majority continues in satisfactory sexual patterns.[16] Surgical treatment of prolapse, however, is associated with risks of sexual dysfunction, with some reports suggesting that up to 50% of women cease coital activity following prolapse repair. Certainly the routine use of posterior colporrhaphy has been called into question given the risks of vaginal narrowing, dyspareunia, and aparenuia. Although these risks are generally assumed to be higher with procedures that remove the vagina, narrow the caliber or alter the axis, these risks have also been reported in abdominal sacrocolpopexy series. These findings strongly reinforce the need to carefully assess sexual function before and after any pelvic intervention, especially prolapse repairs.

Sexual function questionnaires. A variety of questionnaires are available for assessment of sexual function. Researchers should understand the status of such instruments prior to selecting one for their studies. There are instruments specifically designed for postpartum women, couples assessment, women with pelvic floor and many other options. Table 4.2 summarizes these instruments.

CONCLUSION

The clinician's knowledge of vaginal physiology and sexual function is important for optimal care of women with pelvic floor disorders. Researchers should carefully assess their research goals, avoid proxy measures, and rely on validated instruments whenever possible. It is anticipated that our knowledge and treatment options will be further enhanced and refined over the next decade. Interested researchers are urged to master today's literature in preparation for interpreting and planning future studies.

ACKNOWLEDGMENT

The author wishes to thank Rebecca Rogers MD for her assistance in compiling Table 4.2.

Table 4.2 Instruments for assessment of sexual function

Instrument	Content face validity	Domain analysis	Reliability internal consistency	Criterion construct validity	Population used for validation	Item #	?PFD in women?	ICS rating
PISQ 2000 Pelvic organ Prolapse Incontinence Sexual Questionnaire	Expert	Yes (3) — behav-emot, physical, partner	Cronbach> or = K= Item total correlations Test-retest reliability	Validated against age, depression indices, SHF-12 IIQ	180 women with and without pop/ui	31 short=12	Yes	Not rated
SRS 1995 Sabbatsberg Sexual Self Rating Scale	Expert	None	Cronbach alpha .95, item-total Correlations .61-.86, No test-retest	Compared to SF-36, HADS, social class, hormone levels, worse scores in women with vaginal dryness, dyspareunia	40s heterosexual women both with FSD and normals	12	?	Not rated
FSFI 2000 Female Sexual Function Index	Expert and focus group for further analysis	Yes (6) — desire, subjective arousal, lubrication, orgasm, satisfaction and pain	Cronbach's > or =.82 K=.79 to .86	Different for two groups, divergent validity with scale of marital satisfaction, factorial/ discriminate/divergent	131 normals	18 FSAD (21-69 y/o)		
GRISS 1985 The Golombok-Rust Inventory of Sexual Satisfaction	Expert	Yes, (4) — anorgasmia, vaginismus, impotence, and premature ejaculation, avoidance, dissatisfaction and non-sensuality, infrequency and no communication about sex	Chronbach's .61-83, ?half reliability .94.	Therapist's rating, differences between clinical population and normals, correlated with therapists evaluations	Heterosexual couples — 51 clinic couples and 36 normals, 88 sex therapy couples	28	Small study in unwanted sexual activity and DI	Highly recommended Grade A
SHF-12 1988 Sexual History Form	Expert opinion/ focus group further analysis	Yes (6) — desire, subjective arousal, lubrication, orgasm, satisfaction, and pain	Chronbach's > or = .82, K=.92, item total correlations - .18-.85	Other measures correlated significantly .38 to .73 to Locke Wallace MAS, SII total and scale 6, question about sexual satisfaction and sexual drive, 12 women completed the GRISS as well overall score correlated .65, difference between 29 controls, 8 dysfunctional women and 8 partners of dysfunctional men, also correlated with age	27 married women, see above	19	Yes	Not rated

Instrument	Content face validity	Domain analysis	Reliability internal consistency	Criterion construct validity	Population used for validation	Item #	?PFD in women?	ICS rating
IRS 1986 Intimate Relationship Scale	Expert opinion	Yes (3) — personal or emotional, physical, and cognitive or communication	Chronbach's> or = .87, K=.92, item total correlations ->.25, no test-retest reliability	Not done	194 couples — postpartum	12	No	Not rated
BISF-W 1994 Brief Index of Sexual Functioning for Women		Yes (3) — sexual interest desire, sexual activity, and sexual satisfaction; revised to evaluate eight domains: thoughts, desire, arousal, frequency of sexual activity, receptivity/initiation, pleasure orgasm, relationship satisfaction, and problems affecting sexual function		Compared to the Derogatis Sexual Function Interview, able to discriminate between women with surgical menopause and those without limited to assessment of the last 30 days	269 heterosexual and homosexual women ages 20–73, seeking routine gyn care, white, married, healthy women with organic and inorganic causes of sexual dysfunction, past 30 days, surgical menopause	22	No	Recommended
DISF, DISF-SR (PAIS) Derogatis Interview for Sexual Functioning: Related to the Psychosocial Adjustment to Illness Scale	Expert	Yes, sexual cognition and fantasy, sexual arousal, sexual behavior and experiences, orgasm, and sexual drive and relationship. Verimax rotation	Cronbach's alpha = .8 to .93 interrater reliability .81-.86	Compared to the Global adjustment to Illness Scale, the SCL-90R. affect balance scale, and patient's attitudes, information and experiences scale, Alsom compared patients with and without lung cancer: high correlations with this and global adjustment scores (GAIS) .13-.46, able to discriminate between women who screen positive and those who screen negative	Community populations — available in English, Danish, Dutch, French, German, Italian and Norwegian and Spanish, past 30 days including today — renal dialysis, acute burn, hypertension, cardiac, cancer	25 interview and self-administered questionnaire, PAIS domain of six questions	Yes	Recommended
WSFQ Watts Sexual Function Questionnaire						17		Mentioned
SFQ Sexual Function Questionnaire		7 — desire, physical arousal, lubrication, enjoyment, orgasm, pain, partner satisfaction			731 women with sexual dysfunction and 201 women without sexual dysfunction	31	No	Mentioned

Continued

Table 4.2   Instruments for assessment of sexual function—cont'd

Instrument	Content face validity	Domain analysis	Reliability internal consistency	Criterion construct validity	Population used for validation	Item #	?PFD in women?	ICS rating
Plouffe's 1985 Simple Questionnaire	Expert	No — 3 questions only, 4 with Walters — did urinary symptoms interfere with sex?	No	Compared to interview by psychiatrist, sexual dysfunction more common in incontinent subjects	98 sexually active women	31	Yes	Potential
Bristol 1999 BFLUTSsex Female lower urinary tract symptoms	Expert	No — 4 questions only — pain or discomfort due to a dry vagina, whether sex life has been spoiled by urinary symptoms, pain on sexual intercourse, leakage on intercourse. Also asked how much of a problem it is for them.	69.6–91.1%, no Cronbach's alpha testing	Difference between women with PFE and those without although differences disappeared when controlled for baseline data		4	Yes – pelvic floor muscle training, other study	With potential
ASEX Arizona Sexual Experiences Scale	Not explained, BISF	Drive, arousal, vaginal lubrication, orgasm, satisfaction from orgasm — no domain analysis	91 = Cronbach's alpha, Pearson's r = .80 for patients and .89 for controls	Patients reported more dysfunction than controls, correlated with physician-diagnosed sexual dysfunction	38 control subjects and 58 patients with depression	5	No	None

Key: pop/ui, pelvic organ prolapse/urinary incontinence; HADS, Hospital Anxiety and Depression Scale; FSAD, female sexual arousal disorder; DI, detrusor instability; PFE, pelvic floor exercises. The author wishes to gratefully acknowledge Rebecca Rogers, MD for her assistance in compiling Table II.

REFERENCES

1. Hoyte L, et al. Variations in levator ani volume and geometry in women: the application of MR based 3D reconstruction in evaluating pelvic floor dysfunction. Archivos Espanoles de Urologia 2001;54(6): 532–539.
2. Singh K, et al. Three-dimensional magnetic resonance imaging assessment of levator ani morphologic features in different grades of prolapse. Am J Obstet Gynecol 2003;188(4):910–915.
3. Benson JT, McClellan E. The effect of vaginal dissection on the pudendal nerve. Obstet Gynecol 1993;82(3):387–389.
4. Clark M, et al. Monitoring pudendal nerve function during labor. Obstet Gynecol 2001; 97(4): 637–639.
5. Cervero F. Visceral pain—central sensitization. Gut 2000; 47:iv56–iv57.
6. Cruz F, et al. Desensitization of bladder sensory fibers by intravesical capsaicin has long lasting clinical and urodynamic effects in patients with hyperactive or hypersensitive bladder dysfunction. J Urol 1997;157(2):585–589.
7. Lose G, Englev E. Oestradiol-releasing vaginal ring versus oestriol vaginal pessaries in the treatment of bothersome lower urinary tract symptoms. Br J Obstet Gynaecol 2000;107(8):1029–1034.
8. Sell RL, Wells JA, Wypij D. The prevalence of homosexual behavior and attraction in the United States, the United Kingdom and France: results of national population-based samples. Arch Sexual Behav 1995;24(3):235–248.
9. Browne A, Williams KR. Resource availability for women at risk: its relationship to rates of female-perpetrated partner homicide. Paper presented at the American Society of Criminology Annual Meeting, Montreal, Canada, November 11–14 1987.
10. Sherfey MJ. The nature and evolution of female sexuality. New York: Random House; 1972.
11. Hooton T, Roberts P, Stamm W. Effects of recent sexual activity and use of a diaphragm on the vaginal microflora. Clin Infect Dis 1994;19(2):274–278.
12. Klein M, et al. Relationship of episiotomy to perineal trauma and morbidity, sexual dysfunction, and pelvic floor relaxation. Am J Obstet Gynecol 1994;171(3):591–598.
13. Brooks TR. Sexuality in the aging woman. Female Patient 1994;19:63–70.
14. Diokno AC, Brown MB, Herzog IAR. Sexual function in the elderly. Arch Intern Med 1990;150:197–200.
15. Freedman M. Sexuality in post-menopausal women. Menopausal Med 2000;8(4):1–5.
16. Weber AM, et al. Sexual function in women with uterovaginal prolapse and urinary incontinence. Obstet Gynecol 85(4):483–487.
17. Barber MD, et al. Sexual function in women with urinary incontinence and pelvic organ prolapse. Obstet Gynecol 2002;99(2):281–289.
18. Rogers GR, et al. A short form of the Pelvic Organ Prolapse/Urinary Incontinence Sexual Questionnaire (PISW-12). Int Urogynecol J 2003;14(3):164–168.
19. Rogers GR, et al. Sexual function in women with and without urinary incontinence and/or pelvic organ prolapse. Int Urogynecol J 2001;12(6):361–365.
20. American College of Obstetricians and Gynecologists. Sexual dysfunction. ACOG Tech Bull 1995;211:763–772.
21. Laumann EO, Pai KA, Rosen RC. Sexual dysfunction in the United States: prevalence and predictors. JAMA 1999;281(6):537–544.
22. Hite S. The Hite report. New York: Macmillan; 1981.
23. Weber AM, Walters MD, Piedmonte MR. Sexual function and vaginal anatomy in women before and after surgery for pelvic organ prolapse and urinary incontinence. Am J Obstet Gynecol 2000;182(6):1610–1615.
24. Dannecker C, et al. Episiotomy and perineal tears presumed to be imminent: randomized controlled trial. Acta Obstet Gynecol Scand 2004;83(4):364–368.
25. Duerbeck N, Reed K. Episiotomy: a review. Clin Consult Obstet Gynecol 1996;4(4):249–256.
26. Kahn MA, Stanton SL. Posterior colporrhaphy: its effects on bowel and sexual function. Br J Obstet Gynaecol 1997;104(1):82–86.
27. Kenton K, Shott S, Brubaker L. Outcome after rectovaginal fascia reattachment for rectocele repair. Am J Obstet Gynecol 1999;181(6):1360–1363; discussion 1363–1364.
28. Kagan AR., et al. The narrow vagina, the antecedent for irradiation injury. Gynecol Oncol 1976;4(3):291–298.
29. Villasanta U. Complications of radiotherapy for carcinoma of the uterine cervix. Am J Obstet Gynecol 1972;114(6):717–726.
30. Holley RL, et al. Sexual function after sacrospinous ligament fixation for vaginal vault prolapse. J Reprod Med 1996;41(5):355–358.
31. Given FT, Muhlendorf IK, Browning GM. Vaginal length and sexual function after colpopexy for complete uterovaginal eversion. Am J Obstet Gynecol 1993;169(2):284–288.
32. FitzGerald MP. Chronic pelvic pain. Current Women's Health Reports 2003;3(4):327–333.
33. Kumar R, Brant HA, Robson KM. Childbearing and maternal sexuality: a prospective survey of 119 primiparae. J Psychosom Res 1981;25(5):373–383.
34. Homesley HD, et al. Antiestrogenic potency of toremifene and tamoxifen in postmenopausal women. Am J Clin Oncol 1993;16(2):117–122.
35. Hilton P. Urinary incontinence during sexual intercourse: a common, but rarely volunteered symptom. Br J Obstet Gynaecol 1988;95:377–381.
36. Lam GW, et al. Social context, social abstention, and problem recognition correlated with adult female urinary incontinence. Dan Med Bull 1992;39(6):565–570.
37. Nygaard I, Milburn A. Incontinence during sexual activity: prevalence in a gynecologic practice. J Women's Health 1995;4:83–86.
38. Haase P, Skibsted L. Influence of operations for stress incontinence and/or genital descensus on sexual life. Acta Obstet Gynecol Scand 1988;67:659–661.
39. Black NA, et al. Impact of surgery for stress incontinence on the social lives of women. Br J Obstet Gynaecol 1998;105(6):605–612.
40. Basson R. Human sex-response cycles. J Sex Marital Ther 2001;27(1):33–43.
41. Berglund AL, et al. Social adjustment and spouse relationships among women with stress incontinence before and after surgical treatment. Soc Sci Med 1996;42(11):1537–1544.
42. Lemack GE, Zimmern PE. Sexual function after vaginal surgery for stress incontinence: results of a mailed questionnaire. Urology 2000;56(2):223–227.

SECTION 3

Pathophysiology of urinary and anal
incontinence and pelvic prolapse

CHAPTER

Pathophysiology of Stress Urinary Incontinence in Women

5

Firouz Daneshgari and Courtenay Moore

INTRODUCTION

Stress urinary incontinence (SUI) as defined by the International Continence Society (ICS) is the involuntary leakage of urine on effort or exertion, or on sneezing or coughing.[1] It is estimated that SUI affects between 4% and 35% of American women with over 165,000 antiincontinence procedures performed annually in the US.[2,3] Despite recognition of several risk factors—aging, obesity, race, childbirth—related to SUI, the true pathophysiology of SUI remains poorly understood.

Why do we need to understand the pathophysiology of stress urinary incontinence? The high rate of complications and rate of recurrent SUI after surgery suggests that the existing treatment modalities for SUI are not completely successful.

It is estimated that at least one-third of the procedures performed for treatment of SUI are done on patients with recurrent SUI.[4] This estimate is supported by the fact that, over the past few decades, dozens of new antiincontinence procedures have been introduced to improve upon the deficiencies of the previous procedures, a goal that remains elusive.

The relatively high rate of recurrent SUI and the search for more effective anti-SUI treatments attest to the fact that enhanced understanding of the pathophysiology of SUI is central to providing women with better cure rates and ultimately a better quality of life.

If one agrees that the existing treatment modalities for any condition (in this case SUI) are based upon our understanding of the pathophysiology of that disease, the treatment failures could be related, at least in part, to our shortcomings in understanding that pathophysiology. These shortcomings have led, in part, to a lack of successful treatments for SUI. In order to fully understand the pathophysiology of SUI, one must first understand the physiology of continence.

PHYSIOLOGY OF URINARY CONTINENCE

The physiologic factors involved in urinary continence can be divided into *central* and *peripheral* control mechanisms. The *central* control mechanisms include input from the cerebral cortex, midbrain, thoracic, and sacral spinal cord through the autonomic and somatic innervations to the lower urinary tract organs. The *peripheral* control mechanisms involve organs (bladder, urethra), muscles, and bony supporting structures.

Urinary control or urinary continence is the result of a complex and fascinating coordination between the elements of the central and peripheral continence mechanisms. In women, urinary continence during stress (elevations in intraabdominal pressure) is maintained by several mechanisms. First, there is passive transmission of abdominal pressure to the proximal urethra. A guarding reflex involving an active contraction of striated muscle of the external urethral sphincter can transiently help continence.[5,6] However, the abdominal pressure transmitted to the proximal urethra does not account entirely for the increase in urethral pressure.[7] Abdominal pressure is also transmitted through the proximal urethra pressing the anterior wall against the posterior wall. The posterior wall remains rigid if there is adequate pelvic support from muscle and connective tissues. During voiding, the pubourethral ligaments and vaginal connections to pelvic muscles and fascia actively change the position of the bladder neck and proximal urethra. These attachments contain both fascia and smooth muscle.[8] This change in position compresses the urethra against the pubis during bladder filling and straining. Thus, urinary continence results from the combination of passive anatomic coaptation and active muscle tone.

PATHOPHYSIOLOGIC THEORIES

Over the last century a number of investigators have proposed theories on the pathophysiology of SUI in women.

These theories were based on the understanding of the physiology of continence at that time, relying on the observations and investigative works of the researcher. Over the last 100 years, four theories have dominated the literature and thereby the treatment recommendations for SUI. Here, we review the basis for these theories.

Alterations in the urethrovesical axis. The early theories regarding SUI focused on a lack of physical compression and an alteration in urethral position. In 1913, Howard Kelly, a gynecologist from Johns Hopkins, published a surgical technique to treat "a peculiar form of incontinence of urine in women which either follows childbirth or comes on about middle age, and is not associated with any visible lesion of the urinary tract." Kelly found many of these women to have "a gaping internal sphincter orifice which closes sluggishly." In order to correct this defect, Kelly "sutured together the torn or relaxed tissues at the neck of the bladder."[9]

Unlike Kelly, who believed stress incontinence to be caused by an open vesical neck, Bonney believed SUI to result from the loss of normal urethral support and positioning. In 1923, Bonney wrote "Incontinence depends in some way upon a sudden and abnormal displacement of the urethra and the urethrovesical junction immediately behind the pubic symphysis."[9] However, it was not until 1961 that the theory of urethral position was popularized by a Swedish gynecologist, GE Enhorning. Enhorning studied the pressures of the urethra and the bladder in continent and incontinent women. Based on these observations he concluded that for urethral competence, the urethra must be located above the pelvic floor so that pressure transmitted to the bladder is equally transmitted to the urethra, causing a compensatory increase in closure pressure[9] (Fig. 5.1). The theory of SUI due to an alteration in urethral angles prevailed until the late 1970s.

Intrinsic sphincteric deficiency. In 1976, Edward McGuire introduced the alternative concept that SUI was due to something more than an alteration of urethral positioning. "The change in the angle does not explain all the causes of SUI in women."[10] In landmark articles, McGuire introduced the importance of intrinsic sphincter deficiency (ISD) in the pathophysiology of SUI. The first line of evidence for the importance of ISD came from a study on the effects of sacral denervation on urethral and bladder function. In this study sacral nerve rhizotomy leading to denervation of the pudendal nerve, and therefore the external sphincter, was performed on three female paraplegics. Complete sacral denervation resulted in the loss of anal sphincter and urethral skeletal muscular activity, but not the resting urethral smooth muscle tone. Sacral rhizotomy had no effect on the resting urethral pressure or

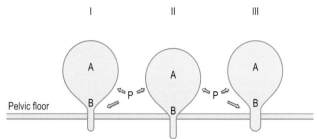

Figure 5.1 Urethral position theory. Increases in intraabdominal pressure (P) are transmitted to the bladder neck and proximal urethra. I. Normal female. Increases in P are transmitted equally to the bladder neck/proximal urethra (B). II. Urethral hypermobility. During increases in P, the bladder neck/proximal urethra (B) descends abnormally to a position outside the abdominal cavity. The pressure within the bladder (A) exceeds the pressure within the bladder neck/proximal urethra (B) and stress urinary incontinence ensues. III. Intrinsic sphincteric deficiency. Here the bladder neck/proximal urethra (B) is adequately supported (there is no descent), but the bladder neck/proximal urethra is nonfunctional, again resulting in stress urinary incontinence. (Reproduced with permission from Gillenwater JY. Adult and pediatric urology. 1996;2, Figure 26A–46 page 1209)

urethral smooth muscle function.[11] Therefore, none of these patients developed SUI. These findings confirmed the importance of urethral smooth muscle in maintaining continence.

In 1980, McGuire observed that during video urodynamics, patients who had failed multiple retropubic operations had a deficient sphincteric mechanism characterized by an open bladder neck and proximal urethra at rest, with minimal or no urethral descent during stress (Fig. 5.2).

These observations led to another landmark article investigating the concept of ISD as the cause of incontinence in 125 women. Maximum urethral pressures (MUP) and the abdominal pressure required to cause stress incontinence or

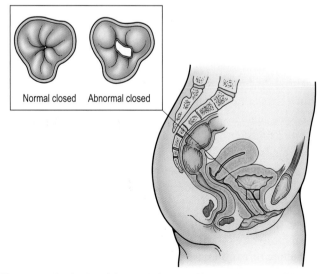

Normal closed   Abnormal closed

Figure 5.2 Intrinsic sphincter deficiency. The urethra is unable to generate enough outlet resistance to retain urine in bladder.

Valsalva leak point pressure (VLLP) were recorded during urodynamics. In these women, there was an inverse correlation between the VLLP required to cause SUI and the severity of incontinence as assessed by the number of pads used. From this, McGuire et al concluded that VLLP was a more sensitive measurement of the severity of incontinence than MUP. Based on VLPP values obtained in this study of women with mild to severe SUI, a new classification system emerged: SUI in patients with a VLPP <60 cmH$_2$O was considered to be the result of ISD, while SUI in patients with a VLLP of >90 cmH$_2$O was considered to be related to an anatomic cause other than ISD. SUI in patients with VLLP between 60 and 90 cmH$_2$O was considered to be due to a combination of anatomic defects and ISD.

Hammock theory.
In 1994, the hammock theory was introduced by Dr John DeLancey, a pioneering gynecologist in studies of pelvic floor structures. From his cadaveric studies, DeLancey described the urethra as lying on a supportive layer composed of the endopelvic fascia and anterior vaginal wall (Fig. 5.3). This supportive layer gains stability through its lateral attachments with the arcus tendineus fascia and the levator ani muscle. Given these cadaveric studies, DeLancey theorized that intraabdominal pressure is transmitted to the bladder neck and proximal urethra, closing the outlet as it is compressed against the rigid support of the pubocervical fascia and anterior vaginal wall (Fig. 5.4).

Integral theory.
In 1990 Almsten and Petros introduced the "integral" theory of SUI and urge incontinence. According to this theory, laxity of the anterior vaginal wall leads to activation of stretch receptors in the bladder neck and proximal urethra, triggering an inappropriate micturition reflex, resulting in detrusor overactivity.[9] The laxity of the vaginal wall also leads to SUI because of a dissipation of urethral closure pressures. Under normal circumstances the anterior pubococcygeus muscle lifts the anterior vaginal wall to compress the urethra, closing the bladder neck by the traction of the underlying vaginal wall in a backward and

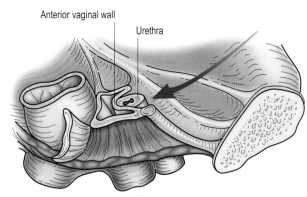

Figure 5.3 Hammock theory. The urethra lies on a supportive layer composed of the endopelvic fascia and the anterior vaginal wall. (Reproduced with permission from Am J Obstet Gynecol 1995, 173(1):346)

downward fashion while the pelvic floor musculature draws the hammock cephalad, closing the bladder neck. Laxity of the pubourethral ligament and anterior vaginal wall causes hypermobility of the bladder neck and dissipation of pressure, resulting in SUI.

FOR AND AGAINST THE THEORIES
Each theory has its proponents as well as opponents. Many researchers have questioned the validity of each theory based on additional studies.

Urethral position theory.
As described above, McGuire's presentation of ISD was one of the first important observations that allowed the scientific community to look beyond the urethrovesical angle as the sole pathophysiologic factor in SUI. In 1986, Fantl also questioned the validity of the urethral position theory. In a study of 84 stress incontinent women, Fantl found that the urethral axis at rest, during bearing down, and in its total excursion was not significantly different between continent and incontinent women.[12] This study proved that the urethral axis alone was not predictive of urethral function. He concluded that "Specific correlation between the urethral axis and its sphincteric function is lacking."[12]

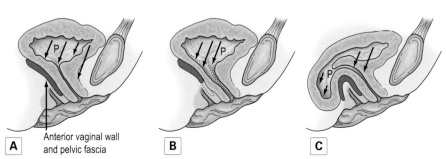

Figure 5.4 Hammock theory. (**A**) The anterior vaginal wall and pelvic fascia act as a hammock, compressing the urethra during increases in intraabdominal pressure (P). (**B**) The loss of the hammock (*dotted lines*) during increases in P leads to the loss of urine into the posterior urethra, resulting in stress urinary incontinence. (**C**) Loss of the hammock, [leading to the presence of a cystourethrocele] may not result in stress incontinence provided the hammock counteracts the effects of P by increasing urethral resistance. (Reproduced with permission from Gillenwater JY. Adult and pediatric urology. 1996;2)

Open bladder neck. Several studies have questioned the importance of an open bladder neck in maintaining continence. Versi et al found that 51% of continent climacteric women had bladder neck incompetence on urodynamics.[13] Similarly, Chapple used ultrasound to note that 21% of continent nulliparous women had an open bladder neck.[14] These studies suggest that the distal urethral sphincter, not the bladder neck or internal sphincter, is responsible for continence. Furthermore, from clinical observations, it appeared that the ISD was almost always the result of neurologic injury, radiation exposure or multiple prior surgeries, with multiple failed SUI operations being the most common cause of ISD,[10] perhaps implying that ISD is the cause of recurrent, but not primary, SUI.

Integral and hammock theories. Proving or disproving the role of the integrity of anatomic support structures in patients with SUI is very difficult. As the evidence for both the integral and hammock theories is derived from cadaveric studies, imaging studies such as dynamic magnetic resonance imaging (MRI) may be the most accurate way to test the validity of these theories in women with SUI.

Currently, no clinical or laboratory studies have demonstrated the significance of the pubourethral ligaments or other supportive elements described in the integral or hammock theories in maintaining continence. Biopsies of the pubourethral ligaments or other tissues involved in the supportive structure have shown no differences in morphology, histochemistry or fine structure between continent and incontinent women.[15]

TREATMENT MODALITIES

Based on the above theories of the pathophysiology of SUI, various treatment options for SUI have evolved over the last century (Table 5.1).

Retropubic suspensions for correction of urethral position. Although there are several retropubic antiincontinence procedures, most are modifications of the

Table 5.1 Treatment for SUI	
Theory	**Treatment modality**
Urethrovesical axis	Retropubic suspensions/Kelly plication
ISD	Bulking agent
Integral theory	TVT/midurethral slings
Hammock theory	Needle suspensions/sling

Marshall-Marchetti-Krantz (MMK) vesicourethral suspension and its later revision, the Burch colpocystourethropexy. These two operations were the most common antiincontinence procedures performed before 1970.[16] Retropubic suspension procedures were based on Enhorning's theory that an alteration in urethral positioning was responsible for SUI. This theory implies that the urethral height within the pelvis determines continence. Based on this assumption, in order to correct SUI the urethra must be restored to an intraabdominal position. In the MMK, the urethral and periurethral vaginal walls are fixed to the periosteum of the posterior pubis. In the Burch procedure, the urethrovaginal tissue is fixed laterally to Cooper's ligaments rather than anteriorly to the pubic symphysis.

Bulking agents for ISD. Use of bulking agents in treatment of SUI is a prime example of how our understanding of the pathophysiology of SUI has led to the creation and application of a treatment modality. Following the introduction of the concept of ISD, a number of bulking agents have been used to correct it.[22] Bulking and injectable agents attempt to restore urethral closure by injecting material periurethrally to provide additional submucosal bulk. This leads to increased mucosal coaptation and therefore increased urethral closure pressure and resistance to passive urine outflow. Despite the attractiveness of the concept, bulking agents have found limited application in treatment of women who otherwise are not candidates for surgical management of their SUI.

Needle suspensions and pubovaginal slings for hammock theory. In order to minimize the invasiveness of abdominal retropubic suspensions, bladder neck needle suspensions were introduced. First developed by Pereyra in 1959, needle suspensions were designed for the correction of SUI associated with a poorly supported, hypermobile urethra by restoring the urethra to a well-supported position.[9] This procedure created a hammock of support at the bladder neck. Over the ensuing years, several modifications were made to the original Pereyra procedure to reduce complication rates.[23,24] However, needle suspensions fell out of favor with the publication of the 1997 American Urological Association Female Stress Urinary Incontinence Clinical Guideline Panel. After reviewing the long-term cure/dry rates (>48 months), the panel concluded that the best surgical procedures for the "cure" of female SUI were the pubovaginal sling and retropubic suspension.[17]

Pubovaginal slings were most commonly used for the treatment of ISD, type III SUI or after a failed previous antiincontinence procedure. In the traditional method of this procedure, a strip of autograft fascia was placed at the bladder neck and fixed across the rectus muscle. In order to make the sling a less invasive procedure, a number of variations were introduced, including use of the vaginal wall instead of autograft tissue, and bone anchor fixation to the symphysis pubis or behind the symphysis rami.

Midurethral slings for integral theory.

The integral theory proposed by Ulmsten and Petros led the way for application of a new generation of antiincontinence procedure: the tension-free vaginal tape (TVT) and other midurethral slings. In this procedure, a piece of sanitized mesh was applied to the midurethral area to compensate for the incompetent pubourethral ligament. Using ultrasound, Petros demonstrated that midurethral suspensions prohibit the hypermobile bladder neck from opening the midurethra.[9] Due to the ease of performance and high success rates, these procedures are among those most commonly performed by gynecologists and urologists worldwide. Furthermore, in order to make the midurethral sling procedures less invasive and more cost effective, a number of variations and products have been introduced to this category of antiincontinence procedures.

ROLE OF "OTHER FACTORS" IN PATHOPHYSIOLOGY OF STRESS URINARY INCONTINENCE

Hopefully it is becoming clear that just as the physiology of the continence mechanism is a complex and multistep process, so is the pathophysiology of SUI. The spectrum of SUI, and its clinical presentations, cannot be explained by the presence of a single risk factor or a single theory. Instead, SUI should be viewed as the result of multiple insults to the female continence mechanism. Several factors place women at an increased risk for damage to the continence mechanism. These risk factors can be divided into categories that predispose, promote, decompensate or incite SUI.[18]

Predisposing risk factors include gender, genetics, race, and collagen and smooth muscle composition. The Norwegian Epidemiology of Incontinence Group (EPINCONT) demonstrated a familial risk of SUI.[19] Women with incontinent mothers or older sisters were at an increased risk of SUI. The same study also found an increase in the prevalence of SUI with aging. The exact changes that occur with aging are unknown. Changes in muscle tone, hormonal status, and innervation due to parturition may be partially responsible for the increased prevalence of SUI in older women.[20] Race has also been implicated in SUI, with white women at an increased risk for SUI compared to black women.[18] Risk factors that promote incontinence consist of lifestyle habits, nutrition, obesity, smoking, menopause, constipation, and medications. Decompensating factors include aging, physical and mental well-being, environment, and medications. Cognitive abnormalities, such as Alzheimer's disease, and physical immobility, such as Parkinson's disease, while not directly causing incontinence, are important comorbid factors that exacerbate the condition.

Childbirth, pelvic or vaginal surgery, pelvic nerve or muscle damage, and radiation are all inciting factors for SUI.

THE TRAMPOLINE THEORY

Since the physiology of continence in women is multifactorial, so is the pathophysiology of SUI. SUI may result from a combination of complex anatomic and physiologic insults to the central and peripheral control mechanisms. Given its complexity, SUI cannot be explained by one theory or a single risk factor. We propose a more comprehensive theory, the "trampoline theory," to encompass all the factors that play a role in SUI.

A trampoline is composed of fabric, springs, and an outer ring. The proper functioning of a trampoline relies upon an intact fabric (LUT tissue), functioning springs (supporting structures of the bladder and urethra) and a strong outer ring (bony pelvis) (Fig. 5.5). Rarely does the malfunction of one element lead to the dysfunction of the entire trampoline. Similarly, it is doubtful that malfunction of any one element of the continence mechanism will result in SUI. If several of the elements malfunction, however, and no other element compensates for the lost function, then the trampoline malfunctions. The same phenomenon may apply to SUI. It is the malfunction of not just one but many elements that ultimately overwhelms the threshold of the continence mechanism and leads to SUI (Fig. 5.6).

The trampoline theory does not present any new scientific information on the pathophysiology of SUI but it does represent a new metaphor that may encourage clinicians

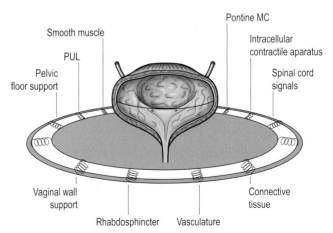

Figure 5.5 Trampoline theory. Intact trampoline: all elements are functioning and there is no stress urinary incontinence.

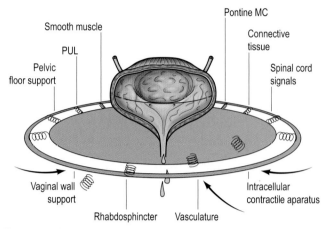

Figure 5.6 Trampoline theory. The malfunction of multiple elements results in stress urinary incontinence.

and investigators to broaden their horizon in regard to the pathophysiology of SUI. This step, in itself, may encourage future investigation of other factors, including the known and many unknown factors related to the pathophysiology of SUI. We need to accelerate investigations into the possible role of factors such as inherent biochemical dysfunction or ischemia, the effects of chronic conditions including diabetes, increased collagenase activities in the pelvic floor, and the effects of antiincontinence procedures, including denervation from vaginal dissection.[21,25] By identifying these factors, we may be able to alter or reduce the impact they have on the continence mechanism, and ultimately create strategies to prevent SUI.

REFERENCES

1. Abrams P, Cardozo L, Fall M, et al. The standardization of terminology of lower urinary tract function: report from the Standardization Sub-committee of the International Continence Society. Am J Obstet Gynecol 2002;187:116.
2. Davis TL, Lukacz ES, Luber KM, et al. Determinants of patient satisfaction after the tension-free vaginal tape procedure. Am J Obstet Gynecol 2004;191:176.
3. Diokno AC, Burgio K, Fultz H, et al. Prevalence and outcomes of continence surgery in community dwelling women. J Urol 2003;170:507.
4. Olsen AL, Smith VJ, Bergstrom JO, et al. Epidemiology of surgically managed pelvic organ prolapse and urinary incontinence. Obstet Gynecol 1997;89:501.
5. Tanagho EA, Meyers FH, Smith DR. Urethral resistance: its components and implications. II. Striated muscle component. Invest Urol 1969;7:195.
6. Enhorning G. Simultaneous recording of intravesical and intra-urethral pressure. A study on urethral closure in normal and stress incontinent women. Acta Chir Scand 1961;Suppl 276: 1.
7. Constantinou CE. Principles and methods of clinical urodynamic investigations. Crit Rev Biomed Eng 1982;7:229.
8. DeLancey JO. Structural aspects of the extrinsic continence mechanism. Obstet Gynecol 1988;72:296.
9. Plzak L 3rd, Staskin D. Genuine stress incontinence theories of etiology and surgical correction. Urol Clin North Am 2002;29:527.
10. Blaivas JG. Incontinence. J Urol 1993;150:1455.
11. McGuire EJ. The effects of sacral denervation on bladder and urethral function. Surg Gynecol Obstet 1977;144:343.
12. Fantl JA, Hurt WG, Bump RC, et al. Urethral axis and sphincteric function. Am J Obstet Gynecol 1986;155:554.
13. Versi E, Cardozo L, Studd J. Distal urethral compensatory mechanisms in women with an incompetent bladder neck who remain incontinent, and the effect of the menopause. Neurourol Urodynamics 1990;9:579

14. Chapple CR, Helm CW, Blease S, et al. Asymptomatic bladder neck incompetence in nulliparous females. Br J Urol 1989;64:357.
15. Petros PE. The pubourethral ligaments—an anatomial and histological study in the live patient. Int Urogynecol J Pelvic Floor Dysfunct 1998;9:154.
16. Stoffel JT, Bresette JF, Smith JJ. Retropubic surgery for stress urinary incontinence. Urol Clin North Am 2002;29:585.
17. Leach GE, Dmochowski RR, Appell RA, et al. Female Stress Urinary Incontinence Clinical Guidelines Panel summary report on surgical management of female stress urinary incontinence. The American Urological Association. J Urol 1997;158:875.
18. Bump RC, Norton PA. Epidemiology and natural history of pelvic floor dysfunction. Obstet Gynecol Clin North Am 1998;25:723.
19. Hannestad YS, Lie RT, Rortveit G, et al. Familial risk of urinary incontinence in women: population based cross sectional study. BMJ 2004;329:889.
20. Luber K. The definition, prevalence, and risk factors for stress urinary incontinence. Rev Urol 2004;6:S3.
21. Hijaz A. Daneshgari. F, Cannon TW, Damaser M. Efficacy of a vaginal sling procedure in a rat model of stress urinary incontinence. J Urol 2004;172(5):2065–2068.
22. Dmochowski R, Appell RA. Advancements in minimally invasive treatments for female stress urinary incontinence: radiofrequency and bulking agents. Curr Urol Rep 2003;4(5):350–355.
23. Stamey TA. Cystoscopic suspension of the vesical neck for urinary incontinence. Surg Gynecol Obstet 1973;136:547–554.
24. Raz S. Modified bladder neck suspension for female stress incontinence. Urology 1981; 17:82–85.
25. Zivkovic F, Tamussino K. Long-term effects of vaginal dissection on the innervations of the striated urethral sphincter. Obstet Gynecol 1996;87(2):257–260.

CHAPTER

Anatomy, Physiology and Pathogenesis of Bladder Overactivity

6

Christopher R Chapple

INTRODUCTION

The lower urinary tract comprises the bladder, the urethra, and the external urethral sphincter or rhabdosphincter, which is integrated in the pelvic floor. In the male, the prostate surrounds the proximal part of the urethra. The bladder consists of three distinct layers: an adventitial layer of connective tissue, which is partly covered by the peritoneum, on the outside, a mucosal layer on the lumen side, and a smooth muscle layer, the detrusor muscle, in between.[1]

Anatomically, the bladder can be divided into three parts: the fundus and the body, the trigone, and the bladder neck. The detrusor muscle of the bladder fundus and body is often described as consisting of three layers, with the muscle fibers oriented longitudinally in the inner and the outer layer and circularly in the middle layer.[2] In fact, the detrusor is an interlacing meshwork of muscle bundles with longitudinally oriented muscle bundles dominating its inner and outer parts.[2]

The smooth muscle of the trigone consists of two layers. The deep trigonal muscle is continuous with the body detrusor muscle. The superficial trigone, on the lumen side of the bladder, is rather thin and consists of muscle bundles with a small diameter. It is continuous with the muscle layers of the intramural part of the ureters and with the smooth muscle of the proximal urethra.[1]

The mucosa that lines the bladder consists of the suburothelial layer and the urothelial epithelium.[1] The former contains connective tissue and a network of blood vessels and smooth muscle cells, as well as a number of cell types currently under evaluation and classified by the term "interstitial cells." The urothelium has a thickness of up to six cell layers. At the trigone, its thickness is limited to two or three layers.

The bladder neck is considerably different in men and women. The smooth muscles in the male bladder neck are oriented circularly and constitute the internal urethral sphincter. They merge with the prostatic musculature. The muscle bundles in the female bladder neck are oriented obliquely or longitudinally and do not constitute a mor-

phologically recognizable sphincter. However, as the female bladder neck normally remains closed until detrusor contractions occur, it behaves like a sphincter and therefore it is also referred to as the internal sphincter.[1] The significance of the contribution of the bladder neck to female continence has been challenged,[3] as it is suggested in many asymptomatic patients to be functionally unimportant.

The striated muscle fibers which constitute the external urethral sphincter are unusually small and are all of the slow-twitch type.[2] As a consequence, this sphincter is capable of sustained contraction over relatively long periods of time and thus contributes to the maintenance of continence. The medial or periurethral parts of the levator ani, the most important component of the pelvic floor, provide an additional occlusive force on the urethral wall.[1] The levator ani consists of cells larger than those in the external sphincter and has the morphologic features of a typical voluntary muscle. The cells are a mixture of slow- and fast-twitch type cells. The latter are capable of responding to fast abdominal pressure increases, such as occur during coughing.

The human pelvic floor contains a relatively large amount of connective tissue, which is probably also of significance for support of the pelvic organs.[1] Additional supportive structures in the male and female are the puboprostatic and the pubourethral ligaments, respectively.[1] These ligaments, which also contain smooth muscle bundles, attach the prostate and the female bladder neck and anterior urethral wall to the symphysis pubis. A good support of the proximal urethra above the level of the pelvic floor is essential for good transmission of abdominal pressure, so that urethral occlusion can be maintained during stress.

The function of the lower urinary tract is to temporarily store a continuously increasing amount of urine at low pressure and expel it under appropriate circumstances. The reservoir function of the bladder is favored by a permanently low intravesical pressure over a wide volume range and a bladder outlet that remains firmly closed, even under conditions of abdominal pressure rises, during the filling phase of the bladder which represents the majority of its activity cycle. Conversely, during voiding, the bladder should be able to develop a sustained contraction of sufficient strength with the bladder outlet offering a low resistance to urinary flow to ensure a ready and residue-free voiding process.

INNERVATION
Efferent innervation.
The lower urinary tract is innervated parasympathetically, sympathetically, and somatically. The efferent parasympathetic nerves originate in the intermediolateral columns of gray matter in the sacral spinal segments S2–4 and run as the pelvic nerves into the pelvic plexus, where they either synapse with postganglionic nerves or run straight to ganglia in the bladder wall where they synapse.[4] These intramural ganglia are mainly located in the adventitia.[2] The third sacral segment is dominant in most humans.[5] The efferent sympathetic nerves originate in the intermediolateral gray columns of the thoracolumbar segments T10–L2. Most fibers synapse in the inferior mesenteric plexus and reach the bladder via the hypogastric nerves. Synapsing may also occur in the paravertebral ganglia and the pelvic ganglia. Some fibers just synapse in the intramural ganglia.

The innervation of the bladder neck is strikingly different in men and women.[5] While the male bladder neck has a rich sympathetic innervation, the female bladder neck is only sparsely supplied with sympathetic nerves. Parasympathetic nerves are present in both sexes.

The somatic nerves that innervate the external urethral sphincter originate in Onuf's nucleus, an area of atypical (that is, unusually small) motoneurons in the anterior horn of the segments S2–4 (mainly S2). These nerves are widely believed to run in the pudendal nerves. Some studies, however, seem to indicate that they run in the pelvic nerves.[4]

Neurotransmission.
The terminal branches of the efferent autonomic nerves run within the smooth muscle bundles.[4] They have a series of swellings called varicosities which contain a number of vesicles which in turn contain neurotransmitters. The arrival of a nerve impulse at a varicosity causes the release of its vesicles, which subsequently release their contents into the muscle bundle. This results in the contraction of a group of muscle cells within that bundle.

Electron microscopically, three types of vesicles can be distinguished: agranular vesicles containing acetylcholine, small dense-cored vesicles containing noradrenaline, and large dense-cored vesicles, the contents of which are yet uncertain. The presence of the latter type reflects the complexity of the autonomic innervation of the bladder. In the traditional description, the parasympathetic nerves release acetylcholine, which acts on muscarinic receptors at the muscle side of the neuromuscular junction, and the sym-pathetic nerves release noradrenaline. However, many more neurotransmitters have been identified. These include amines (such as histamine, serotonin, and dopamine), amino acids (such as GABA), prostaglandins, purines (such as ATP) and several peptides (such as substance P, neuropeptide Y, vasoactive intestinal polypeptide, and endorphins). The exact role of these nonadrenergic, noncholinergic substances is unknown. They possibly modulate the effects of the two classic neurotransmitters.[4]

Afferent innervation.
The afferent fibers of the bladder probably originate from the nerve plexus immediately beneath the mucosa.[2] This so-called suburothelial nerve plexus is relatively sparse in the fundus of the bladder and becomes denser in the direction of the bladder neck. It is most prominent in the trigone. Two types of afferent fibers can be distinguished: small myelinated Aδ fibers and small unmyelinated C fibers. Most likely, the Aδ fibers receive information from mechanoreceptors sensing bladder filling, while the C fibers normally only respond to noxious stimuli.

The afferent fibers run in parasympathetic (pelvic) and sympathetic (hypogastric) nerves. The somatic afferents from the urethra and the pelvic floor run with the pudendal nerve. The afferent fibers run to the spinal segments T10–L2 and S2–4, that is, the same segments from which the efferents to the lower urinary tract depart. Here some of them synapse with efferent neurons, while the remainder ascend the spinal cord to the brainstem and higher centers.[4] Afferent fibers from other sites such as other pelvic organs and the perineal skin run to the same segments where they also synapse with efferent neurons or join ascending pathways. The described neural connections between afferent and efferent fibers enable the performance of the many spinal reflexes playing a role in continence and micturition.[6]

THE NORMAL MICTURITION CYCLE
Voiding phase.
Micturition is a complex process that is normally initiated voluntarily and is continued automatically until the bladder is empty. It is characterized by a sustained contraction of the detrusor muscle and relaxation of the external urethral sphincter. The coordination between the two groups of motoneurons innervating these two muscles, that is, the detrusor motoneurons in S2–4 and the somatic motoneurons in Onuf's nucleus, takes place in an area near the locus ceruleus in the pontine tegmentum by integration of ascending information from the parasympathetic, sympathetic, and somatic nervous systems. This coordinating area is known as Barrington's nucleus, pontine micturition center (PMC) or M region. It is under the control of several higher centers, both of the conscious and

unconscious level. The locations of these centers include the midbrain (periaqueductal gray matter, hypothalamus), basal ganglia (amygdala), cerebral cortex (frontal lobe, cingulate gyrus, insula) and possibly the cerebellum.[7]

The PMC is inhibited until the initiation of voiding. The current theory is that information about the degree of bladder filling is sent from neurons in the lumbosacral cord to the midbrain periaqueductal gray matter (PAG), an area known for its involvement in many vital functions.[8] These afferent signals originate from mechanoreceptors and stretch receptors in the bladder wall, as well as the recently described but poorly understood suburothelial nerve plexus which is also closely approximated to so-called "interstitial" cells which are thought to have an important sensory and integrative function in lower urinary tract control. The PAG, possibly controlled by the hypothalamus, activates the PMC when voiding is considered appropriate.[9] This results in both excitation of the detrusor motoneurons in S2–4 and, via excitation of inhibitory interneurons, inhibition of the moto-neurons in Onuf's nucleus. Because micturition develops automatically once initiated and because of the pathways involved, it is referred to as a spinobulbospinal reflex.

The group of motoneurons in the sacral cord innervating the detrusor muscle is traditionally referred to as the sacral micturition center. As this center does not coordinate micturition in a sense similar to the PMC, this term might need reconsideration.[4] It is, however, likely that the com-pleteness of bladder emptying largely depends on the neural interaction at the level of the sacral cord and peripheral ganglia.[5]

Normal bladder contraction in humans is mediated mainly through stimulation of muscarinic receptors in the detrusor muscle. Atropine resistance, i.e. contraction of isolated bladder muscle in response to electrical nerve stimulation after pretreatment with atropine, has been demonstrated in most animal species but seems to be of little importance in normal human bladder muscle. However, atropine-resistant (nonadrenergic, noncholinergic: NANC) contractions have been reported in normal human detrusor and may be caused by ATP. A significant degree of atropine resistance may exist in morphologically and/or functionally changed bladders, and has been reported to occur in hyper-trophic bladders, interstitial cystitis, neurogenic bladders, and in the aging bladder. The importance of the NANC component to detrusor contraction in vivo, normally, and in different micturition disorders remains to be established.

Muscarinic receptors. Molecular cloning studies have revealed five distinct genes for muscarinic acetylcholine receptors in rats and humans, and it is now generally accepted that five receptor subtypes correspond to these gene products.

Detrusor smooth muscle from various species contains muscarinic receptors of the M_2 ($\sim 2/3$) and M_3 ($\sim 1/3$) subtypes. There is general agreement that M_3 receptors are mainly responsible for the normal micturition contraction whereas the role of the M_2 receptors has not been clarified. In certain disease states, M_2 receptors may contribute to contraction of the bladder.

The muscarinic receptor functions in the bladder may be changed in different disorders, such as outflow obstruction and neurologic disorders. However, it is not always clear what the changes mean in terms of alterations in detrusor function.

Filling phase. The intravesical pressure or, more exactly, its component caused by activity of the detrusor muscle, the so-called detrusor pressure, normally remains low during the filling phase of the micturition cycle. This is not only due to the passive properties of the bladder wall but also involves neurologic mechanisms at several levels.[4,5] Cerebral inhibition of the PMC is probably the main factor.[5] Spinal mechanisms include recurrent inhibition of the detrusor motoneurons in S2–4 by interneurons, the filter action of the parasympathetic ganglia (meaning that impulses are not transmitted when preganglionic activity is low) and increased sympathetic activity inhibiting transmission in the parasympathetic ganglia.[4] Sympathetic inhibition is provoked by afferent activity in the pelvic as well as the pudendal nerves, originating from sensory afferents as described above.[5] There is evidence that the role of the sympathetic nervous system is not limited to local spinal reflexes but involves central pathways: the insular cortex appeared to be activated during bladder filling in volunteers who were not allowed to micturate (it is known that acti-vation of the right insula results in an increased sympathetic tone).[10] However, some controversy exists as to the importance of the sympathetic system.[11]

Continence is maintained at the bladder neck but the neural control of this structure is poorly understood.[5] Perhaps the passive occlusion of the bladder neck resulting from the surrounding collagen and elastic tissue and its muscular and ligamentous suspension is of more importance in the closure mechanism. An incompetent bladder neck does not necessarily lead to incontinence due to the occlu-sion of the distal urethral sphincter (comprising extrinsic and intrinsic components). A crucial role in this occlusion is probably played by the so-called L region, an area located ventrolateral to the PMC.[12] Neurons from this region pro-ject bilaterally to Onuf's nucleus and electrical stimulation of this area induces pelvic floor contraction and elevation of the urethral pressure. Because the L region appeared especially active in volunteers who tried to micturate but, probably because of emotional reasons, were unable to do so, it may be assumed that afferents of this region originate in limbic system-related structures.[12]

PATHOPHYSIOLOGY OF BLADDER OVERACTIVITY

As mentioned above, the detrusor pressure normally remains low during bladder filling. The occurrence of involuntary phasic detrusor contractions during the filling phase of a urodynamic study, spontaneously or on provocation, was previously termed "detrusor instability" (in nonneurogenic cases) or "detrusor hyperreflexia" (in neurogenic cases) by the International Continence Society, but is now referred to as "idiopathic or neurogenic detrusor overactivity" respectively.[13] The changes in terminology are summarized in Box 6.1.

Box 6.1 Terminology	
OUT	**IN**
Detrusor hyperreflexia	Neurogenic detrusor overactivity
Detrusor instability	Idiopathic detrusor overactivity
Motor urgency	None
Sensory urgency	None
Motor urge incontinence	Detrusor overactivity incontinence with urgency
Reflex incontinence	Detrusor overactivity incontinence without sensation
Genuine stress incontinence	Urodynamic stress incontinence

It follows from this subdivision that detrusor overactivity may have several causes. The possible mechanisms causing detrusor overactivity will therefore be discussed under three headings.

Obstructive detrusor overactivity. Bladder outlet obstruction causes increased voiding pressures and a prolonged duration of voiding. It has been hypothesized that this results in ischemic damage to the intramural ganglia and consequently a partial denervation of the detrusor muscle.[14] Experiments have shown that denervation of smooth muscle cells may result in supersensitivity to agonists, increased excitability, and increased electrical coupling. These changes may make the detrusor muscle susceptible to the development of involuntary contractions. It has been argued that the detrusor muscle hypertrophy upon obstruction does not necessarily play a causative role.[14] A somewhat contrasting and more evidence-based explanation comes from the observation of increased levels of nerve growth factor in the bladders of obstructed rats and humans and increased

dimensions of afferent and efferent rat neurons.[15] Additional experiments in rats demonstrated that the structural changes are accompanied by functional changes, at least in the afferents.[16]

Neurogenic detrusor overactivity. Several neurogenic conditions may cause overactivity. Following spinal transsection, there is a period of spinal shock, during which there is a state of flaccidity and areflexia of the body below the level of the lesion due to the withdrawal of the supraspinal influences on the motoneurons. This situation also applies to the PMC and the sacral micturition center. After a highly variable time, reflex activity develops. Such activity is found in the bladder typically after 6–8 weeks, provided the sacral cord has remained intact.[17] It is thought that these reflexes are mediated by unmyelinated C fiber afferents that are present but inactive in the healthy individual, rather than by the Aδ fibers that mediate the normal micturition reflex.[18] The same fibers are held responsible for the overactivity observed in other spinal diseases like multiple sclerosis. The involvement of these fibers has been supported by the successful treatment of patients with intravesical application of the vanilloids capsaicin and resiniferatoxin.[18,19] The effect of capsaicin was found in patients with detrusor overactivity caused by suprapontine pathology.[18]

Theoretically, there is no need to assume a role for segmental reflexes in these cases. Involuntary contractions may develop at any time due to the disruption of the inhibiting influences of suprapontine centers on the PMC. The location of the injury is not only relevant to the pathophysiologic mechanism of the overactivity, but is also of significance for the voiding process. Detrusor–sphincter dyssynergia is to be expected in spinal patients due to the disturbed coordination of the PMC and will be absent in patients with suprapontine lesions.

Idiopathic detrusor overactivity. In many cases, although the etiology is unclear, the cause of idiopathic detrusor overactivity is likely to be neurogenic rather than myogenic, particularly in view of the association between detrusor overactivity and aging. An increased number of putative afferent nerves in the bladder wall of female patients has been reported.[20] Although no effect of intravesical capsaicin on idiopathic detrusor overactivity was found,[18] efficacy was found in 12 patients treated with the more potent analogue resiniferatoxin.[21] This suggests the involvement of the afferent C fibers. The role of nonneurogenic factors can not be excluded, however, as abnormal cell-to-cell communications have been reported in the bladders of patients with idiopathic overactivity.[22]

Drake et al have suggested that whilst traditionally normal bladder function is controlled by the central nervous system (CNS) and any peripheral contribution to bladder control is believed to be small, nevertheless anatomically and functionally such a contribution might exist. They propose that the detrusor muscle is arranged into modules, which are circumscribed areas of muscle active during the filling phase of the micturition cycle. These modules are controlled by a peripheral myovesical plexus, consisting of intramural ganglia and interstitial cells. They suggest that whilst detrusor overactivity is traditionally thought to be a consequence of abnormal expression of the micturition reflex or changes in the properties of the smooth muscle, in fact it results from exaggerated symptomatic expression of peripheral autonomous activity, arising from a shift in the balance of excitation and inhibition in smooth muscle modules.[23]

As mentioned above, detrusor overactivity is characterized by the occurrence of involuntary phasic detrusor contractions during the filling phase of the micturition cycle. Another category of patients comprises those who have overactive bladder symptoms without signs of detrusor overactivity, a condition usually described as "sensory urgency." This term, however, is no longer recommended by the International Continence Society[13] because of the difficulty in characterizing these patients; although, since the same therapeutic options as in detrusor overactivity may successfully be applied in a portion of these patients, a similar pathophysiology may be hypothesized but remains to be proven.

The overactive bladder.

In the most recent report on the standardisation of terminology of lower urinary tract function, the Standardization Subcommittee of the International Continence Society defines the symptoms, signs, and conditions associated with lower urinary tract dysfunction.[13] It has been proposed that the filling symptoms of urgency with or without urge incontinence, usually with increased urinary frequency and nocturia, are indicative of a symptom syndrome called the overactive bladder syndrome (OAB), also known as the urge syndrome and urgency-frequency syndrome.

OAB is a symptom syndrome defined as "Urgency, with or without urge incontinence, usually with frequency and nocturia." These symptoms are suggestive of detrusor overactivity (urodynamically demonstrable involuntary bladder contractions) but can be due to other forms of voiding or urinary dysfunction. These terms can be used if there is no proven infection or other obvious pathology. OAB is therefore clearly distinct from urodynamically proven detrusor overactivity, although the majority of people with OAB are thought to have this underlying diagnosis. The relationship between the symptoms is shown in Figure 6.1.

Urgency is probably the most important symptom in this syndrome; improvements in terms of increased "warning time" of the need to get to the toilet are often mentioned by

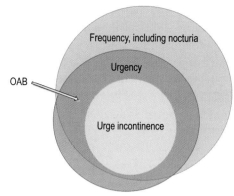

Figure 6.1 The potential interrelationship with the cardinal symptoms of the overactive bladder (urgency, frequency) symptom complex.

patients as the most noticeable response to therapy. Despite its importance, this symptom is difficult to define and hence to quantify. At this juncture it is useful to consider the definition of the various terms applied to the symptoms of the OAB syndrome.

- Urgency: the complaint of a *sudden, compelling desire* to pass urine that is difficult to defer
- Urge incontinence: the complaint of involuntary leakage of urine accompanied or immediately preceded by *urgency*
- Frequency (voiding 8 or more times per day): usually accompanies *urgency* with or without urge incontinence; the patient complains that he/she voids too often by day
- Nocturia: usually accompanies *urgency* with or without urge incontinence: the individual has to wake at night one or more times to void

Clearly, urgency drives the other symptoms of the OAB syndrome (Fig. 6.2).

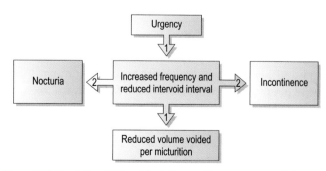

Figure 6.2 The interrelationship between the symptoms of the overactive bladder symptom complex, demonstrating the importance of urgency. 1. Proven direct effect. 2. Effect correlated with urgency but inconsistent due to multifactorial etiology of the symptom.

Various studies have reported a prevalence for this symptom complex of 16–17% in the population.[24] Incontinence occurs in approximately a third of patients and approximately a third of patients have a mixed picture of combined sphincteric weakness and detrusor overactivity.

The diagnostic pathway follows on from the appropriate assessment of any patient as detailed elsewhere.

History

- Questionnaires
- Frequency/volume chart

Urinalysis
Physical examination

- Pelvic Organ Prolapse Quantification (POPQ) system
- Bladder neck mobility
- Sacral reflex integrity/pelvic floor muscle strength

Tests

- Pad test
- Flowmetry/postvoid residual (PVR)
- Urodynamics

In any patient who fails to respond to initial therapy or in the presence of a complex picture, formal cystometry is important as the diagnostic study to demonstrate abnormal detrusor function and/or abnormal bladder sensation.

Specific indications for cystometry include:

- after treatment failure
- prior to invasive therapy
- complicated incontinence
- long-term surveillance of incontinence associated with neurologic disorders.

During cystometry, bladder sensation can also be evaluated. This can be judged at defined points during filling cystometry and must be interpreted in relation to bladder volume at that specific moment and in relation to the patient's symptomatic complaint or sensation. Many patients with overactive bladder syndrome will present with an increased bladder sensation characterized by an early first sensation of bladder filling or an early desire to void. Another pattern may be an early strong desire to void which occurs at low bladder volume and which persists. This can be indicated by the patient as urgency or the sudden compelling desire to void.

Under the previous ICS terminology, individuals in whom these involuntary contractions are demonstrable were said to have "motor urgency" while individuals in whom these are not demonstrable were classified as "sensory urgency." However, the ICS no longer recommends these terms as they are often misused and have little intuitive meaning. Furthermore, it may be simplistic to relate urgency just to the presence or absence of detrusor overactivity when there is usually a concomitant fall in urethral pressure, particularly as it is so difficult to measure urethral pressure accurately. Fluctuations in urethral pressure have been described as the "unstable urethra." However, the significance of these fluctuations remains unclear. Therefore the ICS does not recommend this term. If symptoms are present in association with a decrease in urethral pressure, it is proposed that a description of the events is given.

Provocative maneuvers such as rapid filling, use of cooled or acid medium, postural changes and hand washing may be used during cystometry to provoke detrusor overactivity. However, it should be realized that with this type of provocation, detrusor overactivity may be detected in some asymptomatic individuals. If doubt remains as to the exact behavior of the bladder, ambulatory urodynamics can be used to monitor bladder activity for a prolonged period of time but this remains a nonstandardized technique and is best regarded still as a research tool. Cystometry also permits measurement of cystometric bladder capacity and allows this to be matched to the bladder diary data. Cystometric bladder capacity is the bladder volume at the end of the filling. This is the volume at which the patient feels she can no longer delay micturition because of the strong desire to void. If there is uncontrollable urgency resulting in incontinence, this volume is the volume at which voiding starts.

TREATMENT

Treatment for all forms of incontinence should commence with conservative methods before progressing to more complex surgical procedures. A multidisciplinary approach is important. In the UK, in addition to urologists and gynecologists, continence nurse specialists, physiotherapists, and healthcare professionals in community-based primary care services play a pivotal role in the management and support of incontinent patients. It is important to get an overall picture of the effect of incontinence on the patient's life. General support of the patient with respect to activities of living, pads/special pants, catheters, and appliances forms an important facet in the management of these patients and continence nurses play a vital role in this context.

Behavioral therapy and pharmacotherapy are the mainstays of treatment and there is a continuing search for more effective and selective drugs with minimal side effects. About 50% of patients gain satisfactory benefit from pharmacotherapy. The role of physiotherapy in the treatment of urge incontinence remains unclear as evidenced by systematic review of clinical trials.

Behavioral therapy. This involves the patient drinking less before bed or before a journey, while retraining the bladder to hold on for a longer time. A fluid/volume chart helps with this. Lifestyle interventions such as restriction of diuretics (e.g. caffeine, alcohol) and fluid can be helpful. Most patients have often taken this step before being seen in the clinic. The additive effect of "bladder training" to that seen with pharmacotherapy remains controversial, although logic would support the importance of modifying behavior to augment the therapeutic efficacy of pharmacotherapy.

Pharmacologic treatment. There is currently no group of drugs which can be used with consistently successful results. Many drugs have been tried but the results are often disappointing, due to poor treatment efficacy and/or side effects. There have been many evaluations of the drugs currently used for treatment of OAB. The present review is based on the evaluation made by the Second International Consultation on Incontinence, held in Monaco in 2004.[25] Drugs were evaluated using different types of evidence (Box 6.2). Pharmacologic and/or physiologic efficacy evidence means that a drug has been shown to have desired effects in relevant preclinical experiments or in healthy volunteers (or in experimental situations in patients). Clinical drug recommendations are based on evaluations made using a modification of the Oxford system, in which emphasis is given to the quality of the trials assessed (Box 6.3, Table 6.1).

Drugs used for treatment of bladder overactivity. Detrusor overactivity may be the result of several different mechanisms, both myogenic and neurologic. Most probably, both factors contribute to the genesis of the disease.

An abundance of drugs has been used for the treatment of OAB (Table 6.1). However, for many of them, clinical use is based on the results of preliminary, open studies rather than randomized, controlled clinical trials (RCTs). The

---

Box 6.2   Types of evidence

Pharmacodynamic
   In vitro
   In vivo

Pharmacokinetic
   Absorption
   Distribution
   Metabolism
   Excretion

Physiologic
   Animal models
   Clinical phase I

Clinical
   Oxford guidelines

Box 6.3   ICI assessments: Oxford guidelines (modified)

Levels of evidence

Level 1: randomized controlled clinical trials

Level 2: good-quality prospective studies

Level 3: retrospective "case–control" studies

Level 4: case series

Level 5: expert opinion

Grades of recommendation

Grade A: based on level 1 evidence (= highly recommended)

Grade B: consistent level 2 or 3 evidence (= recommended)

Grade C: level 4 studies or "majority evidence" (= recommended with reservation)

Grade D: evidence inconsistent/inconclusive (= not recommended)

---

antimuscarinics tolterodine and trospium, the drugs with mixed actions, oxybutynin and propiverine, and the vasopressin analog desmopressin were found to fulfill the criteria for level 1 evidence according to the Oxford assessment system and were given grade A recommendations by the International Consultation on Incontinence. More recently, the anticholinergic drugs solifenacin and darifenacin have been introduced and (at the last ICI consultation, as yet unpublished) have also been given a grade A recommendation pending statutory authority approval.

Surgery. Surgery for detrusor overactivity should be reserved only for patients for whom all conservative treatment modalities have failed since all surgical procedures bring with them associated risks and complications. The objective of surgery is to increase the functional bladder capacity and decrease the maximal detrusor pressure, which in turn would prevent incontinence from occurring. In patients with neuropathic bladders, surgery would confer a protection to the upper tract as well.

Cystoplasty involves remodeling of the bladder in order to disrupt its ability to contract and to increase its physical and functional capacity. In contrast, electrical stimulation of the bladder's nerve supply, commonly termed neuromodulation, aims to suppress the reflexes responsible for causing involuntary bladder contractions. Denervation procedures also act on the problematic neural reflexes but do so by temporary or permanent interruption of the reflex pathways. Another option is to completely bypass the bladder as a last resort. Preoperatively patients should be counseled regarding the outcomes of the operation, especially regarding voiding difficulty and the potential use of intermittent self-catheterization.

Numerous approaches have been used to try to overcome unwanted bladder contractions in both the idiopathic and

Table 6.1   Drugs used in the treatment of detrusor overactivity. Assessments according to the Oxford system (modified)

	Level of evidence	Grade of recommendation
Antimuscarinic drugs		
Tolterodine	1	A
Trospium	1	A
Darifenacin	1	A*
Solifenacin	1	A*
Propantheline	2	B
Atropine, hyoscyamine	2	D
Drugs acting on membrane channels		
Calcium antagonists	Under investigation	
Potassium channel openers	Under investigation	
Drugs with mixed actions		
Oxybutynin	1	A
Propiverine	1	A
Dicyclomine	4	C
Flavoxate	4	D
α-adrenoceptor antagonists		
Alfuzosin	4	D
Doxazosin	4	D
Prazosin	4	D
Terazosin	4	D
Tamsulosin	4	D
β-adrenoceptor agonists		
Terbutaline	4	D
Clenbuterol	4	D
Salbutamol	4	D
Antidepressants		
Imipramine	2	C**
Prostaglandin synthesis inhibitors		
Indomethacin	4	C
Flurbiprofen	4	C
Vasopressin analogs		
Desmopressin	1	A***
Other drugs		
Baclofen	2	C****
Capsaicin	2	B
Resiniferatoxin	2	B
Botulinum toxin	2	B

*   Provided approval
**   Should be used with caution
***   Nocturia
**** Intrathecal use

neuropathic populations. Many innovative procedures have enjoyed temporary popularity but then fallen into disuse as unacceptable complications and long-term results emerged. Among the historical footnotes at the present time are bladder transsection, prolonged bladder distension, and selective sacral neurectomy.

The mainstay of current therapy for bladder overactivity is augmentation cystoplasty, using the "clam" technique.[26] Three additional surgical options have been added to this in recent years: bladder autoaugmentation,[27] sacral neuromodulation,[28] and botulinum toxin injection therapy.[29,30]

Whilst a number of surgical techniques have been reported over the years to deal with drug-resistant detrusor overactivity, it is now widely accepted that procedures such as detrusor transsection and transtrigonal phenol injection therapy produce unreliable, short-lived results to the extent that their routine use can no longer be supported.

Augmentation cystoplasty. The principle underlying an augmentation cystoplasty is that by bivalving a functionally overactive bladder and introducing a segment of intestine, it is possible to produce a bladder with an increased functional capacity and a lower end filling pressure.

The two most commonly used intestinal segments are ileum and sigmoid. The sigmoid is usually used in patients where a short small bowel mesentery renders the procedure difficult but it has been suggested that ileum is preferable in that it produces lower reservoir pressures and better compliance. The original technique described for clam cystoplasty is still widely used but modifications to this include opening the bladder in the sagittal plane, which appears equally effective, and opening the bladder as a "star." The star modification can be particularly useful in patients with neurogenic bladder dysfunction (NBD) where the bladder is small and very thickwalled. An alternative surgical technique popularized by McGuire is his modification of the hemi-Kock procedure with a transverse "smile" incision (looking posteriorly) which is fashioned 3 cm above the ureteral orifices, creating an anteriorly based detrusor flap. Most workers find coronal or sagittal bivalving of the bladder to be effective and acceptable provided that adequate opening of the bladder is performed right down to the ureteral orifices both to adequately open the bladder and also prevent "diverticulation" of the cystoplasty segment. There are reports of laparoscopic enterocystoplasty having been undertaken successfully but this remains the province of the enthusiastic pioneer at present.[31]

It must be remembered that this is major surgery and despite adequate preoperative counseling, many patients take some months to adapt to their new bladder and learn to void effectively by abdominal straining. It is important to check on postoperative residuals and intermittent self-

catheterization is necessary for a number of these patients, particularly those with NBD, and it is of interest to review the reported incidence of intermittent self-catheterization which varies from 15% up to 85% of cases. It is evident that a number of factors contribute to the intermittent self-catheterization rate, including the level of residual accepted as tolerable by the supervising urologist and concomitant use of procedures directed at the bladder outflow, either urethral dilation or treatments for stress incontinence. A particular debate centers around the treatment of coexisting stress incontinence at the time of the clam procedure and current opinion remains divided on this matter. Certainly, any measures designed to deal with stress incontinence will increase the rate of intermittent self-catheterization.

Other problems encountered with augmentation cystoplasty include difficulty in voiding, mucus production, infections, and metabolic disorders which are usually mild and subclinical. Provided that patients are counseled preoperatively regarding mucus, this is rarely a problem. Persistent urinary infection can be troublesome, particularly in female patients, and it has been reported to occur in up to 30% of cases with the need for long-term antibiotic therapy in a number of these.

It must be remembered that there are long-term sequelae associated with augmentation cystoplasty and prominent amongst these is bowel disturbance, with increased frequency and looseness of bowel actions and a tendency to incontinent episodes, which occurs in up to a third of patients. Bowel dysfunction following augmentation cystoplasy is thought to be related to the interruption of the normal enterohepatic circulation. Bladder perforations do occur in up to 10% of patients in reported series. It must also be borne in mind that a significant number of patients require long-term intermittent self-catheterization.

At present, lifelong follow-up of these patients is recommended not only because of the above complications but also in view of the suggestion that augmentation cystoplasty predisposes to the subsequent development of malignancy. There exists no convincing evidence to support an association with tumor in the absence of other predisposing factors such as previous tuberculosis or chronic urinary stasis such as that associated with paraplegia.

Augmentation cystoplasty is an effective management option in contemporary practice in children, adolescents, and adults with intractable detrusor overactivity resistant to pharmacotherapy, although most of the reported series have a follow-up of less than 5 years. Nevertheless, it does involve major surgery, there are a number of medium- and long-term complications associated with its use and patients require lifelong monitoring. A proportion of patients are not improved by this procedure. With these observations in mind, alternative therapies have been explored.

Tissue engineering technology may prove to be useful in developing viable alternatives to the currently used bowel segments.[32] It has been shown that the bladder has the ability to repair and remodel itself to a large extent, particularly if provided with suitable support. It appears that the urothelial layer has the ability to regenerate normally but the muscle layer does not fully develop. Recent work in this field has therefore concentrated on finding the most suitable scaffold for native bladder regeneration. In addition, engineering tissue using selective cell transplantation may provide the means for creating new, functional bladder segments. The donor tissue is dissociated into individual cells, which are implanted directly into the host or expanded in tissue culture, attached to a support matrix and reimplanted following expansion. The use of autologous bladder cells eliminates the problems of tissue rejection. Other attempts in the area have looked at the potential for neural ingrowth into bioengineered tissues.

At the present time, these techniques remain experimental. However, initial laboratory studies have shown that such technology holds genuine potential for future advances in the field of reconstructive urology.

Autoaugmentation.

In 1989 Cartwright and Snow reported a surgical technique which they named bladder autoaugmentation.[27] The principle is that the detrusor muscle over the entire dome of the bladder is excised, leaving the underlying bladder urothelium intact. A large epithelial "bulge" is created which functions by augmenting the storage capacity of the bladder. Following excision of the dome detrusor muscle, the lateral margins of the detrusor are fixed bilaterally to the psoas muscles.

An alternative surgical approach which has been explored in case reports is laparoscopic-assisted autoaugmentation but comment on this cannot be made in the absence of adequate numbers of patients and no significant follow-up.[33]

Whilst it is recognized that spontaneous perforation of an augmentation cystoplasty bladder is a very real phenomenon, occurring in up to 10% of cases, it is a particular concern that patients may be at greater risk of a perforation following the autoaugmentation procedure because of the thinness of the mucosa in the bulging "diverticulum" produced by the operation. Certainly evidence in support of this is provided by animal studies where autoaugmentation resulted in a higher risk of perforation occurring, and at lower pressures, than augmentation cystoplasty. To date this complication has not been reported in clinical series.

A possible explanation for this is that there is the ingrowth of fibrous tissue around the mucosal diverticulum with the progress of time and this would certainly correspond to the limited increase in capacity seen following the procedure. This also raises the question as to the durability of this operation if this fibrosis is progressive.

At present, whilst autoaugmentation has a number of attractive features to recommend it, it is clear that the increase in bladder capacity and reduction in detrusor overactivity which results from this procedure are far less pronounced than those achieved with augmentation cystoplasty.

The number of cases reported in the literature is small, with short-term follow-up. Whilst the definite advantage of this technique is the lower incidence of morbidity as compared to conventional augmentation cystoplasty, the question must be posed as to whether this is adequately counterbalanced by the limited efficacy of the procedure and the possibility that the response achieved may not be maintained in the longer term.

Whilst a definite advantage of this procedure is the fact that it is less interventional than augmentation cystoplasty, and with a lower morbidity, the search for less invasive techniques has led to sacral neuromodulation and botulinum toxin injection therapy, providing the opportunity for an organ-preserving and reversible treatment alternative to standard augmentation cystoplasty.

Sacral neuromodulation.

The principle of sacral neuromodulation is to stimulate the sacral plexus, usually the S3 nerve root. The exact mechanism of action of this therapy is as yet poorly defined in view of our relative lack of knowledge about the precise neurologic control of the lower urinary tract. Nevertheless, it is well established that efferent and afferent autonomic and synaptic pathways are interlinked to enable coordinated storage and voiding of urine in conjunction with central nervous control. A likely explanation is that stimulation of the sacral plexus results in afferent stimulation reflexly inhibiting the bladder. An alternative secondary mode of action is that electrical stimulation of the sacral nerve results in contraction of the pelvic floor which further contributes to the efferent feedback. The phenomenon of longer lasting effects even when implants are turned off serves to emphasize that there are aspects of the mechanism of action of this therapy which still remain obscure, no doubt reflecting our limited knowledge in this field.

Treatment of patients by neuromodulation involves a three-stage process of acute stimulation, peripheral nerve evaluation (PNE) with a temporary electrode, and finally a permanent implant. The first implant for human sacral nerve stimulation was performed in 1986 by Schmidt and Tanagho,[28] during research into sacral anterior root stimulation in patients with severe neuropathic voiding problems. Since then a number of conditions refractory to conservative therapy have been treated by neuromodulation, with varying degrees of success. These include motor and sensory detrusor dysfunction, chronic retention in women, and pelvic pain, but treatment of detrusor overactivity has been most widely studied.

Neuromodulation is an adjunct to the surgical treatments available to the patient and all the treatment options, risks, and benefits need to be explained. It does have the advantage of being reversible and does not affect further treatment if unsuccessful. Whilst its mechanism of action is unclear, it seems to have a low morbidity and in the patients who respond to PNE, results appear good although existing studies have a limited follow-up. Disadvantages of the technique are that only 40–50% of patients respond to temporary stimulation. The technique for temporary stimulation is inaccurate due to movements of the temporary electrode and developments in this area include modifications to the electrode and a trend towards placement of a permanent electrode for the PNE which facilitates the second stage of the procedure.

Sacral neuromodulation is well tolerated by patients and surgical complications are rare. However, there is a significant initial failure rate (despite successful preoperative nerve testing) and some patients experience rapid or gradual accommodation to the stimulation and thus lose any lasting benefit. The equipment is costly, an experienced team is necessary to follow up the patients and overall, out of the original patient cohort submitted to PNE, probably only 10–20% obtain a worthwhile long-term result. If initial benefit is lost then reoperation can be considered with a view to placing an electrode in the contralateral foramen. Pain at the site of the generator may also occur and require revision surgery. These problems account for the relatively high reoperation rate of 33%. Despite this, it is an interesting and innovative approach to the management of bladder overactivity and holds promise for the future.

PERCUTANEOUS POSTERIOR TIBIAL NERVE STIMULATION. The PercSANS™ is another nerve stimulation device developed for use in bladder overactivity. Stimulation to the posterior tibial nerve is applied via a thin needle which is inserted 5 cm cephalad from the medial malleolus and just posterior to the margin of the tibia. Correct positioning is confirmed by flexion of the great toes on stimulation.[34] Stimulation is given on an intermittent basis with the needle being reinserted for each treatment period. Clinical use of the technique has shown early promise, with reported success rates of 67–81%. As with the noninvasive neuromodulation techniques, patients appear to require ongoing treatment if they are to maintain benefit,[35] and in a recent report at the EAU, many patients declined long-term therapy because of the need for repeated visits. Again, no significant side effects have been reported.

Botulinum toxin injection therapy. Botulinum toxin is a presynaptic neuromuscular blocking agent inducing selective and reversible muscle weakness for up to several months when injected intramuscularly in small amounts.

The toxin, usually of the A type (although there is a little work with the B subtype), has been used in a number of areas of medicine and more recently has been described by Schurch and colleagues as a therapy for overactive bladder.[30] Whilst the data on many of the indications for the use of this therapy remain preliminary, there is a rapidly accruing evidence base.

Initial therapy with botulinum-A toxin injection has been with neurogenic detrusor overactivity and detrusor–sphincter dyssynergia. It is effective in the treatment of detrusor–sphincter dyssynergia when injected either transurethrally or transperineally. After treatment, external urethral sphincter pressure, voiding pressure, and postvoid residual volume decreased. The effect lasts for 2–9 months depending on the number of injections. The best results have been reported in those patients with multiple sclerosis and incomplete spinal cord injury, patients suffering from neurogenic detrusor overactivity and detrusor–sphincter dyssynergia. Based on initial successful results, the application of botulinum-A toxin injection therapy into the external urethral sphincter has been extended to the treatment of bladder outflow obstruction and also to decrease outlet resistance in patients with an acontractile detrusor. In cases of successful treatment, spontaneous voiding re-occurs and catheterization can be resumed.

Interestingly, in a report of a case of bladder paralysis following wound botulism, Sautter et al noted that wound botulism had been increasingly reported in recent years and that nearly all of these new cases had occurred in injecting drug abusers.[36] They noted that surprisingly and despite the well-known blocking action of the botulinum toxin on the autonomic nerve system, little attention has been paid to changes in the lower urinary tract following acute botulinum toxin poisoning.

Injections of botulinum-A toxin into the detrusor muscle were first reported by Schurch et al to treat neurogenic detrusor overactivity in spinal cord-injured patients[30] and by Schulte-Baukloh et al in children with myelomeningocele.[29] In Schurch et al's initial prospective nonrandomized study carried out at two clinics were 31 patients with traumatic spinal cord injury who emptied the bladder by intermittent self-catheterization. These patients had severe neurogenic detrusor overactivity and incontinence despite a high dose of anticholinergic medication. Long-lasting (mean 9 months) detrusor relaxation was noted to occur after the injection of 300 units of "Botox" (botulinum toxin A). Continence was restored in about 95% of the patients and the use of anticholinergic drugs could be markedly reduced or even stopped.

A retrospective European multicenter study from 10 sites in 231 patients has presented the most extensive experience to date with botulinum-A toxin injections into the detrusor muscle to treat neurogenic incontinence due to detrusor overactivity.[37] Three hundred units of Botox were injected cystoscopically into the detrusor muscle at 30 different locations, while sparing the trigone. By the time of the initial (mean 12 weeks after injection) as well as at the second urodynamic follow-up examinations (mean 36 weeks after injection), the mean cystometric bladder capacity ($P<0.0001$) and the mean reflex volume ($P<0.01$) increased significantly, while the mean voiding pressure ($P<0.0001$) decreased significantly. The mean bladder compliance had increased significantly ($P<0.0001$) by the first follow-up examination and nonsignificantly by the time of the second follow-up. No injection-related complications or toxin-related side effects were reported. The patients considerably reduced their intake or even stopped taking anticholinergic drugs and were satisfied with the treatment.

A subsequent placebo-controlled study has investigated the safety and efficacy of each of two doses of Botox (200 or 300 U) injected into the detrusor for urinary incontinence caused by neurogenic detrusor overactivity of predominantly spinal cord origin.[38] There were significant post-treatment decreases in incontinence episodes from baseline in the two Botox groups ($P</=0.05$) but not in the placebo group. In addition, more patients who received Botox reported no incontinence episodes during at least one posttreatment evaluation period. Positive treatment effects were also reflected by significant improvements in bladder function in the Botox groups, as assessed by urodynamics and patient quality of life. Benefits were observed from the first evaluation at week 2 to the end of the 24-week study. No safety concerns were raised. These authors were able to conclude that intramuscular injections of botulinum toxin A

into the detrusor can provide rapid, well-tolerated, clinically significant decreases in the signs and symptoms of urinary incontinence caused by neurogenic detrusor overactivity during a 24-week study period.

The excellent results of the use of Botox injections into the detrusor in neurogenic detrusor overactivity have subsequently led to this therapy being extended to the treatment of incontinence due to idiopathic detrusor overactivity causing OAB.

Whilst preliminary results have been promising, the most appropriate dosage of the toxin, the dilution it should be administered in and its precise site of injection, both in terms of the depth of injection in the bladder wall and anatomic location in the bladder, remain to be adequately established. Preliminary reports in abstract form have suggested that lower doses of botulinum toxin A may be just as effective as those reported to date, and possibly lower doses may be just as effective in nonneurogenic cases as in neurogenic cases.

Although botulinum toxin is a successful and standard treatment in other areas of medicine, clinical experience of this technique in bladder overactivity remains relatively scarce at present. However, it may be of significant future value in the management of idiopathic bladder overactivity and OAB resistant to pharmacotherapy following on from the reported experience in neurogenic overactivity. There is great interest in this therapeutic modality at present and a number of case studies are being prepared. Clearly, for the future, controlled trials are absolutely essential to establish the potential role of botulinum-A toxin injections in the fields of urology and neurourology.

REFERENCES

1. Dixon JS, Gosling JA. The anatomy of the bladder, urethra and pelvic floor. In: Mundy AR, Stephenson TP, Wein AJ, eds. Urodynamics: principles, practice and application, 2nd edn. New York: Churchill Livingstone; 1994.
2. Dixon J, Gosling J. Structure and innervation in the human. In: Torrens M, Morrison JFB, eds. The physiology of the lower urinary tract. London: Springer-Verlag; 1987.
3. Chapple CR, Helm W, Blease S, et al. Asymptomatic bladder neck incontinence in nulliparous females. Br J Urol 1989;64:357–359.
4. Mundy AR, Thomas PJ. Clinical physiology of the bladder, urethra and pelvic floor. In: Mundy AR, Stephenson TP, Wein AJ, eds. Urodynamics: principles, practice and application, 2nd edn. New York: Churchill Livingstone; 1994.
5. Torrens M. Human physiology. In: Torrens M, Morrison JFB, eds. The physiology of the lower urinary tract. London: Springer-Verlag; 1987.
6. Morrison JFB. Reflex control of the lower urinary tract. In: Torrens M, Morrison JFB, eds. The physiology of the lower urinary tract. London: Springer-Verlag; 1987.
7. Morrison JFB. Bladder control: role of higher levels of the central nervous system. In: Torrens M, Morrison JFB, eds. The physiology of the lower urinary tract. London: Springer-Verlag; 1987.
8. Blok BF, Willemsen AT, Holstege G. A PET study on brain control of micturition in humans. Brain 1997;120:111–121.
9. Nour S, Svarer C, Kristensen JKI, Paulson OB, Law I. Cerebral activation during micturition in normal men. Brain 2000;123:781–789.
10. Blok BFM, Sturms LM, Holstege G. A PET study on cortical and subcortical control of pelvic floor musculature in women. J Comp Neurol 1997;389:535–544.
11. Craggs M, McFarlane J. Neuromodulation of the lower urinary tract. Exp Physiol 1999; 84:149–160.
12. Blok BFM, Holstege G. The central nervous system control of micturition in cats and humans. Behav Brain Res 1998;92:119–125.
13. Abrams P, Cardozo L, Fall M, et al. The standardisation of terminology of lower urinary tract function: report from the Standardisation Sub-Committee of the International Continence Society. Neurourol Urodynam 2002;21:167–178.
14. Brading AF, Turner WH. The unstable bladder: towards a common mechanism. Br J Urol 1994; 73:3–8.
15. Steers WD, Kolbeck S, Creedon D, Tuttle JB. Nerve growth factor in the urinary bladder of the adult regulates neuronal form and function. J Clin Invest 1991;88:1709–1715.
16. Steers WD, Creedon DJ, Tuttle JB. Immunity to nerve growth factor

prevents afferent plasticity following urinary bladder hypertrophy. J Urol 1996;155:379–385.

17. Fam BA, Sarkarati M, Yalla SV. Spinal cord injury. In: Yalla SV, McGuire EJ, Elbadawi A, Blaivas JG, eds. Neurourology and urodynamics: principles and practice. London: Collier Macmillan; 1988.

18. Fowler CJ. Bladder afferents and their role in the overactive bladder. Urology 2002;59 (Suppl 5A):37–42.

19. Dasgupta P, Fowler CJ. Chillies: from antiquity to urology. Br J Urol 1997;80:845–852.

20. Smet PJ, Moore KH, Jonavicius J. Distribution and colocalization of calcitonin gene-related peptide tachykinins and vasoactive intestinal peptide in normal and idiopathic unstable human urinary bladder. Lab Invest 1997;77:37–49.

21. Cruz F. Vanilloid receptor and detrusor instability. Urology 2002;59 (Suppl 5A):51–60.

22. Elbadawi A, Yalla SV, Resnick NM. Structural basis of geriatric voiding dysfunction. III. Detrusor overactivity. J Urol 1993;150:1668–1680.

23. Drake MJ, Mills IW, Gillespie JI. Model of peripheral autonomous modules and a myovesical plexus in normal and overactive bladder function. Lancet 2001;358(9279):401–403.

24. Milsom I, Abrams P, Cardozo L, Roberts RG, Thuroff J, Wein AJ. How widespread are the symptoms of an overactive bladder and how are they managed? A population-based prevalence study. BJU Int 2001;87:760–766.

25. Andersson K-E, Appell R, Cardozo L, et al. Pharmacological treatment of urinary incontinence. In: Abrams P, Cardozo L, Khoury S, Wein A, eds. Incontinence. Plymouth: Health Publication Ltd; 2005.

26. Bramble FJ. The treatment of adult enuresis and urge incontinence by enterocystoplasty. Br J Urol 1992;54:693–696.

27. Cartwright PC, Snow BW. Bladder autoaugmentation: early clinical experience. J Urol 1989; 142:505–507.

28. Schmidt RA. Advances in genitourinary neurostimulation. Neurosurgery 1986;18:1041–1044.

29. Schulte-Baukloh H, Michael T, Schobert J, Stolze T, Knispel HH. Efficacy of botulinum-A toxin in children with detrusor hyperreflexia due to myelomeningocoele: primary results. Urology 2002;59(3):325–327.

30. Schurch B, Stöhrer M, Kramer G, Schmid DM, Gaul G, Hauri D. Botulinum-A toxin for treating detrusor hyperreflexia in spinal cord injured patients: a new alternative to anticholinergic drugs? Preliminary results. J Urol 2000;164:692–697.

31. Elliott SP, Meng MV, Anwar HP, Stoller ML. Complete laparoscopic ileal cystoplasty. Urology 2002;59(6):939–943.

32. Atala A. New methods of bladder augmentation. BJU Int 2000;85(Suppl):24–34.

33. McDougall EM, Clayman RV, Figenshau RS, Pearle MS. Laparoscopic retropubic auto-augmentation of the bladder. J Urol 1995:153:123–126.

34. Govier FE, Scott L, Nitti V, Kreder KJ, Rosenblatt P. Percutaneous afferent neuromodulation for the refractory overactive bladder: results of a multicenter study. J Urol 2001;165:1193–1198.

35. Kohli N, Rosenblatt PL. Neuromodulation techniques for the treatment of the overactive bladder. Clin Obstet Gynecol 2002;45(1):218–232.

36. Sautter T, Herzog A, Hauri D, Schurch B. Transient paralysis of the bladder due to wound botulism. Eur Urol 2001;39(5):610–612.

37. Reitz A, Stöhrer M, Kramer G, et al. European experience of 200 cases treated with botulinum-A toxin injections into the detrusor muscle for urinary incontinence due to neurogenic detrusor overactivity. Eur Urol 2004;45(4):510–515.

38. Schurch B, de Seze M, Denys P, et al. Botox Detrusor Hyperreflexia Study Team. Botulinum toxin type a is a safe and effective treatment for neurogenic urinary incontinence: results of a single treatment, randomized, placebo controlled 6-month study. J Urol 2005;174(1):196–200.

Functional and Overflow Incontinence

7

Catherine E DuBeau

INTRODUCTION

This chapter covers two types of urinary incontinence (UI) which, although less common than urge, stress, or mixed UI in women, have significance for several special populations. *Functional* UI is an extremely important problem in disabled and older persons. *Overflow* UI, which occurs in the setting of a weakened detrusor and/or functional or mechanical bladder outlet obstruction, may occur in women following antiincontinence and other surgery, with marked pelvic organ prolapse, in a small but real number postpartum, with neurologic conditions, and in special subsets of younger women.

FUNCTIONAL INCONTINENCE

Definition. Originally, the term "functional UI" referred to the inability to reach a toilet in time to avoid an "accident" (leakage) due to musculoskeletal or psychologic problems, as distinct from "iatrogenic UI" due to medications. Such problems could act synergistically with preexisting lower urinary tract (LUT) dysfunction. This definition was modified with the introduction of the term "transient incontinence" for UI related to reversible conditions. The mnemonic DIAPPERS recalls the causes of transient UI: delirium, infection, atrophic vaginitis/urethritis, pharmaceuticals, psychologic, endocrine (later, excessive urine output), restricted mobility, and stool impaction.[1] The term "transient," however, could lead to the impression that UI was of recent onset or short-lived, although this was not intended.[1] Others differentiated "acute UI" (sudden onset, usually related to an acute problem or iatrogenic illness), "UI associated with reversible conditions" (e.g. medications, medical illnesses, and mobility problems), and "functional UI" (associated with the inability or lack of motivation to reach a toilet on time). The Agency for Healthcare Policy and Research (AHCPR) Consensus Guideline Panel defined functional UI as that caused or exacerbated by factors outside the lower urinary tract such as impaired cognition and functional abilities (e.g. mobility).[2]

None of the above terms, however, has been codified by the International Continence Society.[3] This situation led the Frail Elderly Committee of the Third International Consultation on Incontinence to use the phrase "UI caused by or contributed to by treatable, potentially reversible conditions"[4] to capture all the elements of "functional" and "transient" UI. This will be the definition used in this chapter. Importantly, this definition implies that functional UI is not an "either/or" classification. In many older persons, UI caused or exacerbated by other conditions coexists with urge, stress, and mixed UI.

Regardless of the terminology used, the concept of UI associated with medical conditions, limited mobility, and medications originates in the recognition that continence does not depend solely on LUT function. Continence requires physical function (mobility to reach a toilet, manual dexterity to remove clothing); mental function (cognition and attention sufficient to recognize bladder filling and find a toilet, and the motivation to stay dry); environmental factors (easy access to toilets); and absence of conditions that alter fluid balance (e.g. congestive heart failure, pedal edema) or any of the above functions. Such factors are most relevant in older persons, although they may affect some younger persons (e.g. toilet access in public places, functional limitations in persons with disability).

Epidemiology. Few studies have examined the population-based prevalence of functional UI. One older clinical study estimated the prevalence of UI associated with confusion, medical, and functional factors to be 5.7% in community-dwelling persons over age 65; however, ascertainment bias was likely because the rate of urge UI was only 5%.[5] In a small series from a geriatric UI clinic, after clinical evaluation 2% (1/45) were thought to have functional UI, using the AHCPR definition.[2] The difficulty with such studies is the presumption that functional UI is a unique entity. In many older women, functional precipitants coexist with other types of UI and lower urinary tract dysfunction.

Table 7.1 Quick office-based evaluation of functional dependence

Tool	Domain	Methods
Timed Up and Go test[62]	Lower extremity impairment	Time in seconds it takes for a patient to rise from a chair, walk 3 meters, turn around and sit again in the chair. Time <20 s: no impairment, 21–29 s: possible impairment; ≥30 s: definite impairment
Arm strength	Upper extremity impairment	Motor strength testing of shoulder, elbow, and wrist extensors and flexors
Geriatric Depression Scale, short form	Depression	15-item test; scores 5 or greater suggest depression; available online[63]

Treatable and potentially reversible conditions contributing to UI

Impaired mobility and functional status. Poor mobility is one of the major correlates of UI in older persons.[6] One typical study found that in community-dwelling women with poor mobility, the odds ratio for UI in those aged 60–84 years was 2.50 (95% CI 1.10–5.68), and in those aged 85 and over it was 7.01 (95% CI 2.57–19.17).[7] Among persons receiving home care, UI was strongly related to physical restraints and environmental barriers, with odds ratios of 3.20 and 1.53, respectively.[8] Nursing home residents with UI have significantly greater functional impairments related to toileting than continent residents.[9] Functional dependence and UI share similar predisposing factors, including upper and lower extremity impairment, sensory impairment, and anxiety/depression.[10] This makes the evaluation of functional impairment in incontinent older persons especially important, because addressing predisposing factors may ameliorate both syndromes. Even seemingly "intractable" UI in severely disabled persons is amenable to interventions that can improve the patient's voiding and/or quality of life.[11]

Environmental restrictions, ranging from distant bathroom locations to physical restraints and difficulty removing clothing, should not be overlooked. Even when the underlying cause of restricted mobility cannot be reversed, use of aids such as urinals, bedside commodes or clothing that is easier to remove may improve or resolve UI. There are now web-based resources to help patients locate public toilets.[12]

A functional evaluation can be done quickly in office settings using short, simple geriatric assessment tools (Table 7.1). Patients with possible or definite impairment should be referred to their primary care physicians or a geriatrician for further evaluation and treatment of the many potentially remediable causes of mobility impairment in older persons (Box 7.1).

Cognitive impairment. The association between cognitive impairment and UI is complex. Certainly, dementing

Box 7.1 Potentially remediable causes of impaired mobility

Physical deconditioning

Arthritis

Postural or postprandial hypotension

Peripheral arteriovascular disease with claudication

Spinal stenosis

Cardiac or pulmonary disease with poor stamina

Poor eyesight

Fear of falling

Stroke

Foot and footwear problems

Drug-induced disequilibrium

Vitamin B12 deficiency

Vestibular disease

Parkinson-type diseases

illnesses frequently affect areas of the cortex important for continence and urine withholding, such as the frontal cortex.[13] However, careful studies of persons with dementia and UI demonstrate that mobility is a stronger correlate of UI than the level of cognitive impairment.[14] Even in severely demented persons, continence or reduced level of UI may be possible if they can say their name and transfer with assistance.[15] Delirium is another type of cognitive impairment, which differs from dementia in that it has an abrupt onset, the symptoms may wax and wane over short periods of time, attention is affected more than memory, and it is precipitated by illness and medications. In delirious patients UI is an epiphenomenon that will resolve once the underlying cause(s) of the confusion are identified and treated.

Urinary tract infection. Urinary tract infections (UTIs) can precipitate UI, presumably through local detrusor and proximal urethral irritation. The diagnosis of UTI in older women, however, is complicated by the high prevalence of asymptomatic bacteriuria, which has not been correlated with UI. Diagnosis should be individualized and clinical, not based solely on urinalysis and culture. Dipstick analysis of leukocyte esterase and nitrite is sensitive but not specific; if negative, a UTI can be safely excluded.[16] Suggested diagnostic criteria for women are >10 WBC/μl and 10^4 cfu/ml.[16] Symptoms such as dysuria, pain, new/worsening UI, hematuria, suprapubic discomfort, costovertebral angle tenderness, and fever should be factored in.[17] Because UTI may present with UI, many experts agree that a trial of antibiotics is warranted if bacteriuria, pyuria, and leukocyte esterase and nitrite are found on the initial evaluation of an incontinent but otherwise asymptomatic woman.[2] The effect of treatment on UI should be monitored and recorded to guide future management.

Medications. Any agent that impairs cognition, mobility, fluid balance, bladder contractility or sphincter function or causes coughing can affect continence (Table 7.2). Many medications may impair several of these functions, e.g. the antipsychotic haloperidol can produce confusion, have extrapyramidal side effects (EPS) making ambulation difficult, and, via its anticholinergic action, impair detrusor contraction and cause stool impaction. At the same time, if a woman with UI who is taking haloperidol has no EPS, a stable gait, no constipation, and a normal PVR, the drug is unlikely to be affecting her continence. The evaluation of all older persons with UI should include a review of all prescribed and over-the-counter medications. Whenever possible, medications which could be exacerbating UI should be decreased or eliminated before adding antiincontinence medication (the principle of "subtract before adding").

Medical conditions. The common medical conditions that may cause or exacerbate UI are listed in Table 7.3. Older women in particular may have several of these conditions. The relationship between the presence of a condition and an individual's UI is not absolute. For instance, the presence of dementia may not have any connection with an individual's UI (see above); nocturnal UI should not be ascribed to LUT causes unless sleep disturbance and nocturnal polyuria are excluded or treated. In all clinical settings, identification of these factors is important because many are readily treatable or remediable, and they contribute to morbidity beyond incontinence.

Table 7.2 Medications potentially impairing continence in older women	
Drug	**Mechanism(s)**
Anticholinergics	Impaired detrusor contractility, retention, delirium, constipation/fecal impaction
Loop diuretics	Rapid diuresis, polyuria, frequency, urgency
Antipsychotics (including atypical agents)	Anticholinergic actions, sedation, impaired mobility, rigidity, constipation/fecal impaction
Sedative/hypnotics	Sedation, disorientation, delirium, impaired mobility, sleep alteration
Narcotic analgesics	Impaired detrusor contractility, retention, delirium, constipation/fecal impaction
α-adrenergic blockers	Stress incontinence
Calcium channel blockers	Impaired detrusor contractility, retention
ACE inhibitors	Stress incontinence from cough
Alcohol	Rapid diuresis, frequency, urgency, sedation, delirium, immobility
Gabapentin	Nocturnal polyuria from pedal edema
Thiazolidinediones	Nocturnal polyuria from pedal edema
Nonsteroidal antiinflammatory agents	Nocturnal polyuria from pedal edema; may impair detrusor contractility
Cholinesterase inhibitors	Possible interference with antimuscarinic treatment

Table 7.3   Medical conditions associated with urinary incontinence

Condition	Mechanism	Comments
Neurologic disease		
Cerebrovascular disease; stroke	DO from damage to cerebral inhibitory centers; impaired sensation to void from interruption of subcortical pathways; impaired function and cognition	UI should be temporally related to the stroke
Delirium	Impaired function and cognition	Evaluate and treat causes of delirium
Dementia	DO from damage to cerebral inhibitory centers; impaired function and cognition	Mobility more important factor than degree of cognitive impairment
Multiple sclerosis	DO, areflexia or sphincter dyssynergia (dependent on level of spinal cord involvement)	Should have high suspicion in young women who present with abrupt UI or retention
Multisystem atrophy	Detrusor and sphincter areflexia from damage to spinal intermediolateral tracts	Occurs in persons with Parkinson's disease and Parkinson-like syndromes
Normal-pressure hydrocephalus	DO from compression of frontal inhibitory centers; impaired function and cognition	UI usually later symptom; may not respond to shunting
Parkinson's disease	DO from loss of inhibitory inputs to pontine micturition center; impaired function and cognition; retention and overflow from constipation	Effect of dopaminergic agents on voiding symptoms uncertain
Spinal cord injury	DO, areflexia or sphincter dyssynergia (dependent on level of injury)	Specialist management essential
Spinal stenosis	DO from damage to detrusor upper motor neurons (cervical stenosis); DO or areflexia (lumbar stenosis)	Case reports of resolution of urinary symptoms after laminectomy
Metabolic disease		
Diabetes mellitus	Detrusor underactivity due to neuropathy, DO, osmotic diuresis with polyuria; altered mental status from hyper- or hypoglycemia; retention and overflow from constipation	Multifactoral multidisciplinary management important
Hypercalcemia	Polyuria; altered mental status	Evaluate underlying cause of hypercalcemia
Vitamin B12 deficiency	Impaired bladder sensation and detrusor underactivity from peripheral neuropathy	Consider in elderly persons with elevated PVR; deficiency may be present without anemia or other neurologic signs
Infectious disease		
Herpes zoster	Urinary retention if sacral dermatomes involved; outlet obstruction from viral prostatitis in men; retention and overflow UI from constipation	
Human immunodeficiency virus	DO, areflexia or sphincter dyssynergia	Anti-HIV medications may also play a role
Neurosyphilis	DO, areflexia or sphincter dyssynergia	Diagnosis by positive RPR or FTA ABS and positive CSF VDRL
Tuberculosis	Inanition and functional impairments	Sterile pyuria found in ≤50% of genitourinary tuberculosis cases

Key: DO=detrusor overactivity; TB=tuberculosis; UI=urinary incontinence, FTA ABS=fluorescent treponemal antibody absorption
Adapted from DuBeau CE. Interpreting the effect of common medical conditions on voiding dysfunction in the elderly. Urol Clin North Am 1996;23(1):11–18

Table 7.3   Medical conditions associated with urinary incontinence—cont'd

Condition	Mechanism	Comments
Psychiatric disease		
Affective and anxiety disorders	Decreased motivation	Should be diagnosis of exclusion
Alcoholism	Functional and cognitive impairment; rapid diuresis and retention in acute intoxication	Long-term effects of alcohol on detrusor function uncertain
Psychosis	Functional and cognitive impairment; decreased motivation	Should be diagnosis of exclusion
Cardiovascular disease		
Arteriovascular disease	Detrusor underactivity or areflexia from ischemic myopathy or neuropathy	Consider in patients with widespread vascular disease
Congestive heart failure	Nocturnal polyuria, impaired mobility from decreased stamina	
Other organ system diseases		
Gastrointestinal disease	Overflow UI from constipation	Address underlying cause of constipation
Musculoskeletal disease	Mobility impairment; DO from cervical myelopathy in rheumatoid arthritis and osteoarthritis	Multifactoral multidisciplinary management important
Peripheral venous insufficiency	Nocturnal polyuria	Treat underlying cause; use support stockings; elevation and attention to sodium intake important
Pulmonary disease	Exacerbation of UI by chronic cough and/or smoking; nocturnal polyuria from obstructive sleep apnea	

The relationship between atrophic vaginitis and urethritis, often considered in postmenopausal women, is discussed in Chapter 25.

OVERFLOW INCONTINENCE AND URINARY RETENTION

Voiding dysfunction and urinary retention are relatively uncommon in women of all ages. Estimates of symptomatic obstruction in women presenting with lower urinary tract symptoms (LUTS) range from 2% to 25%,[18] with 2.7–23% having urodynamic outflow obstruction.[19] Among frail elderly women with incontinence, the prevalence of urodynamic underactive detrusor was nearly 60%, with underactive detrusor or outlet obstruction being the primary cause of UI in 12%.[20]

Definitions

The International Continence Society (ICS) has moved away from the term "overflow incontinence" because it lacks a convincing definition.[3] In this chapter, the following definitions will be used:

- *Overflow incontinence*: leakage associated with either chronic or acute urinary retention. Types of overflow incontinence will be characterized by the associated pathophysiology, when known (e.g. postpartum retention).
- *Dysfunctional voiding*: characterized by an intermittent and/or fluctuating flow rate due to involuntary intermittent contractions of the periurethral striated muscle during voiding in neurologically normal individuals.[3]
- *Chronic urinary retention*: voiding difficulty with nonpainful bladder, which remains palpable or percussable after the patient has passed urine, and a significant postvoiding residual urine volume (generally >300 ml[3]).
- *Acute retention of urine*: generally, a painful, palpable or percussable bladder, in a patient who is unable to pass any urine. Pain may not be a presenting feature in circumstances where sensory afferents may be impaired (e.g. herniated intervertebral disc, postpartum, after epidural anesthesia).[3] The retention volume should be

significantly greater than the expected normal bladder capacity.[3]

There may be complete, partial or no overlap between these conditions. Not every patient with retention will have overflow UI, and patients with chronic urinary retention may have started with an episode of acute retention. The "cut-off" value of 300 ml as a "significant residual" is based on expert opinion, and may not apply well in individual patients (especially older women, because of smaller normal bladder capacity, and any person taking medications that impair detrusor contractility).

Pathophysiology of urinary retention. Urinary retention is the result of impaired detrusor contractility, bladder outlet and/or urethral obstruction to voiding, or a combination of the two.

Impaired detrusor contractility. Detrusor contractility can be affected by intrinsic myogenic damage to detrusor smooth muscle; neurogenic damage; extrinsic factors that impair muscle or nerve function (e.g. medication and anesthesia (see Table 7.2)); and anatomic changes to the bladder wall that decrease the efficiency of smooth muscle contraction (e.g. increased connective tissue). In many cases, the causes are likely multiple, reflecting common or intersecting pathways of injury. For instance, arterial insufficiency (from arteriosclerosis, hypotension, low oxygen states) can cause ischemic-reperfusion injury with patchy denervation, fibrosis, and impaired smooth muscle function.[21] Loss of trophic nerve inputs can lead to smooth muscle degeneration.

Advanced age is associated with impaired detrusor contractility.[22] Understanding age-related changes in the bladder is complicated by a paucity of longitudinal data, variable definitions of "normal," and use of potentially biased (and symptomatic) referral populations. It is difficult to sort out the role of aging, decreased blood flow, poor voiding habits, comorbidity, and central and peripheral nervous system innervation and reflex patterns as determinants of bladder function in older women.[22] The research focus has been urodynamic function, neurohumoral responsiveness of detrusor smooth muscle, and ultrastructure. However, while the key role of the urothelium and afferent systems on micturition is increasingly appreciated, there are extremely scant human data on urothelial changes with age.

Age-related impaired contractility is associated with lower urine flow rates and a small increase (generally <50 ml) in postvoiding residual volume (PVR). Frail older persons may have a combination of poor contractility and detrusor overactivity, a condition termed detrusor hyperactivity with impaired contractility (DHIC).[23] In DHIC, the bladder contraction does not empty the bladder fully, leaving a high PVR (which otherwise is not explained by outlet obstruction). DHIC symptoms include leakage with urgency and increased abdominal pressure, dribbling, frequency, and nocturia, similar to other LUT conditions such as stress UI and obstruction, for which DHIC can be mistaken. Antimuscarinics are not contraindicated to treat urge symptoms in DHIC, but PVR and symptoms should be carefully monitored.

Urethral causes. Potential urethral factors in retention are urethral obstruction/compression (mechanical obstruction) and urethral/pelvic floor overactivity (functional obstruction). The most common types of mechanical obstruction are scarring from previous antiincontinence surgery and severe pelvic organ prolapse. Functional obstruction may result to detrusor–sphincter dyssynergia (from spinal cord injury or insult) or hyperactivity of the urethral striated sphincter.

Central causes. Successful micturition has been associated with increased blood flow to the right inferior frontal gyrus[13] and therefore damage to this area or its blood flow could potentially impair voiding. Ventrolateral areas of the pons are activated in patients who are unable to void on command. These areas are thought to project to Onuf's nucleus in the anterior roots of the sacral cord, which is the motor nucleus for the urethral sphincter.[24] The role of Onuf's nucleus in urethral closure is highlighted by duloxetine, a novel serotonin and norepinephrine reuptake inhibitor which is proposed to decrease stress UI by its action in Onuf's nucleus to facilitate urethral sphincter closure.[25]

Urodynamic diagnosis of obstructed voiding in women. Although well standardized for men, the urodynamic diagnosis of obstruction in women as yet lacks consensus. There is little work validating in women the male obstruction nomograms, which typically incorporate maximum detrusor pressure at maximum flow (Pdet.Qmax) and maximum urine flow rate (Qmax) from simultaneous pressure–flow studies (e.g. the ICS nomogram[3]). Some have suggested that these nomograms cannot be extrapolated to women who have lower voiding Pdet than men.[18]

Several groups have investigated alternative definitions and nomograms. Klijer et al[26] studied 57 women with LUTS, of whom 38% had low Qmax (<10th centile on the Liverpool nomogram[27]). Of these, 53% were classified as obstructed on pressure–flow study (Pdet >40 cmH$_2$O and Qmax <15 ml/s) and 89% by voiding cystourethrography (VCUG). The high prevalence of obstruction was not explained but could be due to poor standardization of VCUG. Chassagne et al[28] compared urodynamic parameters in 135 women with stress UI and 35 with "clinical obstruction" (based on symptoms, exam, and pertinent surgical history). They found Qmax ≤10 ml/s with Pdet.Qmax >10 cmH_2O had 69% sensitivity and 94% specificity for obstruction, and Qmax ≤15 ml/s with Pdet.Qmax >15 cmH_2O had 80% sensitivity and 83% specificity. Lemack and Zimmern[29] found that Qmax ≤11 ml/s and Pdet.Qmax ≥21 cmH_2O had 91.5% sensitivity and 73.6% specificity. They applied these criteria to 108 consecutive women referred for LUTS and found that 20% (n=21) were obstructed (including six with perirurethral fibrosis, four with prolapse, three with previous antiincontinence surgery, and one with idiopathic incomplete retention). However, five "obstructed" women had only detrusor overactivity. One explanation may be that the derivation control group had very low Pdet because of concomitant stress UI.[29]

In a retrospective urodynamic study, Blaivas and Groutz[19] defined a population of obstructed women using:

- free Qmax (uninstrumented flow study) ≤12 ml/s combined with a sustained detrusor contraction and a Pdet.Qmax ≥20 cmH_2O
- radiographic evidence of obstruction in the presence of a sustained detrusor contraction ≥20 cmH_2O and poor Qmax, regardless of free Qmax, and/or
- inability to void with a 7F transurethral catheter in place despite a sustained detrusor contraction of at least 20 cmH_2O.

They constructed a nomogram based on a plot of free Qmax versus Pdet.max (maximum Pdet during voiding). Severe obstruction was defined by Pdet.max >107 cmH_2O and moderate obstruction by Pdet.max between 57 and 107 cmH_2O; mild obstruction (Pdet.max <57cmH_2O) was differentiated from no obstruction by the line of slope 1.0 running from the point (Pdet.max=7 and Qmax=0) to the point (Pdet.max=57 and Qmax=50 ml/s). Compared with their a priori criteria for obstruction, the nomogram was 100% sensitive and 80% specific.

Other proposed urodynamic definitions of outlet obstruction in women include the area under the curve of detrusor pressure during voiding[30] and relative bladder outlet resistance,[31] both of which await further validation as urodynamic parameters.

Specific syndromes of voiding dysfunction in women

Acute retention. Persons with acute retention present with a relatively sudden inability to pass urine and a painful, palpable or percussable bladder. Pain may be absent if sensory afferents are impaired (e.g. with diabetes or herniated disc). Women are less affected than men, with an estimated ratio of 1:13.[32] The causes of acute retention fall into three general categories[33]: events or factors that increase outflow resistance (mechanical or dynamic); interruption of detrusor sensory afferents or motor efferents; and medication-associated bladder overdistension (e.g. opioids, anticholinergics, anesthetics). The literature is replete with case reports of unusual precipitants, such as giant urethral calculus and urethral leiomyoma.[33] Despite Fowler's work described below, recent reviews still cite psychogenic causes in women.[33]

Acute retention should be managed with an indwelling catheter and evaluation and management of possible precipitant and contributory factors, followed by a voiding trial after about one week (perhaps longer for retention volumes over 1 liter).[34] If the voiding trial fails, then further urodynamic investigation is needed (including sphincter EMG). If prolonged catheterization is necessary, suprapubic catheterization should be considered because of its lower risk of catheter-associated infection[35] and urethral trauma.

Postoperative urinary retention. The literature on postoperative voiding problems and retention in women is complicated by the lack of uniform clinical and urodynamic definitions; variability in surgical techniques, anesthesia, and postoperative pain control; small study sizes; contradictory results; and a paucity of multicenter studies. While many basic questions remain unanswered, several general principles regarding risk factors, pathophysiology, and treatment can be stated.

Preoperative factors associated with voiding difficulty and retention include: preexisting voiding dysfunction (such as low flow rate);[36] urodynamic factors (elevated PVR,[37] low voiding Pdet,[38] impaired isometric rise in Pdet and Valsalva voiding[39]); advanced age;[40] and previous postpartum retention or voiding difficulty.[39] Operative factors include total anesthetic dose[38] and longer operative time.[40] Use of shorter acting anesthetic agents has meant that retention is less likely to be precipitated by neuroaxial blockade or general anesthesia.[41] The suggested role of intraoperative fluid volume in causing bladder distension has been contradicted by others,[42] with the exception of high-risk patients with a history of retention.[42]

Postoperative patient-controlled analgesia is significantly associated with retention, even after adjustment for type of agent, dose, and age.[38] Data regarding lower retention rates after herniorrhaphy with local anesthesia[43] suggest that lower abdominal pain may contribute to inability to void, although the mechanism is uncertain.[41] The theory that postoperative pelvic and perineal pain causes reflex sympathetic stimulation of the urethral smooth muscle is belied by the generally poor results in trials of pre- and postoperative α-adrenergic blockade.[44]

Voiding dysfunction after stress UI surgery has been estimated to be as high as 35%. For example, voiding dysfunction after colposuspension has been reported to have a mean rate of 12.5% (range 3–32%), with a mean duration of catheterization of 6–15 days.[45] Postoperative factors contributing to retention may include failure of the sphincter to relax, edema surrounding the vesical neck and urethra, pelvic floor spasm, and obstruction from bladder neck elevation.[46] Age, higher preoperative urethral resistance (Pdet.Qmax/Qmax^2), straining during voiding, and MRI evidence of greater bladder neck elevation and urethral compression (but not urodynamic measures of contractility) have been associated with the number of days of voiding dysfunction following colposuspension.[45] PVR volume was the sole predictor of voiding difficulty following cadaveric sling,[37] and low Qmax was predictive after tension-free vaginal tape.[36] A provocative small study (n=10) used concentric needle EMG studies in women with voiding difficulty following sling and colposuspension procedures. They found persistent urethral activity by EMG during voiding,[46] suggesting that failure of sphincter relaxation contributes to postoperative voiding difficulty.

Treatment of postoperative retention begins with catheter decompression and management of contributory factors, such as constipation. If these measures fail, then intermittent catheterization and/or surgical repair (urethrolysis, sling release) are recommended. The cholinergic agent bethanecol is not effective.[47] The use of botulinum toxin injection into the urethral sphincter for retention after antiincontinence surgery is under investigation.[48]

Postpartum retention.

Depending on the definition, the rate of postpartum retention ranges from 7% to 17.9%.[49] Higher rates generally come from reports with vague definitions of retention ("voiding dysfunction") or which studied only a brief postpartum period. For example, in a review of 19 RCTs of epidural analgesia in labor and delivery, three studies were identified that addressed "impaired voiding," with respective incidence rates of 0–35%, 62–68%, and 28–61%.[50] In other studies rates are much lower: in a large unselected series of 8402 parturients, 0.05% were unable to void until the third postpartum day,[51] and in a retrospective analysis of 11,332 deliveries, immediate retention occurred in 0.45%, 26% of whom were still in retention more than 72 hours postpartum.[49] A 4-year follow-up study found no difference in urinary symptoms, UI or fecal incontinence between women who had a postpartum PVR >150 ml and those who did not.[52] Factors associated with postpartum retention and voiding difficulties include physiologic changes of pregnancy, regional anesthesia, prolonged labor, instrument-assisted vaginal delivery, cesarean delivery, perineal trauma, episiotomy, and primiparity.[49,53,54] Studies of prophylactic interventions have not been done.

Retention from pelvic organ prolapse.

Urinary retention may be a symptom of pelvic organ prolapse (POP).

In severe cases of POP, ureteral obstruction may occur as well.[55] Prevalence rates are difficult to estimate because of variable urodynamic definitions of obstruction and the use of referral populations. In one series of women referred for POP, 72% with grade 3–4 cystocele were obstructed, and obstruction correlated with cystocele grade but not detrusor contractility.[56] In another referral series, 30% of women with POP had PVR >100 ml, and they had lower Qmax and higher PVR than women with UI without POP.[57] Low Qmax (11 ml/s) and high Pdet.Qmax (50 cmH$_2$O) have been observed in women with severe posthysterectomy vault prolapse.[58] Unlike retention, other voiding difficulty symptoms are only weakly associated with prolapse severity.[59] Surgical and pessary treatment to reduce the prolapse in women with retention can be complicated by "unmasking" of stress and urge UI.[56]

"Idiopathic" retention in young women (Fowler's syndrome).

For many years, young women who presented with otherwise unexplained retention were thought to have a primary psychiatric disorder. However, in 1988 Fowler proposed that the cause was increased urethral striated sphincter activity.[60] She also observed that many of these women had features of polycystic ovary syndrome, raising the possibility of an underlying hormonal etiology. Onset is typically between the ages of 15 and 39 (mean 28 years), and is preceded by a potentially "contributory" event (predominantly gynecologic procedures and childbirth) in nearly two-thirds. Presentation is generally with a bladder volume greater than 1 liter and there may be preexisting symptoms of interrupted urine stream.

The specific EMG abnormality in this syndrome has two components: complex repetitive discharges (CRDs) and decelerating bursts (DBs) (the latter described as sounding like "whale songs").[60] The CRD activity is thought to be due to ephaptic (cell to cell) transmission between muscle fibers. The excessive excitability of the muscle membranes is proposed to be similar to that seen in myotonic-like disorders associated with channelopathies. The EMG abnormalities have been associated with maximal urethral sphincter volume on transvaginal ultrasound (2.29+1.62 vs 1.62+.32 cm^3, P<0.001), suggesting work hypertrophy effects. Retention presumably results from the urethral hyperactivity but functional inhibition of the micturition reflex by proprioceptive afferents in the proximal urethra is another possibility. Sacral neuromodulation is effective for restoring voiding in these patients.[60]

"Spurious" retention.

An incorrect diagnosis of urinary retention may be made if ultrasound determination of an elevated PVR is not confirmed by catheterization. Pelvic masses and cysts are usually responsible for such spuriously high ultrasound PVRs.[61]

SUMMARY

Potentially reversible and treatable conditions may contribute to the development or worsening of incontinence in women of all ages, and play an especially significant role in older and frail women. While these contributory factors are rarely the sole cause of incontinence, failure to address them may decrease the effectiveness of other UI treatment. Therefore, knowledge of these factors is imperative for all providers caring for women with UI. Quick assessment of functional dependence is possible even in specialist office settings. Management of these factors, especially those involving medical conditions and medication adjustment, often may require multidisciplinary coordination between specialists and primary care providers.

"Overflow" incontinence and urinary retention are uncommon but relevant problems for particular groups of women. Some of the same reversible conditions that contribute to incontinence also can precipitate or exacerbate retention. Although urethral and detrusor causes of retention in women are increasingly understood, little is known about prevention. Much more needs to be known about treatment for many of the retention syndromes in women. Standardization of the urodynamic definition of obstruction in women will be essential for future research on etiology, evaluation, and clinical care of retention in women.

REFERENCES

1. Resnick NM. Urinary incontinence in the elderly. Med Grand Rounds 1984;3:281–290.
2. Agency for Health Care Policy and Research, Public Health Service. Urinary incontinence in adults: clinical practice guideline. Rockville, MD: US Department of Health and Human Services; 1992. AHCPR Pub Number 92–0038.
3. Abrams P, Cardozo L, Fall M, et al. The standardisation of terminology in lower urinary tract function. Neurourol Urodynam 2002;21:167–178.
4. Ouslander JG. Management of overactive bladder. N Engl J Med 2004;350:786–799.
5. Campbell AJ, Reinken J, McCosh L. Incontinence in the elderly: prevalence and prognosis. Age Ageing 1985;14:65–70.
6. Hunskaar S, Burgio K, Diokno AC, Herzog AR, Hjalmas K, Lapitan MC. Epidemiology and natural history of urinary incontinence. In: Abrams P, Cardozo L, Khoury S, Wein A, eds. Incontinence, 2nd edn. Plymouth, UK: Health Publication Ltd; 2002:165–202.
7. Kok ALM, Voorhorst FJ, Burger CW, Van Houten P, Kenemans P, Janssens J. Urinary and faecal incontinence in community-residing older women. Age Ageing 1992;21:211–215.
8. Landi F, Cesari M, Russo A, et al for the Silvernet HC Study Group. Potentially reversible risk factors and urinary incontinence in frail older people living in community. Age Ageing 2003;32:194–199.
9. Ouslander JG, Morishita L, Blaustein J, Orzeck S, Dunn S, Sayre J. Clinical, functional, and psychological characteristics of an incontinent nursing home population. J Gerontol 1987;42:631–637.
10. Tinetti ME, Inouye SK, Gill TM, Doucette JT. Shared risk factors for falls, incontinence, and functional dependence: unifying the approach to geriatric syndromes. JAMA 1995;273:1348–1353.
11. Ouslander JG. Intractable incontinence in the elderly. BJU Int 2002;85(Suppl 3):72–78.
12. The Bathroom Diaries.™ Clean restrooms around the world, 2006 http://thebathroomdiaries.com
13. Blok BFM, Sturms LM, Holstege G. Brain activation during micturition in women. Brain 1998;121:2033–2042.
14. Skelly J, Flint AJ. Urinary incontinence associated with dementia. J Am Geriatr Soc 1995;43:286–294.
15. Ouslander JG, Schnelle JF, Uman G, et al. Predictors of successful prompted voiding among incontinent nursing home residents. JAMA 1995;273:1366–1370.
16. Hamilton-Miller JMT. Issues in urinary tract infections in the elderly. World J Urol 1999;17:396–401.
17. Nicolle L. Urinary tract infection in geriatric and institutionalized patients. Curr Opin Urol 2002;12:51–55.
18. Groutz A, Blaivas JG. Non-neurogenic female voiding dysfunction. Curr Opin Urol 2002;12:311–316.
19. Blaivas JG, Groutz, A. Bladder outlet obstruction nomogram for women with lower urinary tract symptomatology. Neurourol Urodynam 2000;19:553–564.
20. Resnick NM, Yalla SV, Laurino E. The pathophysiology of urinary incontinence among institutionalized elderly persons. N Engl J Med 1989;320:1–7.
21. Fry CH, Brading AF, Hussain M, et al. Cell Biology. In: Abrams P, Cardozo L, Khoury S, Wein A, ed. Incontinence 2005. Paris: Editions 21. 2005; 313–362.
22. Nordling J. The aging bladder: a significant but underestimated role in the development of lower urinary tract symptoms. Exper Gerontol 2002;37:991–999.
23. Resnick NM, Yalla SV. Detrusor hyperactivity with impaired contractile function: an unrecognized but common cause of urinary incontinence elderly patients. JAMA 1987;257:3076–3081.
24. Fowler CJ. Brain activation during micturition [editorial]. Brain 1998;121:2031–2032.
25. Van Kerrebroeck P. Duloxetine: an innovative approach for treating stress urinary incontinence. BJU Int 2004;94(Suppl 1):31–37.
26. Klijer R, Bar K, Bialek W. Bladder outlet obstruction in women: difficulties in diagnosis. Urol Int 2004;73:6–10.
27. Haylen BT, Law MG, Frazer M, Schulz S. Urine flow rates and residual urine volumes in urogynecology patients. Int Urogynecol J 1999;10:378–383.
28. Chassagne S, Bernier PA, Haab F, Roehrborn CG, Reisch JS, Zimmern PE. Proposed cutoff values to define bladder outlet obstruction in women. Urology 1998;51:408–411.
29. Lemack GE, Zimmern PE. Pressure flow analysis may aid in identifying women with outlflow obstruction. J Urol 2000;163:1823–1828.
30. Cormier L, Ferchaud J, Galas JM, Guillemin F, Mangin P. Diagnosis of female bladder outlet obstruction and relevance of the parameter area under the curve of detrusor pressure during voiding: preliminary results. J Urol 2002;167:2083–2087.
31. Kranse R, von Mastrigt R. Relative bladder outlet obstruction. J Urol 2002;168:565–570.
32. Klarskov P, Andersen JT, Asmussen CF, et al. Acute urinary retention in women: a prospective study of 18 consecutive women. Scand J Urol Nephrol 1987;21:29–31.
33. Choong S, Emberton M. Acute urinary retention. BJU Int 2000;85:186–201.
34. Djavan B, Shariat S, Omar M, et al. Does prolonged catheter

drainage improve the chance of recovering voluntary voiding after acute retention of urine? Eur Urol 1998;33:110.

35. Agency for Healthcare Policy and Research. Making health care safer: a critical analysis of patient safety practices. Available online at: www.ahcpr.gov/clinic/ptsafety/chap15b.htm

36. Hong B, Park S, Kim HS, Myung-Soo C. Factors predictive of urinary retention after a tension-free vaginal tape procedure for female stress urinary incontinence. J Urol 2003;170:852–856.

37. Miller EA, Amundsen CL, Toh KL, Flynn BJ, Webster GD. Preoperative urodynamic evaluation may predict voiding dysfunction in women undergoing pubovaginal sling. J Urol 2003;169:2234–2237.

38. Petros JG, Mallen JK, Howe K, Timm EB, Robillard RJ. Patient-controlled analgesia and postoperative urinary retention. Surg Gynecol Obstet 1993;177:172–175.

39. Nguyen JK. Diagnosis and treatment of voiding dysfunction caused by urethral obstruction after anti-incontinence surgery. Obstet Gynecol Surv 2002;57:468–475.

40. Lamonerie L, Marret E, Deleuze A, Lembert N, Dupont M, Bonnet F. Prevalence of postoperative bladder distension and urinary retention detected by ultrasound measurement. Br J Anaesthesia 2004;92:544–546.

41. Mulroy MM. Hernia surgery, anesthetic technique, and urinary retention—apples, oranges, and kumquats? Regional Anesth Pain Med 2002;27:587–589.

42. Pavlin DJ, Pavlin EG, Fitzgibbon DR, Koerschgen ME, Plitt M. Management of bladder function after outpatient surgery. Anesthesiology 1999;91:42–50.

43. Jensen P, Mikkelsen T, Kehlet H. Postherniorrhaphy urinary retention—effect of local, regional, and general anesthesia: a review. Regional Anesth Pain Med 2002;27:612–617.

44. Watson AJ, Currie I, Jarvis GJ. A prospective placebo controlled double blind randomised study to investigate the use of indoramin to prevent post-operative voiding disorders after surgical treatment for genuine stress incontinence. Br J Obstet Gynaecol 1999;106:270–272.

45. Bombieri L, Freeman RM, Perkins EP, Williams MP, Shaw SR. Why do women have voiding dysfunction and de novo detrusor instability after colposuspension? Br J Obstet Gynaecol 2002;109:402–412.

46. FitzGerald MP, Brubaker L. The etiology of urinary retention after surgery for genuine stress incontinence. Neurourol Urodynam 2001;20:13–21.

47. Hindley RG, Brierly RD, Thomas PJ. Prostaglandin E2 and bethanechol in combination for treating detrusor underactivity. BJU Int 2004;93:89–92.

48. Smith CP, O'Leary M, Erickson J, Somogy GT, Chancellor MB. Botulinum toxin urethral sphincter injection resolves urinary retention after pubovaginal sling operation. Int Urogynecol J 2002;13:55–56.

49. Carley ME, Carley JM, Vasdev GV, et al. Factors that are associated with clinically overt postpartum urinary retention after vaginal delivery. Am J Obstet Gynecol 2002;187:430–433.

50. Mayberry J, Clemmens D, De A. Epidural analgesia side effects, co-interventions, and care of women during childbirth: a systematic review. Am J Obstet Gynecol 2002;186:S81–S93.

51. Groutz A, Gordon D, Eolman I, Jaffa A, Kupferminc MJ, Lessing JB. Persistent postpartum urinary retention in contemporary obstetric practice. Definition, prevalence and clinical implications. J Reprod Med 2001;46:44–48.

52. Yip S-K, Sahota D, Chang AMZ, Chung TKH. Four-year follow-up of women who were diagnosed to have postpartum urinary retention. Am J Obstet Gynecol 2002;187:648–652.

53. Glavind K, Bjork J. Incidence and treatment of urinary retention postpartum. Int Urogynecol J 2003;14:119–121.

54. Ching-Chung L, Shuenn-Dhy C, Ling-Hong T, Ching-Chang H, Chao-Lun C, Po-Jen C. Postpartum urinary retention: assessment of contributory factors and long-term clinical impact. Aust NZ J Obstet Gynaecol 2002;42:365–368.

55. Gomes CM, Rovner ES, Banner MP, Ramchandani P, Wein AJ. Simultaneous upper and lower urinary tract obstruction associated with severe genital prolapse: diagnosis and evaluation with magnetic resonance imaging. Int Urogynecol J 2001;12:144–146.

56. Romanzi LJ, Chaikin DC, Blaivas JG. The effect of genital prolapse on voiding. J Urol 1999;161:581–586.

57. Coates KW, Harris RL, Cundiff GW, Bump RC. Uroflowmetry in women with urinary incontinence and pelvic organ prolapse. Br J Urol 1997;80:217–221.

58. Wall LL, Hewitt JK. Urodynamic characteristics of women with complete posthysterectomy vaginal vault prolapse. Urology 1994;44:336–341.

59. Ellerkmann RM, Cundiff GW, Melick CF, Nihira MA, Leffler K, Bent AE. Correlation of symptoms with location and severity of pelvic organ prolapse. Am J Obstet Gynecol 2001;185:1332–1337.

60. DasGupta R, Fowler CJ. The management of female voiding dysfunction: Fowler's syndrome—a contemporary update. Curr Opin Urol 2003;13:293–299.

61. Tan TL, Ding YY, Lieu PK. False positive findings in the ultrasound assessment of postvoid residual urine volume [letter]. Age Ageing 2003;32:356.

62. Podsiadlo D, Richardson S. The timed "Up & Go": a test of basic functional mobility for frail elderly persons. J Am Geriatr Soc 1991;39:142–148.

63. 15-item Geriatric Depression Scale. Available online at: www.stanford.edu/~yesavage/Testing.htm.

Pathophysiology of Anal Incontinence

8

Christine Norton

INTRODUCTION

Bowel continence involves many different factors, many of which are as yet imperfectly understood.[1] Often there is not a single "cause" for an individual patient's symptoms. For many people the cause of incontinence will be an interaction of colonic motility (propulsive forces), rectal sensation and compliance, anal sphincter function, stool consistency, cognitive and physical abilities to respond appropriately, and a physical and social environment conducive to continence. "Continence" implies an individual's ability to comply with a society's arbitrary rules for acceptable toilet-related behavior, and as such is both a neuromuscular and social skill.[2] Onset of symptoms is often gradual, with a thin line dividing, for example, urgency and frank incontinence: it is therefore necessary to determine not only the history of the symptoms but also the trigger for presentation for healthcare at a particular point in time. It is important to understand the combination of factors which apply for each individual in order to plan an effective intervention. This chapter will review the most usual causes. A summary of common causes is given in Table 8.1.[3]

The causes discussed in this chapter are by no means mutually exclusive and for many people these conditions coexist, with the combination precipitating frank fecal incontinence. For example, a woman might sustain some insult to the anal sphincter during childbirth but be continent until she also develops irritable bowel syndrome, has anal surgery or passes the menopause. Or sphincter weakness from obstetric causes may be compounded by years of straining due to an evacuation difficulty, by repeated heavy lifting or by obesity. The person with minor symptoms may become incontinent when a medication makes the stool looser or peripheral neuropathy secondary to diabetes mellitus blunts rectal and anal sensation.

There are several different ways of classifying fecal incontinence, with no universally accepted definitions as yet. For example, some authors have classified it according to the

Table 8.1 Common causes of fecal incontinence in adults	
Primary problem	**Common causes**
1. **Anal sphincter or pelvic floor damage**	Obstetric trauma Iatrogenic (e.g. hemorrhoidectomy, anal stretch, lateral sphincterotomy) Idiopathic degeneration Direct trauma or injury (e.g. impalement) Congenital anomaly
2. **Gut motility/stool consistency**	Infection Inflammatory bowel disease Irritable bowel syndrome Pelvic irradiation Diet Emotions/anxiety
3. **Anorectal pathology**	Rectal prolapse Anal or rectovaginal fistula Hemorrhoids or skin tags
4. **Neurologic disease**	Spinal cord injury Multiple sclerosis Spina bifida, sacral agenesis
5. **Secondary to degenerative neurological disease**	Alzheimer's disease or environmental (see below)
6. **Impaction with overflow "spurious diarrhea"**	Institutionalized or immobile elderly people Severe constipation in children
7. **"Lifestyle" and environmental**	Poor toilet facilities Inadequate care/nonavailable assistance Drugs with gut side effects Frailty and dependence Chronic straining? Obesity?
8. **Idiopathic**	Unknown cause

Reproduced from reference 3, by permission.

consistency of the incontinence (solid, liquid or gas).[4] Others have emphasized the difference between urge and passive stool loss.[5]

DEFINITIONS

There is no universally recognized definition of anal or fecal incontinence. An international committee has proposed the following.[6]

- Anal incontinence (AI) is the involuntary loss of flatus, liquid or solid stool that is a social or hygienic problem.
- Fecal incontinence (FI) is the involuntary loss of liquid or solid stool that is a social or hygienic problem.

There is no agreement as to the frequency, volume or impact on the patient that should constitute a clinical problem.

OVERLAP WITH URINARY SYMPTOMS

Increasingly, the pelvic floor and its associated nerves and structures are being seen as a whole and the relationship between symptoms and the interrelatedness of interventions is being appreciated. Anal incontinence is common and underreported in women with urinary incontinence, with approximately one-quarter of urinary incontinent patients admitting AI.[7] Conversely, over 50% of women presenting with FI also admit urinary leakage (Norton, unpublished data).[8] There is a known association between urinary and fecal incontinence from many epidemiologic studies[9-11] but whether there is a common neuromuscular or functional cause has yet to be determined. Women with coexisting urinary and fecal incontinence are more likely to have a urodynamic diagnosis of detrusor instability than genuine stress incontinence, suggesting possible neurologic, motility or anxiety disorders may be the common link rather than the pelvic floor.[7] There is an association between idiopathic detrusor instability and the irritable bowel syndrome.[12] Other studies have found that 28% of women investigated for stress urinary incontinence have anal incontinence (only 1% for solid stool)[13] and 21% of consecutive urogynecology referrals had some fecal incontinence.[14] Both of these studies found an association with constipation. This symptom seems to be rarely spontaneously volunteered[15] and urologists and urogynecologists probably should be encouraged to inquire routinely.

ANAL SPHINCTER OR PELVIC FLOOR DAMAGE

As outlined in Chapter 3, there are two sphincters involved in maintaining fecal continence: the smooth muscle internal sphincter is largely responsible for resting tone in the anus and thus passive stool retention;[16] the striated external sphincter is responsible for voluntarily augmenting resting tone with a squeeze to enable stool retention during an urge to defecate.[17] Either or both of these sphincters can sustain damage or be weakened. Whether this actually leads to frank incontinence will be partly dependent upon stool consistency and gut motility. The role of the pelvic floor in maintaining fecal continence and how weakness might contribute to incontinence or a strong pelvic floor might help to prevent leakage to compensate for anal sphincter weakness remain to be defined.

Obstetric trauma to the anal sphincters. It is a common assertion that obstetric trauma to the anal sphincters is the most prevalent cause of fecal incontinence. However, the consistent finding in major epidemiologic studies of equal rates of FI in men as in women[18,19] must cast doubt on this presumption.

Until the advent of the anal ultrasound, it was assumed that the primary mechanism of obstetric trauma was damage to the pudendal nerve (often termed "neuropathic" or "idiopathic" FI in the colorectal literature). Stretching of this nerve during vaginal delivery was thought to lead to some nonreversible damage, which could even be progressive over time.[20] Once anal ultrasound became available and sphincter disruption could be easily visualized,[21,22] trauma was thought to be more directly mechanical muscle damage and the term "neuropathic incontinence" fell out of favor. The truth probably lies in varying combinations of muscle and nerve damage.

Known risk factors for obstetric damage include first baby, instrumental delivery (especially forceps), a large infant, an abnormal presentation, and prolonged second stage of labor.[22,23] Precipitate delivery may also be a factor. Midline episiotomy is associated with increased risk of anal tear and subsequent symptoms.[24]

Third-degree tears occur in 1–2% of vaginal deliveries and are associated with the same risk factors.[25-27] Symptoms of altered continence have been found in 30–80% of women in the early years after repair of a recognized third-degree tear. It is not known what happens to initially asymptomatic women in the longer term. Clinically, many women present in the fourth to sixth decade of life with symptoms of FI, a history of difficult childbirth, and visible sphincter damage on anal ultrasound. Training in recognition and repair is improving and it is now generally accepted that this is a specialized procedure that should be done by a senior member of the obstetric team in an operating theater with regional or general anesthesia. An overlapping, rather than end-to-end repair may give better results.[26,28] Whether this policy will lead in future to a reduction in the proportion of women who experience symptoms of AI after repaired third-degree tear remains to be seen.

Iatrogenic damage to the anal sphincters

Colorectal surgery. Hemorrhoidectomy has been found to be associated with a variable rate of subsequent AI. One report followed up 507 patients by postal questionnaire on average 6 years after surgery. A total of 33% (139/507) reported anal incontinence, including 72 who were incontinent of gas only, 56 who were incontinent to liquid feces, and 11 who were incontinent to solid feces.[29] Other reports of surgical treatment for hemorrhoids list a lower incidence of FI.[30] Some patients are found to have clear disruption to the internal anal sphincter on ultrasound examination. With other patients there is no visible sphincter damage and it is unclear if symptoms relate to altered sensation or to an impaired mucosal seal as anal cushions are replaced with scar tissue. It is not clear how far this relates to surgical technique, and whether newer techniques such as stapled hemorrhoidectomy are associated with fewer symptoms. Banding and sclerotherapy for hemorrhoids seem to carry a lower risk but are not appropriate for more advanced hemorrhoids. The practice of anal stretch has fallen into disrepute because of subsequent problems with fecal incontinence.[31]

There is an increasing tendency to attempt to avoid creation of a stoma when a patient needs all or part of the large bowel removed. Resection of the rectum for rectal cancer is often preferred by patients as an alternative to living with a colostomy, but those with a low resection may find continence compromised. Creation of a coloanal pouch may be associated with lower incidence of FI (estimated at 18%) according to some authors[32,33] but others[34] reported a rate of 49% FI following coloanal anastomosis. The mechanism for this may be a combination of reduced capacity, reduced rectal compliance and possibly damage to the sensory and/or motor function of the anus during resection.

Patients with disease which necessitates surgical removal of the colon, such as severe ulcerative colitis or familial adenomatous polyposis (FAP), often undergo anastomosis of the small bowel to the rectum or anus (ileo-anal anastomosis), or fashioning of an ileo-anal internal pouch ("restorative proctocolectomy"). This usually results in frequent and fairly fluid bowel actions, possibly with urgency, and some patients find their ability to control this unreliable. Many also experience passive soiling, especially at night. Postoperatively, 25–35% of these patients have daytime FI[35-38] and 32–52% have nocturnal FI.[35,36] There is controversy as to whether better continence is achieved with differing surgical techniques (e.g. stapling vs hand sewing the anastomosis for an ileo-anal pouch).

Lateral sphincterotomy (deliberate division of the distal internal anal sphincter) has long been a surgical option for a nonhealing anal fissure in order to reduce anal pressures and allow healing. Subsequent soiling and poor control of flatus are common,[39] especially in women who have a shorter internal anal sphincter and in whom the entire length of the sphincter is often inadvertently divided. In a series of 585 patients with chronic anal fissures treated with sphincterotomy, 45% developed FI at some point in their recovery. However, this tended to improve with time from surgery, and at follow-up an average of 72 months after surgery, 11% reported FI.[40] Increased use of "chemical sphincterotomy" (e.g. glycerin trinitrate (GTN)[41] or diltiazem), with surgery reserved for the most severe or resistant cases, may lead to fewer future problems.

Radiation. Patients who have undergone radiotherapy secondary to a pelvic malignancy (bowel, anus, uterus or cervix) may have degeneration of the anal sphincters, especially the internal anal sphincter. Symptoms may be exacerbated if the radiation has also given rise to a radiation proctitis with loose stool, reduced rectal capacity, and hypersensitivity of rectal mucosa. Modern radiotherapy techniques attempt to minimize accidental bowel damage but some patients who had radiotherapy some decades ago can experience severe persisting symptoms.[42,43]

Gynecological surgery. There is some evidence that surgical solutions for one pelvic floor problem may unmask another and cause it to become symptomatic, or even possibly create new problems by distorting the pelvic anatomy or disrupting the nerve supply. For example, repairing a vaginal prolapse may unmask a tendency to urinary or fecal incontinence as the prolapse was actually supporting a cystocele or rectocele. Colposuspension as a treatment for urinary incontinence is known to create new symptoms of prolapse in a proportion of patients. Repair of a rectocele corrects the anatomic defect for three-quarters of women undergoing posterior colporrhaphy but there is not a clear relationship between anatomic defect and dysfunction. Repair of a rectocele has been found to create de novo fecal incontinence in 7% in one series, with some patients also reporting new sexual dysfunction (9%), rectal evacuation difficulties (11%), and poor control of flatus.[44] Other authors have reported new FI.[45]

Hysterectomy has been found in retrospective studies to change bowel function,[46] with over one-third of women reporting newly decreased bowel frequency or difficulty with evacuation. It is postulated that the associated factors might include damage to the hypogastric nerve plexus during surgery, hormonal changes or a common thread of chronic abdominal discomfort and anxiety in polysymptomatic women. Only 59% of women report normal bowel function prior to hysterectomy.[47] It may be that the surgery disrupts the pelvic nerve plexus and structural support to the bladder. However, often the primary reason for hysterectomy is pelvic floor dysfunction and so it may be a symptom rather than a cause of the problem.[48]

Idiopathic degeneration of the anal sphincters.

It seems that sometimes the internal anal sphincter may degenerate and become very thin, for reasons as yet unknown.[49] This thin atrophic sphincter often has a low resting closure pressure and the patient complains of passive seepage of stool. It is not known whether degeneration can also affect the external anal sphincter, although clinically it is often reported as appearing atrophic on anal ultrasound or magnetic resonance imaging. It is not known if the mechanism for this is neurologic, mechanical or a combination.

Direct trauma or injury to the anal sphincters.

There is some debate about the role of sexual use or abuse of the anus as a cause of fecal incontinence. Some evidence suggests that unwanted or forced anal sex can cause direct anal sphincter injury[50] but most people also have some psychosocial problems after such an event, which could contribute to symptoms.[51] Consenting sexual use of the anus may not be associated with symptoms.[52]

Direct trauma can occur as a result of road traffic or impalement injuries. If damage is severe, it is usual to divert the fecal stream into a stoma to allow healing of a sphincter repair.

Congenital anomaly.

Developmental abnormalities are relatively common and can lead to a variety of presentations, from a simple imperforate anus, where a membrane prevents passage of meconium after birth, to an ectopic anus which does not open through the sphincters, or an opening in the perineum or vaginal (a cloaca). Most are picked up in childhood but occasionally an adult will present with a previously undiagnosed anomaly. Repair of congenital anomalies in childhood does not always result in good continence[53,54] and many patients will experience psychosocial difficulties related to FI ongoing into adult life.[55]

GUT MOTILITY/STOOL CONSISTENCY

Diarrhea or loose stool is much harder to control than formed stool and there is a consistently reported association between loose stools and FI in the general population[56,57] and in nursing home residents.[58,59] FI is more prevalent in people with irritable bowel syndrome[60] and conditions in which diarrhea predominates[61-63] than in the general population. Excessive exercise can also precipitate diarrhea-associated FI.[64] Volume, speed of transit, and consistency interact to provide increased frequency and a sensation of urgency which, if severe or no toilet is available, can overwhelm even normal sphincters at times. It may also be more difficult to distinguish loose stool from flatus, causing either unnecessary toilet visits or accidents when stool is passed with flatus.

Diarrhea itself has many possible causes, the more common of which include infective gastroenteritis, inflammatory bowel disease (ulcerative colitis and Crohn's disease), irritable bowel syndrome (where it may alternate with bouts of constipation), after surgery where a substantial amount of large bowel has been removed (e.g. for carcinoma or inflammatory bowel disease), after radiotherapy for any pelvic tumor, and as a side effect of some drugs (notably antibiotics). Some people develop diarrhea in response to intolerance of an element in their diet (e.g. people with celiac disease in response to gluten). Anxiety leads to frequent loose bowel actions for some people. Many people with fecal incontinence clinically present with frequent loose stools. It is often not clear if this is the "cause" of their problem or a result of the anxiety created by this condition. If the individual with diarrhea also has some sphincter damage for any of the reasons outlined above, then control can be very precarious.

ANORECTAL PATHOLOGY

There are many minor anal conditions, such as hemorrhoids and skin tags, which can make anal cleaning difficult and may lead to passive soiling with stool or mucus. There are also some more major conditions, such as rectal prolapse and anal fistula, which can impair continence.[65]

NEUROLOGIC DISEASE

A more detailed discussion of this subject is given in two reviews.[66,67] Over 60% of people with a spinal cord injury are incontinent at times and for 11%, this is at least weekly.[68] An upper motor neuron lesion will tend to result in a reflex bowel, with continence if bowel emptying can be stimulated before reflex emptying occurs. A lower motor neuron lesion will usually result in a flaccid bowel and patulous anus. One study interviewed in considerable depth 115 people who had a spinal cord injury at least 9 months previously. It was found that time taken for toileting was positively associated with higher scores for depression and anxiety, and bowel management was rated as more of a problem than bladder, body image, spasticity or skin care, and almost as problematic as access, dependence, and sexual function.[68]

Multiple sclerosis (MS) is associated with bowel dysfunction (incontinence and/or constipation) in over two-thirds of individuals, with half reporting accidents in the previous 3 months and a quarter leaking at least once per week.[69] The mechanism for this incontinence is not clear and probably varies with the individual's lesions. There is a correlation of fecal incontinence with degree of disability, duration of disease, and bladder symptoms.[70] However, 25% of those with even mild MS report some fecal incontinence.[71]

Long-standing diabetics may suffer chronic diarrhea and there is evidence that some also have an internal sphincter neuropathy and impaired sensation, which makes fecal incontinence much more likely in this group.[72] Other neurologic diseases, such as spina bifida, also have a profound effect on bowel sensation and control.

Care should be taken when reading the literature on this subject as the term "neurogenic incontinence" is often used in the specialized colorectal literature to denote fecal incontinence associated with pudendal nerve damage during childbirth and does not refer to that caused by major neurologic disease or injury. Many people with impaired sensory or motor function of the bowel and its sphincters will tread a delicate balance between fecal incontinence and constipation: anything done to help one of these problems may precipitate the other. Clinically, many patients prefer constipation as a socially more acceptable condition than incontinence.

SECONDARY TO DEGENERATIVE NEUROLOGIC DISEASE

Fecal incontinence is common in elderly people with Alzheimer's disease or other dementias.[73,74] The cause of this seems to be a complex interaction of neurologic impairment, causing a loss of sensation and ability to control the bowel, interacting with loss of intellectual function and social awareness of the need for continence, and in some cases the lack of physical ability to cope with bowel function.[74] Individuals who are also immobile easily become constipated with subsequent fecal impaction (see below). In institutional settings, this may be compounded by staff shortages, poor toilet facilities, dehydration, poor diet or lack of individualized care.

CONSTIPATION

There is a well-recognized association between severe constipation with fecal impaction and incontinence, either of solid stool or of liquid stool often referred to as "spurious diarrhea," particularly amongst the frail elderly population in institutional care. In children with encopresis, this is the primary mechanism of soiling.[75] However, the mechanism for this incontinence remains somewhat obscure. It has often been suggested that impaction of the rectum causes anal relaxation but anal resting and squeeze pressures have been found to be similar in impacted individuals as in age-matched nonimpacted controls. There is, however, a reduction in sensation, and in the volume of rectal distension needed to elicit internal sphincter relaxation via the rectoanal inhibitory response, and some loss of the anorectal angle in incontinent individuals. It is unclear which of these

mechanisms is cause or effect of impaction or subsequent incontinence. It may be that once impaction is present (possibly caused by a combination of immobility, low fluid and fiber intake, drug side effects, confusion, lack of privacy, and many other factors), lack of sensation makes it difficult to contract the external sphincter appropriately to prevent leakage when the internal sphincter relaxes in response to rectal distension.[76,77]

Some women with severe pelvic floor weakness seem to have a tendency to a combined difficulty with evacuation and passive loss of formed stool, although the mechanisms for this syndrome have yet to be defined. A common factor in the genesis of pelvic floor problems may be chronic straining with perineal descent from constipation, with subsequent pelvic floor damage (direct or neurologic)[78,79] resulting in prolapse or urinary or fecal incontinence. Straining at stool by young women has been found to be associated with later prolapse and stress urinary incontinence.[80] Clinically, many older women presenting with fecal incontinence give a history of previous long-standing constipation but this has not been documented in the literature.

"LIFESTYLE" AND ENVIRONMENTAL FACTORS

Unlike urinary incontinence, little work has been done on defining which additional factors might contribute to fecal incontinence. There is a suggestion that obesity increases the risk of FI but whether this is a direct effect or is mediated by unhealthy eating, poorer muscle tone as a result of less exercise and lesser health awareness is unknown. Extra weight may impair the blood flow or nerves to the pelvic floor and this may be reversible.[48]

Smoking might in theory contribute to FI as nicotine can stimulate distal gut peristalsis and a chronic cough might put stress upon the pelvic floor, but empirical data are lacking.

Individuals who have physical or mental impairments may have their ability to maintain continence impaired by an adverse physical or social environment. This is particularly relevant to those in institutional settings. Environmental factors include toilet facilities which are inaccessible or lack privacy so that the person avoids using the toilet; carers who are not sensitive to the individual's needs and bowel habit; clothes which are difficult to manipulate in a hurry; and other factors which vary with the abilities of the individual. The toilet itself may be too high, leaving the feet dangling and making abdominal effort to assist defecation difficult. Or it may be too low, making sitting and rising difficult for those with immobile hips. A social environment in which staff are always overworked and harassed may lead the individual to repeatedly ignore the call to stool, in the hope of finding a quieter time later, and eventually lead to the impaction described above. Even those who are not frail but have urgency may find their continence compromised by a lack of available public toilet facilities.

Caffeine stimulates the bowel.[81] Artificial sweeteners act as an osmotic laxative. Many people report sensitivities to a variety of foods which precipitate intestinal hurry.

Many drugs have listed possible direct or indirect effects on the gut. Some will cause constipation, others diarrhea, or either in different people. A careful drug history will include all prescription, over-the-counter or "herbal" preparations, with possible gastrointestinal effects considered.

Frailty and dependence on others will mean that the individual's ability to maintain continence is influenced by the availability and attitudes of carers. These may be conducive to continence or may make good bowel control very difficult. Immobility has been consistently found to be associated with fecal incontinence in institutionalized older people.[58,82]

IDIOPATHIC

There is a group of patients in whom no "cause" for the symptom of fecal incontinence can at present be identified. There is a need for much better understanding of the mechanisms of continence and incontinence and probably development of new investigative techniques to aid in definition of the full range of causative mechanisms.

REFERENCES

1. Pemberton JH, Swash M, Henry MM, eds. The pelvic floor. Edinburgh: Harcourt Health Sciences; 2002.
2. Norton C. Nurses, bowel continence, stigma and taboos. J Wound Ostomy Cont Nurs 2004; 31(2):85–94.
3. Norton C, Chelvanayagam S. Bowel continence nursing. Beaconsfield: Beaconsfield Publishers; 2004.
4. Jorge JM, Wexner SD. Etiology and management of fecal incontinence. Dis Colon Rectum 1993;36(1):77–97.
5. Kamm MA. Faecal incontinence: clinical review. BMJ 1998;316:528–532.
6. Norton C, Whitehead WE, Bliss DZ, Metsola P, Tries J. Conservative and pharmacological management of faecal incontinence in adults. In: Abrams P, Khoury S, Wein A, Cardozo L, eds. Incontinence (Proceedings of the Third International Consultation on Incontinence). Plymouth: Health Books; 2005.
7. Khullar V, Damiano R, Toozs-Hobson P, Cardozo L. Prevalence of faecal incontinence among women with urinary incontinence. Br J Obstet Gynaecol 1998;105:1211–1213.
8. Norton C. Biofeedback and nursing management for adults with faecal incontinence (unpublished PhD thesis). King's College, London, 2001.
9. Fornell EU, Wingren G, Kjolhede P. Factors associated with pelvic floor dysfunction with emphasis on urinary and fecal incontinence and genital prolapse: an epidemiological study. Acta Obstet Gynecol Scand 2004;83:383–389.
10. Roberts RO, Jacobsen SJ, Reilly WT, et al. Prevalence of combined fecal and urinary incontinence: a community-based study. J Am Geriat Soc 1999;47(7):837–841.
11. Edwards NI, Jones D. The prevalence of faecal incontinence in older people living at home. Age Ageing 2001;30:503–507.
12. Monga AK, Marrero JM, Stanton SL, Lemieux M-C, Maxwell JD. Is there an irritable bladder in the irritable bowel syndrome? Br J Obstet Gynaecol 1997;104:1409–1412.
13. Leroi AM, Weber J, Menard J-F, Touchais J-Y, Denis P. Prevalence of anal incontinence in 409 patients investigated for stress urinary incontinence. Neurourol Urodynam 1999;18:579–590.
14. Soligo M, Salvatore S, Monti C, et al. Faecal incontinence in women with urinary tract disorders. Jerusalem: International Continence Society; 1998.
15. Gordon D, Groutz A, Goldman G, et al. Anal incontinence: prevalence among female patients attending a urogynecologic clinic. Neurourol Urodynam 1999;18:199–204.
16. Frenckner B, Euler CV. Influence of pudendal block on the function of the anal sphincters. Gut 1975;16:482–489.
17. Engel AF, Kamm MA, Bartram CI, Nicholls RJ. Relationship of symptoms in faecal incontinence to specific sphincter abnormalities. Int J Colorectal Dis 1995;10:152–155.
18. Perry S, Shaw C, McGrother C, et al. The prevalence of faecal incontinence in adults aged 40 years or more living in the community. Gut 2002;50:480–484.
19. Drossman DA, Li Z, Andruzzi E, Temple RD, Talley NJ, Thompson WG. U.S. householder survey of functional gastrointestinal disorders. Dig Dis Sci 1993;38(9):1569–1580.
20. Snooks SJ, Swash M, Henry MM, Setchell M. Risk factors in childbirth causing damage to the pelvic floor. Br J Surg 1985;72(Suppl):S15–S17.
21. Law PJ, Kamm MA, Bartram CI. Anal endosonography in the investigation of faecal incontinence. Br J Surg 1991;78:312–314.
22. Damon H, Henry L, Bretones S, Mellier G, Minaire Y, Mion F. Postdelivery anal function in primiparous females: ultrasound and manometric study. Dis Colon Rectum 2000;43(4):472–477.
23. Norton C. Faecal incontinence following pregnancy. In: Maclean AB, Cardozo L, eds. Incontinence in women. London: RCOG Press; 2002:352–365.
24. Signorello LB, Harlow BL, Chekos AK, Repke JT. Midline episiotomy and anal incontinence: retrospective cohort study. BMJ 2000;320:86–90.
25. Sultan AH, Kamm MA, Hudson CN, Bartram CI. Third degree obstetric and sphincter tears: risk factors and outcome of primary repair. BMJ 1994;308:887–891.
26. Sultan AH. Third degree tears. In: Maclean AB, Cardozo L, eds. Incontinence in women. London: RCOG Press; 2002.
27. Gjessing H, Backe B, Sahlin Y. Third degree obstetric tears; outcome after primary repair. Acta Obstet Gynecol Scand 1998;77(7):736–740.
28. Sultan AH, Monga AK, Kumar D, Stanton SL. Primary repair of obstetric anal sphincter rupture using the overlap technique. Br J Obstet Gynaecol 1999;106(4):318–323.
29. Johannsson HO, Graf W, Pahlman L. Long-term results of haemorrhoidectomy. Eur J Surg 2002;168(8-9):485–489.
30. Khan S, Pawlak SE, Eggenberger JC, Lee CS, Szilagy EJ, Wu JS. Surgical treatment of hemorrhoids: prospective, randomized trial comparing closed excisional hemorrhoidectomy and the Harmonic Scalpel technique of excisional hemorrhoidectomy. Dis Colon Rectum 2001; 44(6):845–849.
31. Snooks SJ, Henry MM, Swash M. Faecal incontinence after anal dilatation. Br J Surg 1984;71:617–618.
32. Hildebrandt U, Lindemann W, Ecker KW, Walter P. [The colo-anal

pouch: indications, function and results]. Zentralbl Chir 1994; 119(12):886–891.

33. Barrier A, Martel P, Dugue L, Gallot D, Malafosse M. [Direct and reservoir colonic-anal anastomoses. Short and long term results.] Annales Chirurgiae 2001;126(1):18–25.

34. Paty PB, Enker WE, Cohen AM, Minsky BD, Friedlander-Klar H. Long-term functional results of coloanal anastomosis for rectal cancer. Am J Surg 1994;167(1):90–94.

35. Tiainen J, Matikainen M. Health-related quality of life after ileal J-pouch-anal anastomosis for ulcerative colitis: long-term results. Scand J Gastroenterol 1999;34(6):601–605.

36. McIntyre P, Pemberton JH, Wolff BG, Beart RW, Dozois RR. Comparing functional results one year and ten years after ileal pouch-anal anastomosis for chronic ulcerative colitis. Dis Colon Rectum 1994;37(4):303–307.

37. Hewett PJ, Stitz R, Hewett MK. Comparison of the functional results of restorative proctocolectomy for ulcerative colitis between the J and W configuration ileal pouches with sutured ileoanal anastomosis. Dis Colon Rectum 1995;38(6):567–572.

38. Fazio VW, O'Riordain MG, Lavery IC, et al. Long-term functional outcome and quality of life after stapled restorative proctocolectomy. Ann Surg 1999;230(4):575–584.

39. Khubchandani I, Reed JF. Sequelae of internal sphincterotomy for chronic fissure in ano. Br J Surg 1989;76:431–434.

40. Nyam DC, Pemberton JH. Long-term results of lateral internal sphincterotomy for chronic anal fissure with particular reference to incidence of fecal incontinence. Dis Colon Rectum 1999; 42(10):1306–1310.

41. Watson SJ, Kamm MA, Nicholls RJ, Phillips RK. Topical glyceryl trinitrate in the treatment of chronic anal fissure. Br J Surg 1996;83(6):771–775.

42. Birnbaum EH, Myerson RJ, Fry RD, Kodner IJ, Fleshman JW. Chronic effects of pelvic radiation therapy on anorectal function. Dis Colon Rectum 1994;37(9):909–915.

43. Iwamoto T, Nakahara S, Mibu R, Hotokezaka M, Nakano H, Tanaka M. Effect of radiotherapy on anorectal function in patients with cervical cancer. Dis Colon Rectum 1997; 40:693–697.

44. Kahn MA, Stanton SL. Posterior colporrhaphy: its effects on bowel and sexual function [see comments]. Br J Ostet Gynaecol 1997;104(1):82–86.

45. Van Dam JH, Huisman WM, Hop WC, Schouten WR. Fecal continence after rectocele repair: a prospective study. Int J Colorectal Dis 2000;15(1):54–57.

46. Taylor T, Smith AN, Fulton PM. Effect of hysterectomy on bowel function. BMJ 1989; 299:300–301.

47. Van Dam JH, Gosselink MJ, Drogendijk AC, Hop WCJ, Schouten WR. Changes in bowel function after hysterectomy. Dis Colon Rectum 1997;40:1342–1347.

48. Bump RC, Norton PA. Epidemiology and natural history of pelvic floor dysfunction. Obstet Gynecol Clin North Am 1998;25:723–746.

49. Vaizey CJ, Kamm MA, Bartram CI. Primary degeneration of the internal anal sphincter as a cause of passive faecal incontinence. Lancet 1997;349:612–615.

50. Engel AF, Kamm MA, Bartram CI. Unwanted anal penetration as a physical cause of faecal incontinence. Eur J Gastroenterol Hepatol 1995;7:65–67.

51. Berkelmans I, Leroi AM, Weber J, Denis P. Faecal incontinence with transitory absence of anal contraction in two sexually or physically abused women. Eur J Gastroenterol Hepatol 1996; 8(3):235–238.

52. Chun AB, Rose S, Mitrani C, Silvestre AJ, Wald A. Anal sphincter structure and function in homosexual males engaging in anoreceptive intercourse. Am J Gastroenterol 1997;92(3):465–468.

53. Rintala R. Faecal continence and quality of life in adult patients with an operated low anorectal malformation. J Pediatr Surg 1992;27(7):902–905.

54. Rintala RJ, Lindahl H. Is normal bowel function possible after repair of intermediate and high anorectal malformations? J Pediatr Surg 1995;30(3):491–494.

55. Cavet J. People don't understand: children, young people and their families living with a hidden disability. London: National Children's Bureau; 1998.

56. Kalantar JS, Howell S, Talley NJ. Prevalence of faecal incontinence and associated risk factors: an underdiagnosed problem in the Australian community? Med J Aust 2002;176(2):54–57.

57. Walter S, Hallbook O, Gotthard R, Bengmark M, Sjodahl R. A population-based study on bowel habits in a Swedish community: prevalence of faecal incontinence and constipation. Scand J Gastroenterol 2002;37(8):911–916.

58. Johanson JF, Irizarry F, Doughty A. Risk factors for fecal incontinence in a nursing home population. J Clin Gastroenterol 1997;24(3):156–160.

59. Nelson R, Furner S, Jesudason V. Fecal incontinence in Wisconsin nursing homes: prevalence and associations. Dis Colon Rectum 1998;41(10):1226–1229.

60. Drossman DA, Sandler RS, Broom CM, McKee DC. Urgency and fecal soiling in people with bowel dysfunction. Dig Dis Sci 1986;31(11):1221–1225.

61. Bliss DZ, Johnson S, Savik K, Clabots CR, Gerding DN. Fecal incontinence in hospitalized patients who are acutely ill. Nurs Res 2000;49(2):101–108.

62. Mintz ED, Weber JT, Guris D, Puhr N, Wells JG, Yashuk JC. An outbreak of Brainerd diarrhea among travelers to the Galapagos Islands. J Infect Dis 1998;177(4):1041–1045.

63. Kyne L, Merry C, O'Connell B, Kelly A, Keane C, O'Neill D. Factors associated with prolonged symptoms and severe disease due to Clostridium difficile. Age Ageing 1999; 28(2):107–113.

64. Lustyk MK, Jarrett ME, Bennett JC, Heitkemper MM. Does a physically active lifestyle improve symptoms in women with irritable bowel syndrome? Gastroenterol Nurs 2001; 24(3):129–137.

65. Buchanan G, Cohen R. Common ano-rectal conditions. In: Norton C, Chelvanayagam S, eds. Beaconsfield: Beaconsfield Publishers; 2004.

66. Coggrave M, Wiesel P, Norton C, Brazzelli M. Bowel management for adults with neurological disease or injury (Cochrane review). Cochrane Library, Issue 2. Chichester: John Wiley; 2004.

67. Wiesel P, Bell S. Bowel dysfunction: assessment and management in the neurological patient. In: Norton C, Chelvanayagam S, eds. Bowel continence nursing. Beaconsfield: Beaconsfield Publishers; 2004.

68. Glickman S, Kamm MA. Bowel dysfunction in spinal-cord-injury patients. Lancet 1996; 347(9016):1651–1653.

69. Hinds JP, Eidelman BH, Wald A. Prevalence of bowel dysfunction in multiple sclerosis. Gastroenterology 1990;98:1538–1542.

70. Wiesel P, Norton C, Glickman S, Kamm MA. Pathophysiology and management of bowel dysfunction in multiple sclerosis. Eur J Gastroenterol Hepatol 2001;13:1–8.

71. Hinds JP, Wald A. Colonic and anorectal dysfunction associated with multiple sclerosis. Am J Gastroenterol 1989;84(6):587–595.

72. Schiller LR, Santa Ana C, Schmulen AC, Hendler RS, Harford WV, Fordtran JS. Pathogenesis of faecal incontinence in diabetes mellitus. N Engl J Med 1982;307:1666–1671.

73. Stokes G. Psychological approaches to bowel care in older people with dementia. In: Potter J, Norton C, Cottenden A, eds. Bowel care in older people. London: Royal College of Physicians; 2002: 97–109.

74. Harari D. Epidemiology and risk factors for bowel problems in frail older people. In: Potter J, Norton C, Cottenden A, eds. Bowel care in older people. London: Royal College of Physicians; 2002.

75. Clayden GS, Hollins G. Constipation and faecal incontinence in childhood. In: Norton C, Chelvanayagam S, eds. Bowel continence nursing. Beaconsfield: Beaconsfield Publishers; 2004.

76. Read NW, Abouzekry L. Why do patients with faecal impaction have faecal incontinence? Gut 1986;27:283–287.

77. Barrett JA. Faecal incontinence and related problems in the older adult. London: Edward Arnold; 1993.

78. Snooks SJ, Barnes PRH, Swash M, Henry MM. Damage to the innervation of the pelvic floor musculature in chronic constipation. Gastroenterology 1985;89:977–981.

79. Lubowski DZ, Swash M, Nicholls RJ. Increases in pudendal nerve terminal motor latency with defecation straining. Br J Surg 1988;75:1095–1097.

80. Spence-Jones C, Kamm MA, Henry MM. Bowel dysfunction: a pathogenic factor in uterovaginal prolapse and urinary stress incontinence. Br J Obstet Gynaecol 1994;101:147–152.

81. Brown SR, Cann PA, Read NW. Effect of coffee on distal colon function. Gut 1990; 31:450–453.

82. Chassagne P, Landrin I, Neveu C, et al. Fecal incontinence in the institutionalized elderly: incidence, risk factors, and prognosis. Am J Med 1999;106(2):185–190.

Pathophysiology of Pelvic Organ Prolapse

Muriel K Boreham, Clifford Y Wai and Joseph I Schaffer

...It is brought about moreover through holding the breath, or leaping, and from lifting a weight, or from a blow...But it has also occurred through mental stress...or when the approach of enemies was announced, or when women were exposed to severe storms at sea... (Soranus *Gynecology*, 100 AD)

INTRODUCTION

Pelvic organ prolapse is a global health concern affecting adult women of all ages. The prevalence of prolapse is unknown. In one widely quoted study, the lifetime risk of a woman undergoing surgery for prolapse or incontinence was 11%.[1] However, a study by Swift et al of 1004 women aged 18–83, presenting for routine annual gynecologic exam, revealed the distribution of pelvic organ support by Pelvic Organ Prolapse Quantification (POPQ) staging to be: stage 0, 24%; stage 1, 38%; stage 2, 35%; stage 3, 3%.[2] These data are similar to those found in 27,342 women who participated in the Women's Health Initiative Hormone Replacement Therapy Clinical Trial (WHI), where approximately 40% had some form of prolapse.[3]

The discrepancy between the percentage of women undergoing surgery for prolapse and those found to have it on a routine exam may be due to the fact that this condition is often asymptomatic. Since patients do not report symptoms, an objective prolapse examination is not performed and thus treatment is not instituted. It is clear that the magnitude of this problem has been underestimated. If emphasis is placed on careful evaluation of symptoms and directed prolapse physical examination, it is likely that the true scope of this condition will be uncovered.

In this chapter, we will discuss the pathophysiology of pelvic organ prolapse with emphasis on risk factors, anatomy, and mechanisms of prolapse.

RISK FACTORS

There have been many postulated risk factors for pelvic organ prolapse including pregnancy, vaginal childbirth, aging, chronically increased intraabdominal pressure, menopause, hypoestrogenism, trauma, genetic factors, race, musculoskeletal diseases, chronic diseases, smoking, and prior surgery. It is likely that the etiology of pelvic organ prolapse is multifactoral and results from a combination of risk factors which vary from patient to patient. It is the rare patient in whom prolapse can be attributed to one independent risk factor.

Vaginal childbirth is the risk factor which has been most frequently associated with pelvic organ prolapse. In the Pelvic Organ Support Study (POSST), increasing parity was associated with advancing prolapse.[2] The risk of prolapse increased 1.2 times with each vaginal delivery. In the Oxford Family Planning Study, women with two deliveries were 8.4 times more likely to have surgery for prolapse compared to women with no deliveries.[4] Carley reported an increase in prolapse with one vaginal delivery (odds ratio 4.7) while in nulliparous women the risk was decreased (odds ratio 0.13).[5] In a case–control study comparing Turkish women who had surgery for prolapse and/or incontinence with those who did not have surgery for these conditions, women with four or more vaginal deliveries had 11.7 times the risk of suffering prolapse or incontinence.[6]

Age appears to be a risk factor for pelvic organ prolapse. In the POSST study, there was a 100% increased risk of prolapse for each decade of life.[2] Olsen found that the cumulative incidence of primary operations for prolapse and incontinence increased from 0.1% in the 20–29 age group to 11.1% in the 70–79 age group.[1] Aging is a complex process and the increase in prolapse may be due to the combination of physiologic aging, hypoestrogenism, and an increased incidence of age-related degenerative and organic diseases.

Chronically increased intraabdominal pressure is believed to be a clinically relevant factor in the pathogenesis of prolapse. This condition is not well defined but may be due to obesity, chronic constipation, chronic coughing or repetitive heavy lifting.

Numerous studies have identified obesity as an independent risk factor for stress urinary incontinence.[7-10] However, the association between obesity and the development of pelvic organ prolapse is less clear. In some studies, increased body mass index has been associated with pelvic organ prolapse[3] but other studies have failed to support this finding.[11] Heavy lifting has also been implicated in the pathogenesis of prolapse. A Danish study found that nursing assistants who were exposed to repetitive heavy lifting were at increased risk of undergoing surgery (odds ratio 1.6) for prolapse when compared with the general population.[12]

Cigarette smoking and chronic obstructive pulmonary disease (COPD) have also been associated with the development of pelvic organ prolapse but there are few data to support this proposed relationship.[1,5,13] Although it is postulated that chronic repetitive increases in intraabdominal pressure, i.e. chronic cough, might lead to prolapse, no clear mechanism has been determined. It is possible that tobacco abuse, with the inhaled chemical compounds, and not chronic coughing may cause changes that lead to pelvic organ prolapse.

VAGINAL SUPPORT ANATOMY

It has been proposed that the vagina has three levels of support.[14] Level I support suspends the upper portion of the vagina (parametria), level II attaches the midvagina to the pelvic side walls (paracolpium), and level III fuses the distal vagina to adjacent structures (Fig. 9.1). Defects in these three levels of support result in anterior, apical, and posterior vaginal wall prolapse (Table 9.1).

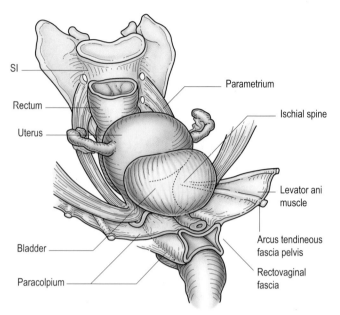

Figure 9.1 Level I and level II vaginal support structures.

Apical support is lost when the uterosacral/cardinal ligament complex (level I) fails. Whether this is due to attenuation, smooth muscle or connective tissue dysfunction, or actual breaks in the visceral fascia that makes up the ligaments is unknown.[14] Loss of apical support is frequently associated with small bowel herniation into the vaginal wall (enterocele). Classic teaching is that enteroceles form when the small bowel comes directly into contact with the vaginal epithelium. If this were the case, by definition, a defect or weakness in the vaginal wall would have to be present. However, Tulikangas et al demonstrated that the vaginal adventitia and muscularis are indeed intact in women with enteroceles.[15] Although controversy exists regarding the vaginal wall changes, clinical impression suggests that enterocele is the result of weakness or discontinuity of the fibromuscular layer in the region of the apex. Small bowel can also dissect into the anterior vaginal wall and appear

Table 9.1	Levels of support		
Level	Structure	Function	Resulting defect
I	Uterosacral-cardinal ligament complex	Suspension of apex	Apical prolapse
II	Attachment to ATFP Anterior/posterior fibromuscular vaginal wall	Supports bladder Prevents bulging of bladder and rectum	Paravaginal defect Cystocele/rectocele
III	Fusion of distal vagina to perineal body	Distal vaginal attachment	Perineal descent, distal rectocele
Adapted from reference 14, with permission			

on physical examination to be a cystocele. Similarly, small bowel frequently herniates into the posterior vaginal wall and appears as a rectocele. Large bowel may also dissect into the vaginal apex, creating a sigmoidocele. This is generally associated with a redundant sigmoid colon.

Anterior vaginal wall prolapse is thought to be caused by transverse, central, and paravaginal defects. Transverse defects occur when the apex of the vagina loses level I support.[14] The vaginal wall has several layers including epithelium, muscularis, and adventitia. The muscularis and adventitia are termed the "fibromuscular layer." It is proposed that central defects occur secondary to breaks in the central portion of the fibromuscular layer. Finally, paravaginal defects occur when the lateral vaginal walls become detached from the arcus tendineus fascia pelvis.[16] Many women have a combination of defects that must each be addressed during reconstructive surgery.

Posterior vaginal wall prolapse is also believed to be due to deficiencies in the fibromuscular layer. The rectovaginal septum, or Denonvillier's fascia, attaches to the perineal body and is only present in the most distal 2–3 cm of the vagina.[17] Detachment of the rectovaginal septum from the perineal body is recognized as one type of rectocele (distal transverse separation) and is generally addressed with a defect-specific rectocele repair.[18,19] This type of defect may be associated with perineal descent and it is possible that poor episiotomy repair, or episiotomy itself, may contribute to the formation of a distal rectocele. Similar to anterior wall defects, rectoceles may also arise from midline or lateral defects in the fibromuscular layer of the vagina.

BONY SUPPORT ANATOMY

The final component of pelvic support is the bony pelvis. The pelvis is composed of four bones: two innominates, the sacrum, and the coccyx. The pelvic bones provide a protective cage around the pelvic organs and participate in support through muscle and connective tissue attachments (Fig. 9.2).[20] Women with a narrower arch are more likely to suffer posterior compartment injuries during vaginal delivery, whereas women with a wider arch are more likely to have anterior injuries.[20] From this observation, pelvimetry has been investigated to describe pelvic characteristics that predispose to prolapse. In a case–control study, women with prolapse were found to have a larger transverse inlet diameter compared with women without prolapse.[21]

THEORY OF PROLAPSE DEVELOPMENT

It is postulated that pelvic organ support is maintained by complex interactions between levator ani muscles, the vagina, and connective tissue of the pelvic floor. However, the mechanisms by which the levator ani supports the vaginal wall and how these mechanisms fail during the development of prolapse have not been fully delineated. A major problem facing researchers is difficulty in modeling the complex interactions between the levator ani, nerves, and connective tissue that contribute to the development of pelvic organ prolapse.

When the levator ani muscle has normal tone and the vagina has adequate depth, the upper vagina lies nearly horizontal in the standing female. This creates a "flap-valve"

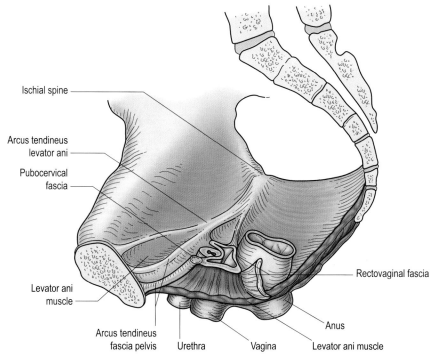

Figure 9.2 Muscle and connective tissue to the bony pelvis.

Ischial spine

Arcus tendineus levator ani

Pubocervical fascia

Levator ani muscle

Arcus tendineus fascia pelvis

Urethra

Vagina

Rectovaginal fascia

Anus

Levator ani muscle

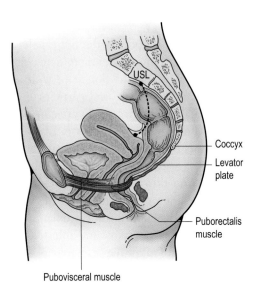
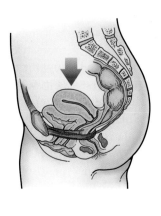

Figure 9.3 Normal levator plate with flap-valve effect.

effect in which the upper vagina is compressed against the levator plate during periods of increased intraabdominal pressure (Fig. 9.3). It is theorized that when the levator ani muscle loses tone, it drops from a horizontal to a semi-vertical position, causing a widened or open genital hiatus that predisposes the pelvic viscera to prolapse (Fig. 9.4).[22] Without adequate levator ani support, the visceral fascial attachments of the pelvic contents are placed on tension and are thought to stretch and eventually fail.

Mechanism of levator ani damage. Skeletal muscle is a dynamic tissue that is constantly remodeling and regenerating. A heterogeneous population of fibers with different functions allows skeletal muscle to adapt to different situations, such as stretch and mechanical load. It is thought that damage to the levator ani muscles occurs due to direct injury to the muscle tissue or through damage to its nerve supply. Labor and vaginal delivery have the potential to cause this type of damage. It is unclear what effect other pathologic conditions, such as chronically increased intra-abdominal pressure, have on the levator ani muscle.

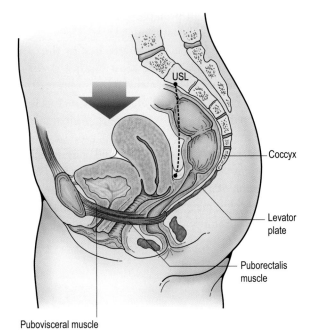

Figure 9.4 Weakened pelvic floor with widened genital hiatus predisposing to prolapse.

Direct injury. Direct injury to the levator ani muscles is believed to occur during the second stage of labor. The muscle undergoes significant stretch as the fetal head distends the pelvic floor. It has been shown through computer-simulated models that the medial pubococcygeus muscles undergo the most stretch.[23] Tunn et al described the levator ani muscle after vaginal delivery in 14 women.[24] They found the urogenital and levator hiatus areas to be increased immediately postpartum compared with repeat scans 2 weeks later. This suggests the levator ani actually remodels and recovers in some women after vaginal delivery. This appears to be true functionally as well, in that post-partum women have been found to have decreased pelvic floor muscle strength after delivery with return of function

by 10 weeks.[25] However, it is also likely that in some cases permanent stretch injury occurs. Evidence for this is suggested by the clinical observation that multiparous women have a widened genital hiatus when compared to nulliparous women.

In the developing world, prolonged and obstructed labor causes ischemic injury with resultant fistulae.[26] In a less extreme situation, it is possible that during second-stage labor, the vagina and levator ani muscle may be deprived of oxygen and undergo necrotic changes. If the injury is severe enough, the muscle tissue may be so devascularized that it becomes severely atrophied or nonfunctional. In Tunn's small series, one woman showed complete unilateral loss of the iliococcygeal muscle 6 months after vaginal delivery.[24]

The levator ani is a skeletal muscle composed mainly of slow oxidative (type I) fibers. Changes seen in slow-twitch muscle following denervation include muscle necrosis with resultant atrophy and fibrosis. A study of 45 premenopausal cadavers showed that fibrosis of the levator ani (especially the ventral portion) increases with increasing parity and in nulliparous women these changes increased with age. However, there was no evidence of neurologic damage in either group.[27]

Neurologic injury. In addition to anatomic studies, pudendal nerve terminal motor latencies (PNTML) and electromyography (EMG) have been used to investigate neural damage after vaginal delivery. There is evidence that pudendal neuropathy is associated with vaginal delivery.[28] In addition, chronic straining to achieve defecation has been associated with pelvic muscle denervation.[29-31] The excess straining and perineal descent that occur can cause stretching of the pudendal nerve and result in neuropathy.[32] However, there is little proof that pudendal neuropathy is associated with the development of prolapse.

It is proposed that stretch injury of the pudendal nerve occurs during the second stage of labor because the nerve is fixed as it exits Alcock's canal.[33] Snooks et al found evidence of prolonged pudendal nerve latency in 80% of primigravid women after childbirth, but most resolved by 6 months after delivery.[31] Although a number of these women will develop urinary or fecal incontinence, only a small fraction will actually experience the clinical problem of prolapse.

In fact, Heit et al did not find evidence of denervation when studying fiber distribution in levator ani of women with prolapse.[34] This may be explained by understanding the levator ani nerve supply. The predominant innervation is derived solely from efferent branches of sacral nerve roots 2–4 through the pelvic nerve complex with no contribution from the pudendal nerve.[35]

EMG is more sensitive to subtle neuropathy than PNTML and has the additional advantage of allowing distinction between acute and chronic nerve damage. Weidner et al established the feasibility of quantitative EMG in the levator ani of nulliparous women.[36] Although quantitative EMG of the anal sphincter after vaginal delivery has been performed, postpartum nerve injury in the levator ani has yet to be investigated with EMG.[37]

Nerve injury is a suspected, but unproven, risk factor for pelvic organ prolapse. Further research is necessary to delineate the role it plays in the pathophysiology of this condition.

Mechanism of vaginal wall injury. The vaginal wall is composed of squamous epithelium, smooth muscle muscularis, and adventitia. All elements are embedded in an extracellular matrix that includes collagen and elastin fibers and smooth muscle. Abnormalities of any of these components may contribute to vaginal dysfunction and the development of pelvic organ prolapse.

Site-specific defects. The site-specific defect theory is based on the premise that tears in the "endopelvic fascia" surrounding the vaginal wall allow herniation of the pelvic organs.[38] The association of pelvic organ prolapse with vaginal delivery is consistent with this theory. However, study of the microscopic anatomy of the vaginal wall indicates that endopelvic fascia may not exist as a specific anatomic tissue, but rather represents the fibromuscular layer of the vaginal wall (i.e. vaginal muscularis and adventitia) (Fig. 9.5).[39,40]

Although most are in agreement that vaginal delivery predisposes women to pelvic organ prolapse, there is little agreement regarding the changes in the pelvic musculature and vaginal wall that result in prolapse. Nichols and Randall propose an attenuation of the vaginal wall without loss of fascial attachments. They term prolapse of this type *distension* cystocele or rectocele.[20] Anterior and posterior wall defects due to loss of attachment of the lateral vaginal wall to the pelvic side wall are described as *displacement*

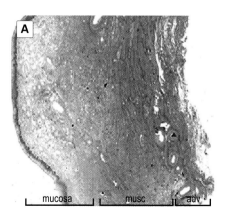

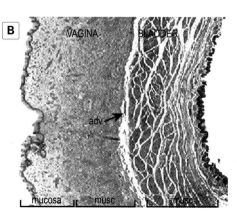

Figure 9.5 Cross-sections of anterior vaginal wall obtained at time of hysterectomy (**A**) were compared with cadaveric specimens (**B**). Biopsy specimens obtained at the time of operation contained vaginal mucosa, muscularis (*musc*), and adventitial (*adv*) layers. Vaginal mucosa consists of squamous epithelium and lamina propria. The vaginal muscularis is separated from the bladder wall musculature only by a loose framework of collagen fibers (adventitia) and no discrete endopelvic fascia. The adventitia of the anterior vaginal wall approximates the bladder muscularis. Sections are stained with hematoxylin and eosin (original magnification 5×).

(paravaginal) cystocele or rectocele.[38,41] It is reported that in the distension-type prolapse, the vaginal wall looks smooth and without rugae, due to attenuation, whereas in the displacement-type prolapse, vaginal rugae will be visible. Both types of defects could result from the stretching that occurs during the second stage of labor.

Smooth muscle dysfunction. Abnormalities in the anatomy, physiology, and cellular biology of smooth muscle in the vaginal wall may contribute to the pathophysiology of pelvic organ prolapse. For example, smooth muscle fibers arising from the vaginal wall attach to the levator ani complex[41] and dysfunction of this smooth muscle may affect the attachment of the lateral vagina to the pelvic side wall. Additionally, it has been shown that the fraction of smooth muscle in the muscularis of the anterior and posterior vaginal wall apex in women with prolapse is decreased compared with women without prolapse.[39] A decreased smooth muscle content of the round ligament in women with pelvic organ prolapse has also been described.[42]

The cellular processes that effect these changes in the vaginal wall during the pathogenesis of pelvic organ prolapse are unknown. Currently, it is not known whether changes in smooth muscle content are a result of the mechanical forces imposed on the prolapsed tissues or if decreased amounts of muscularis smooth muscle have a role in the development of this disorder. Decreased content of differentiated smooth muscle in the vaginal wall of women with pelvic organ prolapse may be secondary to mechanical forces imposed on prolapsed vaginal tissues or to denervation of the vaginal tissues during vaginal delivery. Nevertheless, decreased fraction of smooth muscle in the muscularis of prolapsed vaginal tissues may impair vaginal tone.

Connective tissue problems.

The connective tissue of the pelvis is composed of collagen, elastin, smooth muscle, and microfibers which are anchored in an extracellular matrix of polysaccharides. The connective tissue in which the pelvic organs are invested provides much of the anatomic support of the pelvis and its contents. There is evidence to suggest that abnormalities of connective tissue and connective tissue repair may predispose women to prolapse.[43,44] For example, Norton found that women with joint hypermobility were found to have a higher prevalence of genital prolapse (cystocele, rectocele, and uterine/vaginal vault prolapse) compared to women with normal joint mobility. Women with connective tissue disorders such as Ehlers–Danlos or Marfan's syndrome are more likely to develop pelvic organ prolapse[43] and urinary incontinence.[45] In a small case series studying symptoms of prolapse in patients with connective tissue disorders, one-third of women with Marfan's syndrome and three-quarters of those

with Ehlers–Danlos syndrome reported a history of pelvic organ prolapse.[45]

Collagen is one of the main constituents of pelvic connective tissue. There are many types of collagen described but types I and III are the most prevalent in pelvic tissues. Type I collagen fibers are usually well organized and are associated with ligamentous tissue. Type III collagen is common in the loose areolar tissue which makes up the vaginal wall adventitia and surrounds the pelvic organs. Quantitative or qualitative deficiencies in collagen have been associated with the development of pelvic organ prolapse.

Decreased collagen content is found in women with stress urinary incontinence and pelvic organ prolapse. When compared to women with good pelvic organ support, those with prolapse were found to have less total collagen in their pubocervical fascia as well as a weaker type of collagen.[46,47] This may be secondary to increased collagen turnover or breakdown. Site-specific analysis of collagen in prolapsing tissue has found structural, biochemical, and quantitative differences in collagen content.[48,49]

The fascia and connective tissues of the pelvic floor may also lose strength with aging and loss of neuroendocrine signaling in pelvic tissues.[44] Estrogen deficiency can affect the biomedical composition, quality, and quantity of collagen. Estrogen can affect collagen content by increasing synthesis or decreasing breakdown. Exogenous estrogen supplementation has been found to increase the skin collagen content in postmenopausal women who are estrogen deficient.[50]

Conclusions.

Pelvic organ prolapse is a common condition that can severely impact upon quality of life. It is likely to become more common as the population ages in the coming years. Epidemiologic studies point to vaginal delivery as the strongest risk factor, although the etiology is often multifactorial. The pathophysiologic mechanisms of prolapse have not been fully elucidated but it is likely that damaged or malfunctioning skeletal muscle, smooth muscle, connective tissue, and nerves all play a role in the progression of this disease.

FUTURE RESEARCH DIRECTIONS

Much is still unknown regarding the pathophysiology of pelvic organ prolapse. Current theories do not adequately explain why a gravida 0 can develop pelvic organ prolapse, whereas a gravida 9 may have excellent pelvic organ support. Similarly, we cannot always explain why one patient develops recurrence after repair of all support defects, while another patient with the same repair has a permanent cure.

The most successful approach to pelvic organ prolapse may ultimately be prevention. Therefore, future research should focus on identifying modifiable risk factors. Vaginal delivery is the most obvious risk factor which has the potential to be modified. Future research should try to identify specific aspects of the birthing process which can be modified to decrease the incidence of prolapse and pelvic floor dysfunction. In addition, methods must be developed to follow patients over long periods of time. Whether it is studying the effects of vaginal delivery 20 years later or assessing how durable surgical repairs are over time, we must find ways to follow the progress of pelvic organ support.

In the realm of basic science, there is much to be learned about the pathophysiology of pelvic organ prolapse. The pelvic floor has not been a major area of focus for basic science researchers and a more thorough understanding of the molecular and cellular mechanisms that mediate defective support of the pelvic viscera is needed. Clinical researchers will need to collaborate with basic science colleagues to answer the fundamental questions of pathophysiology.

REFERENCES

1. Olsen A, Smith VJ, Bergstrom JO, et al. Epidemiology of surgically managed pelvic organ prolapse and urinary incontinence. Obstet Gynecol 1997;89:501–506.
2. Swift S, Woodman P, O'Boyle A, et al. Pelvic Organ Support Study (POSST): the distribution, clinical definition and epidemiology of pelvic organ support defects. Am J Obstet Gynecol 2005;192:795–806.
3. Hendrix SL, Clark A, Nygaard I, et al. Pelvic organ prolapse in the Women's Health Initiative: gravity and gravidity. Am J Obstet Gynecol 2002;186:1160–1166.
4. Mant J, Painter R, Vessey M. Epidemiology of genital prolapse: observations from the Oxford Family Planning Association study. Br J Obstet Gynaecol 1997;104:579–585.
5. Carley ME, Turner RJ, Scott DE, et al. Obstetric history in women with surgically corrected adult urinary incontinence and pelvic organ prolapse. J Am Assoc Gynecol Laparosc 1999;6:85–89.
6. Erata YE, Kilic B, Guclu S, et al. Risk factors for pelvic surgery. Arch Gynecol Obstet 2002;267:14–18.
7. Dwyer PL, Lee ETC, Hay DM. Obesity and urinary incontinence in women. Br J Obstet Gynaecol 1988;95:91–96.
8. Wingate L, Wingate MB, Hassanein R. The relation between overweight and urinary incontinence in postmenopausal women: a case control study. J North Am Menopause Soc 1994;1:199–203.
9. Brown JS, Seeley DG, Fong J. Urinary incontinence in older women: who is at risk? Obstet Gynecol 1996;87:715–721.
10. Burgio KL, Matthews KA, Engel BT. Prevalence, incidence and correlates of urinary incontinence in healthy, middle-aged women. J Urol 1991;146:1255–1259.
11. Nygaard I, Bradley C, Brandt D for the Women's Health Initiative. Pelvic organ prolapse in older women: prevalence and risk factors. Obstet Gynecol 2004;104:489–497.
12. Jorgensen S, Hein HO, Gyntelberg F. Heavy lifting at work and risk of genital prolapse and herniated lumbar disc in assistant nurses. Occup Med (Lond) 1994;44:47–49.
13. Gilpin SA, Gosling JA, Smith AR, et al. The pathogenesis of genitourinary prolapse and stress incontinence of urine: a histological and histochemical study. Br J Obstet Gynaecol 1989;96:15–23.
14. DeLancey JOL. Anatomic aspects of vaginal eversion after hysterectomy. Am J Obstet Gynecol 1992;166:1717–1724.
15. Tulikangas PK, Walters MD, Brainard JA, et al. Enterocele: is there a histologic defect? Obstet Gynecol 2001;98:634–637.
16. DeLancey JOL. Fascial and muscular abnormalities in women with urethral hypermobility and anterior vaginal wall prolapse. Am J Obstet Gynecol 2002;187:93–98.
17. DeLancey JOL. Structural anatomy of the posterior pelvic compartment as it relates to rectocele. Am J Obstet Gynecol 1999;180:815–823.
18. Cundiff GW, Weiner AC, Visco AF, et al. An anatomic and functional assessment of the discrete defect rectocele repair. Am J Obstet Gynecol 1998;179:1451–1457.
19. Porter WE, Steele A, Walsh P, et al. The anatomic and functional outcomes of defect-specific rectocele repairs. Am J Obstet Gynecol 1999;181:1353–1358.
20. Nichols DH, Randall CL. Types of genital prolapse. In: Nichols DH, Randall CL, eds. Vaginal surgery, 3rd edn. Baltimore: Williams and Wilkins; 1989.
21. Sze EH, Kohli N, Miklos JR, et al. Computed tomography comparison of bony pelvis dimensions between women with and without genital prolapse. Obstet Gynecol 1999;93:229–232.
22. Berglas B, Rubin IC. Study of the supportive structures of the uterus by levator myography. Surg Gynecol Obstet 1953;97:677–692.
23. Lien KC, Mooney B, DeLancey JO, et al. Levator ani muscle stretch induced by simulated vaginal birth. Obstet Gynecol 2004;103:31–40.
24. Tunn R, DeLancey JOL, Howard D, et al. MR imaging of levator ani muscle recovery following vaginal delivery. Int Urogynecol J 1999;10:300–307.
25. Peschers UM, Schaer GN, DeLancey JO, et al. Levator ani function before and after childbirth. Br J Obstet Gynaecol 1997;104:1004–1008.
26. Wall LL. Obstetric fistulas in Africa and the developing world: new efforts to solve an age-old problem. Women's Health Issues 1996;6:229–234.
27. Dimpfl T, Jaeger C, Mueller-Gelber WM, et al. Myogenic changes of the levator ani muscle in premenopausal women: the impact of vaginal delivery and age. Neurourol Urodynam 1998;17:197–205.
28. Snooks SJ, Swash M, Mathers SE, et al. Effect of vaginal delivery on the pelvic floor: a 5-year follow-up. Br J Surg 1990;77:1358–1360.
29. Jones PN, Lubowski DZ, Swash M, et al. Relation between perineal descent and pudendal nerve damage in idiopathic faecal incontinence. Int J Colorectal Dis 1987;2:93–95.
30. Lubowski DZ, Swash M, Nicholls RJ, et al. Increase in pudendal nerve terminal motor latency with defaecation straining. Br J Surg 1988;75:1095–1097.
31. Snooks SJ, Barnes PR, Swash M, et al. Damage to the innervation of the pelvic floor musculature in chronic constipation. Gastroenterology 1985;89:977–981.
32. Kiff ES, Swash M. Slowed conduction in the pudendal nerves in idiopathic (neurogenic) faecal incontinence. Br J Surg 1984;71:614–616.
33. Benson JT, Walters MD. Neurophysiology of the lower urinary tract. In: Walters MD, Karram MM, eds. Urogynecology and reconstructive pelvic surgery, 2nd edn. St Louis: Mosby; 1999.
34. Heit J, Benson JT, Russell B, et al. Levator ani muscle in women with genitourinary prolapse: indirect assessment by muscle histopathology. Neurourol Urodynam 1996;15:17–29.
35. Barber MD, Bremer RE, Thor KB, et al. Innervation of the female levator ani muscles. Am J Obstet Gynecol 2002;187:64–71.

36. Weidner AC, Sanders DB, Nandedkar SD, et al. Quantitative electromyographic analysis of levator ani and external anal sphincter muscles of nulliparous women. Am J Obstet Gynecol 2000;183:1249–1256.

37. Gregory WT, Lou JS, Stuyvesant A, et al. Quantitative electromyography of the anal sphincter after uncomplicated vaginal delivery. Obstet Gynecol 2004;104:327–335.

38. Richardson AC, Lyon JB, Williams NL. A new look at pelvic relaxation. Am J Obstet Gynecol 1976;126:568–573.

39. Boreham MK, Miller RT, Schaffer JI, et al. Smooth muscle myosin heavy chain and caldesmon expression in the anterior vaginal wall of women with and without pelvic organ prolapse. Am J Obstet Gynecol 2001;185:944–952.

40. Weber AM, Walter MD. Anterior vaginal prolapse: review of anatomy and techniques of surgical repair. Obstet Gynecol 1997;89:311–318.

41. DeLancey JOL, Starr RA. Histology of the connection between the vagina and levator ani muscles. Implications for urinary tract function. J Reprod Med 1990;35:765–771.

42. Ozdegirmenci O, Karslioglu Y, Dede S, et al. Smooth muscle fraction of the round ligament in women with pelvic organ prolapse: a computer-based morphometric analysis. Int Urogynecol J 2005;16:39–43.

43. Norton PA, Baker JE, Sharp HC, et al. Genitourinary prolapse and joint hypermobility in women. Obstet Gynecol 1995;85:225–228.

44. Smith ARB, Hosker GL, Warrell DW. The role of partial denervation of the pelvic floor in the aetiology of genitourinary prolapse and stress incontinence of urine. A neurophysiological study. Br J Obstet Gynecol 1989;96:24–28.

45. Carley ME, Schaffer JI. Urinary incontinence and pelvic organ prolapse in women with Marfan or Ehlers Danlos syndrome. Am J Obstet Gynecol 2000;182:1021–1023.

46. Jackson SR, Avery NC, Tariton JF, et al. Changes in metabolism of collagen in genitourinary prolapse. Lancet 1996;347:1658–1661.

47. Makinen J, Soderstrom KO, Kiilholma P, et al. Histologic changes in the vaginal connective tissue of patients with and without uterine prolapse. Arch Gynecol 1986;239:17–20.

48. Boreham MK, Wai CY, Miller RT, et al. Morphometric analysis of smooth muscle in the anterior vaginal wall of women with pelvic organ prolapse. Am J Obstet Gynecol 2002;187:56–63.

49. Boreham MK, Wai CY, Miller RT, et al. Morphometric properties of the posterior vaginal wall in women with pelvic organ prolapse. Am J Obstet Gynecol 2002;187:1501–1508.

50. Brincat M, Moniz CF, Studd JWW, et al. Sex hormone and skin collagen content in postmenopausal women. BMJ 1983;287:1337–1338.

SECTION 4

Diagnostic evaluation

Diagnostic Evaluation of Urinary Incontinence

Christopher R Chapple and Philippe E Zimmern

INTRODUCTION

The lower urinary tract comprises the bladder and urethra and should be considered as a single functioning vesico-urethral unit required to adequately store urine as well as empty efficiently. Dysfunction occurs when there is break-down of these fundamental tasks, resulting in storage and/or voiding symptoms, urinary retention or incontinence. The bladder tends to be an "unreliable witness," its symptoms often being nonspecific and neither diagnosing the under-lying dysfunction nor paralleling the severity of the underlying functional disorder.

The customary evaluation of patients with both storage and voiding dysfunction includes an in-depth history and physical examination, as well as appropriate laboratory studies. Endoscopy and radiography provide useful struc-tural information and are used when clinically indicated. Urodynamic studies provide the only objective functional tests of bladder and urethral function and are a valuable adjunct to the investigation of patients with lower urinary tract dysfunction. Urodynamics, when properly selected and accurately interpreted, provides healthcare professionals with an improved diagnostic capability useful in formulating treatment strategies, educating patients, and ultimately improving therapeutic outcome. The results of urodynamics should not be interpreted as a free-standing study but in conjunction with the clinical presentation. Although the interpretation of urodynamics can be complex on occasion, in the majority of cases the indications for urodynamic investigation are evident and its application provides an essential complement to the modern practice of urology, gynecology, and associated specialties.

EVALUATION OF URINARY INCONTINENCE

In any patient presenting with incontinence, it is essential to carry out a complete evaluation of the patient, both subjective and objective. It is imperative that the exact functional derangement is defined and the precise etiologic factors are identified. This is particularly important when

there is more than one abnormality present, since incorrect treatment may aggravate symptoms rather than cure them. A careful balance should be struck between the treatment modality to be chosen and the patient's expectations. In addition to a clear history, a full examination, physical, uro-dynamic and, where appropriate, utilizing imaging, should be performed.

History. The most helpful classification of potential causes of incontinence is based on etiology.

1. Sphincter failure (stress incontinence)
2. Bladder overactivity (urgency incontinence)
3. Anatomic anomalies, e.g. uretero-/vesico-/urethro-vaginal fistulae
4. Overflow incontinence
5. Temporary causes, e.g. infection, immobility, fecal impaction
6. Functional disorders

It is important to remember that more than one condition can and often does coexist. Furthermore, reported symp-toms are not specific to any underlying abnormality; for example, urgency and frequency may be described by patients with sphincter failure or bladder overactivity. It is not unusual for patients to present with a combination of urge and stress. When both symptoms are present, the incontinence is called *mixed*, which is especially common in older women. Often, however, one symptom (urge or stress) is more bothersome to the patient than the other. Identifying the most bothersome symptom is important in targeting diagnostic and therapeutic interventions.

Salient features within the history include:

- onset and duration of leakage
- type of leakage (triggering events)
- severity of leakage and degree of bothersomeness
- impact of leakage on quality of life
- pad usage

- storage symptoms
- voiding symptoms
- nature of previous incontinence or prolapse surgery, if any
- other significant symptoms.

Whatever the cause of the incontinence, it is vital to assess the impact it has on the patient's lifestyle. The severity of the problem can be established by asking about the frequency of incontinent episodes and the number and type of protection used (e.g. pads worn per day).

Stress leakage may occur with any activity that results in a rise in intraabdominal pressure, most commonly coughing, sneezing or laughing, getting up from a chair or walking. Symptoms are usually better at rest so nocturia is not characteristic, nor are stress incontinence symptoms expected at night.

With urgency incontinence, patients complain of a loss of voluntary control of bladder activity and micturition resulting in urgency, urgency incontinence, frequency, nocturia, and nocturnal enuresis.[2] They often describe triggers such as cold weather, hand washing and "key in the door," when they are able to inhibit micturition for some time only to leak as they enter the house. Sometimes the trigger for overactive bladder contractions may be associated with a rise in intraabdominal pressure, e.g. coughing or sneezing, in which case the patient may appear to be describing stress incontinence. The reduced interval time between the urgency sensation and the occurrence of incontinence is what typically bothers the patient, giving her the sense that she has no "control" over her bladder.

With dribbling incontinence, many patients complain of "being wet all the time." It is important to establish to what extent this is a figure of speech. Continual leakage of urine is uncommon and is usually associated with overflow incontinence. Rarely there is an anatomic abnormality such as a fistula. Occasionally there may be gross genuine stress incontinence with a wide-open bladder neck resulting in continuous leakage of urine. Overflow incontinence occurs when the bladder is chronically overdistended. In both men and women, decreased bladder sensation resulting in incomplete voiding may be a consequence of a neurologic deficit, for example in multiple sclerosis or diabetic neuropathy.

Many women with severe prolapse recall that as the prolapse worsened (no doubt by producing urethral kinking), their stress incontinence symptoms improved or even completely disappeared. Certainly reduction of a vaginal prolapse during examination by the clinician can unmask so-called occult incontinence in many clinically continent patients with severe prolapse.

Assessment. Self-administered questionnaires may be used to elicit both symptoms and impact on quality of life, and several are available that have been validated with psychometric testing. An example of a simple symptom questionnaire is the Urogenital Distress Inventory Short Form (UDI-6) which has been validated in older adult males and females. Out of the myriad available quality of life questionnaires, the incontinence-specific King's Health Questionnaire has been widely validated, is commonly used, and is available in 27 languages.

The Bristol Female-LUTS Questionnaire also continues to receive attention as demonstrated by a recent randomized, crossover study comparing the responses to the same questionnaire administered twice in 114 women with lower urinary tract symptoms (LUTS) attending a tertiary urogynecology clinic.[24] In one group, the questionnaire was mailed 1 week before urodynamic studies (UDS) took place and administered a second time by direct interview on the day of UDS, whereas in the second group, the questionnaire was administered at the time of UDS and then mailed 1 week later. Although response rates were not surprisingly lower on postal questionnaires, there were more questions having a predictive value on UDS findings of stress urinary incontinence (SUI) and detrusor overactivity when self-completed over interview directed. Nonetheless, the authors concluded that "no symptom had a high enough specificity and sensitivity to replace urodynamic testing."

The International Consultation on Incontinence (ICI) has recently developed the ICIQ which is a disease-specific quality of life questionnaire with a large number of disease area-associated modules which are currently under development and evaluation. The International Consultation on Incontinence Questionnaire-Short Form (ICIQ-SF) has five questions and has been promoted by the World Health Organization as an "easy-to-use" urinary incontinence assessment tool. In a recent study, 64 women consulting for urinary incontinence completed the questionnaire three times, twice during the same visit, by self-administration and physician interview, then at home 1 week later. The study was powered to detect a minimal difference of 2.5 between the mean scores on patient and physician administration. Of 64 patients enrolled, 59 sent back the questionnaire at 1 week, and no difference was observed between home and physician-administered scores.[18]

For assessing quality of life related to urinary incontinence, several questionnaires are now available including the I-QOL,[36] the SEAPI-QMM,[33] which has been recently validated and was designed in the same way as a TNM classification, the IIQ-Short Form 7 Item,[35] and the Contilife[5] originally designed in France. These self-administered questionnaires are available for general use, have been for the most part translated into many languages, and can help both researchers and clinical practitioners.

Questionnaires are sometimes developed for younger or middle-aged patients. A recent study in women over 65 years old presenting for routine care and with no urologic symptoms established the baseline "background" noise to be expected when interpreting the scores of the UDI-6 and AUA-7 questionnaires in older patients. Of note, a score of 1 on a scale from 0 (none) to 3 (severe) for most questions was common even in these individuals without urologic complaints.[34]

Can questionnaire score help to distinguish between stress and urgency mechanisms? The MESA Questionnaire was designed to separate out these two conditions using a set of specific questions oriented more towards stress or urge. Depending on the response level for these questions, a score for stress can be obtained and compared to the score for urge, thus helping to categorize patients with pure stress or stress-predominant leakage, or predominant urge. This questionnaire was used as a screening tool in two recent NIH-sponsored trials as part of the Urinary Incontinence Treatment Network.[12]

Questionnaires have been studied for their predictive value. For example, Lemack and Zimmern found that a high response (2 or 3) for question 3 of the UDI-6 questionnaire highly correlated to the urodynamic finding of SUI, whereas this correlation was weaker for question 2 on urgency in regard to urodynamic detrusor overactivity.[26]

Questionnaires such as the UDI-6 have been studied to compare patient and physician perception of the severity and bother of the patient's symptoms. It appears that physicians frequently underestimate the patient symptomatology, even after a detailed one-on-one interrogation and history taking. Therefore, interviewer bias can lead to an underestimation of patient's bother and offer a more optimistic impression of a patient outcome after surgery, for example, than if the information came from a self-administered questionnaire.[30]

Several questionnaires in other areas such as sexual function, fecal incontinence, pelvic organ prolapse, general health, and mental status are beyond the scope of this chapter.

Although the role of questionnaires is rapidly expanding, some being directed at symptom specificity, others at bother or impact on quality of life,[13] a universally adopted, clear, short, and simple instrument is still lacking for routine clinical practice. Such progress would aid in comparing outcomes in reported series on urinary incontinence all over the world.

Physical examination. After recording height and weight, the examination should start with an inspection of the abdomen for scars indicating prior surgeries, palpation of the flank for masses and the lower abdomen for a distended bladder. Inspection of the perineum may detect skin changes such as excoriations due to incontinence and the use of pads or diapers, or fungal erythematous areas in the labial creases. After placement of a half-blade speculum over the posterior vaginal wall, the anterior vaginal wall is inspected and the patient is asked to cough and strain to demonstrate SUI.[32] The degree of urethral mobility with straining is also noted using either the POP-Q value of Aa located at 3 cm proximal to the external urinary meatus (level of bladder neck) or a lubricated Q-tip inserted in the urethra (Q-tip test).[10,23] If the cough test fails in supine position, it should be repeated later in the standing position. However, when successful, it often indicates an element of sphincteric deficiency.[28] A cough followed by leakage indicates that the cough triggered a detrusor contraction.

The presence of prolapse involving the anterior, apical, and posterior compartments should be documented and possibly shown to the patient with a mirror. The half-blade speculum is turned superiorly to elevate the anterior vaginal wall and permit the visualization of the posterior vaginal wall.[32] The Baden-Walker halfway method[6] and the POP-Q classification[8,19] are recommended to grade the severity of the prolapse(s). Examination in standing position may help detect an enterocele and/or an apical descent.[7]

Other important findings include the estrogen status of the vaginal walls, any signs of vaginal infection, scars from prior vaginal repair procedures, pelvic or ovarian masses by bimanual examination, pelvic floor muscle strength, and a rectal examination to assess anal tone and a possible rectocele. A neurologic examination, including inspection of the lower back, perineal as well as perianal sensation testing, and lower extremity reflexes, is also recommended. In patients with suspected neurologic deficits, a more complete neurologic investigation is needed.

Although the low lithotomy position and the birthing chair are frequently used to examine women, some practitioners prefer to carry out the vaginal examination with the patient lying in the left lateral position using a Simms speculum and asking the patient to "bear down" or "cough" to objectively demonstrate stress leakage of urine and assess the degree of bladder neck mobility and uterovaginal prolapse.

Once the history, assessment, and physical examination have been conducted, the next step is to decide on further testing(s).[17] However, before proceeding with any imaging or urodynamic studies, it is important to remember that a urinary tract infection, although an uncommon cause of incontinence, will aggravate any existing urinary symptoms and may also invalidate the results of other investigations performed. Therefore the presence of urinary tract infection should always be checked for prior to investigation. The confirmation of recurrent infections may also alter the type and priority of investigations performed or lead to a temporary recommendation for low-dose daily antibiotic prophylaxis to allow the scheduling and implementation of these tests without concern for a recurrent infection.

VOLUME VOIDED CHARTS

The urodynamic value of the simple voided volume chart is often overlooked, an important omission since this is a natural volumetric urodynamic record of bladder function. The volume/frequency chart is a simple noninvasive tool used in the evaluation of patients with voiding dysfunction, and in particular, in those with increased urinary frequency and incontinence.[3]

Volume/frequency charts help define severity of symptoms and add objectivity to the history. One can readily diagnose increased urinary frequency secondary to high urinary output and from physiologic nocturnal diuresis. A record of fluid intake helps identify an easily treatable cause of urinary frequency. The recommended daily fluid intake of 6–8 glasses of fluids (1 glass= 8 ounces, 1 ounce=30 ml, so nearly 2 liters for all fluids/day) is often misconstrued by the patient as the doctor's recommendation to drink 6–8 glasses of water daily in addition to the basic fluid needs. This excessive fluid intake frequently results in frequency and urgency and may worsen urinary incontinence. It is important to review these simple guidelines with the patient and discover if her craving for fluids is not prompted by a sensation of dry mouth, by the desire to avoid constipation, a fear of another bladder infection, or a special diet to lose weight. The average maximum voided volume represents the patient's functional capacity, knowledge of which is useful to know to prevent overfilling of the bladder during cystometry.

A normal bladder fills to a volume approximating its functional capacity and the chart records a series of sizable (300–500 ml) and fairly consistent volumes.

An overactive bladder contracts at variable degrees of distension before full capacity, erroneously informing the patient that it is full, resulting in urinary frequency and low and varying voided volumes.

In addition, frequency/volume charts provide important feedback to the practitioner and patient necessary to objectively evaluate the effectiveness of any therapies used in the treatment of the urinary dysfunction.

Technique. The patient is instructed to record fluid intake and the time and volume of each void for 3–7 days. Episodes of incontinence and the use of pads can also be recorded. In bladder drill the patient will be instructed to *hold on* to their urine up to a fixed time parameter, such as hourly, and then void, recording volumes voided and incontinent episodes, gradually increasing the time between voids accordingly until an acceptable voiding pattern is achieved.

Practical points. In sensory frequency resulting from hypersensitive bladder states due to urine infection, trigonitis or a condition such as interstitial cystitis, the symptoms and voided volume chart often vary considerably from week to week.

It is essential not to base therapy on the results of such investigations alone. In particular, it is essential to exclude another etiology for bladder symptoms, such as neoplasia, carcinoma in situ or intravesical stones, before proceeding with therapy.

Comment. The voided volume chart may provide information that is helpful in both the assessment and treatment of bladder dysfunction. It is particularly useful in providing a form of biofeedback during bladder retraining. It is important, however, not to overinterpret the results obtained but to use them in combination with other forms of urodynamic and urologic assessment.

PAD TESTING

The subjective assessment of incontinence is often difficult to interpret and does not reliably indicate degree of abnormality. Not all patients who complain of urinary incontinence are in fact incontinent during a cystometric examination. Pad testing is a simple, noninvasive objective method for detecting and quantifying urine leakage.[22,25,27]

The quantification of urine loss. To obtain a representative result, especially in subjects with variable or intermittent urinary incontinence, the test should occupy as long a period as possible, in circumstances which should approximate those of everyday life, yet be as practical as possible in the available circumstances and be carried out in a standardized fashion.

Technique. On the basis of pilot studies performed in various centers, we would recommend a 1-hour test period during which a series of standard activities are carried out. This test can be extended by further 1-hour periods if the result of the first test is not considered representative by either the patient or the investigator. Alternatively, the test can be repeated having filled the bladder to a defined volume.

The total amount of urine lost during the test period is determined by weighing a collecting device such as a nappy, absorbent pad or condom appliance. A nappy or pad should be worn inside waterproof underpants or should have a waterproof backing. Care should be taken to use a collecting device of adequate capacity. Immediately before the test begins, the collecting device is weighted to the nearest gram.

Typical test schedule

1. Test is started without the patient voiding.
2. The pre-weighed collecting device is put on and the first 1-hour test period begins.
3. The subject drinks 500 ml sodium-free liquid within a short period (maximum 15 min), then sits or rests.

4. Half hour period: subject walks, including stair climbing equivalent to one flight up and down.

5. During the remaining period, the subject performs the following activities:
   - standing up from sitting, 10 times
   - coughing vigorously, 10 times
   - running on the spot for 1 minute
   - bending to pick up small object from floor, 5 times
   - wash hands in running water for 1 minute.

6. At the end of the 1-hour test the collecting device is removed and weighed.

7. If the test is regarded as representative, the subject voids and the volume is recorded. Otherwise the test is repeated preferably without voiding.

If the collecting device becomes saturated or filled during the test it should be removed and weighed, and replaced by a fresh device. The activity programmed may be modified according to the subject's physical ability.

Practical points

Interpretation. The total weight of urine lost during the test period is taken to be equal to the gain in weight of the collecting device(s). An increase in the weight of the pad of less than 1 g in 1 hour is not considered a sign of incontinence since a weight gain of up to 1 g may be due to weighing errors, sweating or vaginal discharge. Evaporation is not important. The test should not be performed during a menstrual period and the patient may influence the test result by voluntarily voiding. A negative result should be interpreted with caution; the test may need to be repeated or supplemented with a longer test. The reproducibility of the 1-hour pad test is relatively poor.

If substantial variations from the usual test schedule occur, this should be recorded so that the same schedule can be used on subsequent occasions.

Voiding. In principle, the subject should not void during the test period. If the patient experiences urgency, then she should be persuaded to postpone voiding and to perform as many of the activities in point 5 as possible in order to detect leakage. Before voiding, the collection device is removed for weighing. If inevitable voiding cannot be postponed then the test is terminated. The voided volume and the duration of the test should be recorded. For subjects not completing the full test, the results may require separate analysis or the test may be repeated after rehydration.

Normal values. The hourly pad weight increase in continent women varies from 0.0 to 2.1 g/h, averaging 0.26 g/h. With the 1-hour ICS pad test, the upper limit (99% confidence limit) has been found to be 1.4 g/h.

Longer test at home. Home pad tests lasting 24–48 hours are superior to the 1-hour test in detecting urinary incontinence. The normal upper limit in a 24-hour test is 8 g. Though longer tests are better at screening for incontinence, they are less practical and more cumbersome.

Variations. Coloration of the urine with oral Pyridium before performing pad testing can help differentiate between vaginal discharge and urinary incontinence.

Additional procedures intended to give information of diagnostic value are permissible provided they do not interfere with the basic test. For example, additional changes and weighing of the collecting device can give information about the timing of urine loss. An electronic recording nappy may be used so that the timing is recorded directly.

Comment. This type of study is easy to conduct and interpret and provides a great deal of useful information. The weight of urine lost during the test is measured and recorded in grams. A loss of less than 1 g is within experimental error and the patient should be regarded as essentially dry. However, the objective quantification of incontinence by pad test remains under scrutiny due to its practicality, repeatability, and inability to discriminate between stress and urgency urinary incontinence.

With regard to practicality, the feasibility of mailing pad tests from home was investigated prospectively using a variety of commercially available pad brands.[14] All pads were saturated with a known volume, sealed in a plastic bag, sent by first-class mail ($4/envelope), and re-weighed upon arrival 7 days later and again at 14 days. The weights did not differ significantly from urine-soaked control pads at 14 days after mailing, and the volume lost ranged from 1 to 2 g on average between day 0 and day 14.

It can be concluded that at this stage, the home and/or office pad test belongs to the repertoire of pre- and/or postoperative outcome measures in clinical research studies on urinary incontinence. Its role in routine clinical practice remains undetermined.[15]

FLOW RATE

Technique. The patient is asked to pass their urine into a flow meter which gives a graphical representation of the urine flow rate over time. Characteristic flow rate patterns are seen in obstruction but many flow rates are equivocal and should be interpreted with caution. Both poor detrusor function and obstruction cause a reduction in flow rate. Furthermore, detrusor pressure may initially increase to overcome obstruction so that any reduction in flow rate is masked.

The urinary flow rate is measured with a flow meter which is a device that measures and indicates a quantity of fluid (volume or mass) passed per unit time. The measurement is expressed in ml/s. Patients should be instructed to void normally with a comfortably full bladder and be provided with as much privacy as possible to remove the inhibitory effects of the testing environment.

Practical points. The important factors to consider when interpreting a flow rate are the rate and pattern, in particular whether the flow is continuous or intermittent. A number of characteristic tracings have been reported but the definition of normal remains debated in women. Flow rates are dependent upon bladder volume and age. In carrying out a urinary flow rate, particular attention needs to be paid to certain factors as they can influence the result obtained.

- Voided volumes of less than 150–200 ml can lead to erroneous results and should be repeated. High voided volumes >600 ml may lower flow rates by overstretching the bladder, resulting in decreased detrusor contractility.
- If possible, the patient should be in favorable surroundings and should not be stressed unduly.
- Whether the patient is voiding standing, bending backwards, forwards, to the side, or half-standing.
- Whether the flow rate is a so-called "free flow rate" occurring after natural filling or after mechanical filling at the end of a urodynamic testing or following, for example, a retrograde bladder filling as part of a stress test or an office cystoscopy.

BLADDER ULTRASOUND OR BLADDER SCAN

Ultrasound is combined with a flow rate to provide more detailed information on bladder function. This is a routine investigation for all patients with voiding disorders seen as outpatients; an alternative is to measure the residual by catheterization.

Technique. The full bladder is scanned, the patient voids into a flow meter in private and a postvoiding scan is carried out to assess bladder residual. Interpretation of the flow rate takes into account the factors mentioned above. Any form of ultrasound probe allowing adequate visualization of the bladder is used. The patient should be scanned at the time that they feel "full," thereby providing an idea of the functional bladder capacity. Similarly, the patient should be scanned as soon after voiding as possible in order to provide accurate assessment of the true bladder residual.

Practical points. Ensure that the patient has a subjectively full bladder prior to carrying out the study to provide a representative result. Make sure that the study is carried out in circumstances where the patient is relaxed, so as not to introduce error into the results obtained.

Comment. This test provides data on bladder capacity, flow rate, and postvoiding residual, producing a more detailed assessment of the lower urinary tract function than a flow rate alone.[16] It can be carried out easily with little specialized equipment, is noninvasive and does not use ionizing radiation. It is of particular value in the follow-up of patients attending clinics, for instance with a hypocontractile detrusor following surgery for the relief of obstruction or where it is suspected that voiding efficiency may have been compromised, e.g. after a repair procedure for stress incontinence.

FURTHER DIAGNOSTIC EVALUATION OF PATIENTS
Urodynamic assessment
When should urodynamic testing be performed?
Women with a history of pure stress urinary incontinence associated with urethrovesical hypermobility and no prior history do not necessarily require urodynamic evaluation prior to surgery for stress incontinence.[37,38] However, a diagnosis made on the basis of history alone will not exclude detrusor overactivity in up to 25% of cases. Urodynamic assessment is therefore an important preoperative requisite in women with stress incontinence, particularly those who have other associated abnormalities or risk factors identified from their history and physical examination that may complicate the presentation and thereby influence treatment.[1,4] These include:

- women with significant overactive bladder symptoms or mixed stress/urgency incontinence[11]
- those with recurrent incontinence following previous surgery
- patients with associated neurologic disease, and those whose presentation suggests predominantly intrinsic sphincter deficiency.

Women who are dysfunctional voiders with high postvoid residual urine volumes are considered at higher risk of postoperative retention and should be urodynamically evaluated. Pure urgency incontinence not responding to behavioral and pharmacologic management is also an indication for study.

All symptomatic patients with neuropathic bladder dysfunction should undergo urodynamics, and preferably videourodynamics, in order to accurately characterize the detrusor and sphincteric abnormalities, and to help identify patients who are at renal risk from their lower tract abnormality. More sophisticated electrophysiologic studies are useful in the diagnosis of neuropathic bladder. The most commonly studied patients are those with multiple sclerosis, stroke, diabetes, Parkinson's disease, and spinal cord injury.

Cystometry, with or without video.

The majority of urodynamic units do not have the benefit of fluoroscopically equipped facilities. In the assessment of the majority of patients presenting with urinary incontinence, frequency and/or urgency simple cystometry provides all of the necessary information. Synchronous cystography and cystometry recordings are most important in the assessment of complex cases, particularly where previous surgery has failed, since this investigation allows a combined anatomic and functional evaluation of lower urinary tract function. Nevertheless, it must be remembered that simple cystourethrography can be carried out in all x-ray departments and can provide true, high-quality, lateral views of the urethra during voiding.[31,39]

In equivocal or more complex cases, detailed urodynamic investigation is necessary. *Cystometry* is the method by which the pressure/volume relationship of the bladder is measured. The term cystometry is usually taken to mean the measurement of detrusor pressure during controlled bladder filling and subsequent voiding with measurement of the synchronous flow rate (filling and voiding cystometry). In *simple cystometry* the intravesical (total bladder) pressure is measured while the bladder is filled. It is not accurate as it assumes that the detrusor pressure approximates the intravesical pressure. However, as the bladder is an intraabdominal organ, the detrusor pressure is subject to changes in the intraabdominal pressure which may lead to inaccurate diagnoses. *Subtracted cystometry* involves the measurement of both the intravesical and the intraabdominal pressure simultaneously. Electronic subtraction of the latter from the former enables the detrusor pressure to be determined. Cystometry helps characterize detrusor function by assessing bladder compliance, sensation, stability, and capacity.

If appropriate radiologic facilities exist, the bladder can be filled with contrast media, thus allowing simultaneous screening of the bladder and outflow tract during filling and voiding to be conducted (*cystourethrography*). When these two procedures are combined, this results in the gold standard investigation, the *videocystometrogram* or videourodynamic study. Radiologic screening provides valuable additional anatomic information on the appearance of the bladder, the presence of vesicoureteric reflux, the degree of support to the bladder base during coughing, and by itself is more than adequate for the diagnosis of sphincteric competence and/or the level of any outflow obstruction in the lower urinary tract on the voiding phase. This information, along with the accompanying pressure flow tracings, can be recorded on a videotape, allowing subsequent review and discussion.

The majority of patients can be adequately investigated using the simpler urodynamic techniques described, including simple cystometry. Videocystometry is, however, essential for the adequate assessment of complex cases where equivocal results have been obtained from simpler investigations, for the definition of neuropathic disorders, and in situations where there has been an apparent failure of a previous surgical procedure.

Technique for videocystometrography/cystometry.

The detrusor pressure is estimated by the automatic subtraction of rectal pressure (as an index of intraabdominal pressure) from the total bladder pressure (intravesical pressure), thus removing the influence of artefacts produced by abdominal straining. During this study, notice is taken of the initial bladder residual, the bladder volume at the time of the patient's first sensation of filling, the final tolerated bladder volume, and the final residual volume after voiding. All systems are zeroed at atmospheric pressure. For external transducers, the reference point is the level of the superior edge of the symphysis pubis. For catheter-mounted transducers, the reference point is the transducer itself.

Patients, excluding those with indwelling catheters, are asked to void into a flow meter to allow measurement of a free flow rate. Next, a fluid-filled rectal catheter is introduced into the rectum, the end of the tube being protected with a fingerstall to prevent fecal blockage (a slit is cut in this to prevent tamponade producing artefactual results during the study). With the patient in the supine position, the external urethral meatus is cleaned with antiseptic solution. A 10 Ch Nelaton filling catheter with a 1 mm diameter saline-filled plastic pressure catheter inserted into the subterminal site hole is gently inserted into the bladder and the two catheters then disengaged. The bladder is filled via the 10 F catheter, which is removed prior to the voiding phase, leaving the fine catheter in situ. Alternatively a 6, 7 or 8 F dual-lumen catheter can be used which avoids the need to use two catheters and then disengage them. The bladder can be drained of urine and this initial residual volume recorded. Allternatively the study can be carried out by filling on top of the initial residual and calculating the residual at the end of the study by subtraction.

The two pressure measurement lines are then connected to the transducers incorporated in the urodynamic apparatus. The lines are flushed through, great care being taken to exclude all air bubbles from both the tubing and transducer chambers. Contrast medium or saline (in a "nonvideo" study) at room temperature is then instilled into the bladder at a predetermined rate under the control of a peristaltic pump. Medium and fast fill (50–100 ml/min) is used routinely, although slower filling rates (10–25 ml/min) approaching the physiologic range are mandatory in the assessment of the neuropathic bladder.

It is our practice to fill the bladder initially in the supine position and the volume at first sensation of filling is noted. When the subject first experiences discomfort, the radiographic table is tipped towards the standing position and subsequent bladder filling discontinued when at the maximum tolerated capacity. During bladder filling, the patient is asked to consciously suppress bladder contraction and may be asked to cough or heel bounce. The patient is then turned to the oblique position relative to the x-ray machine and asked to void into the flow meter provided.

In units where a tipping table is not available, the study can be carried out in the sitting or standing position initially but it is important to subsequently stand the patient upright at the end of the study to assess postural detrusor overactivity and to determine whether there is stress incontinence. In the absence of radiologic screening, this is assessed with the patient standing with legs slightly apart and squatting.

Throughout the study, continuous rectal pressure, total bladder pressure, and electronically subtracted detrusor pressure (total bladder pressure minus rectal pressure) measurements are sampled at a predetermined rate (usually 1 Hz) and the results shown on the video display unit or stored to disk or polygraph chart recorder, depending on the equipment in use.

Videodynamics provides an excellent method of evaluating the urethral outlet in female patients with urinary incontinence. With the patient standing quietly and partially obliqued, the bladder neck position may be abnormally low, below the level of the upper third of the symphysis pubis, signifying loss of pelvic floor support in patients with hypermobile urethras/anatomic stress incontinence. Coughing or Valsalva maneuvers cause these vesicourethral units to descend and leak. With termination of the increased intra-abdominal pressure, the bladder neck quickly "springs back" to its original position, terminating leakage. The semilateral/oblique position enables the bladder neck to be distinguished from a dependent cystocele and it also helps to evaluate the size and functional significance of the cystocele.

Beaking or funneling of the bladder neck probably represents a normal finding, is common in continent females, but should be distinguished from a rectangular-shaped incompetent bladder neck common in patients with intrinsic sphincter deficiency (ISD). Typically, patients with pure ISD as the cause of their incontinence demonstrate severe leakage with minimal intraabdominal pressure increases and minimal urethrovesical hypermobility. The urethra does not spring back but appears to remain open and continue leaking even after the stress event. Patients often have both bladder neck hypermobility and ISD and experience is necessary in order to interpret their relative functional significance. Cystourethrography via the adjacent x-ray screening apparatus allows the synchronous display of pressure and flow and also radiographic data relating to bladder morphology, e.g. diverticula, vesicoureteric reflux and the appearances of the bladder outlet and urethra, to be displayed alongside the numerical data on a video display unit.

Practical points. Since a number of variations in technique are currently available, the following points deserve specific consideration.

TYPE OF CATHETER
- *Fluid-filled catheter*: specify number of catheters, single or multiple lumens, type of catheter, size of catheter.
- *Catheter tip transducer*: specifications vary between manufacturers; these catheters tend to be expensive and rather too fragile for routine use.

MEASURING EQUIPMENT. A number of commercial urodynamic systems are currently available. These vary greatly in terms of sampling rate, associated computer software back-up, and price. A major problem with existing computer programs is the ease with which they record artefacts which can then bias the results of the subsequent automatic data analysis. The investigator is strongly advised not to rely upon the computer-generated data sheets but to use an appropriate standardized reading sheet which allows interpretation of the urodynamic findings by the investigator.

TEST MEDIUM (LIQUID OR GAS). This is obviously not applicable to catheter tip transducers. The advantage of equipment using gas as a medium is that it can be more compact and is therefore more easily portable. A major drawback with gas cystometry is its susceptibility to artefact being introduced by changes in the temperature of the gaseous medium, a far less important consideration when fluid is used.

POSITION OF PATIENT (E.G. SUPINE, SITTING OR STANDING) TYPE OF FILLING. This may be by diuresis or catheter. Filling by catheter may be continuous or incremental; the precise filling rate should be stated (see below). When the incremental method is used, the volume increment should be stated.

CONTINUOUS OR INTERMITTENT PRESSURE MEASUREMENT. Continuous pressure measurement is of greatest use in clinical practice. For example, in patients with a suprapubic catheter and no urethral access, staged measurement of pressures can be carried out through the suprapubic catheter.

WHO CARRIES OUT THE STUDY AND HOW? DATA QUALITY. It is essential that urodynamic studies are carried out or supervised by experienced investigators.

- Always take a clinical history of the patient before carrying out the study and counsel the patient before they attend on the day and at the start of the study as to the nature of the test.
- Make sure the urodynamic equipment is regularly serviced and calibrate the transducers on a regular basis.
- Make sure that the lines are zeroed at the start of the study, check subtraction is perfect before starting the study with a detrusor pressure between 0 and 5 cmH$_2$O, and every minute during the study ask the patient to cough and verify that the rectal and vesical pressure lines track together in their response. If in doubt about artefact, repeat the study.
- Choose the correct filling rate for the study, e.g. normal filling at 50 ml/min and slower filling at 10–20 ml/min for neuropaths and patients with a reduced functional capacity.

LEAK POINT PRESSURE. The abdominal pressure or vesical pressure at which leakage occurs is a major problem because there is no standard technique with regard to:

- catheter caliber
- presence of prolapse
- bladder volume at which the leakage is measured
- Valsalva versus cough
- straining (contraction/relaxation of pelvic floor)
- absolute measurement or relative measurement compared to baseline
- no defined threshold values for treatment decision.

The literature abounds with contradictory reports as to whether there is any correlation between urethral pressure and leak point pressure.[9,20]

Our experience would support the use of graduated coughs as a means of assessing leakage, ideally coupled with cystourethrography or videocystometry. Basically, both tests suffer limitations. Since women leak with stress efforts in their everyday life and not with Valsalva, the Valsalva leak point pressure serves at best as a surrogate marker of sphincter competency. For the urethral pressure profile, the methodology imposed by the test (passive measurement, supine position) negates the real-life effect of the stress component over a presumably deficient sphincter.

Comment. Before starting to fill the bladder, the residual urine may be measured. However, the removal of a large volume of residual urine may alter detrusor function, especially in neuropathic disorders. Certain cystometric parameters may be significantly altered by the speed of bladder filling.

During cystometry it is taken for granted that the patient is awake, unanesthetized, and neither sedated nor taking drugs that affect bladder function. Any variations from this ideal must be taken into account when interpreting results.

In a small group of women who present with incontinence, urinary leakage cannot be demonstrated either clinically or radiographically. Conventional testing can be repeated or continuous ambulatory urodynamic monitoring considered if available.

Definitions. A number of definitions have been applied to standardize the interpretation of cystometry and in particular to enable the free exchange of comparable clinical and scientific data.[2]

TROUBLESHOOTING PRESSURE FLOW URODYNAMICS

It is important to be aware of a number of clinical scenarios which can be a source of confusion and lead to errors in the interpretation of results.

Poor subtraction. The rectal and bladder lines are not functioning properly.

Remedy: ask the patient to cough at the start of the study and every minute during the study to check the subtraction. If cough transmission on one or other line appears inadequate, flush out lines to clear air bubbles. Failing all else, replace the measurement catheter and if no better, suspect transducer error (rare).

Negative rectal pressure. A negative rectal pressure adds to the total bladder pressure and therefore the subtracted bladder pressure (detrusor pressure) may be higher than the total bladder pressure.

Remedy: adequate calibration of lines at the start of the study and avoidance of air bubbles; a fingercot placed around the rectal line to prevent blockage by stool material and with a slit cut in it to prevent tamponade when flushing out the line.

Cough/giggle overactivity. Be aware of this entity; an uncommon but well-documented abnormality which can be important as a cause of symptoms in women.

After contraction. A potential cause of confusion. It is not well understood and its true significance remains unclear.

Isometric pressure contraction (piso). Obtained as a spike of pressure when asking the patient to inhibit micturition and perform a "stop test." Previously said to be a sign of detrusor "power." Not particularly useful or of diagnostic value.

COMPLEX URODYNAMIC INVESTIGATION

The current techniques available for the investigation of urethral sphincteric dysfunction are far from satisfactory. Urethral pressure profilometry, although useful in the assessment of sympatholytic agents in drug trials, is not appropriate as a diagnostic technique. The dynamic evaluation of urethral sphincter function by the use of anal or skin-mounted electrodes is inaccurate. Accurate electromyographic evaluation of the urethral sphincter is possible with a concentric needle electrode but it is a painful investigation and cannot be carried out during voiding.

URETHRAL PRESSURE MEASUREMENT

At rest, the urethra is closed and this must be recognized when interpreting the results of urethral pressure studies. The urethral pressure and the urethral closure pressure are therefore idealized concepts which represent the ability of the urethra to prevent leakage. In current urodynamic practice, the urethral pressure is measured by a number of different techniques which do not always yield consistent values. Not only do the values differ with the method of measurement but there is often lack of consistency for a single method. For example, the effect of catheter rotation when urethral pressure is measured by a catheter-mounted transducer and the considerable artefacts which automatically result from the introduction of any catheter into the urethra.

Technique. Measurements may be made at one point in the urethra over a period of time or at several points along the urethra consecutively, forming a *urethral pressure profile* (UPP).

At rest, the UPP denotes the intraluminal pressure along the length of the urethra. All systems are zeroed at atmospheric pressure. For external transducers, the reference point is the superior edge of the symphysis pubis. For catheter-mounted transducers, the reference point is the transducer itself. Intravesical pressure should be measured to exclude a simultaneous detrusor contraction. The subtraction of intravesical pressure from urethral pressure produces the *urethral closure pressure profile*.

Intraluminal urethral pressure may be measured:

- at rest (the *storage phase*), with the bladder at any given volume: *resting urethral pressure profile*
- during coughing or straining: *stress urethral pressure profile*.

Ambulatory urodynamics. This form of cystometry overcomes some of the problems associated with conventional urodynamics. The equipment is portable, allowing the subject to move freely and void in private. In addition, the patient fills her bladder spontaneously after drinking a fluid load. As the technique is not adequately standardized with no internationally accepted diagnostic criteria, it is best regarded as a research tool at present, particularly since some studies have reported involuntary detrusor contractions in up to 70% of apparently normal subjects.

Urethral pressure profilometry. Although UPP has the potential to be highly informative, the test has multiple problems, the most significant being the large overlap in values obtained from normal and symptomatic patients. UPP does not discriminate SUI from other urinary disorders, provide a measurement of the severity of the condition or predict a return to normal following successful intervention.

Abdominal leak point pressures. Abdominal leak point pressure (ALPP) is defined as the vesical pressure at leakage during abdominal stress in the absence of detrusor contraction. The abdominal stress may be induced by a cough (CLPP) or a Valsalva maneuver (VLPP), with the two stressors differing physiologically in particular with regard to the rate and nature of pressure rise seen. Whilst higher abdominal pressures can be achieved with CLPP, the VLPP is better controlled and less variable.[21] Generally, CLPP is used for patients who do not leak during VLPP measurement. The pressure at which the urine is expelled can be measured visually, fluoroscopically, by flowmetry or by electrical conductance.

Although the concept of ALPP as a method of investigating incontinence is empirically sound, its value is limited by a lack of standardized methodology. Variations occur in the type of catheter (transurethral, rectal, vagina), catheter caliber, bladder volume, and patient position. The exact baseline used during the test also varies (e.g. zero level or the level at which the pressure just starts to rise), which can make a dramatic difference to the ALPP value. For ALPP to be a valid test, it is assumed that the transurethral catheter used does not obstruct the urethra or alter coaptation, straining or coughing does not distort the urethra, and no pelvic relaxation or contraction occurs. However, it is difficult to know whether these are actually occurring during the test, which is a major drawback.

Few data are available on the magnitude of the change in ALPP post-SUI treatment, and how this correlates with cure, improvement or failure. One general finding is that VLPP does not change significantly if the treatment fails. For example, following suburethral sling operations in 30 women, VLPP increased significantly after a successful operation (mean change: 61.1 cmH$_2$O; $P<0.001$) but not after failure (mean change: 9.7 cmH$_2$O, $P=0.226$).[29]

Neurophysiologic evaluation. The electrical activity of action potentials of depolarizing striated muscle fibers in the urethra can be studied with electromyography using surface or needle electrodes. Results must be interpreted in the light of symptoms and other investigations. This remains a research tool but has provided valuable insight into the pathophysiology and the effect of treatment on various conditions.

REFERENCES

1. Abrams P. Urodynamics. Second Edition. London: Springer-Verlag; 1997.
2. Abrams P, Cardozo L, Fall M, et al. The standardisation of terminology of lower urinary tract function: report from the Standardisation Sub-committee of the International Continence Society. Neurourol Urodynam 2002;21:167–178.
3. Addla S, Adeyouju A, Neilson D. Assessment of reliability of 1-day, 3-day and 7-day frequency volume charts. Eur Urol 2004; 2(Suppl):30.
4. Agency for Health Care Policy and Research. Clinical practice guideline: urinary incontinence in adults. U.S. Department of Health and Human Services Rockville, Maryland. AHCPR Publication No. 96–0682: 1996.
5. Amarenco G, Arnould B, Carita P, Haab F, Labat JJ, Richard F. European psychometric validation of the CONTILIFE: a Quality of Life questionnaire for urinary incontinence. Eur Urol 2003;43:391–404.
6. Baden WF, Walker TA. Physical diagnosis in the evaluation of vaginal relaxation. Clin Obstet Gynecol 1972;15:1055–1069.
7. Barber MD, Lambers A, Visco AG, Bump RC. Effect of patient position on clinical evaluation of pelvic organ prolapse. Obstet Gynecol 2000;96:18–22.
8. Bump RC, Mattiasson A, Bo K, et al. The standardization of terminology of female pelvic organ prolapse and pelvic floor dysfunction. Am J Obstet Gynecol 1996;175:10–17.
9. Bump RC, Norton PA, Zinner NR, Yalcin I. Mixed urinary incontinence symptoms: urodynamic findings, incontinence severity, and treatment response. Obstet Gynecol 2003;102:76–83.
10. Crystle CD, Charme LS, Copeland WE. Q-tip test in stress urinary incontinence. Obstet Gynecol 1971;38:313–315.
11. Digesu GA, Khullar V, Cardozo L, Salvatore S. Overactive bladder symptoms: do we need urodynamics? Neurourol Urodynam 2003; 22:105–108.
12. Diokno AC, Brock BM, Brown MB, Herzog AR. Prevalence of urinary incontinence and other urological symptoms in the noninstitutionalized elderly. J Urol 1986;136:1022–1025.
13. Donovan J, Badia X, Corcos J, et al. Symptom and quality of life assessment. In: Abrams P, Cardozo L, Khoury S, Wein A, eds. Incontinence: Second WHO International Consultation on Incontinence. Plymouth: Health Publications Ltd; 2002.
14. Flisser AJ, Figueroa J, Bleustein CB, Panagopoulos G, Blaivas JG. Pad test by mail for home evaluation of urinary incontinence. Neurourol Urodynam 2004;23:127–129.
15. Gilleran JP, Zimmern P. An evidence-based approach to the evaluation and management of stress incontinence in women. Curr Opin Urol 2005;15:236–243.
16. Goode PS, Locher JL, Bryant RL, Roth DL, Burgio KL. Measurement of postvoid residual urine with portable transabdominal bladder ultrasound scanner and urethral catheterization. Int Urogynecol J Pelvic Floor Dysfunct 2000;11:296–300.
17. Gordon D, Groutz A. Evaluation of female lower urinary tract symptoms: overview and update. Curr Opin Obstet Gynecol 2001;13:521–527.
18. Hajebrahimi S, Corcos J, Lemieux MC. International consultation on incontinence questionnaire short form: comparison of physician versus patient completion and immediate and delayed self-administration. Urology 2004;63:1076–1078.
19. Hall AF, Theofrastous JP, Cundiff GW, et al. Interobserver and intraobserver reliability of the proposed International Continence Society, Society of Gynecologic Surgeons, and American Urogynecologic Society pelvic organ prolapse classification system. Am J Obstet Gynecol 1996;175:1467–1470.
20. Hilton P, Stanton SL. Urethral pressure measurement by microtransducer: the results in symptom-free women and in those with genuine stress incontinence. Br J Obstet Gynaecol 1983;90:919–933.
21. Homma Y. The clinical significance of the urodynamic investigation in incontinence. BJU Int 2002;90:489–497.
22. Jorgensen L, Lose G, Thunedborg P. Diagnosis of mild stress incontinence in females: 24-hour pad weighing test versus the one-hour test. Neurourol Urodynam 1987;6:165–166.
23. Karram MM, Bhatia NN. The Q-tip test: standardization of the technique and its interpretation in women with urinary incontinence. Obstet Gynecol 1988;71:807–811.
24. Khan MS, Chaliha C, Leskova L, Khullar V. The relationship between urinary symptom questionnaires and urodynamic diagnoses: an analysis of two methods of questionnaire administration. Br J Obstet Gynaecol 2004;111:468–474.
25. Kromann-Andersen B, Jakobsen H, Andersen JT. Pad-weighing tests: a literature survey on test accuracy and reproducibility. Neurourol Urodynam 1989;8:237–242.
26. Lemack GE, Zimmern PE. Identifying patients who require urodynamic testing before surgery for stress incontinence based on questionnaire information and surgical history. Urology 2000;55:506–511.
27. Lose G, Rosenkilde P, Gammelgaard J, Schroeder T. Pad-weighing test performed with standardized bladder volume. Urology 1988;32:78–80.
28. McLennan MT, Bent AE. Supine empty stress test as a predictor of low valsalva leak point pressure. Neurourol Urodynam 1998;17:121–127.
29. Petrou SP, Broderick GA. Valsalva leak-point pressure changes after successful and failed suburethral sling. Int Urogynecol J Pelvic Floor Dysfunct 2002;13:299–302.
30. Rodriguez LV, Blander DS, Dorey F, Raz S, Zimmern P. Discrepancy in patient and physician perception of patient's quality of life related to urinary symptoms. Urology 2003;62:49–53.
31. Showalter PR, Zimmern PE, Roehrborn CG, Lemack GE. Standing cystourethrogram: an outcome measure after anti-incontinence procedures and cystocele repair in women. Urology 2001;58:33–37.
32. Shull BL. Clinical evaluation of women with pelvic support defects. Clin Obstet Gynecol 1993;36:939–951.
33. Stothers L. Reliability, validity, and gender differences in the quality of life index of the SEAPI-QMM incontinence classification system. Neurourol Urodynam 2004;23:223–228.
34. Svatek R, Roche V, Thornberg J, Zimmern P. Normative values for the American Urological Association Symptom Index (AUA-7) and short form Urogenital Distress Inventory (UDI-6) in patients 65 and older presenting for non-urological care. Neurourol Urodynam 2005;24:606–610.
35. Uebersax JS, Wyman JF, Shumaker SA, McClish DK, Fantl JA. Short forms to assess life quality and symptom distress for urinary incontinence in women: the Incontinence Impact Questionnaire

and the Urogenital Distress Inventory. Continence Program for Women Research Group. Neurourol Urodynam 1995;14:131–139.

36. Wagner TH, Patrick DL, Bavendam TG, Martin ML, Buesching DP. Quality of life of persons with urinary incontinence: development of a new measure. Urology 1996;47:67–71.

37. Weber AM, Taylor RJ, Wei JT, Lemack G, Piedmonte MR, Walters MD. The cost-effectiveness of preoperative testing (basic office assessment vs. urodynamics) for stress urinary incontinence in women. BJU Int 2002;89:356–363.

38. Weidner AC, Myers ER, Visco AG, Cundiff GW, Bump RC. Which women with stress incontinence require urodynamic evaluation? Am J Obstet Gynecol 2001;184:20–27.

39. Lemack G, Zimmern P. Voiding cystourethrography and magnetic resonance imaging of the lower urinary tract. In: Corcos J, Schick E, eds. The urinary sphincter. New York: Marcel Dekker; 2001.

Diagnostic Evaluation of Anal Incontinence

Christine Norton

INTRODUCTION

Assessment of anal incontinence (AI) or fecal incontinence (FI) includes a detailed bowel history,[1] inspection of the bowel by radiology or endoscopy to exclude major bowel pathology, anorectal physiology studies,[2] and an endoanal ultrasound study[3] to define any structural or functional abnormality of the anorectum. Anorectal physiology tests and anal ultrasound are not widely available at present. Consideration must be given to the possibility of serious bowel pathology in anyone with a change in bowel habit, and a colonoscopy is usually the investigation of choice. A history, physical examination, and tests are used in combination to determine cause/s and contributing factors for fecal incontinence in each individual. No one of these tests alone gives a diagnosis or a clear pathway for treatment.

ACTIVE CASE FINDING

Fecal incontinence is perceived by many as an embarrassing, even humiliating condition. Therefore, there is a reluctance to admit to symptoms or to present for help.[4,5] This places the onus upon health professionals to actively ask about symptoms in patients with known risk factors, including patients with urinary incontinence, pelvic organ prolapse, and neurologic disorders. However, it cannot be assumed that all people with symptoms desire intervention.

HISTORY

A detailed history of symptoms, related conditions, and lifestyle factors is essential to understanding the patient's condition. Box 11.1 gives an example of a checklist.[6] This assessment takes time to perform in detail. The assessing healthcare professional needs to be sensitive to the difficulty and lack of an appropriate vocabulary many patients experience when voicing their symptoms.

Diaries and symptom questionnaires. In contrast to urinary incontinence, relatively little work has been done on development and validation of patient questionnaires and diaries for FI.[7] Traditionally, many treatment studies have reported results using changes in composite scores as the primary endpoint. Box 11.2 gives a commonly used example.[8] Others are also in use[9,10] but none has been subject to rigorous validation. More recently, attempts have been made to construct questionnaires based on patient experiences and to evaluate quality of life[11-13] but results from these have not yet been widely reported.

A diary can give a useful record of the pattern of bowel activity (Fig. 11.1).

PHYSICAL EXAMINATION

General. General assessment will include the patient's overall state of health, mobility, and cognitive function. Dexterity and mobility may determine ability to use the toilet independently or to perform effective perianal cleaning after defecation. Minor degrees of soiling can be a simple matter of limited arm reach and obese buttocks, making complete removal of stool difficult. Even minor traces of fecal matter can cause perianal irritation and soreness and stain the underwear, leading to an odor and hygiene problem. Formal mental testing may be indicated if dementia is suspected.

Obesity has been found to be a risk factor for FI. Estimation of the patient's body mass index may indicate that weight reduction interventions are warranted.

Anorectal examination. Box 11.3 gives a summary of possible findings from an anorectal examination.[9] The patient's inability to remove clothing and take up position for the examination may indicate difficulty with independent toileting in a hurry.

Inspection. Cursory inspection may reveal evidence of soiling or poor hygiene, local soreness and previous injuries or scars. Skin tags (often a sign of a chronic anal fissure or hemorrhoids) or scars can make hygiene difficult. Third-

Box 11.1 Fecal incontinence assessment checklist

Main Complaint

Duration of symptoms/trigger for onset:

Usual bowel pattern: Any recent change?

Usual stool consistency: 1. Lumps
2. Lumpy sausage
3. Cracked sausage
4. Soft smooth sausage
5. Soft blobs
6. Fluffy, mushy
7. Watery, no pieces

Fecal incontinence

How often?   How much?

Urgency?   Time can defer for:

Urge incontinence: Never/Seldom/Sometimes/Frequently

Difficulty wiping: Yes ☐ No ☐ Sometimes ☐

Postdefecation soiling: Yes ☐ No ☐ Sometimes ☐

Passive soiling: Yes ☐ No ☐ Sometimes ☐
Events causing?

Amount of flatus: Control of flatus: Good ☐ Variable ☐
Poor ☐

Ability to distinguish stool/flatus? Yes ☐ No ☐

Abdominal pain relieved by defecation?

Other pain?

Rectal bleeding?

Mucus?

Nocturnal bowel problems?

Evacuation difficulties

Straining?

Incomplete evacuation?

Need to digitate anally, vaginally or to support the perineum?

Painful defecation?

Other factors

Bloating?

Sensation of prolapse?

Pads/pants?

Bowel medication?   Other current medication:

Past Medical History (include psychologic)

History of depression/antidepressants?

Physical or social difficulties with toilet access?

Previous bowel treatments and results

Obstetric history: Parity: Difficult deliveries or heavy babies?

Dietary influences:

Smoker?

Weight/Height/Body Mass Index

Fluids (caffeine)

Skin problems

Bladder problems

Effect on lifestyle/relationships/emotional/psychologic effect

Examination and results of anal ultrasound and anorectal physiology studies

Note: in clinical practice this assessment tool is laid out over three pages. From reference 6, with permission.

Box 11.2 St Mark's Hospital fecal continence score

Total score

	Never	Rarely	Sometimes	Usually	Always
		<1 mth	<1 week	<1 day	daily
Solid	0	1	2	3	4
Liquid	0	1	2	3	4
Gas	0	1	2	3	4
Lifestyle	0	1	2	3	4

	No	Yes
Need to wear a pad/plug/change underwear for soiling	0	2
Taking constipating medicines	0	2
Lack of ability to defer defecation for 15 minutes	0	4

From reference 8, with permission.

degree hemorrhoids may leak mucus or blood, as may a perianal fistula. The perineum may be attenuated or even absent in a cloacal deformity (congenital or secondary to obstetric or other trauma). Previously undetected congenital anorectal anomalies may be found, even in adults. Inspection of the lower back for sacral dimples may lead to a suspicion of occult spina bifida.

Occasionally other perianal conditions such as warts or dermatitis may be found. In cases of major sphincter damage or neuropathy, examination may reveal an anus which is completely patulous at rest. In less severe cases, minor traction at the anal verge will cause a profound anal relaxation with associated FI. Some patients have a "funnel-shaped" anus after previous anal surgery.[14] This can lead to trapping of soft stool at the end of defecation which is not wiped away with routine cleaning and subsequently stains the underwear.

SECTION 4 Diagnostic evaluation

St Mark's Hospital Bowel Diary

Name _____ Week beginning _____

Key ▦ ✓ = bowels open in toilet ☐ ✓ = bowel accident
P = pad/pants change

Special instructions
Please tick in the shaded column each time you open your bowels in the toilet.
Please tick in the white column each time you have a bowel accident or leakage.
Write P if you need to change a pad or pants.

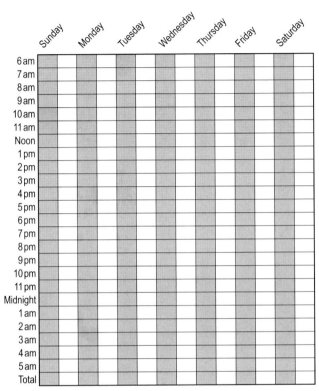

Figure 11.1 Example of a bowel diary.

Box 11.3 Physical examination results

Inspection	Anal canal length
Perineal soiling	Anorectal anomalies
Scars	Puborectalis tone and motion
Anal closure	Rectal content
Muscular defect	Soft tissue scarring
Loss of perineal body	Rectocele
Rectal prolapse	Intussusception
Muscular contraction	Rectovaginal fistula
Perineal descent	
Anal skin reflex to pinprick	**Endoscopy**
Anatomic anorectal pathology	Intussusception
Hemorrhoids	Solitary rectal ulcer
Skin tags	Scarring
Fistula	Mucosal defects
Mucosal ectropion	Neoplasm
Fissure	Inflammation
Others	Inflammatory bowel disease
Palpation	Infectious colitis
Resting tone	Others
Squeeze tone	Fistula
Sphincter defects	

From reference 9, with permission.

often have an internal and external component. Prolapsing hemorrhoids may only be evident on straining. Third-degree hemorrhoids are evident on inspection of the anus.

Rectal prolapse. It is notable that some patients with a frank prolapse are unaware of it. Patients reporting symptoms which might relate to a rectal prolapse (a sensation of the rectum protruding, needing to "push something back" after defecation or vigorous exercise, dragging, obstructed defecation, loss of formed stool without sensation in the absence of major neurologic diesase, or copious mucus leakage) should be examined with this possibility in mind. Few rectal prolapses are visible with the patient at rest and even upon bearing down or straining in the left lateral position, a prolapse may be easily missed. The patient may be reluctant to push strongly for fear of passing flatus or stool. By far the best position to examine for prolapse is with the patient squatting or sitting on the toilet. The patient should be left in privacy and instructed to strain maximally for 1–2 minutes. The examiner then leans the patient forward on the toilet and inspects for visible protrusion of the rectal mucosa. It is usual to report findings as partial or circumferential, and mucosal or full-thickness prolapse, with an estimation of the length of the prolapse beyond the anal verge.

Digital examination. Digital anal and rectal examination may indicate a low resting pressure in the anus, with very little resistance to finger insertion, suggesting internal anal sphincter weakness. The patient is then asked to squeeze on the examining finger and this may show a very uncoordinated response, or a weak squeeze pressure or rapid fatigue of that squeeze. However, findings should be interpreted with caution as examiner estimate of pressures shows a poor correlation with those measured objectively during manometry. It may also be possible to detect a low rectal lesion or a rectocele, or rectal loading in older and disabled patients.

Proctoscopy. Proctoscopic examination may reveal hemorrhoids, an anal fissure, prolapse of the rectal mucosa or other anal lesions. After insertion of the proctoscope, the central introducer of the proctoscope is withdrawn, allowing visualization of any hemorrhoids which will bulge into the anal lumen in the 3, 7, and 11 o'clock positions, and as the instrument is withdrawn their extent is noted. Hemorrhoids

Neurologic examination. Cursory evaluation of sensation and reflexes may indicate deficiencies which warrant more formal neurologic evaluation. Bowel problems can be the first symptoms of multiple sclerosis or other spinal disorders.[15,16]

Endoscopy. Patients with FI associated with an unexplained change in bowel habit may need exclusion of a malignancy or other bowel pathology such as inflammatory bowel disease or diverticular disease. This is particularly important if there is associated rectal bleeding, weight loss, anemia, and/or a strong family history in a patient over 55 years old. Colonoscopy is the investigation of choice, although barium enema may be more easily available in some centers and CT "virtual colonoscopy" is rapidly developing. In skilled hands and with good bowel preparation, complete views of the entire mucosa as far as the terminal ileum are achieved in the majority of cases.

Many patients are very concerned that their symptoms may herald a sinister bowel condition and even if the findings are negative, are greatly reassured on being told that symptoms are "benign," especially if they have had personal experience of friends or relatives with bowel cancer, which is today the second most common malignancy in western Europe. Solitary rectal ulcer syndrome may be visualized in patients who are chronically straining.

ANORECTAL PHYSIOLOGY TESTING

There is a variety of tests which are often performed together and usually referred to together as anorectal testing. Different laboratories will perform different combinations, often to very different protocols, with little standardization and no generally established normal ranges in most cases.[17] Unlike urodynamic testing, where international consensus has been developed on terminology and methods, this usually means that each set of tests has to be interpreted in the light of local norms and in the knowledge of the protocol used.[18]

Traditionally, the patient is positioned in the left lateral position with knees bent throughout these tests, which are normally performed sequentially. It is not usual to give any bowel preparation prior to the tests.

Manometry. Various different equipment is available for measuring anal pressures. Solid state, a single air- or water-filled micro balloon, or single- or multiple-channel (usually four or eight channels) water-perfused systems are all in use. Many are linked to computerized recording and interpretation systems. Any digital or instrumental examination of the anus is avoided for 20–30 minutes prior to manometry as this can affect the results (for example, manometry should not be done immediately after anal ultrasound or proctoscopy).[19]

The anal probe is inserted through the anal canal into the rectum (over 6 cm insertion will ensure that the anal margin is cleared). The probe is then gradually withdrawn, usually in 0.5 cm stages, and the resting pressure in the anal canal noted. This will enable an estimation of total functional anal length (the distance between first pressure rise as the probe leaves the rectum and enters the upper anus, until it reaches the anal verge and pressure is equal to atmospheric pressure). Resting pressure is mostly contributed by the internal anal sphincter and anal blood flow. Low pressure may indicate IAS weakness or disruption as seen on ultrasound and is usually associated with symptoms of passive fecal soiling.[20] It is usual to report the maximum resting pressure.

The probe is then reinserted and squeeze increments over resting pressure are recorded. This may just be at the point of maximal resting pressure or, more usually, a squeeze profile, with squeeze effort recorded at 0.5 cm intervals in the anal canal. It is usual to report the maximum squeeze increment over baseline resting pressure, usually repeated several times to check consistency. It is important to check that the patient is not straining or bearing down instead of squeezing as this can result in an artefactual high pressure. An endurance squeeze (ability to hold a squeeze before fatigue)[20] and a cough reflex may also be recorded (pressure increment above resting pressure during a forceful cough, reflecting reflex activity of the EAS). Figure 11.2 shows a typical manometric record. It is technically possible to perform ambulatory monitoring of manometric pressures but the clinical significance of findings has yet to be determined.[18]

Vector manometry uses computer manipulation of the readings from a multichannel anal probe to construct a three-dimensional reconstruction of an anal pressure profile (Fig. 11.3). This can be especially useful for anal mapping where no anal ultrasound is available and can help to identify occult sphincter injuries.[21]

Rectal sensation to distension. Rectal sensitivity to filling is usually tested using a rectal balloon which is seated just inside the rectum and gradually distended with air or water. The patient is asked to note the first sensation of rectal filling, when an urge to defecate is experienced and then when maximum tolerable volume is reached. The volume in the balloon is recorded at each point. The results will vary with the compliance of the balloon employed and whether air or water is used.

While exact values are not significant, the test may indicate a hypersensitive or very low-volume noncompliant rectum if all volumes are very low. If the volume for first sensation is above that expected, there may be a neuropathy. Some biofeedback protocols are designed to address delayed first sensation and aim to enable the patient to detect rectal

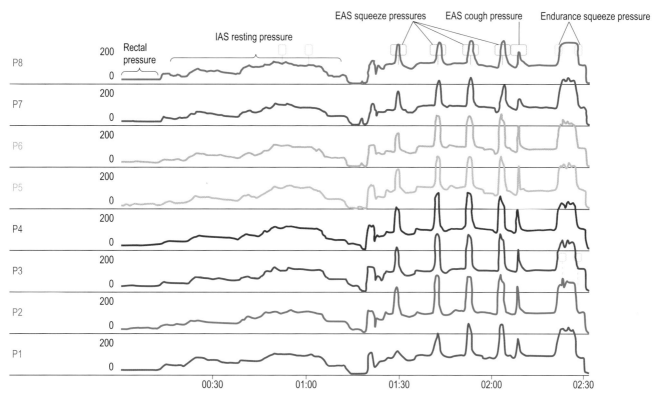

Figure 11.2 Typical manometric record.

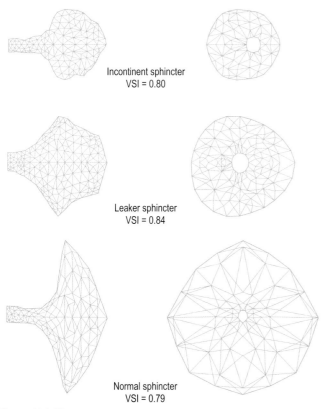

Figure 11.3 Vector manometry.

contents at progressively lower volumes[22,23] (see Chapter 16 for more details). High volumes at all three points may indicate a megarectum. Absent sensation is usually a marker for a major neurologic disorder. Filling of the balloon is usually stopped at 500 ml if no sensation is elicited.

Rectoanal inhibitory reflex. The normal response to rectal filling of sufficient volume is reflex anal relaxation. This is to allow the "sampling" described in Chapter 3. Absence of this reflex is a strong indication that Hirschsprung's disease may be present. An alternative is major neuropathy.

To perform this test, both a rectal distension balloon and an anal pressure probe are positioned. The rectal balloon is rapidly inflated and deflated with 50 ml of air (or a larger volume if this produces no response) and the anal pressure is observed. Normally, there should be a momentary reflex pressure rise (contraction of the EAS) followed by an inhibition and fall in anal pressure, which usually lasts 5–10 seconds until it recovers its resting value (Fig. 11.4). This response can be profound and prolonged in neuropathy but its presence excludes Hirschsprung's disease.

Balloon expulsion test. A rectal balloon is inflated with air or water, either to a preset volume or until the patient experiences an urge to defecate. The patient is then instructed to attempt to expel the balloon in simulation of

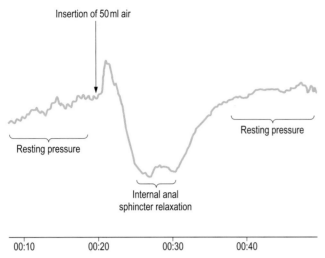

Figure 11.4 Rectoanal inhibitory reflex.

defecation and observed for coordination of this defecatory effort. Some patients will demonstrate massive straining effort but with no movement of the balloon; a few will have a true "paradoxic contraction" or "anismus" of the puborectalis and anal sphincter,[24] suggesting that FI may be secondary to an evacuatory difficulty with incomplete rectal emptying. Alternatively the balloon may be expelled with little or no effort at all, suggesting minimal sphincter resistance, or rectal prolapse may be observed during the expulsion effort.

Barostat compliance testing. Compliance testing measures rectal distensibility, the ability of the rectum to hold a larger volume of stool at a given pressure. A normal rectum is compliant, with an increase in volume resulting in little or no pressure rise.[17] If compliance is poor, urgency and frequency may result.[25] The barostat machine distends a rectal balloon in a controlled ramping of volume and measures the pressure–volume relationship (compliance curve).

EMG. Surface EMG is not validated for assessment of anorectal function.[25] EMG mapping of the anal sphincter via needle electrodes is a sensitive measure of EAS and puborectalis function and denervation[25] and was once the best way to detect sphincter dysfunction or defects. However, it is painful for the patient and is largely superseded by anal ultrasound, except as a research tool.

Electrosensitivity testing. A ring electrode mounted on a tube is inserted into the anal canal and a low-frequency current is gradually switched up until the patient can feel it. This threshold is recorded. Several trials are usually made to ensure consistency and to overcome any learning effect. This is then repeated at a higher frequency in the rectum. If there is stool in the rectum, recording may not be accurate

and it is occasionally necessary to ask the patient to empty the rectum and repeat the test if an abnormal result is obtained. High sensory thresholds are often a marker for hindgut denervation.[19]

Pudendal nerve terminal motor latency (PNTML). A specially constructed finger electrode is worn and used to stimulate the pudendal nerve during rectal examination. The time from stimulation until reflex contraction of the anus is measured electronically. It was once thought that a prolonged latency time related to neurologic damage, often as a consequence of childbirth, and that this could predict response to treatments such as surgery. Delayed or prolonged latency time was taken as a surrogate marker for pudendal nerve injury.[18] However, the test is very open to operator variation and is not supported by neurophysiologic theory. Thirty-one percent of patients with bilateral neuropathy have normal sphincter function and 49% of those with normal PNTML have reduced squeeze pressures.[26]

Expert opinion does not support the validity or reliability of this test[18,25] and its use is decreasing. However, it is still widely quoted, especially in outcome studies.

Saline retention test. This test involves infusing up to 1500 ml of saline into the rectum via a catheter and observing the volume infused when the patient first experiences anal leakage of the saline.[27] The test does discriminate continent from incontinent people both in rectal volumes tolerated and the detection of leakage.[27] It is less used than formerly.

Perineal descent. Especially after childbirth, women may have a lax perineum, which may be associated with either FI or evacuation difficulty. It is possible to measure the position of the perineum at rest, relative to bony landmarks, and during bearing down or straining to measure the degree of movement by using a specially constructed perineometer.

ANAL ULTRASOUND

The advent of endoanal ultrasound has revolutionized both understanding and investigation of FI.[28,29] Manometry may offer little extra information where ultrasound is available.[30] The images have been validated both with EMG sphincter mapping[31] and histologically.[32] Interrater and intrarater variability can be a problem.[33,34] Although the initial investment in equipment is costly, the test itself is relatively quick and simple, taking 5–10 minutes. Except in cases of clear sphincter rupture, it would now not be considered ethical in many setting to proceed to secondary anal sphincter repair without this test.[3] However, interpretation of the images is not always straightforward and remains a skilled procedure requiring expert training, with interpretation being very operator dependent.[35]

No preparation is needed prior to the procedure. It is usual to examine the patient in the prone position, as a lateral position can artificially distort the symmetry of the image. The ultrasound probe is inserted into the rectum and then slowly withdrawn. Standard axial imaging of the anal canal with a 10 MHz mechanical rotated crystal gives a 360° image of the typical four-layer pattern of the sphincters. The image is seen in real time and is usually recorded for later review or printing. Several structures can be seen quite clearly (Fig. 11.5).

The subepithelial layer is moderately reflective. The internal anal sphincter shows as a dark well-defined low reflective ring. Its diameter can be accurately measured. Normally the IAS thickens with age so that the normal diameter of 1–2 mm in young adults increases to 2–3 mm in middle age and over 3 mm in older adults.[36] Idiopathic degeneration of the internal sphincter[37] can be diagnosed by an abnormally thin IAS for the patient's age. Abnormal anal distension may result in a completely fragmented IAS, as after an anal stretch. Iatrogenic surgical injury, such as following sphincterotomy or hemorrhoidectomy, may show as a single defect in the IAS. Damage resulting from past or present anal sepsis may also be defined.

The longitudinal layer is a complex structure with a large fibroelastic[38] and muscle component, the latter formed from the puboanalis as well as the longitudinal muscle of the rectum.

The external anal sphincter shows as light bands of muscle surrounding the IAS. The external sphincter is better defined in men than women, in whom it tends to be similar in reflectivity to the longitudinal layer. It is then distinguished only by interface reflections between muscle/fat planes either side. High in the anal canal, the puborectalis shows as an incomplete symmetric muscle ring, especially in women. Care is needed not to misdiagnose this normal anatomy of a shorter sphincter anteriorly than posteriorly as a high EAS defect. For the distal two-thirds of the anal canal, the EAS should form a complete ring. The transverse perineii fuse anterior with the sphincter in women, whereas in men they remain separate.[39] EAS disruption or scarring can be visualized and accurately located (Fig. 11.6). Muscle quality or degeneration can also be suspected, although this is better quantified objectively on MRI (see below).

A probe designed for transvaginal examination may be used in women to image the sphincters from the perineum.[40] Three-dimensional anal ultrasound uses computer reconstruction to give 3D images of anal structures. At present this is largely a research tool.[41]

MAGNETIC RESONANCE IMAGING

Magnetic resonance imaging can be used as an alternative or adjunct to anal ultrasound.[29] Dedicated endoanal coils are

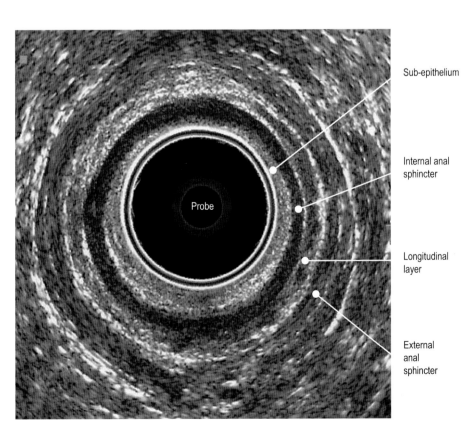

Figure 11.5 Normal anal ultrasound.

Sub-epithelium

Internal anal sphincter

Probe

Longitudinal layer

External anal sphincter

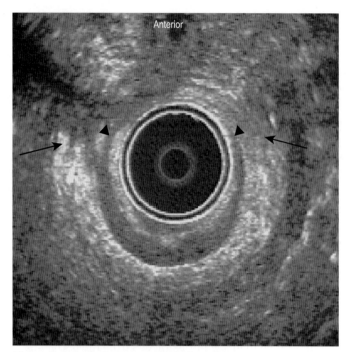

Figure 11.6 Anal ultrasound—EAS disruption.

not widely available but could be used with any magnet. The coil is inserted with the patient in the left lateral position, then the patient is turned supine and the coil wedged in position with sandbags. The total examination time is about 20 minutes. During a sequence, which takes up to 5 minutes, the patient must remain still as any movement degrades the image.

T2-weighted sequences in axial, coronal, and sagittal planes are acquired. The smooth muscle of the internal sphincter is higher in intensity than striated muscle of the external sphincter. Fat is much brighter than either. This gives the major advantage of the MRI: the clarity with which the quality of the external sphincter may be assessed. MRI is superior to ultrasound in diagnosis of perianal sepsis and in quantifying external anal sphincter muscle degeneration.[42,43] Poor-quality muscle as diagnosed on MRI has been found to be associated with poor results from anal sphincter repair.[44] However, interobserver reproducibility may not be as good as for anal ultrasound.[33,43]

Dynamic MRI allows visualization of all pelvic organs and the pelvic floor and puborectalis in motion, such as during straining.[25]

PROCTOGRAPHY

A defecating proctogram can be used to define the extent and possible significance of a rectocele and to look for intrarectal or intraanal intussusception of the rectal mucosa, or rectal prolapse.[29]

The rectum is catheterized and filled with 120 ml of barium paste. The small bowel is opacified with a dilute barium suspension (taken 30 minutes before the procedure). The patient is then seated on a radiotranslucent commode and asked to pass the barium in simulated defecation with screening from the side (Fig. 11.7). Ability to retain the paste prior to defecation may be impaired in severe sphincter

Figure 11.7 Proctogram.

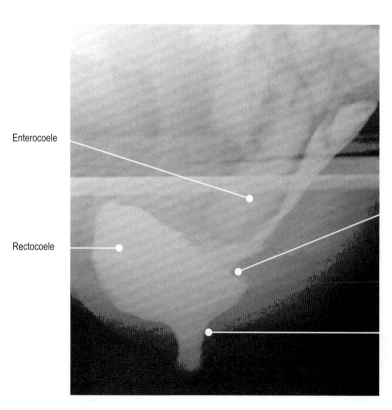

dysfunction. The anorectal angle can be assessed at rest and during defecation. At rest, the anorectal junction is at the level of the ischial tuberosities and the anal canal is closed. Normal function is indicated by relaxation of the puborectalis with opening of the anal canal and rapid and complete evacuation within 30 seconds. During evacuation, the anorectal angle widens as the anorectal junction descends and the anal canal opens. At the end of evacuation, pelvic floor tone returns and the puborectalis pulls the anorectal junction upwards and forwards, back to the resting position.

Slow evacuation (less than two-thirds evacuated within 30 seconds) with poor opening of the anal canal is typical of anismus.[45] A rectocele is measured from the anterior margin of the anal canal to the anterior aspect of the rectocele. This is common and usually asymptomatic. An anterior bulging greater than 3 cm, with paste in a rectocele, is considered significant if this does not empty completely at the end of evacuation. In this situation, the patient is asked to apply digital pressure to the perineum or the posterior vaginal wall. If the rectocele then empties completely, this usually indicates that a satisfactory result would be obtained from surgical rectocele repair. Complete rectal prolapse will usually already have been diagnosed on clinical examination, but more minor degrees can be visualized. However, the clinical significance of mucosal prolapse is controversial.

FURTHER TESTS

Depending on the patient's history, persistent loose stool may indicate that a stool sample should be checked for infection or parasites. A lactose tolerance breath test can detect lactose malabsorption and a hydrogen breath test can detect bacterial overgrowth in the gut.[46] Laxative abuse may also be checked. Blood tests may be indicated when an over- or underactive thyroid or other metabolic disturbance needs to be excluded, and for celiac disease. The need for a more general gastroenterologic opinion should be considered.

REFERENCES

1. Norton C, Chelvanayagam S. A nursing assessment tool for adults with fecal incontinence. J Wound Ostomy Cont Nurs 2000;27:279–291.
2. Pemberton JH. Anorectal and pelvic floor disorders: putting physiology into practice. J Gastroenterol Hepatol 1990;5(Suppl 1):127–143.
3. Law PJ, Kamm MA, Bartram CI. Anal endosonography in the investigation of fecal incontinence. Br J Surg 1991;78:312–314.
4. Leigh RJ, Turnberg LA. Fecal incontinence: the unvoiced symptom. Lancet 1982;1:1349–1351.
5. Johanson JF, Lafferty J. Epidemiology of fecal incontinence: the silent affliction. Am J Gastroenterol 1996;91(1):33–36.
6. Norton C, Chelvanayagam S. Bowel continence nursing. Beaconsfield: Beaconsfield Publishers; 2004.
7. Donovan J, Bosch R, Gotoh M, al. Assessment of symptoms and quality of life. In: Abrams P, Cardozo L, Wein A, Khoury S, eds. Incontinence. Plymouth: Health Books; 2005.
8. Vaizey CJ, Carapeti EA, Cahill JA, Kamm MA. Prospective comparison of fecal incontinence grading systems. Gut 1999;44:77–80.
9. Jorge JM, Wexner SD. Etiology and management of fecal incontinence. Dis Colon Rectum 1993;36(1):77–97.
10. Pescatori M, Anastasio G, Bottini C, Mentasti A. New grading and scoring for anal incontinence. Dis Colon Rectum 1992;35:482–487.
11. Bugg GJ, Kiff ES, Hosker G. A new condition-specific health-related quality of life questionnaire for the assessment of women with anal incontinence. Br J Obstet Gynaecol 2001; 108:1057–1067.
12. Rockwood TH, Church JM, Fleshman JW, et al. Patient and surgeon ranking of the severity of symptoms associated with fecal incontinence: the fecal incontinence severity index. Dis Colon Rectum 1999;42:1525–1532.
13. Rockwood TH, Church JM, Fleshman JW, et al. Fecal incontinence quality of life scale. Dis Colon Rectum 2000;43:9–17.
14. Buchanan G, Cohen R. Common ano-rectal conditions. In: Norton C, Chelvanayagam S, eds. Bowel continence nursing. Beaconsfield: Beaconsfield Publishers; 2004.
15. Hinds JP, Eidelman BH, Wald A. Prevalence of bowel dysfunction in multiple sclerosis. Gastroenterology 1990;98:1538–1542.
16. Lawthom C, Durdey P, Hughes T. Constipation as a presenting symptom of multiple sclerosis. Lancet 2003;362:958.
17. Byrne PJ. Indications for gastrointestinal physiological assessment. In: Duthie GS, Gardiner A, eds. Physiology of the gastrointestinal tract. London: Whurr Publishers; 2004: 1–14.
18. Diamant NE, Kamm MA, Wald A, Whitehead WE. AGA technical review on anorectal testing techniques. Gastroenterology 1999;116(3):735–760.
19. Nicholls T. Anorectal physiology investigation techniques. In: Norton C, Chelvanayagam S, eds. Bowel continence nursing. Beaconsfield: Beaconsfield Publishers; 2004.
20. Marcello PW, Barrett RC, Coller JA, et al. Fatigue rate index as a new measure of external sphincter function. Dis Colon Rectum 1998;41:336–343.
21. Perry RE, Blatchford GJ, Christiansen MA, Thorso AG, Attwood SEA. Manometric diagnosis of anal sphincter injuries. Am J Surg 1990;159:112–117.
22. Chiarioni G, Bassotti G, Stranganini S, Vantini I, Whitehead WE, Stegagnini S. Sensory retraining is key to biofeedback therapy for formed stool incontinence. Am J Gastroenterol 2002;97:109–117.
23. Whitehead WE, Engel BT, Schuster MM. Perception of rectal distension is necessary to prevent fecal incontinence. Adv Physiol Sci 1980;17:203–209.
24. Preston DM, Lennard-Jones JE. Anismus in chronic constipation. Dig Dis Sci 1985; 30(5):413–418.
25. Bharucha AE. Outcome measures for fecal incontinence: anorectal structure and function. Gastroenterology 2004;126:S90–S98.
26. Hill J, Hosker G, Kiff ES. Pudendal nerve terminal motor latency measurements: what they do and do not tell us. Br J Surg 2002;89:1268–1269.
27. Read NW, Harford WV, Schmulen AC, Read M, Santa Ana C, Fordtran JS. A clinical study of patients with fecal incontinence and diarrhoea. Gastroenterology 1979;76:747–756.
28. Law PJ, Bartram CI. Anal endosonography: technique and normal anatomy. Gastrointest Radiol 1989;14:349–353.
29. Bartram CI, DeLancey JO. Imaging pelvic floor disorders. Berlin: Springer-Verlag; 2003.
30. De Leeuw JW, Vierhout ME, Struijk PC, Auwerda HJ, Bac DJ,

Wallenburg CS. Relationship of anal endosonography and manometry to anorectal complaints. Dis Colon Rectum 2002;45:1004–1010.

31. Burnett SJ, Speakman CTM, Kamm MA, Bartram CI. Confirmation of endosonographic detection of external anal sphincter defects by simultaneous electromyographic mapping. Br J Surg 1991;78:448–450.

32. Sultan AH, Kamm MA, Talbot IC, Nicholls RJ, Bartram CI. Anal endosonography for identifying external sphincter defects confirmed histologically. Br J Surg 1994;81:463–465.

33. Gold DM, Halligan S, Kmiot WA, Bartram CI. Intraobserver and interobserver agreement in anal endosonography. Br J Surg 1999;86:371–375.

34. Enck P, Heyer T, Gantke B, et al. How reproducible are measures of the anal sphincter muscle diameter by endoanal ultrasound? Am J Gastroenterol 1997;92:293–296.

35. Bartram CI, Sultan AH. Anal endosonography in fecal incontinence. Gut 1995;37:4–6.

36. Frudinger A, Halligan S, Bartram CI, Price AB, Kamm MA, Winter R. Female anal sphincter: age-related differences in asymptomatic volunteers with high-frequency endoanal US. Radiology 2002;224(2):417–423.

37. Vaizey CJ, Kamm MA, Bartram CI. Primary degeneration of the internal anal sphincter as a cause of passive fecal incontinence. Lancet 1997;349:612–615.

38. Lunniss PJ, Phillips RK. Anatomy and function of the anal longitudinal muscle. Br J Surg 1992;79(9):882–884.

39. Williams AB, Bartram CI, Halligan S, Marshall MM, Nicholls RJ, Kmiot WA. Endosonographic anatomy of the normal anal canal compared with endocoil magnetic resonance imaging. Dis Colon Rectum 2002;45(2):176–183.

40. Stewart LK, Wilson SR. Transvaginal sonography of the anal sphincter: reliable, or not? Am J Roentgenol 1999;173(1):179–185.

41. Gold DM, Bartram CI, Halligan S, Humphries KN, Kamm MA, Kmiot WA. Three-dimensional endoanal sonography in assessing anal canal injury. Br J Surg 1999;86(3):365–370.

42. Rociu E, Stoker J, Eijkemans MJ, Schouten WR, Lameris JS. Fecal incontinence: endoanal US versus endoanal MR imaging. Radiology 1999;212(2):453–458.

43. Malouf AJ, Halligan S, Williams A, Bartram C, Dhillon S, Kamm MA. Prospective assessment of interobserver agreement for endoanal MRI in fecal incontinence. Abdom Imag 2001;26:76–78.

44. Briel JW, Stoker J, Rociu E, Lameris JS, Hop WC, Schouten WR. External anal sphincter atrophy on endoanal magnetic resonance imaging adversely affects continence after sphincteroplasty. Br J Surg 1999;86(10):1322–1327.

45. Halligan S, Malouf A, Bartram CI, Marshall M, Hollings N, Kamm MA. Predictive value of impaired evacuation at proctography in diagnosing anismus. Am J Roentgenol 2001; 177(3):633–636.

46. Vasani JP, Tsai HH. Breath testing and its interpretation. In: Duthie GS, Gardiner A, eds. Physiology of the gastrointestinal tract. London: Whurr Publishers; 2004: 58–72.

SECTION 4 Diagnostic evaluation

Diagnosis of Pelvic Organ Prolapse

Michael K Flynn and Cindy L Amundsen

INTRODUCTION

In an age in which imaging modalities are used to diagnose an ever-increasing number of medical conditions, pelvic organ prolapse (POP) remains one of the few conditions that continue to be diagnosed primarily by the patient's history and physical examination. POP is a very complex condition ranging from an asymptomatic bulge into the vaginal canal to complete uterine procidentia.

The diagnosis of POP can be complicated by several factors. There is an absence of a clear universally accepted definition of normal and abnormal pelvic support. While a trained practitioner can easily identify anatomically perfect pelvic support and a lay person can easily identify procidentia as pathologic, the clinical significance of more mild POP remains unclear. Indeed, many question whether the anatomic stage I or stage II POP is truly abnormal as it may occur in up to 50% of asymptomatic women presenting for routine gynecologic care.[1] Besides the absence of universally accepted definitions of POP, the symptoms of POP are often vague and difficult to correlate with objective findings. Finally, POP is often associated with dysfunction in the bladder or rectum and distinguishing symptoms due to POP from symptoms due to dysfunction in those systems can be exceedingly difficult, particularly if the symptoms are out of proportion to the degree of prolapse observed.

Despite these limitations in the diagnosis of prolapse, POP clearly exists and in many cases is amenable to repair. When diagnosing POP, one should both identify the affected areas of pelvic support and characterize the severity of the defect and associated symptoms in each compartment.

The vagina is divided into three areas of distinct support: the anterior, apical, and posterior compartments. The anterior and posterior compartments may be further divided into proximal and distal segments. These distinctions are based on the nature of the anatomic support for each compartment as well as the nature of symptoms associated with support defects in each compartment. The compartment involved along with the severity of the anatomic defect and the associated symptoms generally determine how the prolapse is treated.

The severity of the anatomic defect can be measured objectively with quantification systems such as the Pelvic Organ Prolapse Quantification (POP-Q) system. Because POP is not associated with significant morbidity or mortality, symptom severity is determined with changes in the patient's quality of life and can be quantified with validated disease-specific quality of life (QOL) questionnaires. Once the defects and symptoms have been identified, severity characterized and associated pelvic organ functions assessed, POP can be diagnosed and treated appropriately.

QUANTIFICATION OF PROLAPSE: THE POP-Q SYSTEM

Before discussing the clinical evaluation of POP, it is worth reviewing the system used to quantify POP. Until the mid 1990s most surgeons used the Baden Walker system for classification of severity of POP.[2] In 1996 Bump et al published the International Continence Society's Pelvic Organ Prolapse Quantification (POP-Q) system designed to objectively measure the degree of prolapse in the anterior, apical, and posterior vaginal compartments.[3] This is now the recognized classification system for prolapse staging for the International Continence Society, American Urogynecologic Society, and the Society of Gynecologic Surgeons.

Figure 12.1 shows the classic schematic diagram of the different measurements taken for the POP-Q system as described by Bump et al, superimposed on a sagittal view of the female pelvis to better demonstrate the significance of each point and their relationships to important anatomic structures.[4] The system emphasizes the use of terms referring to the vaginal compartments (anterior, posterior, and apical) as opposed to the traditional terms (cystocele, enterocele, and rectocele) because the latter implies that the corresponding organs are involved without any ancillary evidence. For instance, it is not uncommon for a posterior

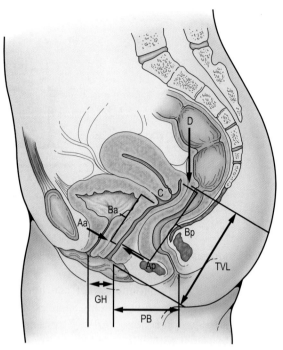

Figure 12.1 Nine measurements are used to evaluate pelvic organ support. This drawing demonstrates stage 0 prolapse. See text for explanation of the definitions of each point (Reproduced with permission from Prietto NM, Luber K, Nayen C. OBS Management 2003; May:80–95[14].)

vaginal wall defect to be called a rectocele without showing that the organ filling the defect is not small bowel or other structure. Using references to the vaginal compartments avoids this potential error.

The figure shows the nine measurements (Aa, Ba, C, D, Ap, Bp, GH, PB, and TVL) that comprise the POP-Q. The anterior compartment is characterized by Aa and Ba, the vaginal apex by C and D, and the posterior compartment by Ap and Bp. GH, PB, and TVL represent the genital hiatus, perineal body, and total vaginal length respectively. We recommend performing these measurements with the patient either in the supine position or at a 45° angle seated in a birthing chair. Ideally, these points are taken at the point of maximal prolapse, which is best achieved with the patient performing a Valsalva maneuver. An instrument such as a sponge forceps, marked in 1 cm increments, facilitates obtaining these measurements. All measurements of the vaginal compartments are made using centimeters in relation to the hymeneal ring, with negative values reflecting maximal descent above the hymen and positive numbers reserved for prolapse beyond the hymen. The points are defined as follows.

Aa: a fixed point on the midline of the anterior vaginal wall that is 3 cm proximal to the urethral meatus. Once this point has been identified, its relationship to the hymen at maximal prolapse is measured. By definition, it is −3 in a patient with perfect support and +3 when completely prolapsed.

Ba: a floating point located between Aa and C. It is defined as the point between Aa and C that prolapses the lowest at maximal strain. In an anatomically normal woman, it is equal to Aa or −3 and in a woman with complete procidentia, is equal to point C. This site is best located by placing the posterior blade of a bivalve speculum in the vagina against the posterior vaginal wall, taking care to avoid blocking descent of the cervix or vaginal cuff.

Ap: a fixed point 3 cm from the hymen in the midline of the posterior vaginal wall. Once this point is identified, its relationship to the hymen during Valsalva is measured. By definition, Ap is −3 in the absence of prolapse and +3 when completely prolapsed.

Bp: a floating point that is identified in a manner identical to Ba except that it is in reference to the posterior vaginal wall. By definition, Bp is equal to Ap or −3 in the absence of posterior compartment prolapse and equal to point C in the patient with complete procidentia.

C: refers to the most dependent edge of the cervix or the vaginal cuff in patients with posthysterectomy prolapse.

D: refers to the posterior fornix in the patient who still has a cervix. This measurement is eliminated in the post-hysterectomy patient. This point is crucial in the distinction of cervical elongation from uterine prolapse.

TVL: is the total vaginal length. The prolapsed vagina is placed back in the pelvis and the greatest length from the apex to the hymen is measured.

GH: the distance from the posterior midline hymen to the middle of the urethral meatus.

PB: the distance from the posterior midline hymen to the midanal opening.

POP-Q staging. Once the POP-Q measurements have been obtained, the prolapse can be staged. The POP-Q measurements are divided into the anterior, posterior, and apical compartments and each compartment staged separately as follows.

Stage 0: is near-perfect anatomic support with no prolapse. It is demonstrated by Aa, Ba, Ap, and Bp all equal to −3 and no more than 2 cm difference between TVL and C.

Stage I: defined as any value of Aa, BA, Ap, Bp or C greater than −1 (i.e. prolapse is present but no point is lower than 1 cm above the hymen).

Stage II: defined as the leading edge of prolapse being within 1 cm of the hymen. It may be 1 cm above the hymen or extend to 1 cm beyond the hymen.

Stage III: defined as the leading edge of the prolapse being greater than 1 cm beyond the hymen but the difference between C and TVL is greater than 2 cm.

Stage IV: the difference between C and TVL is less than 2, indicating complete vaginal eversion.

The significance of the stages is yet to be proven as a reliable scale for POP severity. For instance, stage I prolapse may represent normal for many women.[1,5,6] However, the staging system clearly describes increasingly severe anatomic prolapse along an ordinal scale. This may be more useful in the quantification of differences between preoperative and postoperative prolapse as well as for the assessment of changes in POP severity over time.

OBTAINING A CLINICAL HISTORY OF A PATIENT WITH PELVIC ORGAN PROLAPSE

As with any medical condition, the evaluation of the patient begins with a thorough history designed to elicit the nature and severity of the patient's chief complaint. Patients with POP most commonly complain of either pelvic or vaginal pressure or else of "something bulging" out of the vagina.[7,8] The symptom of pelvic pressure is present in 60–75% of patients with demonstrable POP.[9,10] However, while this is a common complaint in patients with POP, it correlates weakly with the severity of prolapse and does not correlate at all with prolapse from a specific compartment.[9] The complaint of protrusion from the vagina is less common than that of pelvic pressure but is better correlated with increasingly anatomically severe prolapse.[9,10] Historically, clinicians have attributed other symptoms such as pelvic pain or low back pain to POP but recent studies have shown that the symptoms are neither specific nor sensitive for POP.[5,9-11]

When a patient presents complaining of pressure or a bulge, clinicians should inquire about the specific characteristics of the symptoms. In particular, details should be obtained concerning the onset and duration of the symptoms as well as the absence or presence of any associated pain or bowel, bladder or sexual dysfunction. If the symptoms vary with activity (walking, standing or lifting), position (sitting, standing or lying down), diet, bowel activity or intercourse, the details should be documented. If the patient complains of a protrusion, how far out does the mass protrude from the vagina? Is it visible? Does it need to be replaced for complete bowel or bladder empting (splinting)? How do these symptoms affect her life and ability to participate in social activities? If a clinician is not administering one of the disease-specific QOL questionnaires, he or she should completely explore and document the effect of the prolapse on the patient's social and emotional well-being.

The clinician should also specifically inquire about symptoms associated with the pelvic organs, including the bowel, bladder, and vagina. In particular, the respective function of these organs, including urine storage and emptying, fecal and flatal storage and evacuation and sexual function, should be systematically explored. It is very common to find symptoms associated with these organ functions in patients with POP and the astute clinician will systematically explore

these systems for evidence of dysfunction when evaluating a patient with POP.[9,12-16] Patients should be asked about symptoms of stress and urge urinary incontinence (urgency, frequency or urinary leakage). Should the patient acknowledge urinary leakage, she should be evaluated for incontinence and the reader is referred to Chapter 10 for further information on this.

Stress urinary incontinence may correlate with mild stage I or II anterior prolapse but is often absent in advanced prolapse.[9,17] Other urinary symptoms that may relate to POP include signs of difficulty with voiding such as urinary hesitancy, intermittent flow, a weak urinary stream, the sensation of incomplete emptying, needing to replace the bulge into the vagina (splinting) to empty the bladder or need to change positions on the commode to empty the bladder. Unfortunately, while these symptoms may be present in up to 50% of patients with POP, they surprisingly do not correlate well with anterior compartment defects. In fact, several studies have indicated that isolated apical and posterior defects may significantly affect urinary flow and bladder emptying[9,10,13,17] so such symptoms should not be considered indicative of an anterior defect. In addition, one must be aware that these urinary symptoms may be caused by dysfunction of the bladder itself rather than the vaginal prolapse.

The clinician should also explore symptoms of defecatory and sexual dysfunction. The most common defecatory symptom associated with POP is constipation.[9,10] Unfortunately, it is not clear whether constipation precedes prolapse or if it is a result of the prolapse. Most authors feel that long-standing constipation plays a role in the etiology of prolapse but can also be exacerbated by the prolapse.[18,19] Fecal or flatal incontinence is occasionally found in association with POP, particularly in those patients with distal posterior or perineal defects.[9,14] The reader is referred to Chapter 11 for details on the proper evaluation of anal incontinence. Other symptoms that may suggest defecatory problems include the need to splint the vagina to empty the bowels, incomplete evacuation or digital evacuation of stool. These symptoms do not correlate well with a specific anatomic compartment, although they tend to be found in conjunction with posterior or apical defects.[9,19,20]

Finally, sexual activity is often impaired in this group and up to 40% of patients will not be sexually active due to the prolapse.[12] Inquiring about sexual activity is an important part of the assessment of quality of life and the reason for any abstinence from sexual activity should be sought. Even if the patient is sexually active, she should be asked about dyspareunia or other difficulties with intercourse.

POP is not generally associated with marked morbidity or mortality but is associated with a significant decrease in quality of life. Therefore questions concerning this should be asked. Recently, two questionnaires, the Pelvic

Floor Distress Inventory (PFDI) and Pelvic Floor Impact Questionnaire (PFIQ), have been validated for use in the assessment of POP.[21] These questionnaires, shown in Boxes 12.1 and 12.2, may not be diagnostic per se of POP but can be used as a measure of the impact that POP is having on the patient and they do correlate with severity of the prolapse.[21]

Patients with POP have a high incidence of prior prolapse repairs and the past surgical history should specifically comment on the details concerning prior urologic, gynecologic or hernia surgeries. Reports of prior diagnostic procedures, operative notes, and discharge summaries should be requested and reviewed if available.

Finally, as with all medical conditions, a thorough past medical history should be obtained. The past medical history and review of systems should also specifically characterize any medical conditions that may be relevant to the management of POP. In addition, because POP tends to occur in older populations, there is a greater prevalence of cardiovascular, pulmonary, renal, and cognitive disorders that may dramatically affect the patient's surgical risk profile and alter available therapies.

PHYSICAL EXAMINATION OF THE PELVIC ORGAN PROLAPSE PATIENT

As with any patient evaluation, the physical examination should include a complete evaluation of organ systems outside the pelvis. The prevalence of POP increases with age and is often managed surgically. Attention needs to be paid to screening for signs of cardiovascular, pulmonary,

---

Box 12.1   Short form: Pelvic Floor Impact Questionnaire 7-item. Patients are asked to select the best answer to each question

Name _____

Has your prolapse affected your:
1) Ability to do household chores (cooking, housecleaning, laundry)?
   ☐ Not at all ☐ Mildly ☐ Moderately ☐ Severely

2) Physical recreation such as walking, swimming or other exercises?
   ☐ Not at all ☐ Mildly ☐ Moderately ☐ Severely

3) Entertainment activities (movies, church)?
   ☐ Not at all ☐ Mildly ☐ Moderately ☐ Severely

4) Ability to travel by car or bus more than 30 minutes from home?
   ☐ Not at all ☐ Mildly ☐ Moderately ☐ Severely

5) Participation in social activities outside your home?
   ☐ Not at all ☐ Mildly ☐ Moderately ☐Severely

6) Emotional health (nervousness, depression)?
   ☐ Not at all ☐ Mildly ☐ Moderately ☐ Severely

7) Feeling frustrated?
   ☐ Not at all ☐Mildly ☐Moderately ☐Severely

Box 12.2   Short form: Pelvic Floor Distress Inventory 22-item. For each question, patients fill in the blank with each phrase underneath the question. The same multiple-choice responses (not at all, mildly, moderately, severely) used for the PFIQ-7 are used for the PFDI-22

POPDI—6

Do you usually _____, and if so how much are you bothered by:
1. experience pressure in the lower abdomen
2. experience heaviness or dullness in the abdomen or genital area
3. have a bulge or something falling out that you can see or feel in the vaginal area
4. have to push on the vagina or around the rectum to have or complete a bowel movement
5. experience a feeling of incomplete bladder emptying
6. have to push up on a bulge in the vaginal area with your fingers to start or complete urination

CRADI—8

_____, and if so how much are you bothered by:
1. Do you usually feel you need to strain too hard to have a bowel movement
2. Do you usually feel you have not completely emptied your bowels at the end of bowel movement
3. Do you usually lose stool beyond your control if your stool is well formed
4. Do you usually lose stool beyond your control if your stool is loose or liquid
5. Do you usually lose gas from the rectum beyond your control
6. Do you usually have pain when you pass your stool
7. Do you usually experience a strong sense of urgency and have to rush to the bathroom to have a bowel movement
8. Does part of your bowel ever pass through the rectum and bulge outside during or after a bowel movement

UDI—8

Do you usually have _____, and if so how much are you bothered by:
1. frequent urination
2. leakage related to feeling of urgency
3. leakage related to activity, coughing or sneezing
4. leakage when you go from sitting to standing
5. small amounts of urine leakage (that is, drops)
6. difficulty emptying the bladder
7. pain or discomfort in the lower abdomen or genital area
8. pain in the middle of your lower abdomen as your bladder fills

---

renal, and cognitive disorders common in this group. If any signs or symptoms of significant disease are found in these systems, formal consultations from appropriate specialists should be considered.

Because POP is a problem confined primarily to the pelvis, the pelvic examination is the single most important objective evaluation of prolapse. Instruments that are helpful in the assessment of prolapse include a bivalve speculum, sponge forceps marked in 1 cm increments, and cotton swabs. With the patient in the lithotomy position, one can begin with the assessment of the vulva and perineum. Initial evaluation begins with an overall examination of scarring and any gross visual deformity of normal vulvar structures. This should include an assessment of the estrogenization of the patient's tissue as well as the presence of masses such as urethral diverticulum, Bartholin gland or Gartner's duct cysts that can be mistaken for prolapse. At this time, the external measurements of the POP-Q system, GH and PB, can be obtained.

A neurologic examination of the vulva and perineum is also performed at this time. Using the cotton swab, sensory function is assessed, paying particular attention to the sacral dermatomes. The following sacral reflexes should be tested. The *anal reflex* is triggered by stroking the skin lateral to the anus, which results in a reflexive contraction of the anus in women with an intact reflex. The *bulbocavernosus reflex* is triggered by gentle tapping or squeezing of the clitoris and results in the contraction of the bulbocavernosus muscle. These reflexes can be absent in many neurologically intact women so while their presence is reassuring, their absence is not diagnostic of a nerve injury.[22] However, any asymmetry may represent a neurologic deficit that may require further evaluation.

Once the neurologic evaluation is complete, a bivalve speculum will allow for assessment of the cervix and upper vagina which should be examined for lesions or other signs of pathology. Formal objective assessment of prolapse is typically performed at this point, beginning with the apex. Point C can be measured if the cervix or vaginal cuff is easily visualized and its descent not obstructed by the speculum. With the speculum partly withdrawn to avoid obstructing descent and the patient performing a Valsalva, points C and D can be measured. With the speculum removed, the sponge clamp is inserted into the vagina until the head is in the posterior fornix, to allow for measurement of total vaginal length.

Assessment of the anterior wall begins with a visual inspection of the urethra and urethral meatus. The presence of urethral prolapse, caruncle, diverticulum or a Skene's gland cyst should be noted. The evaluation for prolapse is best done with a Graves speculum disassembled and the posterior blade used to isolate compartments. With the posterior blade of the speculum inserted to the vaginal apex, gentle pressure against the posterior wall allows for isolation of the anterior compartment. The anterior wall is examined for evidence of prolapse and any descent is measured using the POP-Q system discussed above. When assessing point Ba, the speculum blade should be partly withdrawn to be sure that the vaginal apex comes to its lowest point.

After measurements of the anterior wall are complete, the posterior blade of the speculum is removed, rotated 180° and reinserted against the anterior vaginal wall. This effectively isolates the posterior wall to allow for measurements of points Ap and Bp. Again, any defects or bulges are described and points Ap and Bp are measured similarly to the anterior wall.

During the POP-Q examination, it is important not only to determine the compartment involved but also to assess the nature of the defect. An important principle of prolapse surgery is site-specific repair and focal defects can be detected when the patient performs a Valsalva maneuver. Anterior wall defects tend to appear either as smooth-walled defects or as well-ruggaed defects: the smoothwalled epithelium suggests a midline defect whereas the well-ruggaed prolapsed vagina with a sagging vaginal sulcus suggests either a paravaginal defect or an apical detachment of the pubocervical fascia. Some clinicians will open the sponge clamp and place a head in either fornix. If the vagina prolapses with Valsalva, this suggests a midline defect but if there is no descent, a paravaginal defect is more likely. Finally, some clinicians will perform a Q-tip test to assess for urethral hypermobility. While some may perform this in the assessment of urinary incontinence, its utility in the evaluation of prolapse is minimal and it is not used routinely. In the posterior wall, defects are most commonly a detachment of the perineal body from the rectovaginal septum, typically leaving a distal linear defect perpendicular to the axis of the vagina. However, this defect can also be midline or lateral and it is important to form an opinion of the nature of the defect.

While many surgeons will try to identify site-specific defects prior to going to the operating room, it is important to remember that this does not replace a careful intra-operative examination. It is not uncommon for the intra-operative examination to reveal a different defect from that diagnosed preoperatively, particularly paravaginal defects.[23]

A bimanual examination performed at this time gives the clinician an ideal opportunity to assess for undiagnosed site-specific defects. In addition to the typical assessments of pelvic tenderness, masses and other pathology, with fingers palpating the vaginal supports, the clinician can assess for site-specific defects as the patient performs a Valsalva. While there are no data to support the diagnosis of site-specific defects using this technique, it allows the clinician to gain an overall impression of the nature of the patient's pelvic support and to detect possible defects not noted during the POP-Q examination. A rectovaginal examination allows for the assessment of defects posteriorly. In addition, at times small bowel can be felt entering this space, suggesting the presence of an enterocele. Any defects should be documented and then confirmed and repaired intraoperatively.

While performing a bimanual examination, many clinicians will evaluate the tone and strength of the pelvic floor. This subjective assessment is done by placing one or two fingers in the vagina and asking the patient to contract her pelvic floor. The tone, symmetry, and duration of the contraction should be noted and subjectively graded. The finding of asymmetry, absent tone or short duration suggests a possible neuromuscular impairment.

ANCILLARY STUDIES IN THE PATIENT WITH PELVIC ORGAN PROLAPSE

There are a multitude of diagnostic procedures that may be performed for the evaluation of POP and pelvic floor dysfunction. However, the majority are performed to evaluate the function of the bladder or rectum and few are actually useful for the evaluation of POP alone. Some practitioners will perform urodynamics in the absence of urinary incontinence in cases of severe POP, particularly with significant anterior wall prolapse. The goal of urodynamics in this setting is to detect occult stress incontinence that may manifest in 30–70% of patients after POP repair unless a continence procedure is performed.[24,25] Should the patient show signs of stress incontinence when the prolapse is placed in the vagina, many surgeons recommend a continence procedure at the time of POP repair.[24-26] Other studies that may be performed to assess defecatory dysfunction include anal manometry and endoanal ultrasound. The decision to perform these tests is based on the presence of either constipation or fecal/flatal incontinence rather than for evaluation of prolapse and the reader is referred to Chapter 11 for further information on these studies.

One study that is well established for the evaluation of POP is defecography or fluoroscopic cystoproctography. Besides its low cost and use in diagnosing POP, it also provides some information on anorectal function. In the evaluation of POP, this study is typically done to distinguish between an enterocele and rectocele or to detect unsuspected enteroceles or sigmoidoceles. It may also be performed as part of the evaluation of constipation, incomplete fecal emptying or rectal prolapse. In any patient with defecatory symptoms disproportionate to the pelvic examination, defecography can greatly aid in the diagnosis.

Successful defecography requires the opacification of the rectum, small bowel, and vagina. The patient's rectum is filled retrograde with barium paste. A small amount of barium is placed in the vagina to highlight the mucosa. The patient also drinks oral contrast to opacify the small bowel. Under fluoroscopy, a sequence of images is captured. The first image shows the patient at rest. The second image has the patient squeezing her pelvic floor. This should result in visible elevation of the pelvic floor and a measurable change in the anorectal angle. While contracting her pelvic floor, the patient then performs a Valsalva maneuver for the third image. On this image, if the small bowel descends into the pelvis beyond the ischial spines, it is highly suggestive of an enterocele. The patient is then asked to evacuate her bowels and the fourth and fifth images include those taken during

emptying and after the patient has emptied as much as possible. On these images, enteroceles and rectoceles can be seen. Figures 12.2 and 12.3 show the appearance of an enterocele and a rectocele respectively as seen as part of a typical defecography study. Finally, for the sixth image, the patient is asked to strain or perform a Valsalva, which can reveal rectal prolapse.

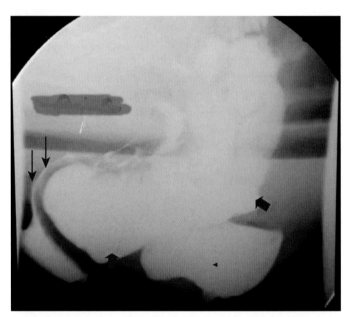

Figure 12.2 Enterocele. This image shows the patient performing a Valsalva procedure. The small arrows show the outline of the vagina. The large arrows show the small bowel filling the space between the vagina and rectum. The arrowhead shows the rectum filled with contrast.

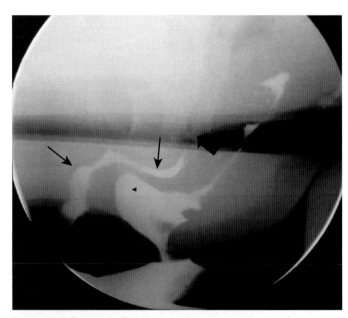

Figure 12.3 Rectocele. This image shows the patient performing a Valsalva procedure. The small arrows show the outline of the vagina. The large arrows show the small bowel which remains above the vagina. The arrowhead shows the rectum filled with contrast bulging into the distal vagina.

Because "normal" encompasses a wide range of results, there are no absolute values that are considered diagnostic for POP. The assessment of a defecography involves both objective and subjective criteria and it should be used as an aid in diagnosing POP rather than as a definitive measure of POP.

Concerns about radiation exposure with defecography and the cumbersome nature of the study have led to the examination of other imaging modalities for POP. Recently researchers have begun to explore magnetic resonance imaging to diagnose POP. The potential advantages over fluoroscopy include better visualization of independent pelvic organs and tissues. This can allow for the potential diagnosis of not only enteroceles but also site-specific defects.[27,28] However, for the evaluation of POP, MRI is limited due to the supine position of the patient and the static nature of the study. While this modality appears promising, it remains experimental and there is no literature supporting its use over defecography.

AREAS FOR FUTURE RESEARCH IN THE DIAGNOSIS OF PELVIC ORGAN PROLAPSE

There exists great opportunity for further research into the diagnosis of POP. Clearly, the most pressing need is a reliable definition of POP which would need to incorporate objective anatomic criteria with a reproducible measure of symptom severity. There is also great scope to explore imaging modalities for use in the diagnosis of POP. Dynamic MRI shows some promise for identifying site-specific defects within prolapsing compartments as well as enteroceles but additional studies are needed.[28]

REFERENCES

1. Swift SE. The distribution of pelvic organ support in a population of female subjects seen for routine gynecologic health care. Am J Obstet Gynecol 2000;183(2):277–285.
2. Baden WF, Walker TA. Genesis of the vaginal profile: a correlated classification of vaginal relaxation. Clin Obstet Gynecol 1972:15;1048–1054.
3. Bump RC, Mattiasson A, Bo K, et al. The standardization of terminology of female pelvic organ prolapse and pelvic floor dysfunction. Am J Obstet Gynecol 1996;175(1):10–17.
4. Prietto NM, Luber K, Nager C. Simple yet thorough office evaluation of pelvic floor disorders. OBG Management 2003;May:80–95.
5. Swift SE, Tate SB, Nicholas J. Correlation of symptoms with degree of pelvic organ support in a general population of women: what is pelvic organ prolapse? Am J Obstet Gynecol 2003;189(2):372–379.
6. Samuelsson EC, Victor FTA, Tibblin G, Svardsudd KF. Signs of genital prolapse in a Swedish population of women 20 to 59 years of age and possible related factors. Am J Obstet Gynecol 1999;180(2):299–305.
7. Nichols DH. Enterocele and massive eversion of the vagina. In: Thompson JD, Rock SA (eds). Telinde's Operative gynecology 7th ed. Philadelphia: Lippincott; 1992: 855–887.
8. Addison WA, Livengood CH, Parker RT. Posthysterectomy vaginal vault prolapse with emphasis on management by transabdominal sacral colpopexy. Postgrad Obstet Gynecol 1988; 8:1–11.
9. Ellerkmann RM, Cundiff GW, Melick CF, et al. Correlation of symptoms with location and severity of pelvic organ prolapse. Am J Obstet Gynecol 2001;186(6):1332–1338.
10. Mouritsen L, Larsen JP. Symptoms, bother and POPQ in women referred with pelvic organ prolapse. Int Urogynecol J 2003;14:122–127.
11. Heit M, Culligan P, Rosenquist C, Shott S. Is pelvic organ prolapse a cause of pelvic or low back pain? Obstet Gynecol 2002;99(1):23–28.
12. Barber MD, Visco AG, Wyman JF, et al. Sexual function in women with urinary incontinence and pelvic organ prolapse. Obstet Gynecol 2002;99(2):281–289.
13. Dietz HP, Haylen BT, Vancaillie TG. Female pelvic organ prolapse and voiding function. Int Urogynecol J 2002;13:284–288.
14. Meshia M, Buonaguidi A, Pifarotti P, et al. Prevalence of anal incontinence in women with symptoms of urinary incontinence and genital prolapse. Obstet Gynecol 2002;100(4):719–723.
15. Fialkow MF, Gardella C, Melville J, et al. Posterior vaginal wall defects and the relation to measures of pelvic floor neuromuscular function and posterior compartment symptoms. Am J Obstet Gynecol 2002;187(6):1443–1489.
16. Eva UF, Gun W, Preben K. Prevalence of urinary and fecal incontinence and symptoms of genital prolapse in women. Acta Obstet Gynecol Scand 2003;82:280–286.
17. Marinkovic SP, Stanton SL. Incontinence and voiding difficulties associated with prolapse. J Urol 2004;171(3):1021–1028.
18. Spence-Jones C, Kamm MA, Henry MM, et al. Bowel dysfunction: a pathogenic factor in uterovaginal prolapse and urinary incontinence. Br J Obstet Gynaecol 1994;101;147–152.
19. Weber AM, Walters MD, Ballard LA, Booher DL, Piedmonte MR. Posterior vaginal prolapse and bowel function. Am J Obstet Gynecol 1998;179(6 Pt 1):1446–1449.
20. Weber AM, Abrams P, Brubaker L, et al. The standardization of terminology for researchers in female pelvic floor disorders. Int Urogynecol J 2001;12:178–186.
21. Barber MD, Kuchibhatla MN, Pieper CF, Bump RC. Psychometric evaluation of 2 comprehensive condition-specific quality of life instruments for women with pelvic floor disorders. Am J Obstet Gynecol 2001;185(6):1388–1395.
22. Walters M. Evaluation of urinary incontinence. In: Walters M, Karram M, eds. Urogynecology and reconstructive pelvic surgery, 2nd edn. Philadelphia: Mosby; 1999: 45–53.
23. Barber MD, Cundiff GW, Weidner AC, Coates KW, Bump RC, Addison WA. Accuracy of clinical assessment of paravaginal defects in women with anterior wall prolapse. Am J Obstet Gynecol 1999;181(1):87–90.
24. Barnes NM, Dmochowski RR, Park R, Nitti V. Pubovaginal sling and pelvic prolapse repair in women with occult stress urinary incontinence: effect on postoperative emptying and voiding symptoms. Urology 2002;59(6):856–860.
25. Bergman A, Koonings PP, Ballard CA. Predicting postoperative urinary incontinence development in women undergoing operation for genitourinary prolapse. Am J Obstet Gynecol 1988;158(5):1171–1175.
26. Meschia M, Pifarotti P, Spennacchio M, et al. A randomized comparison of tension-free vaginal tape and endopelvic fascia plication in women with genital prolapse and occult stress incontinence. Am J Obstet Gynecol 2004;190:609–613.
27. Cortes E, Reid WMN, Singh K, Berger L. Clinical examination and dynamic magnetic resonance imaging in vaginal vault prolapse. Obstet Gynecol 2004;103(1):41–46.
28. Pannu HK. Magnetic resonance imaging of pelvic organ prolapse. Abdomin Imag 2002;27:660–673.

SECTION 5

Treatment of urinary incontinence
(excluding fistula and diverticulum)

Pharmacologic Treatment

Karl-Erik Andersson

INTRODUCTION

Bladder control disorders can roughly be classified as disturbances of filling/storage or disturbances of emptying. Failure to store urine may lead to various forms of incontinence (mainly urgency and stress incontinence) and failure to empty can lead to urinary retention, which may result in overflow incontinence. A disturbed filling/storage function can, at least theoretically, be improved by agents which decrease detrusor activity, increase bladder capacity, and/or increase outlet resistance.[1] To describe disturbances of bladder function with symptoms of urgency, frequency and incontinence, the International Continence Society recently suggested the term "overactive bladder (OAB) syndrome,"[2] defined as the symptoms of urgency, with and without urgency incontinence, usually with frequency and nocturia. In many cases of OAB, involuntary detrusor contractions (detrusor overactivity: DO) can be demonstrated by cystometry.

Many drugs have been tried to treat the different forms of voiding dysfunction (Table 13.1). The present drug recommendations are based on evaluations made by the Third International Consultation on Incontinence, held in Monaco in 2004 (Box 13.1).[3] The terminology used is that recommended by the International Continence Society.[2]

ANTIMUSCARINIC (ANTICHOLINERGIC) DRUGS

Rationale for use. Antimuscarinics block, more or less selectively, muscarinic receptors (Fig. 13.1). The common view is that in OAB/DO, the drugs act by blocking the muscarinic receptors on the detrusor muscle, which are stimulated by acetylcholine released from activated cholinergic (parasympathetic) nerves. Thereby, they decrease the ability of the bladder to contract. However, antimuscarinic drugs act mainly during the storage phase, decreasing urgency and increasing bladder capacity, and during this phase there is normally no parasympathetic input to the lower urinary tract.[4] Furthermore, antimuscarinics are

Table 13.1 Drugs used in the treatment of detrusor overactivity. Assessments according to the Oxford system (modified)

Drug	Level of evidence	Grade of recommendation
Antimuscarinic drugs		
Tolterodine	1	A
Trospium	1	A
Solifenacin	1	A
Darifenacin	1	A
Propantheline	2	B
Atropine, hyoscyamine	3	C
Drugs with mixed actions		
Oxybutynin	1	A
Propiverine	1	A
Dicyclomine	3	C
Flavoxate	2	D
Antidepressants		
Imipramine	3	C
α-AR antagonists		
Alfuzosin	3	C
Doxazosin	3	C
Prazosin	3	C
Terazosin	3	C
Tamsulosin	3	C
β-AR agonists		
Terbutaline	3	C
Salbutamol	3	C
COX inhibitors		
Indomethacin	2	C
Flurbiprofen	2	C
Other drugs		
Baclofen*	3	C
Capsaicin**	2	C
Resiniferatoxin**	2	C
Botulinum toxin***	2	B
Estrogen	2	C
Desmopressin****	1	A

* intrathecal; ** intravesical; *** bladder wall; **** nocturia

Box 13.1 ICI assessments 2004: Oxford guidelines (modified)

Levels of evidence

Level 1: Systematic reviews, metaanalyses, good-quality randomized controlled clinical trials (RCTs)

Level 2: RCTs, good-quality prospective cohort studies

Level 3: Case–control studies, case series

Level 4: Expert opinion

Grades of recommendation

Grade A: Based on level 1 evidence (highly recommended)

Grade B: Consistent level 2 or 3 evidence (recommended)

Grade C: Level 4 studies or "majority evidence" (optional)

Grade D: Evidence inconsistent/inconclusive (no recommendation possible)

usually competitive antagonists. This implies that when there is a massive release of acetylcholine, as during micturition, the effects of the drugs should be decreased, otherwise the reduced ability of the detrusor to contract would eventually lead to urinary retention. High doses of antimuscarinics can produce urinary retention but in the dose range needed for beneficial effects in OAB/DO, there is little evidence for a significant reduction of the voiding contraction.

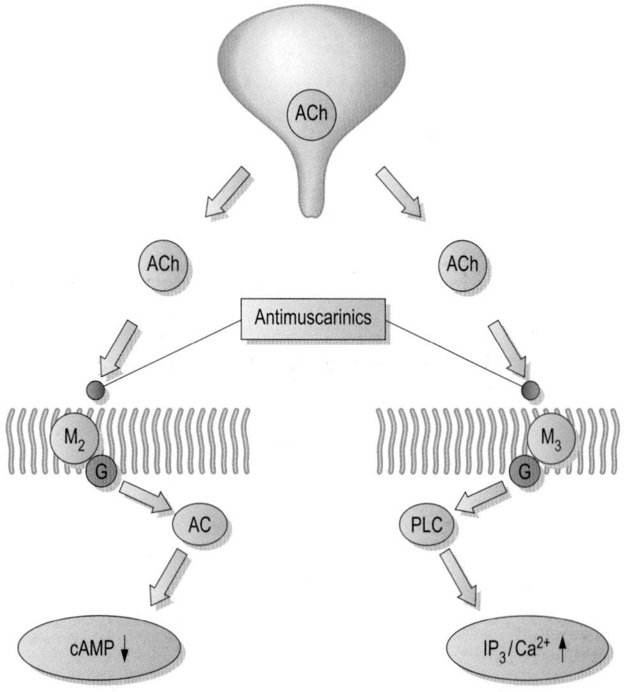

Figure 13.1 The effects of released acetylcholine (ACh), acting at muscarinic M_2 and M_3 receptors in the detrusor, will be blocked by antimuscarinics.

The question is whether there are other sites of action of antimuscarinics that can contribute to their beneficial effects in the treatment of OAB/DO.[5] Muscarinic receptors are found on bladder urothelial cells where their density can be even higher than in detrusor muscle and suburothelially. The role of the urothelium in bladder activation has attracted much interest.[6] It has been suggested that the muscarinic receptors located on the urothelium or on structures in the lamina propria (interstitial cells, afferent nerves) can influence micturition (Fig. 13.2).[5] However, this has not yet been established.

Pharmacology. Generally, antimuscarinics can be divided into tertiary and quaternary amines.[7] They differ with regard to lipophilicity, molecular charge, and even molecular size. Tertiary compounds generally have higher lipophilicity and molecular charge than quaternary agents. Atropine, tolterodine, oxybutynin, propiverine, darifenacin, and solifenacin are tertiary amines. They are generally well absorbed from the gastrointestinal tract and should theoretically be able to pass into the central nervous system (CNS), dependent on their individual physicochemical properties. High lipophilicity, small molecular size, and low charge will increase the ability to pass the blood–brain barrier. Quaternary ammonium compounds, like propantheline and trospium, are not well absorbed, pass into the CNS to a limited extent, and have a low incidence of CNS side effects. They still produce well-known peripheral antimuscarinic side effects, such as accommodation paralysis, constipation, tachycardia, and dryness of mouth.

Many antimuscarinics (all currently used tertiary amines) are metabolized by the P450 enzyme system to active and/or inactive metabolites.[7] The most commonly involved P450 enzymes are CYP2D6 and CYP3A4. The metabolic conversion creates a risk for drug–drug interactions, resulting in either reduced (enzyme induction) or increased (enzyme inhibition, substrate competition) plasma concentration/effect of the antimuscarinic and/or interacting drug. Antimuscarinics secreted by the renal tubules (e.g. trospium) may theoretically be able to interfere with the elimination of other drugs using this mechanism.

Antimuscarinics are still the most widely used treatment for urgency and urgency incontinence.[5] However, currently used drugs lack selectivity for the bladder and action on other organ systems may result in side effects, which limit their usefulness. For example, all antimuscarinic drugs are contraindicated in untreated narrow-angle glaucoma. One way of avoiding many of the antimuscarinic side effects is to administer the drugs intravesically. However, this is practical only in a limited number of patients.

Current antimuscarinic drugs: individual drug profiles. Many drugs with antimuscarinic properties have

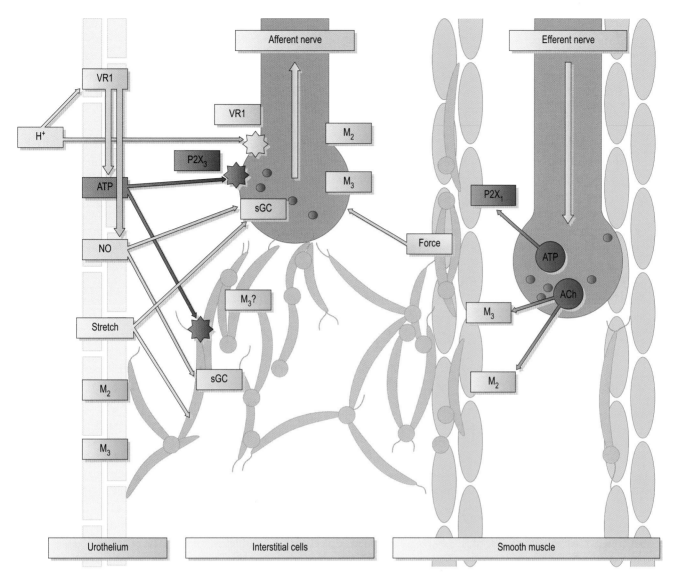

Figure 13.2 Nondetrusor and detrusor muscarinic receptor sites (M_2, M_3) in the bladder where antimuscarinics may act.

been tried for treatment of OAB. For many of them, documentation of effects is not based on RCTs satisfying currently required criteria, and some drugs can be considered as obsolete (e.g. emepronium). Information on some of these drugs can be found elsewhere.[8]

"Pure" antimuscarinics

Atropine. Atropine (dl-hyoscyamine) is rarely used for treatment of OAB/DO because of its systemic side effects. However, in patients with neurogenic DO, intravesical atropine may be effective for increasing bladder capacity without causing any systemic adverse effects, as shown in open pilot trials.[3]

Propantheline. Propantheline bromide is a quaternary ammonium compound, nonselective for muscarinic receptor subtypes, which has a low (5–10%) and individually varying

biologic availability. It is metabolized (metabolites inactive) and has a short half-life (less than 2 h).[9] It is usually given in a dose of 15–30 mg four times daily but to obtain an optimal effect, individual titration of the dose is necessary, and often higher dosages. Controlled randomized trials have demonstrated a positive but varying response.[3,10]

Although the effect of propantheline on OAB/DO has not been well documented in controlled trials satisfying today's standards, it can be considered effective and may, in individually titrated doses, be clinically useful.

Trospium. Trospium chloride is a quaternary ammonium compound with antimuscarinic actions and no selectivity for muscarinic receptor subtypes. Its biologic availability is less than 10%.[11] Trospium is expected to cross the blood–brain barrier to a limited extent and seems to have no negative cognitive effects.[11-13] The drug has a plasma half-life of approximately 20 h and is mainly (60%) eliminated unchanged in the urine. It is not metabolized by the cytochrome P450 enzyme system.

Several RCTs have documented positive effects of trospium both in neurogenic DO[14,15] and nonneurogenic DO.[16-19] Zinner et al treated 523 patients with symptoms associated with OAB and urgency incontinence with 20 mg trospium twice daily or placebo in a 12-week, multicenter, parallel, double-blind, placebo-controlled trial.[20] Dual primary endpoints were change in average number of toilet voids and change in urge incontinent episodes per 24 hours. Secondary efficacy variables were change in average volume per void, voiding urge severity, urinations during day and night, time to onset of action and change in Incontinence Impact Questionnaire. Trospium significantly decreased average frequency of toilet voids and urge incontinent episodes compared to placebo. It significantly increased average volume per void and decreased average urge severity and daytime frequency. All effects occurred by week 1 and all were sustained throughout the study. Nocturnal frequency decreased significantly by week 4 and Incontinence Impact Questionnaire scores improved at week 12. Trospium was well tolerated. The most common side effects were dry mouth (21.8%), constipation (9.5%), and headache (6.5%).

Trospium is a well-documented alternative for treatment of OAB/DO and seems to be well tolerated.

Tolterodine. Tolterodine has no selectivity for muscarinic receptor subtypes but is claimed to have functional selectivity for the bladder over the salivary glands.[21,22] It is rapidly absorbed and extensively metabolized (CYP2D6). The major active metabolite has a similar pharmacologic profile to the mother compound[23] and significantly contributes to the therapeutic effect of tolterodine.[24,25] Both tolterodine and its metabolite have plasma half-lives of 2–3 h but the effects on the bladder seem to be more long-lasting than would be expected from the pharmacokinetic data. The relatively low lipophilicity of tolterodine implies limited propensity to penetrate into the CNS, which may explain a low incidence of cognitive side effects.[26,27]

Tolterodine is available as immediate-release (IR; 1 or 2 mg, twice-daily dosing) and extended-release (ER) forms (2 or 4 mg, once-daily dosing). The ER form seems to have advantages over the IR form in terms of either efficacy or tolerability.[28]

Several RCTs on patients with OAB/DO (both idiopathic and neurogenic DO) have documented a significant reduction in micturition frequency and number of incontinence episodes.[26,27] Comparative RCTs such as the OBJECT (Overactive Bladder: Judging Effective Control and Treatment) and the OPERA (Overactive Bladder: Performance of Extended Release Agents) studies have further supported its effectiveness.

The OBJECT trial compared oxybutynin ER 10 mg once daily with tolterodine IR 2 mg twice daily in a 12-week randomized, double-blind, parallel-group study including 378 patients with OAB.[29] Participants had between seven and 50 episodes of urge incontinence per week and 10 or more voids in 24 hours. The outcome measures were the number of episodes of urge incontinence, total incontinence, and micturition frequency at 12 weeks adjusted for baseline. At the end of the study, extended-release oxybutynin was found to be significantly more effective than tolterodine in each of the main outcome measures adjusted for baseline. Dry mouth, the most common adverse event, was reported by 28% and 33% of participants taking oxybutynin ER and tolterodine IR, respectively. Rates of CNS and other adverse events were low and similar in both groups. The authors concluded that oxybutynin ER was more effective than tolterodine IR and that the rates of dry mouth and other adverse events were similar in both treatment groups.

In the OPERA study, oxybutynin ER at 10 mg/d or tolterodine ER at 4 mg/d were given for 12 weeks to women with 21–60 urge incontinence episodes per week and an average of 10 or more voids per 24 hours.[30] Episodes of incontinence episodes (primary endpoint), total (urge and nonurge) incontinence, and micturition were recorded in 24-h urinary diaries at baseline and at weeks 2, 4, 8, and 12 and compared. Adverse events were also evaluated. Improvements in weekly urge incontinence episodes were similar for the 790 women who received oxybutynin ER (n=391) or tolterodine ER (n=399). Oxybutynin ER was significantly more effective than tolterodine ER in reducing micturition frequency, and 23.0% of women taking oxybutynin ER reported no episodes of urinary incontinence compared with 16.8% of women taking tolterodine ER. Dry mouth, usually mild, was more common with oxybutynin ER. Adverse events were generally mild and occurred at low rates, with both groups having similar discontinuation of treatment due to adverse events. The conclusions were that reductions in weekly urge incontinence and total incontinence episodes were similar with the two drugs. Dry mouth was more common with oxybutynin ER but tolerability was otherwise comparable, including adverse events involving the central nervous system.

Tolterodine, in both the immediate- and extended-release forms, has a well-documented effect in OAB/DO. It is well tolerated and is currently, together with oxybutynin, first-line therapy for patients with this disorder.

Darifenacin. Darifenacin is a tertiary amine with moderate lipophilicity, well absorbed from the gastrointestinal tract after oral administration and extensively metabolized by the liver by the cytochrome P450 isoforms CYP3A4 and CYP2D6. The metabolism of darifenacin by CYP3A4 suggests that coadministration of a potent inhibitor of this enzyme (e.g. ketoconazole) may lead to an increase in the circulating concentration of darifenacin.[31] Darifenacin has been developed as a controlled-release formulation, which allows once-daily dosing. Recommended dosages are 7.5 and 15 mg/d.

Darifenacin is a selective muscarinic M_3 receptor antagonist. In vitro, it is selective for human cloned muscarinic M_3 receptors relative to M_1, M_2, M_4 or M_5 receptors. Theoretically, drugs with selectivity for the M_3 receptor can be expected to have clinical efficacy in OAB/DO with reduction of the adverse events related to the blockade of other muscarinic receptor subtypes.[32] However, the clinical efficacy and adverse effects of a drug are dependent not only on its profile of receptor affinity but also on its pharmacokinetics, and on the importance of muscarinic receptors for a given organ function.

The clinical effectiveness of darifenacin has been documented in several RCTs.[33,34] Haab et al reported a multicenter, double-blind, placebo-controlled, parallel-group study which enrolled 561 patients with OAB symptoms for >6 months.[33] Darifenacin 7.5 mg and 15 mg had a rapid onset of effect, with significant improvement compared with placebo being seen for most parameters at the first clinic visit (week 2). This effect was sustained through week 12. At this time the number of incontinence episodes per week was reduced from baseline by 67.7% with darifenacin 7.5 mg and 72.8% with darifenacin 15 mg, compared with 55.9% with placebo. Darifenacin 7.5 mg and 15 mg, respectively, were significantly superior to placebo for improvements in micturition frequency, bladder capacity, frequency of urgency, severity of urgency, and number of incontinence episodes leading to a change in clothing or pads. The most common adverse events were mild-to-moderate dry mouth and constipation. However, no patients withdrew from the study as a result of dry mouth and discontinuation related to constipation was rare (0.6% placebo versus 0.9% darifenacin). There were no reports of blurred vision and the CNS and cardiac safety profile was comparable to placebo.

Darifenacin has a well-documented effect in OAB/DO and the adverse event profile seems acceptable.

Solifenacin (YM-905).
Solifenacin (YM905) is a tertiary amine, well absorbed from the gastrointestinal tract (absolute bioavailability 90%). It undergoes significant hepatic metabolism involving the cytochrome P450 enzyme system (CYP3A4). The mean terminal half-life is approximately 50 hours.[35,36]

Solifenacin has some selectivity for M_3 receptors (10–20 fold) over M_2 receptors.[37]

The efficacy, safety, and tolerability of solifenacin in adult patients with OAB have been documented both in large-scale early trials[38] and in several pivotal phase 3 studies. In one of these RCTs,[39] a total of 1077 patients were randomized to 5 mg solifenacin, 10 mg solifenacin, tolterodine (2 mg b.i.d.) or placebo. Compared with placebo (−8%), mean micturitions/24 h were significantly reduced with solifenacin 10 mg (−20%), solifenacin 5 mg (−17%), and tolterodine (−15%). Episodes of urgency and incontinence were significantly reduced in patients treated with solifenacin 5 mg and 10 mg; tolterodine produced smaller, nonsignificant reductions in these endpoints. Mean volume voided per micturition was significantly increased. Solifenacin was well tolerated, with few patients discontinuing treatment. Incidences of dry mouth were 4.9% with placebo, 14.0% with solifenacin 5 mg, 21.3% with solifenacin 10 mg, and 18.6% with tolterodine 2 mg b.i.d.

Solifenacin has a well-documented effect in OAB/DO and the adverse event profile seems acceptable.

Antimuscarinics with "mixed" actions. Some drugs used to treat OAB/DO have been shown to have more than one mechanism of action. They all have a more or less pronounced antimuscarinic effect and, in addition, an often poorly defined "direct" action on bladder muscle. For several of these drugs, the antimuscarinic effects can be demonstrated at much lower drug concentrations than the direct action, which may involve blockade of voltage-operated Ca^{2+} channels. Most probably, the clinical effects of these drugs can be explained mainly by an antimuscarinic action.

Oxybutynin.
Oxybutynin is a tertiary amine that is well absorbed but undergoes extensive upper gastrointestinal and first-pass hepatic metabolism via the cytochrome P450 system (CYP3A4) into multiple metabolites. The plasma half-life of oxybutynin is approximately 2 hours but with wide interindividual variation.[40,41] The primary metabolite, N-desethyloxybutynin, has pharmacologic properties similar to the parent compound[42] but occurs in much higher concentrations after oral administration.[41] It has been implicated as the major cause of the side effect of dry mouth associated with the administration of oxybutynin. It seems reasonable to assume that the effect of oral oxybutynin to a large extent is exerted by the metabolite.

Oxybutynin has several pharmacologic effects, some of which seem difficult to relate to its effectiveness in the treatment of DO. It has both an antimuscarinic and a direct muscle relaxant effect and, in addition, local anesthetic actions. The latter effects may be of importance when the drug is administered intravesically but probably play no role when it is given orally. Most probably, when given systemically, oxybutynin acts mainly as an antimuscarinic drug. Oxybutynin was shown to have slightly higher affinity for muscarinic M_1 and M_3 receptors than for M_2 receptors[43] but the clinical significance of this is unclear.

Oxybutynin is available in immediate-release, extended-release, and transdermal preparations. The latter allow once-daily dosing and have demonstrated potential advantages over the immediate-release form in terms of either efficacy and/or tolerability.

The immediate-release form of oxybutynin (OXY-IR) is recognized for its efficacy but also for frequently occurring adverse effects.[44] The commonly recommended dose (5 mg × 3) is unnecessarily high in some patients and a starting dose of 2.5 mg × 2 with consequent dose titration seems to reduce the number of adverse effects. In general, the new formulations of oxybutynin offer patients efficacy roughly equivalent to that of OXY-IR and the advantages of these formulations (extended-release, transdermal) lie in improved dosing schedules and side effect profile.[29,30,45,46]

Extended-release oxybutynin (OXY-ER) offers dosage flexibility between 5 and 30 mg/d and a transdermal preparation (OXY-TDS) offers a twice-weekly dosing regimen. The efficacy of OXY-IR is well documented.[46] A comparison of OXY-TDS with OXY-IR demonstrated a statistically equivalent reduction in daily incontinent episodes (66% for OXY-TDS and 72% for OXY-IR) but much less dry mouth (38% for OXY-TDS and 94% for OXY-IR). Dmochowski et al compared OXY-TDS to placebo and extended-release tolterodine.[47] Both drugs equivalently and significantly reduced daily incontinence episodes and increased the average voided volume but extended-release tolterodine was associated with a significantly higher rate of antimuscarinic adverse events. The primary adverse event for OXY-TDS was application site reaction pruritus in 14% and erythema in 8.3%, with nearly 9% feeling that the reactions were severe enough to withdraw from the study, despite the lack of systemic problems.

Oxybutynin in its different formulations has a well-documented efficacy in the treatment of OAB/DO and is, together with tolterodine, first-line treatment for patients with this disorder.

Propiverine. Propiverine has been shown to have combined antimuscarinic and calcium antagonistic actions. The drug is rapidly absorbed but has a high first-pass metabolism, and its biologic availability is about 50%.[48] Propiverine is an inducer of hepatic cytochrome P450 enzymes in rats in doses about 100 times above the therapeutic doses in man.[49] Several active metabolites are formed;[50,51] most probably, these metabolites contribute to the clinical effects of the drug but their individual contributions have not been clarified. The half-life of the mother compound is about 11–14 h.

Propiverine has been shown to have beneficial effects in patients with DO in several investigations. Thüroff et al collected nine randomized studies on a total of 230 patients and found reductions in frequency (30%) and micturitions per 24 h (17%), a 64 ml increase in bladder capacity, and a 77% (range 33–80%) subjective improvement.[10] Side effects

were found in 14% (range 8–42%). In patients with neurogenic DO, controlled clinical trials have demonstrated propiverine's superiority over placebo.[52] Propiverine also increased bladder capacity and decreased maximum detrusor contractions. Controlled trials comparing propiverine, flavoxate, and placebo[53] and propiverine, oxybutynin, and placebo[54,55] have confirmed the efficacy of propiverine and suggested that the drug may have equal efficacy to and fewer side effects than oxybutynin.

Madersbacher et al compared the tolerability and efficacy of propiverine (15 mg t.i.d.), oxybutynin (5 mg b.i.d.), and placebo in 366 patients with urgency and urge incontinence in a randomized, double-blind placebo-controlled clinical trial.[55] Urodynamic efficacy of propiverine was judged similar to that of oxybutynin but the incidence and severity of dry mouth were judged less with propiverine than with oxybutynin. In a double-blind, multicenter, placebo-controlled, randomized study, Dorschner et al investigated the efficacy and cardiac safety of propiverine in 98 elderly patients (mean age 68 years), suffering from urgency, urge incontinence or mixed urge–stress incontinence.[56] After a 2-week placebo run-in period, the patients received propiverine (15 mg t.i.d.) or placebo (t.i.d.) for 4 weeks. Propiverine caused a significant reduction of the micturition frequency (from 8.7 to 6.5) and a significant decrease in episodes of incontinence (from 0.9 to 0.3 per day). The incidence of adverse events was very low (2% dryness of the mouth under propiverine: two out of 49 patients). Resting and ambulatory electrocardiograms indicated no significant changes.

Propiverine has a documented beneficial effect in the treatment of DO and seems to have an acceptable side effect profile. Its complex pharmacokinetics with several active, not very well-characterized metabolites needs more attention.

Flavoxate. The main mechanism of action of flavoxate has not been established. The drug is well absorbed and oral bioavailability appeared to be close to 100%.[6] Flavoxate is extensively metabolized and its plasma half-life was found to be 3.5 h.[57] A main metabolite (3-methylflavone-8-carboxylic acid, MFCA) has been shown to have low pharmacologic activity.[58,59]

The clinical effects of flavoxate in patients with DO and frequency, urgency and incontinence have been studied in both open and controlled investigations but with varying rates of success.[60] Stanton compared emepronium bromide and flavoxate in a double-blind, crossover study of patients with idiopathic detrusor overactivity and reported improvement rates of 83% and 66% after flavoxate or emepronium bromide, respectively, both administered as 200 mg three times daily.[61] In another double-blind, crossover study comparing flavoxate 1200 mg/day with oxybutynin 15 mg daily in 41 women with idiopathic motor or sensory urgency, and utilizing both clinical and urodynamic criteria, Milani et al found both drugs effective.[62] No difference in efficacy was found between them but flavoxate had fewer and milder side effects. Other investigators comparing the effects of flavoxate with those of placebo have not been able to show any beneficial effect of flavoxate at dosages up to 400 mg three times daily.[63-65] In general, few side effects have been reported during treatment with flavoxate. On the other hand, its efficacy, compared to other therapeutic alternatives, is not well documented.

DRUGS ACTING ON MEMBRANE CHANNELS

Calcium antagonists.
There have been few clinical studies of the effects of calcium antagonists in patients with DO. Naglie et al evaluated the efficacy of nimodipine for geriatric urge incontinence in a randomized, double-blind, placebo-controlled crossover trial.[66] Thirty mg nimodipine was given twice daily for 3 weeks in older persons with DO and chronic urge incontinence. A total of 86 participants with a mean age of 73.4 years were randomized. The primary outcome was the number of incontinent episodes, as measured by the self-completion of a 5-day voiding record. Secondary outcomes included the impact of urinary incontinence on quality of life measured with a modified incontinence impact questionnaire and symptoms, as measured by the AUA symptom score. In the 76 participants completing the study (88.4%), there was no significant difference in the number of incontinent episodes with nimodipine versus placebo. Scores on the incontinence impact questionnaire and the AUA symptom score were not significantly different with nimodipine versus placebo, and the authors concluded that treatment of geriatric urge incontinence with 30 mg nimodipine twice daily was unsuccessful.

Available information does not suggest that systemic therapy with calcium antagonists is an effective way to treat OAB/DO.

Potassium channel openers.
Theoretically, K^+ channel openers may be active during the filling phase of the bladder, abolishing DO with no effect on normal bladder contraction. Several types of K^+ channel openers have been effective in animal models[67,68] but clinically, the effects have not been encouraging. At the present time, there is no evidence from RCTs to suggest that K^+ channel openers represent a treatment alternative for OAB/DO.

α-Adrenoceptor antagonists.
Even though it is well known that α-AR antagonists can ameliorate lower urinary tract symptoms in men with BPH,[69] there are no controlled clinical trials showing that they are an effective alternative in the treatment of bladder overactivity in this patient category. In an open label study, Arnold evaluated the clinical and pressure–flow effects of tamsulosin 0.4 mg once daily in patients with lower urinary tract symptoms (LUTS) caused by benign prostatic obstruction (BPO).[70] He found that tamsulosin produced a significant decrease in detrusor pressure, increase in flow rate and a symptomatic improvement in patients with LUTS and confirmed obstruction. α-AR antagonists have been used to treat patients with neurogenic DO[8,71] but the success has been moderate.

Although α-AR antagonists may be effective in selected cases of DO, convincing effects documented in RCTs are lacking. In women, these drugs may produce stress incontinence.[72]

β-Adrenoceptor agonists.
In isolated human bladder, nonsubtype selective β-AR agonists like isoprenaline have a pronounced inhibitory effect and administration of such drugs can increase bladder capacity in man.[73] However, the β-ARs of the human bladder were shown to have functional characteristics typical of neither β_1- nor β_2-ARs, since they could be blocked by propranolol but not by practolol or metoprolol (β_1) or butoxamine (β_2).[74,75] Both normal and neurogenic human detrusors were shown to express β_1-, β_2-, and β_3-AR mRNAs, and selective β_3-AR agonists effectively relaxed both types of detrusor muscle.[76-78] Thus, it seems that the atypical β-AR of the human bladder may be the β_3-AR.

Favorable effects on DO were reported in open studies with selective β_2-AR agonists such as terbutaline.[79] In a double-blind investigation, clenbuterol 0.01 mg three times daily was shown to have a good therapeutic effect in 15 of 20 women with DO.[80] Other investigators, however, have not been able to show that β-ARs agonists represent an effective therapeutic principle in elderly patients with DO[81] or in young patients with myelodysplasia and DO.[82] Whether or not β_3-AR stimulation will be an effective way of treating the OAB/DO has yet to be shown in controlled clinical trials.

ANTIDEPRESSANTS

Several antidepressants have been reported to have beneficial effects in patients with DO.[83,84] However, imipramine is the only drug that has been widely used clinically to treat this disorder.

Imipramine has complex pharmacologic effects, including marked systemic antimuscarinic actions[85] and blockade of the reuptake of serotonin and noradrenaline[86] but its mode of action in DO has not been established.[87] Even though it is generally considered that imipramine is a useful drug in the treatment of DO, no good-quality RCTs that document this have been retrieved.

It has long been known that imipramine can have favorable effects in the treatment of nocturnal enuresis in children, with a success rate of 10–70% in controlled trials.[87,88] It is well established that therapeutic doses of tricyclic antidepressants, including imipramine, may cause serious toxic effects on the cardiovascular system (orthostatic hypotension, ventricular arrhythmias). Imipramine prolongs QTc intervals and has an antiarrhythmic (and proarrhythmic) effect similar to that of quinidine.[89,90] Children seem particularly sensitive to the cardiotoxic action of tricyclic antidepressants.[85]

The risks and benefits of imipramine in the treatment of voiding disorders do not seem to have been assessed. Very few studies have been performed during the last decade.[87] No good-quality RCTs have documented that the drug is effective in the treatment DO. However, a beneficial effect has been documented in the treatment of nocturnal enuresis.

CYCLO OXYGENASE (COX) INHIBITORS

Cardozo et al performed a double-blind controlled study of 30 women with DO using the COX inhibitor flurbiprofen at a dosage of 50 mg three times daily.[91] The drug was shown to have favorable effects, although it did not completely abolish DO. There was a high incidence of side effects (43%) including nausea, vomiting, headache, and gastrointestinal symptoms. Palmer studied the effects of flurbiprofen 50 mg × 4 versus placebo in a double-blind, crossover trial of 37 patients with idiopathic DO (27% of the patients did not complete the trial).[92] Active treatment significantly increased maximum contractile pressure, decreased the number of voids and decreased the number of urgent voids compared to baseline. Indomethacin 50–100 mg daily was reported to give symptomatic relief in patients with DO, compared with bromocriptine in a randomized, single-blind, crossover study.[93] The incidence of side effects was high, occurring in 19 of 32 patients. However, no patient had to stop treatment because of side effects.

The few controlled clinical trials on the effects of COX inhibitors in the treatment of DO, and the limited number of drugs tested, make it difficult to evaluate their therapeutic value. No new information has been published during the last decade.

VASOPRESSIN ANALOGS

Desmopressin. Desmopressin (1-desamino-8-D-arginine vasopressin; DDAVP) is a synthetic vasopressin analog with a pronounced antidiuretic effect but practically lacking vasopressor actions.[94]

Several controlled, double-blind investigations have shown intranasal administration of desmopressin to be effective in the treatment of nocturnal enuresis in children.[95] The dose used in most studies has been 20 μg intranasally at bedtime. However, the drug is orally active, even if the bioavailability is low (less than 1% compared to 2–10% after intranasal administration), and its efficacy in primary nocturnal enuresis in children and adolescents has been documented in randomized, double-blind, placebo-controlled studies.[96,97]

In RCTs, oral desmopressin has proved to be effective in the treatment of nocturia in men[98] and women.[99] In the study of Lose et al, 144 patients were randomly assigned to groups (desmopressin, n=72; placebo, n=72).[99] For desmopressin, 33 (46%) patients had a 50% or greater reduction in nocturnal voids against baseline levels compared with five (7%) patients receiving placebo ($P<0.001$). The mean number of nocturnal voids, duration of sleep until the first nocturnal void, nocturnal diuresis, and ratios of nocturnal per 24 hours and nocturnal per daytime urine volumes changed significantly in favor of desmopressin versus placebo ($P<0.001$). In the dose titration phase, headache (22%), nausea (8%), and hyponatremia (6%) were reported.

Even if side effects are uncommon during desmopressin treatment, there is a risk of water retention and hyponatremia. The results of a systematic review and metaanalysis revealed an incidence of desmopressin-induced hyponatremia of 7.6%.[100] In elderly patients, it was recommended that serum sodium should be measured before and after a few days of treatment.[101]

Desmopressin is a well-documented therapeutic alternative in pediatric nocturnal enuresis, and is effective also in adults with nocturia with polyuric origin.

BACLOFEN

Baclofen is considered to depress monosynaptic and polysynaptic motoneurons and interneurons in the spinal cord by acting as a GABA agonist, and has been used in voiding disorders, including DO secondary to lesions of the spinal cord.[3] The drug may also be an alternative in the treatment of idiopathic DO.[102] However, published experience with the drug is limited. Intrathecal baclofen may be useful in patients with spasticity and bladder dysfunction, and increase bladder capacity.[103]

CAPSAICIN AND RESINIFERATOXIN (VANILLOIDS)

The rationale for intravesical instillations of vanilloids is based on the involvement of C fibers in the pathophysiology of conditions such as bladder hypersensitivity and neurogenic DO. In the healthy human bladder, C fibers carry the response to noxious stimuli but they are not implicated in the normal voiding reflex. After spinal cord injury, major neuroplasticity appears within bladder afferents in several mammalian species, including man. C-fiber bladder afferents proliferate within the suburothelium and become sensitive to bladder distension. Those changes lead to the emergence of a new C fiber-mediated voiding reflex, which is strongly involved in spinal neurogenic DO. Improvement of this condition by defunctionalization of C-fiber bladder afferents with intravesical vanilloids has been widely demonstrated in humans and animals.

Capsaicin. Cystometric evidence that capsaicin-sensitive nerves may modulate the afferent branch of the micturition reflex in humans was originally presented by Maggi et al, who instilled capsaicin (0.1–10 μM) intravesically in five patients with hypersensitivity disorders, with attenuation of their symptoms a few days after administration.[104] Intravesical capsaicin, given in considerably higher concentrations (1–2 mM) than those administered by Maggi et al, has since been used with success in neurologic disorders such as multiple sclerosis, or traumatic chronic spinal lesions.[3,8,105,106]

Resiniferatoxin (RTX). The beneficial effect of RTX has been demonstrated in several studies.[9,106-110]

De Seze et al compared the efficacy and tolerability of nonalcohol capsaicin (1 mM) vs RTX (100 nM) in 10% alcohol in a randomized, double-blind, parallel groups study in 39 spinal cord-injured adult patients with neurogenic DO (hyperreflexia).[106] Efficacy (voiding chart and cystomanometry) and tolerability were evaluated during a 3-month follow-up. On day 30, clinical and urodynamical improvement was found in 78% and 83% of patients with capsaicin versus 80% and 60% with RTX, respectively, without a significant difference between the two treated groups. The benefit remained in two-thirds of the two groups on day 90. There were no significant differences with regard to the incidence, nature or duration of side effects in capsaicin- versus RTX-treated patients. The data suggested that capsaicin and RTX are equally efficient for relieving the clinical and urodynamic symptoms of neurogenic DO, and that glucidic capsaicin is as well tolerated as ethanolic RTX.

Available information (including data from RCTs) suggests that both capsaicin and RTX may have useful effects in the treatment of neurogenic DO. There may be beneficial effects also in nonneurogenic DO in selected cases refractory to antimuscarinic treatment but further RCT-based documentation is required. RTX is an interesting alternative to capsaicin but the drug is currently not in clinical development owing to formulation problems.

BOTULINUM TOXIN (BTX)
Seven immunologically distinct antigenic subtypes of botulinum toxin have been identified: A, B, C1, D, E, F, and G. Types A and B are in clinical use in urology but most studies have been performed with botulinum toxin type A. There are three commercially available products:

- Botox®, Allergan, Irvine CA: BTX-A$_1$
- Dysport®, Ipsen, Berkshire, UK: BTX-A$_1$
- Myobloc™ Neurobloc™, Dublin/Princeton, NJ: BTX-B$_1$.

It is important not to use these products interchangeably as they have very different dosing and side effect profiles.

On a weight basis, botulinum toxin is the most potent naturally occurring substance known. The toxin blocks the release of acetylcholine and other transmitters from presynaptic nerve endings interacting with the protein complex necessary for docking vesicles.[111-113] This results in decreased muscle contractility and muscle atrophy at the injection site. The produced chemical denervation is a reversible process and axons are regenerated in about 3–6 months. The botulinum toxin molecule cannot cross the blood–brain barrier and therefore has no CNS effects.

There are many open label and a few double-blind studies and reports describing positive outcomes after treatment with BTX in many urologic conditions including: detrusor striated sphincter dyssynergia (DSD), neurogenic DO (detrusor hyperreflexia) pelvic floor spasticity, and possibly BPH and interstitial cystitis.[113,114] However, toxin injections may also be effective in refractory idiopathic DO.[115]

Preliminary studies look very promising with BTX-A but it seems too early to tell whether the same results will be seen with BTX-B. The safety of these products appears satisfactory. A good response appears to occur within 1 week and lasts from 6 to 9 months before reinjection is necessary. It remains to be seen whether this treatment will be cost-effective for all the diseases currently being studied.

DRUGS USED FOR TREATMENT OF STRESS INCONTINENCE
The pharmacologic treatment of SUI (Table 13.2) aims at increasing intraurethral closure forces by increasing tone in the urethral smooth and striated muscles. Several drugs may contribute to such an increase[116] but limited efficacy or side effects have often limited their clinical use.

α-Adrenoceptor agonists. Several drugs with agonistic effects on α-ARs have been used in the treatment of SUI. However, ephedrine and norephedrine (phenylpropanol amine; PPA) seem to have been the most widely used.[3] The original 1992 Agency for Healthcare Policy and Research Guideline reported eight randomized controlled trials with PPA, 50 mg twice daily for SUI in women. Percent cures

Table 13.2 Drugs used in the treatment of stress incontinence. Assessments according to the Oxford system (modified)

Drug	Level of evidence	Grade of recommendation
Duloxetine	1	A
Imipramine	3	D
Clenbuterol	3	C
Methoxamine	2	D
Midodrine	2	C
Ephedrine	3	D
Norephedrine (phenylpropanolamine)	3	D
Estrogen	2	D

(all figures refer to percent effect on drug minus percent effect on placebo) were listed as 0% to 14%, percent reduction in continence as 19–60%, and percent side effects and percent dropouts as 5–33%, and 0–4.3% respectively. A recent Cochrane review evaluated randomized or quasi-randomized controlled trials, which included an adrenergic agonist in at least one arm.[117] There were 11 trials which utilized PPA, two which utilized midodrine, and two which utilized clenbuterol. There was "weak evidence" to suggest that use of an adrenergic agent was better than placebo treatment.

Ephedrine and PPA lack selectivity for urethral α-ARs and can increase blood pressure and cause sleep disturbances, headache, tremor, and palpitations.[3] Kernan et al reported the risk of hemorrhagic stroke to be 16 times higher in women less than 50 years of age who had been taking PPA as an appetite suppressant (statistically significant) and three times higher in women who had been taking the drug for less than 24 hours as a cold remedy (not statistically significant).[118] There was no increased risk in men. PPA has been removed from the market in the United States.

Numerous case reports of adverse reactions due to ephedra alkaloids exist and some have suggested that sale of these compounds as a dietary supplement be restricted or banned.[119] In December 2003, the US Food and Drug Administration decreed such a ban, a move which has survived legal appeal.

Midodrine and methoxamine stimulates α_1-ARs with some degree of selectivity. According to the RCTs available, the effectiveness of these drugs is moderate and the clinical usefulness seems to be limited by adverse effects.[117,120,121]

Attempts have been made to develop agonists with selectivity for the human urethra. Musselman et al reported on a phase 2 randomized crossover study with Ro 115-1240, a peripherally active selective $\alpha_{1A/1L}$ adrenoceptor partial agonist, in 37 women with mild to moderate SUI.[122] A moderate, positive effect was demonstrated but also side effects curtailing further development of the drug.

β-Adrenoceptor antagonists. The theoretical basis for the use of β-AR antagonists in the treatment of stress incontinence is that blockade of urethral β-ARs may enhance the effects of noradrenaline on urethral α-ARs. However, there are no RCTs documenting that these drugs are a treatment alternative.

Other drugs. Several other drugs with varying mechanisms of action have been used in the treatment of stress incontinence.

Imipramine. Gilja et al reported in an open study on 30 women with stress incontinence that imipramine, 75 mg daily, produced subjective continence in 21 patients and increased mean maximal urethral closure pressure (MUCP) from 34 to 48 mmHg[123] A 35% cure rate was reported by pad test and, in an additional 25%, a 50% or more improvement.

Lin et al assessed the efficacy of imipramine (25 mg imipramine three times a day for 3 months) as a treatment in 40 women with genuine stress incontinence.[124] A 20-minute pad test, uroflowmetry, filling and voiding cystometry, and stress urethral pressure profile were performed before and after treatment. The efficacy of successful treatment was 60% (95% CI 44.8–75.2). No RCTs on the effects of imipramine seem to be available.

Clenbuterol. Yasuda et al described the results of a double-blind, placebo-controlled trial with clenbuterol in 165 women with SUI.[125] Positive statistical significance was achieved for subjective evaluation of incontinence frequency, pad usage per day, and overall global assessment. The positive effects were suggested to be a result of an action on urethral striated muscle and/or the pelvic floor muscles.

Ishiko et al investigated the effects of clenbuterol on 61 female patients with stress incontinence in a 12-week randomized study, comparing drug therapy to pelvic floor exercises and a combination of drug therapy and pelvic floor exercises.[126] The frequency and volume of stress incontinence and the patient's own impression were used as the basis for the assessment of efficacy. The improvement of incontinence was 76.9 %, 52.6 %, and 89.5 % in the respective groups. Further well-designed RCTs documenting the effects of clenbuterol are needed to adequately assess its potential as a treatment for stress incontinence.

Duloxetine. Duloxetine hydrochloride is a combined norepinephrine and serotonin reuptake inhibitor, which has been shown to significantly increase sphincteric muscle activity during the filling/storage phase of micturition in the cat acetic acid model of irritated bladder function.[132-134] Bladder capacity was also increased in this model, both effects mediated centrally through both motor efferent and sensory afferent modulation.[130] The sphincteric effects were reversed by α_1-adrenergic (prazosin) and 5-HT-2 serotonergic (LY 53857) antagonism, while the bladder effects were blocked by nonselective serotonergic antagonism (methiothepin), implying that both effects were mediated by temporal prolongation of the actions of serotonin and norepinephrine in the synaptic cleft.[130] Duloxetine is lipophilic, well absorbed, and extensively metabolized (CYP2D6). Its plasma half-life is approximately 12 h.[131]

There are several RCTs documenting the effects of duloxetine in SUI.[132-134] Dmochowski et al enrolled a total of 683 North American women 22–84 years old in a double-blind, placebo-controlled study.[132] The case definition included a predominant symptom of SUI with a weekly incontinence episode frequency (IEF) of 7 or greater, the absence of predominant symptoms of urge incontinence, normal diurnal and nocturnal frequency, a bladder capacity of 400 ml or greater, and a positive cough stress test and stress pad test. After a 2-week placebo lead-in period, subjects were randomly assigned to receive placebo (339) or 80 mg duloxetine daily (344), as 40 mg twice daily, for 12 weeks. Primary outcome variables included IEF and an incontinence quality of life questionnaire. Mean baseline IEF was 18 weekly and 436 subjects (64%) had a baseline IEF of 14 or greater. There was a significant decrease in IEF with duloxetine compared with placebo (50% vs 27%) with comparably significant improvements in quality of life (11.0 vs 6.8). Of subjects on duloxetine, 51% had a 50–100% decrease in IEF compared with 34% of those on placebo ($P<0.001$). These improvements with duloxetine were associated with a significant increase in the voiding interval compared with placebo (20 vs 2 minutes) and they were observed across the spectrum of incontinence severity. The discontinuation rate for adverse events was 4% for placebo and 24% for duloxetine ($P<0.001$), with nausea the most common reason for discontinuation (6.4%). Nausea, which was also the most common side effect, tended to be mild to moderate and transient, usually resolving after 1 week to 1 month. Of the 78 women who experienced treatment emergent nausea while taking duloxetine, 58 (74%) completed the trial. The authors concluded that duloxetine 40 mg twice daily improved incontinence and quality of life.

Similar results were reported by Millard et al,[134] studying the effects of duloxetine 40 mg. b.i.d. versus placebo in 458 women in four continents outside North America, and by van Kerrebroeck et al[133] investigating 494 European and Canadian women.

The effectivness of duloxetine for treatment of SUI is well documented. Adverse effects occur but seem tolerable.[135]

ESTROGENS FOR STRESS INCONTINENCE

The role of estrogen in the treatment of stress incontinence has been controversial, even though there are a number of reported studies.[3]

Two metaanalyses examined the use of estrogens to treat all causes of incontinence in postmenopausal women.[136,137] Of 166 articles identified which were published in English between 1969 and 1992, only six were controlled trials and 17 uncontrolled series.[136] The results showed that there was a significant subjective improvement for all patients and those with genuine stress incontinence. However, assessment of the objective parameters revealed that there was no change in the volume of urine lost. Maximum urethral closure pressure did increase significantly but this result was influenced by only one study showing a large effect.

In the second metaanalysis, Sultana and Walters reviewed eight controlled and 14 uncontrolled prospective trials and included all types of estrogen treatment.[137] They also found that estrogen therapy was not an efficacious treatment of stress incontinence but may be useful for the often associated symptoms of urgency and frequency.

Estrogen when given alone therefore does not appear to be an effective treatment for stress incontinence. However, several studies have shown that it may have a role in combination with other therapies. In a randomized trial, Ishiko et al compared the effects of the combination of pelvic floor exercise and estriol (1 mg/day) in 66 patients with postmenopausal stress incontinence.[138] Efficacy was evaluated every 3 months based on stress scores obtained from a questionnaire. They found a significant decrease in stress score in mild and moderate stress incontinence patients in both groups 3 months after the start of therapy and concluded that combination therapy with estriol plus pelvic floor exercise was effective and capable of serving as first-line treatment for mild stress incontinence.

Reviews of recent literature agree that "estrogen therapy has little effect in the management of urodynamic stress incontinence..."[139,140]

ESTROGENS FOR URGENCY INCONTINENCE

Estrogen has been used to treat postmenopausal urgency and urgency incontinence for many years but there have been few controlled trials performed to confirm that it is of benefit. A double-blind multicenter study of 64 postmenopausal women with the "urge syndrome" failed to show efficacy.[141] Another RCT from the same group, using 25 mg estradiol implants, confirmed the previous findings and, furthermore, found a high complication rate in the estriol-treated patients (vaginal bleeding).[142]

Grady et al determined whether postmenopausal hormone therapy improves the severity of urinary incontinence in a randomized, blinded trial among 2763 postmenopausal women younger than 80 years with coronary disease and intact uteri.[143] The study included 1525 participants who reported at least one episode of incontinence per week at baseline. Participants were randomly assigned to 0.625 mg of conjugated estrogens plus 2.5 mg of medroxyprogesterone acetate in one tablet daily (n=768) or placebo (n=757) and were followed for a mean of 4.1 years. Severity of incontinence was classified as improved (decrease of at least two episodes per week), unchanged (change of at most one episode per week) or worsened (increase of at least two episodes per week). The results showed that incontinence improved in 26% of the women assigned to placebo compared with 21% assigned to hormones, while 27% of the placebo group worsened compared with 39% of the hormone group (P=0.001). This difference was evident by 4 months of treatment and was observed for both urge and stress incontinence. The number of incontinent episodes per week increased an average of 0.7 in the hormone group and decreased by 0.1 in the placebo group (P<0.001). The

authors concluded that daily oral estrogen plus progestin therapy was associated with worsening urinary incontinence in older postmenopausal women with weekly incontinence, and did not recommend this therapy for the treatment of incontinence. It cannot be excluded that the progestogen component may influence the effects found in this study.

Estrogen has an important physiologic effect on the female lower urinary tract and its deficiency is an etiologic factor in the pathogenesis of a number of conditions. However, the use of estrogens alone to treat urinary incontinence has given disappointing results. This apparently contrasts with the conclusions of a recent Cochrane review that "Oestrogen treatment can improve or cure incontinence and the evidence suggests that this is more likely to occur with urge incontinence."[144] Even though estrogen therapy may be of benefit for the irritative symptoms of urinary urgency, frequency, and urge incontinence, this effect may result from reversal of urogenital atrophy rather than a direct action on the lower urinary tract function.[140]

REFERENCES

1. Wein AJ. Neuromuscular dysfunction of the lower urinary tract and its treatment. In: Campbell MF, Walsh PC, Retik AB, eds. Campbell's urology, 8th edn. Philadelphia: WB Saunders; 2002.
2. Abrams P, Cardozo L, Fall M, et al. The standardisation of terminology of lower urinary tract function: report from the Standardisation Sub-committee of the International Continence Society. Neurourol Urodynam 2002;21(2):167–178.
3. Andersson K-E, Appell R, Cardozo L, et al. Pharmacological treatment of urinary incontinence. In: Abrams P, Cardozo L, Khoury S, Wein A, eds. Incontinence. Third International Consultation on Incontinence. France: Editions 21; 2005.
4. Morrison J, Steers WD, Brading A, et al. Neurophysiology and neuropharmacology. In: Abrams P, Khoury S, Wein A, eds. Incontinence. Second International Consultation on Incontinence. Plymouth, UK: Health Publications Ltd; 2002: 85–161.
5. Andersson K-E. Antimuscarinics for treatment of overactive bladder. Lancet Neurol 2004;3(1):46–53.
6. Andersson K-E. Bladder activation: afferent mechanisms. Urology 2002;59(5 Suppl 1):43–50.
7. Guay DR. Clinical pharmacokinetics of drugs used to treat urge incontinence. Clin Pharmacokinet 2003;42(14):1243–1285.
8. Andersson K-E. Current concepts in the treatment of disorders of micturition. Drugs 1988;35:477.
9. Beermann B, Hellstrom K, Rosen A. On the metabolism of propantheline in man. Clin Pharmacol Ther 1972;13(2):212–220.
10. Thuroff JW, Chartier-Kastler E, Corcus J, et al. Medical treatment and medical side effects in urinary incontinence in the elderly. World J Urol 1998;16(Suppl 1):S48–61.
11. Füsgen I, Hauri D. Trospium chloride: an effective option for medical treatment of bladder overactivity. Int J Clin Pharmacol Ther 2000;38(5):223–234.
12. Todorova A, Vonderheid-Guth B, Dimpfel W. Effects of tolterodine, trospium chloride, and oxybutynin on the central nervous system. J Clin Pharmacol 2001;41(6):636–644.
13. Wiedemann A, Füsgen I, Hauri D. New aspects of therapy with trospium chloride for urge incontinence. Eur J Geriatr 2002;3:41–45.
14. Stöhrer M, Bauer P, Giannetti BM, Richter R, Burgdorfer H, Murtz G. Effect of trospium chloride on urodynamic parameters in

patients with detrusor hyperreflexia due to spinal cord injuries: a multicentre placebo controlled double-blind trial. Urol Int 1991;47:138–143.
15. Madersbacher H, Stöhrer M, Richter R, Burgdorfer H, Hachen HJ, Murtz G. Trospium chloride versus oxybutynin: a randomized, double-blind, multicentre trial in the treatment of detrusor hyperreflexia. Br J Urol 1995;75(4):452–456.
16. Allousi S, Laval K-U, Eckert R. Trospium chloride (Spasmo-lyt) in patients with motor urge syndrome (detrusor instability): a double-blind, randomised, multicentre, placebo-controlled study. J Clin Res 1998;1:439–451.
17. Cardozo L, Chapple CR, Toozs-Hobson P, et al. Efficacy of trospium chloride in patients with detrusor instability: a placebo-controlled, randomized, double-blind, multicentre clinical trial. BJU Int 2000;85(6):659–664.
18. Jünemann KP, Al-Shukri S. Efficacy and tolerability of trospium chloride and tolterodine in 234 patients with urge-syndrome: a double-blind, placebo-controlled multicentre clinical trial. Neurourol Urodynam 2000;19:488–489.
19. Halaska M, Ralph G, Wiedemann A, Primus G, Ballering-Bruhl B, Hofner K, Jonas U. Controlled, double-blind, multicentre clinical trial to investigate long-term tolerability and efficacy of trospium chloride in patients with detrusor instability. World J Urol 2003;20(6):392–399.
20. Zinner N, Gittelman M, Harris R, Susset J, Kanelos A, Auerbach S, Trospium Study Group. Trospium chloride improves overactive bladder symptoms: a multicenter phase III trial. J Urol 2004;171(6 Pt 1):2311–2315.
21. Stahl MM, Ekstrom B, Sparf B, Mattiasson A, Andersson KE. Urodynamic and other effects of tolterodine: a novel antimuscarinic drug for the treatment of detrusor overactivity. Neurourol Urodynam 1995;14(6):647–655.
22. Nilvebrant L, Andersson KE, Gillberg PG, Stahl M, Sparf B. Tolterodine—a new bladder-selective antimuscarinic agent. Eur J Pharmacol 1997;327(2-3):195–207.
23. Nilvebrant L, Gillberg PG, Sparf B. Antimuscarinic potency and bladder selectivity of PNU-200577, a major metabolite of tolterodine. Pharmacol Toxicol 1997;81(4):169–172.

24. Brynne N, Stahl MMS, Hallén B, Edlund PO, Palmér L, Höglund P, Gabrielsson J. Pharmacokinetics and pharmacodynamics of tolterodine in man: a new drug for the treatment of urinary bladder overactivity. Int J Clin Pharmacol Ther 1997;35:287–295.

25. Brynne N, Dalen P, Alvan G, Bertilsson L, Gabrielsson J. Influence of CYP2D6 polymorphism on the pharmacokinetics and pharmacodynamics of tolterodine. Clin Pharmacol Ther 1998;63:529–539.

26. Hills CJ, Winter SA, Balfour JA. Tolterodine. Drugs 1998; 55:813–820.

27. Clemett D, Jarvis B. Tolterodine: a review of its use in the treatment of overactive bladder. Drugs Aging 2001;18(4):277–304.

28. Van Kerrebroeck P, Kreder K, Jonas U, Zinner N, Wein A, Tolterodine Study Group. Tolterodine once-daily: superior efficacy and tolerability in the treatment of the overactive bladder. Urology 2001;57(3):414–421.

29. Appell RA, Sand P, Dmochowski R, et al, for the Overactive Bladder: Judging Effective Control and Treatment Study Group. Prospective randomized controlled trial of extended-release oxybutynin chloride and tolterodine tartrate in the treatment of overactive bladder: results of the OBJECT Study. Mayo Clin Proc 2001;76(4):358–363.

30. Diokno AC, Appell RA, Sand PK, et al, for the OPERA Study Group. Prospective, randomized, double-blind study of the efficacy and tolerability of the extended-release formulations of oxybutynin and tolterodine for overactive bladder: results of the OPERA trial. Mayo Clin Proc 2003;78(6):687–695.

31. Kerbusch T, Wahlby U, Milligan PA, Karlsson MO. Population pharmacokinetic modelling of darifenacin and its hydroxylated metabolite using pooled data, incorporating saturable first-pass metabolism, CYP2D6 genotype and formulation-dependent bioavailability. Br J Clin Pharmacol 2003;56(6):639–652.

32. Andersson K-E. Potential benefits of muscarinic M_3 receptor selectivity. Eur Urol Suppl 2002;1 (4):23–28.

33. Haab F, Stewart L, Dwyer P. Darifenacin, an M3 selective receptor antagonist, is an effective and well-tolerated once-daily treatment for overactive bladder. Eur Urol 2004;45(4):420–429.

34. Chapple CR. Darifenacin is well tolerated and provides significant improvement in the symptoms of overactive bladder: a pooled analysis of phase III studies. J Urol 2004;171(Suppl): 130 (abstract 487).

35. Kuipers M, Tran D, Krauwinkel W, Abila B, Mulder H. Absolute bioavailability of YM905 in healthy male volunteers. A single-dose randomized, two-period crossover study. Paper presented at the 32nd International Continence Society Annual Meeting, Heidelberg, Germany, August 2002.

36. Smulders R, Tan H, Krauwinkel W, Abila B, van Zitjveld J. A placebo-controlled, dose-rising study in healthy male volunteers to evaluate safety, tolerability, pharmacokinetics and pharmacodynamics of single oral doses of YM905. Paper presented at the 32nd International Continence Society Annual Meeting, Heidelberg, Germany, August 2002.

37. Ikeda K, Kobayashi S, Suzuki M, et al. M(3) receptor antagonism by the novel antimuscarinic agent solifenacin in the urinary bladder and salivary gland. Naunyn Schmiedebergs Arch Pharmacol 2002;366(2):97–103.

38. Chapple CR, Arano P, Bosch JL, De Ridder D, Kramer AE, Ridder AM. Solifenacin appears effective and well tolerated in patients with symptomatic idiopathic detrusor overactivity in a placebo- and tolterodine-controlled phase 2 dose-finding study. BJU Int 2004;93(1):71–77.

39. Chapple CR, Rechberger T, Al-Shukri S, et al, for the YM-905 Study Group. Randomized, double-blind placebo- and tolterodine-controlled trial of the once-daily antimuscarinic agent solifenacin in patients with symptomatic overactive bladder. BJU Int 2004;93(3):303–310.

40. Douchamps J, Derenne F, Stockis A, Gangji D, Juvent M, Herchuelz A. The pharmacokinetics of oxybutynin in man. Eur J Clin Pharmacol 1988;35:515–520.

41. Hughes KM, Lang JCT, Lazare R, et al. Measurement of oxybutynin and its N-desethyl metabolite in plasma, and its application to pharmacokinetic studies in young, elderly and frail elderly volunteers. Xenobiotica 1992;22:859–869.

42. Waldeck K, Larsson B, Andersson K-E. Comparison of oxybutynin and its active metabolite, N-desethyl-oxybutynin, in the human detrusor and parotid gland. J Urol 1997;157:1093–1097.

43. Norhona-Blob L, Kachur JF. Enantiomers of oxybutynin: in vitro pharmacological characterization at M1, M2 and M3 muscarinic receptors and in vivo effects on urinary bladder contraction, mydriasis and salivary secretion in guinea pigs. J Pharmacol Exp Ther 1991;256:562–567.

44. Andersson KE, Chapple CR. Oxybutynin and the overactive bladder. World J Urol 2001;19(5):319–323.

45. Dmochowski RR, Davila GW, Zinner NR, et al, for the Transdermal Oxybutynin Study Group. Efficacy and safety of transdermal oxybutynin in patients with urge and mixed urinary incontinence. J Urol 2002;168(2):580–586.

46. Siddiqui MA, Perry CM, Scott LJ. Oxybutynin extended-release: a review of its use in the management of overactive bladder. Drugs 2004;64(8):885–912.

47. Dmochowski RR, Sand PK, Zinner NR, et al, for the Transdermal Oxybutynin Study Group. Comparative efficacy and safety of transdermal oxybutynin and oral tolterodine versus placebo in previously treated patients with urge and mixed urinary incontinence. Urology 2003;62(2):237–242.

48. Madersbacher H, Mürz G. Efficacy, tolerability and safety profile of propiverine in the treatment of the overactive bladder (non-neurogenic and neurogenic). World J Urol 2001;19:324–335.

49. Walter R, Ullmann C, Thummler D, Siegmund W. Influence of propiverine on hepatic microsomal cytochrome p450 enzymes in male rats. Drug Metab Dispos 2003;31(6):714–717.

50. Haustein KO, Huller G. On the pharmacokinetics and metabolism of propiverine in man. Eur J Drug Metab Pharmacokinet 1988;13(2):81–90.

51. Muller C, Siegmund W, Huupponen R, et al. Kinetics of propiverine as assessed by radioreceptor assay in poor and extensive metabolizers of debrisoquine. Eur J Drug Metab Pharmacokinet 1993;18(3):265–272.

52. Stöhrer M, Madersbacher H, Richter R, Wehnert J, Dreikorn K. Efficacy and safety of propiverine in SCI-patients suffering from detrusor hyperreflexia: a double-blind, placebo-controlled clinical trial. Spinal Cord 1999;37:196–200.

53. Wehnert J, Sage S. Comparative investigations to the action of Mictonorm (propiverin hydrochloride) and Spasuret (flavoxat hydrochloride) on detrusor vesicae. Z Urol Nephrol 1989; 82:259–263.

54. Wehnert J, Sage S. Therapie der Blaseninstabilität und Urge-Inkontinenz mit Propiverin hydrochlorid (Mictonorm®) und Oxybutynin chlorid (Dridase®): eine randomisierte Cross-over-Vergleichsstudie. Akt Urol 1992;23:7–11.

55. Madersbacher H, Halaska M, Voigt R, Alloussi S, Hofner K. A placebo-controlled, multicentre study comparing the tolerability and efficacy of propiverine and oxybutynin in patients with urgency and urge incontinence. BJU Int 1999;84:646–651.

56. Dorschner W, Stolzenburg JU, Griebenow R, et al. Efficacy and cardiac safety of propiverine in elderly patients: a double-blind, placebo-controlled clinical study. Eur Urol 2000;37:702–708.

57. Sheu MT, Yeh GC, Ke WT, Ho HO. Development of a high-performance liquid chromatographic method for bioequivalence study of flavoxate tablets. J Chromatogr B Biomed Sci Appl 2001;751(1):79–86.

58. Cazzulani P, Pietra C, Abbiati GA, et al. Pharmacological activities of the main metabolite of flavoxate 3-methylflavone-8-carboxylic acid. Arzneimittelforschung 1988;38(3):379–382.

59. Caine M, Gin S, Pietra C, Ruffmann R. Antispasmodic effects of flavoxate, MFCA, and REC 15/2053 on smooth muscle of human prostate and urinary bladder. Urology 1991;37(4):390–394.

60. Ruffmann R. A review of flavoxate hydrochloride in the treatment of urge incontinence. J Int Med Res 1988;16:317–330.

61. Stanton SL. A comparison of emepronium bromide and flavoxate hydrochloride in the treatment of urinary incontinence. J Urol 1973;110:529–532.

62. Milani R, Scalambrino S, Milia R, et al. Double-blind crossover comparison of flavoxate and oxybutynin in women affected by urinary urge syndrome. Int Urogynecol J 1993;4:3–8.

63. Briggs KS, Castleden CM, Asher MJ. The effect of flavoxate on uninhibited detrusor contractions and urinary incontinence in the elderly. J Urol 1980;123: 665–666.

64. Chapple CR, Parkhouse H, Gardener C, Milroy EJG. Double-blind, placebo-controlled, cross-over study of flavoxate in the treatment of idiopathic detrusor instability. Br J Urol 1990;66: 491–494.

65. Dahm TL, Ostri P, Kristensen JK, et al. Flavoxate treatment of micturition disorders accompanying benign prostatic hypertrophy: a double-blind placebo-controlled multicenter investigation. Urol Int 1995;55:205–208.

66. Naglie G, Radomski SB, Brymer C, Mathiasen K, O'Rourke K, Tomlinson G. A randomized, double-blind, placebo controlled crossover trial of nimodipine in older persons with detrusor instability and urge incontinence. J Urol 2002;167(2 Pt 1):586–590.

67. Andersson K-E. Clinical pharmacology of potassium channel openers. Pharmacol Toxicol 1992;70(4):244–254.

68. Andersson KE, Arner A. Urinary bladder contraction and relaxation: physiology and pathophysiology. Physiol Rev 2004;84(3):935–986.

69. Andersson K-E. Alpha-adrenoceptors and benign prostatic hyperplasia: basic principles for treatment with alpha-adrenoceptor antagonists. World J Urol 2002;19(6):390–396.

70. Arnold EP. Tamsulosin in men with confirmed bladder outlet obstruction: a clinical and urodynamic analysis from a single centre in New Zealand. BJU Int 2001;87(1):24–30.

71. Abrams P, Amarenco G, Bakke A, et al, for the European Tamsulosin Neurogenic Lower Urinary Tract Dysfunction Study Group. Tamsulosin: efficacy and safety in patients with neurogenic lower urinary tract dysfunction due to suprasacral spinal cord injury. J Urol 2003;170(4 Pt 1):1242–1251.

72. Dwyer PL, Teele JS. Prazosin: a neglected cause of genuine stress incontinence. Obstet Gynecol 1992;79:117–121.

73. Andersson K-E. Pharmacology of lower urinary tract smooth muscles and penile erectile tissues. Pharmacol Rev 1993;45(3):253–308.

74. Nergårdh A, Boreus LO, Naglo AS. Characterization of the adrenergic beta-receptor in the urinary bladder of man and cat. Acta Pharmacol Toxicol (Copenh) 1977;40(1):14–21.

75. Larsen JJ. Alpha and beta-adrenoceptors in the detrusor muscle and bladder base of the pig and beta-adrenoceptors in the detrusor muscle of man. Br J Pharmacol 1979;65(2):215–222.

76. Igawa Y, Yamazaki Y, Takeda H, et al. Functional and molecular biologic evidence for a possible beta3-adrenoceptor in the human detrusor muscle. Br J Pharmacol 1999;126:819–825.

77. Igawa Y, Yamazaki Y, Takeda H, et al. Relaxant effects of isoproterenol and selective beta3-adrenoceptor agonists on normal, low compliant and hyperreflexic human bladders. J Urol 2001;165:240–244.

78. Takeda M, Obara K, Mizusawa T, et al. Evidence for beta3-adrenoceptor subtypes in relaxation of the human urinary bladder detrusor: analysis by molecular biologic and pharmacological methods. J Pharmacol Exp Ther 1999;288:1367–1373.

79. Lindholm P, Lose G. Terbutaline (Bricanyl) in the treatment of female urge incontinence. Urol Int 1986;41(2):158–160.

80. Grüneberger A. Treatment of motor urge incontinence with clenbuterol and flavoxate hydrochloride. Br J Obstet Gynaecol 1984;91:275–278.

81. Castleden CM, Morgan B. The effect of β-adrenoceptor agonists on urinary incontinence in the elderly. Br J Clin Pharmacol 1980;10:619–620.

82. Naglo AS, Nergårdh A, Boreus LO. Influence of atropine and

83. isoprenaline on detrusor hyperactivity in children with neurogenic bladder. Scand J Urol Nephrol 1981;15(2):97–102.

83. Martin MR, Schiff AA. Fluphenazine/nortriptyline in the irritative bladder syndrome: a double-blind placebo-controlled study. Br J Urol 1984:56:178–179.

84. Lose G, Jorgensen L, Thunedborg P. Doxepin in the treatment of female detrusor overactivity: a randomized double-blind crossover study. J Urol 1989:142:1024–1026.

85. Baldessarini KJ. Drugs in the treatment of psychiatric disorders. In: Gilman AG, Goodman LS, Rall TW, Murad F, eds. The pharmacological basis of therapeutics, 7th edn. New York: MacMillan Publishing; 1985.

86. Maggi CA, Borsini F, Lecci A, et al. The effect of acute and chronic administration of imipramine on spinal and supraspinal micturition reflexes in rats. J Pharmacol Exp Ther 1989:248:278–285.

87. Hunsballe JM, Djurhuus JC. Clinical options for imipramine in the management of urinary incontinence. Urol Res 2001:29:118–125.

88. Glazener CM, Evans JH, Peto RE. Tricyclic and related drugs for nocturnal enuresis in children. Cochrane Database Syst Rev 2003;(3):CD002117.

89. Bigger JT, Giardina EG, Perel JM, Kantor SJ, Glassman AH. Cardiac antiarrhythmic effect of imipramine hydrochloride. N Engl J Med 1977:296:206–208.

90. Giardina EG, Bigger JT Jr, Glassman AH, Perel JM, Kantor SJ. The electrocardiographic and antiarrhythmic effects of imipramine hydrochloride at therapeutic plasma concentrations. Circulation 1979:60:1045–1052.

91. Cardozo LD, Stanton SL, Robinson H, Hole D. Evaluation on flurbiprofen in detrusor instability. Br Med J 1980:280:281–282.

92. Palmer J. Report of a double-blind crossover study of flurbiprofen and placebo in detrusor instability. J Int Med Res 1983;11(Suppl 2):11–17.

93. Cardozo LD, Stanton SL. A comparison between bromocriptine and indomethacin in the treatment of detrusor instability. J Urol 1980:123:399–401.

94. Andersson K-E, Bengtsson B, Paulsen O. Desamino-8-D-Arginine vasopressin (DDAVP): pharmacology and clinical use. Drugs of Today 1988:24:509.

95. Glazener CM, Evans JH. Desmopressin for nocturnal enuresis in children. Cochrane Database Syst Rev 2002;(3):CD002112.

96. Janknegt RA, Zweers HMM, Delaere KPJ, Kloet AG, Khoe SGS, Arendsen HJ. Oral desmopressin as a new treament modality for primary nocturnal enuresis in adolescents and adults: a double-blind, randomized, multicenter study. J Urol 1997:157:513–517.

97. Skoog SJ, Stokes A, Turner KL. Oral desmopressin: a randomized double-blind placebo controlled study of effectiveness in children with primary nocturnal enuresis. J Urol 1997:158:1035–1040.

98. Mattiasson A, Abrams P, Van Kerrebroeck P, Walter S, Weiss J. Efficacy of desmopressin in the treatment of nocturia: a double-blind placebo-controlled study in men. BJU Int 2002;89(9):855–862.

99. Lose G, Lalos O, Freeman RM, van Kerrebroeck P, for the Nocturia Study Group. Efficacy of desmopressin (Minirin) in the treatment of nocturia: a double-blind placebo-controlled study in women. Am J Obstet Gynecol 2003;189(4):1106–1113.

100. Weatherall M. The risk of hyponatremia in older adults using desmopressin for nocturia: a systematic review and meta-analysis. Neurourol Urodynam 2004;23(4):302–305.

101. Rembratt A, Norgaard JP, Andersson KE. Desmopressin in elderly patients with nocturia: short-term safety and effects on urine output, sleep and voiding patterns. BJU Int 2003;91(7):642–646.

102. Taylor MC, Bates CP. A double-blind crossover trial of baclofen: a new treatment for the unstable bladder syndrome. Br J Urol 1979:51:504–505.

103. Bushman W, Steers WD, Meythaler JM. Voiding dysfunction in patients with spastic paraplegia: urodynamic evaluation and response to continuous intrathecal baclofen. Neurol Urodynam 1993:12:163–170.

104. Maggi CA, Barbanti G, Santicioli P, et al. Cystometric evidence

that capsaicin-sensitive nerves modulate the afferent branch of micturition reflex in humans. J Urol 1989;142(1):150–154.

105. Cruz F. Mechanisms involved in new therapies for overactive bladder. Urology 2004;63(3 Suppl 1):65–73.

106. De Seze M, Wiart L, de Seze MP, et al. Intravesical capsaicin versus resiniferatoxin for the treatment of detrusor hyperreflexia in spinal cord injured patients: a double-blind, randomized, controlled study. J Urol 2004;171(1):251–255.

107. Kim JH, Rivas DA, Shenot PJ, et al. Intravesical resiniferatoxin for refractory detrusor hyperreflexia: a multicenter, blinded, randomized, placebo-controlled trial. J Spinal Cord Med 2003;26(4):358–363.

108. Kuo HC. Effectiveness of intravesical resiniferatoxin in treating detrusor hyper-reflexia and external sphincter dyssynergia in patients with chronic spinal cord lesions. BJU Int 2003;92(6):597–601.

109. Watanabe T, Yokoyama T, Sasaki K, Nozaki K, Ozawa H, Kumon H. Intravesical resiniferatoxin for patients with neurogenic detrusor overactivity. Int J Urol 2004;11(4):200–205.

110. Giannantoni A, Di Stasi SM, Stephen RL, Bini V, Costantini E, Porena M. Intravesical resiniferatoxin versus botulinum-A toxin injections for neurogenic detrusor overactivity: a prospective randomized study. J Urol 2004;172(1):240–243.

111. Yokoyama T, Kumon H, Smith CP, Somogyi GT, Chancellor MB. Botulinum toxin treatment of urethral and bladder dysfunction. Acta Med Okayama 2002;56(6):271–277.

112. Smith CP, Franks ME, McNeil BK, et al. Effect of botulinum toxin A on the autonomic nervous system of the rat lower urinary tract. J Urol 2003;169(5):1896–1900.

113. Smith CP, Chancellor MB. Emerging role of botulinum toxin in the management of voiding dysfunction. J Urol 2004;171(6 Pt 1):2128–2137.

114. Leippold T, Reitz A, Schurch B. Botulinum toxin as a new therapy option for voiding disorders: current state of the art. Eur Urol 2003;44(2):165–174.

115. Rapp DE, Lucioni A, Katz EE, O'Connor RC, Gerber GS, Bales GT. Use of botulinum-A toxin for the treatment of refractory overactive bladder symptoms: an initial experience. Urology 2004;63(6):1071–1075.

116. Zinner NR, Koke SC, Viktrup L. Pharmacotherapy for stress urinary incontinence: present and future options. Drugs 2004;64(14):1503–1516.

117. Alhasso A, Glazener CM, Pickard R, N'Dow J. Adrenergic drugs for urinary incontinence in adults. Cochrane Database Syst Rev 2003;(2):CD001842.

118. Kernan WN, Viscoli CM, Brass LM, et al. Phenylpropanolamine and the risk of hemorrhagic stroke. N Engl J Med 2000;343(25):1826–1832.

119. Bent S, Tiedt TN, Odden MC, Shlipak MG. The relative safety of ephedra compared with other herbal products. Ann Intern Med 2003;138(6):468–471.

120. Radley SC, Chapple CR, Bryan NP, Clarke DE, Craig DA. Effect of methoxamine on maximum urethral pressure in women with genuine stress incontinence: a placebo-controlled, double-blind crossover study. Neurourol Urodynam 2001;20(1):43–52.

121. Weil EH, Eerdmans PH, Dijkman GA, et al. Randomized double-blind placebo-controlled multicenter evaluation of efficacy and dose finding of midodrine hydrochloride in women with mild to moderate stress urinary incontinence: a phase II study. Int Urogynecol J Pelvic Floor Dysfunct 1998;9(3):145–150.

122. Musselman DM, Ford AP, Gennevois DJ, et al. A randomized crossover study to evaluate Ro 115-1240, a selective alpha1A/1L-adrenoceptor partial agonist in women with stress urinary incontinence. BJU Int 2004;93(1):78–83.

123. Gilja I, Radej M, Kovacic M, Parazajdes J. Conservative treatment of female stress incontinence with imipramine. J Urol 1984;132:909–911.

124. Lin HH, Sheu BC, Lo MC, Huang SC. Comparison of treatment outcomes for imipramine for female genuine stress incontinence. Br J Obstet Gynaecol 1999:106:1089–1092.

125. Yasuda K, Kawabe K, Takimoto Y, et al, for the Clenbutrol Clinical Research Group. A double-blind clinical trial of a β_2-adrenergic agonist in stress incontinence. Int Urogynecol J 1993:4:146–151.

126. Ishiko O, Ushiroyama T, Saji F, et al. beta(2)-Adrenergic agonists and pelvic floor exercises for female stress incontinence. Int J Gynaecol Obstet 2000;71:39–44.

127. Thor KB, Katofiasc MA. Effects of duloxetine, a combined serotonin and norepinephrine reuptake inhibitor, on central neural control of lower urinary tract function in the chloralose-anesthetized female cat. J Pharmacol Exp Ther 1995;274(2):1014–1024.

128. Katofiasc MA, Nissen J, Audia JE, Thor KB. Comparison of the effects of serotonin selective, norepinephrine selective, and dual serotonin and norepinephrine reuptake inhibitors on lower urinary tract function in cats. Life Sci 2002;71(11):1227–1236.

129. Thor KB, Donatucci C. Central nervous system control of the lower urinary tract: new pharmacological approaches to stress urinary incontinence in women. J Urol 2004;172(1):27–33.

130. Fraser MO, Chancellor MB. Neural control of the urethra and development of pharmacotherapy for stress urinary incontinence. BJU Int 2003;91(8):743–748.

131. Sharma A, Goldberg MJ, Cerimele BJ. Pharmacokinetics and safety of duloxetine, a dual-serotonin and norepinephrine reuptake inhibitor. J Clin Pharmacol 2000;40(2):161–167.

132. Dmochowski RR, Miklos JR, Norton PA, et al, for the Duloxetine Urinary Incontinence Study Group. Duloxetine versus placebo for the treatment of North American women with stress urinary incontinence. J Urol 2003;170(4 Pt 1):1259–1263.

133. van Kerrebroeck P, Abrams P, Lange R, et al, for the Duloxetine Urinary Incontinence Study Group. Duloxetine versus placebo in the treatment of European and Canadian women with stress urinary incontinence. Br J Obstet Gynaecol 2004;111(3):249–257.

134. Millard RJ, Moore K, Rencken R, Yalcin I, Bump RC, for the Duloxetine Urinary Incontinence Study Group. Duloxetine vs placebo in the treatment of stress urinary incontinence: a four-continent randomized clinical trial. BJU Int 2004;93(3):311–318.

135. Viktrup L, Pangallo BA, Detke MJ, Zinner NR. Urinary side effects of duloxetine in the treatment of depression and stress urinary incontinence. Prim Care Companion J Clin Psychiatry 2004;6(2):65–73.

136. Fantl JA, Cardozo L, McClish DK. Estrogen therapy in the management of urinary incontinence in postmenopausal women: a meta-analysis. First report of the Hormones and Urogenital Therapy Committee. Obstet Gynecol 1994:83:12–18.

137. Sultana CJ, Walters MD. Estrogen and urinary incontinence in women. Maturitas 1990:20:129–138.

138. Ishiko O, Hirai K, Sumi T, Tatsuta I, Ogita S. Hormone replacement therapy plus pelvic floor muscle exercise for postmenopausal stress incontinence. A randomized, controlled trial. J Reprod Med 2001:46:213–220.

139. Al-Badr A, Ross S, Soroka D, Drutz HP. What is the available evidence for hormone replacement therapy in women with stress urinary incontinence? J Obstet Gynaecol Can 2003;25(7):567–574.

140. Robinson D, Cardozo LD. The role of estrogens in female lower urinary tract dysfunction. Urology 2003;62(4 Suppl 1):45–51.

141. Cardozo L, Rekers H, Tapp A, et al. Oestriol in the treatment of postmenopausal urgency: a multicentre study. Maturitas 1993:18:47–53.

142. Rufford J, Hextall A, Cardozo L, Khullar V. A double-blind placebo-controlled trial on the effects of 25 mg estradiol implants on the urge syndrome in postmenopausal women. Int Urogynecol J Pelvic Floor Dysfunct 2003;14(2):78–83.

143. Grady D, Brown JS, Vittinghoff E, Applegate W, Varner E, Snyder T. Postmenopausal hormones and incontinence: the Heart and Estrogen/Progestin Replacement Study. Obstet Gynecol 2001:97:116–120.

144. Moehrer B, Hextall A, Jackson S. Oestrogens for urinary incontinence in women. Cochrane Database Syst Rev 2003;(2):CD001405.

Pelvic Floor Muscle Training

Kari Bø

INTRODUCTION

In 1948 Kegel[1] was the first to report pelvic floor muscle training (PFMT) to be effective in treatment of female urinary incontinence (UI). In spite of his reports of cure rates of >84%, surgery soon became the first choice of treatment and not until the 1980s was there renewed interest in conservative treatment. This interest may have developed because of higher awareness among women about incontinence and health and fitness activities, cost of surgery, and morbidity, complications, and relapses reported after surgical procedures.

Although several consensus statements based on systematic reviews have recommended conservative treatment and especially PFMT as the first choice of treatment for UI,[2-5] many surgeons seem to regard minimally invasive surgery, especially the tension-free vaginal tape procedure (TVT), as a better first-line option than PFMT. The scepticism about PFMT may be based on inappropriate knowledge of exercise science and physical therapy, beliefs that there is insufficient evidence for the effect of PFMT or that evidence for long-term effect is lacking or poor, and that women are not motivated to perform PFMT regularly. The aim of this chapter is to report evidence-based knowledge on the above-mentioned points related to PFMT for UI.

METHODS

Only outcomes from randomized controlled trials (RCT) are included in this chapter. A computerized search on PubMed, studies, data, and conclusions from the Clinical Practice Guideline (AHCPR, USA),[2] the Second International Consultation on Incontinence (ICI),[3] and the Cochrane Library of Systematic Reviews[4,6] have been used as background sources. Physical therapy techniques to treat stress urinary incontinence (SUI) and urge incontinence include PFMT with or without biofeedback, electrical stimulation and cones.[3,4] Since SUI and urge incontinence are different conditions that most likely need different treatment approaches, evidence for the different physical therapy interventions will be analyzed separately for each of these conditions.

EFFECTIVENESS OF PHYSICAL THERAPY INTERVENTIONS FOR URINARY INCONTINENCE

The gold standard research design to evaluate the effect of an intervention (surgery, pharmaceutical, training) is a RCT. However, there are high- and low-quality RCTs. High methodology quality is judged on concealment of treatment allocation, blinding of assessors, sufficient sample size (based on power calculation if possible), use of reproducible and valid outcome measurements, and handling of drop-outs and low adherence (intention to treat analysis).

Equally important but less covered in textbooks of statistics and research methodology is the quality of the intervention (high standard surgery, experienced surgeons, theory based and high-quality conducted PFMT). Many ineffective or even harmful treatments can appear in a RCT of high methodology quality. These research challenges are the same when conducting RCTs in surgery and PFMT, and the quality of studies of both surgery and PFMT has been judged to be varied.[4,7]

However, there is an additional problem with PFMT studies. Several research groups have shown that >30% of women are not able to voluntary contract the PFM at their first consultation, even after thorough individual instruction.[8-11] Hay-Smith et al[4] reported that in only 15 of 43 RCTs on the effect of PFM training for SUI, UI and mixed incontinence was the ability to contract checked before training started. A common mistake is to contract other muscles such as abdominals, gluteals, and hip adductor muscles instead of the PFM.[12] In addition, Bump et al[11] showed that as many as 25% of women may strain instead of squeeze and lift. If women are straining instead of performing a correct contraction, the training may harm and not improve PFM function. Proper assessment of ability to contract the PFM is therefore mandatory (Fig.14.1).

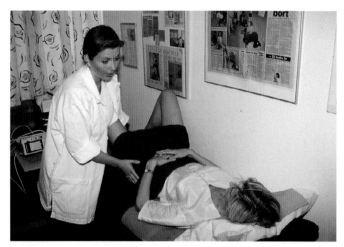

Figure 14.1 Thorough instruction and evaluation of ability to contract the pelvic floor muscles are mandatory before training can start.

STRESS URINARY INCONTINENCE

The numerous reports by Kegel with >80% cure rate comprised uncontrolled studies with the inclusion of a variety of incontinence types and no measurement of urinary leakage before and after treatment. However, since then, several RCTs have demonstrated that PFM exercise is more effective than no treatment[13,14] to treat SUI.[13,15-19] In addition, a number of RCTs have compared PFM training alone with the use of vaginal resistance devices, biofeedback or vaginal cones.[4] Out of 43 RCTs, only one did not show any significant effect of PFM training on urinary leakage.[4] Interestingly, in this study there was no check of the women's ability to contract, adherence to the training protocol was poor and the placebo group contracted gluteal muscles and external rotators of the hips, activities that may give co-contractions of the PFM.[12,20]

Combined improvement and cure rates. As for surgery[7] and pharmacology studies,[21] a combination of cure and improvement measures is often reported. Currently, there is no consensus on what outcome measure to choose as the gold standard for cure (urodynamic diagnosis, no leakage episodes, ≤2 g of leakage on pad test, tests with standardized bladder volume, 1 hour, 24 hour, 48 hour, women's report, etc.).[22] Subjective cure/improvement rates of PFM training reported in RCTs on both SUI and urge incontinence vary between 56% and 70%.[3-5]

Cure rates for SUI. It is often reported that PFM training is more commonly associated with improvement of symptoms, rather than a total cure. However, in several RCTs cure has been reported. In a study by Bø et al,[23] cure rate was defined as conversion of negative to positive closure pressure during cough, and a cure rate of 60% was found. This corresponded with the number of women reporting to be continent or almost continent. In newer RCTs, short-term cure rates of 44–70%, defined as <2 g of leakage on different pad tests, have been found after PFM training.[15,16,18,24-26] The highest cure rates were shown in two single-blind RCTs in which women had thorough individual instruction by a trained physical therapist (PT), combined training with biofeedback or electrical stimulation, and had close follow-up every second week. Adherence was high and drop-out was low.[25,26]

The most effective program. Because of use of different outcome measures and instruments to measure PFM function and strength, it is impossible to combine results between studies and difficult to conclude which training regimen is the more effective. Also the exercise dosage (type of exercise, frequency, duration, and intensity) varies significantly between studies.[3,4]

Bø et al[23] have shown that training with an instructor is significantly more effective than home exercise. In this study individual assessment and teaching of correct contraction was combined with strength training in groups in a 6-month training program.[18,23] The women were randomized to either an intensive training program consisting of seven individual sessions with a PT, combined with 45 minutes weekly PFM training classes, and three sets of 8–12 contractions per day at home or the same program without the weekly intensive exercise classes. The results showed a much better improvement in both muscle strength and incontinence in the intensive exercise group. Sixty percent were reported to be continent/almost continent in the intensive exercise group compared to 17% in the less intensive group. A significant reduction of urinary leakage, measured by pad test with standardized bladder volume, was only demonstrated in the intensive exercise group.

This study demonstrated that a huge difference in outcome can be expected according to the intensity and follow-up of the training program and very little effect can be expected after training without close follow-up. It is worth noting that the significantly less effective group in this study had seven visits with a skilled PT and that adherence to the home training program was high. Nevertheless, the effect was only 17%. More intensive training has also been shown to be more effective in two other RCTs.[27,28] There is a dose–response issue in all sorts of training regimens.[29] Hence, one reason for the disappointing effects shown in some clinical practices or research studies may be insufficient training stimulus and low dosage. If low-dosage programs are chosen as one arm in a RCT comparing PFM training with other methods, PFM training is bound to be less effective.

Training with biofeedback. Biofeedback has been defined as "a group of experimental procedures where an external sensor is used to give an indication of bodily processes, usually with the purpose of changing the measured quality."[30] Biofeedback equipment has been developed within the area of psychology, mainly for measurement of sweating, heart rate, and blood pressure during different forms of stress. Kegel[1] always based his training protocol on thorough instruction of correct contraction using vaginal palpation and clinical observation. He combined PFM training with use of vaginal squeeze pressure measurement as biofeedback during exercise. Today, a variety of biofeedback apparatus is commonly used in clinical practice to assist with PFM training (Fig. 14.2).

In urology or urogynecology textbooks, the term "biofeedback" is often used to indicate a method different from PFM training. However, biofeedback is not a treatment on its own; it is an adjunct to training, measuring the response from a single PFM contraction. In the area of PFM training, both vaginal and anal surface EMG and urethral and vaginal squeeze pressure measurements have been utilized with the purpose of making the patients more aware of muscle function, and to enhance and motivate patients' effort during training.[3,4]

Since Kegel first presented his results, several RCTs have shown that even PFM training without biofeedback is more effective than no treatment for SUI.[4,13,14,18,26] In women with stress or mixed incontinence, all but one RCT have failed to show any effect of adding biofeedback to the training protocol. In the study of Glavind et al,[27] a positive effect was demonstrated. However, this study was confounded by a difference in training frequency, and the effect might be due to a double training dosage, the use of biofeedback, or both. The results support the studies concluding that there is a dose–response issue in PFM training.[23,28,31]

Since PFM training is effective without biofeedback, a large sample size may be needed to show any beneficial effect of adding biofeedback to an effective training protocol. In most of the published studies comparing PFMT with PFMT combined with biofeedback, the sample sizes are small and type II error may have been the reason for negative findings.[3,4] However, in the two largest RCTs published, no additional effect was demonstrated from adding biofeedback.[3,4,25]

Many women may not like to undress, lock the room, and insert a vaginal or rectal device in order to exercise.[32] On the other hand, some women find it motivating to use biofeedback to control and enhance the strength of the contractions when training. Any factor that may stimulate high adherence and intensive training should be recommended in order to enhance the effect of a training program.

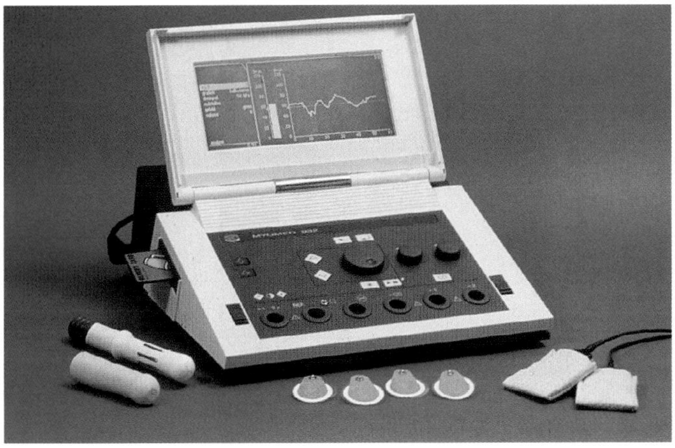

Cones. Vaginal cones, developed by Plevnik[4] in 1985, are weights that are placed in the vagina above the levator plate[6] (Fig. 14.3). The theory behind the use of cones in strength training is that the PFM are contracted reflexively or voluntary when the cone is perceived as slipping out. The weight of the cone is supposed to give a training stimulus and make the women contract harder with progressive weight.

It has been concluded that training with vaginal cones is more effective than no treatment.[3,6] Five RCTs have been found comparing PFMT with and without vaginal cones for SUI.[18,33-36] Bø et al[18] found that PFMT was significantly more effective than training with cones both to improve muscle strength and reduce urinary leakage. In the four other studies there were no differences between PFMT with and without cones.[35] Cammu & Van Nylen[35] reported very low compliance and therefore did not recommend use of cones. Also, in the study of Bø et al,[18] women in the cone group had great motivational problems. Laycock et al[36] had a total drop-out rate of 33% in their study.

The use of cones can be questioned from an exercise science perspective. Holding the cone for as long as 15–20 minutes, as recommended, might cause decreased blood supply, decreased oxygen consumption, muscle fatigue and

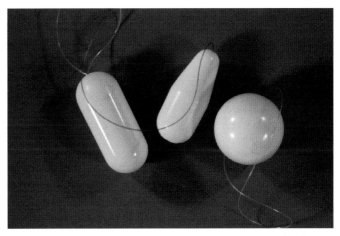

Figure 14.2 Some types of apparatus on the market have EMG and pressure measurement equipment to measure pelvic floor muscle function and can be used as biofeedback. This apparatus can also provide numerous selections of electrical stimulation parameters.

Figure 14.3 Cones for pelvic floor muscle training, available in several shapes and weights.

pain, and contraction of other muscles instead of the PFM. In addition, many women report that they dislike using cones.[35] On the other hand, the cones may add benefit to the training protocol if used in a different way: the subjects can be asked to contract around the cone and simultaneously try to pull it out in lying or standing position, repeating this 8–12 times in three series per day. In this way, general strength training principles are followed and progression can be added to the training protocol. Arvonen et al[37] used "vaginal balls" and followed general strength training principles. They found that training with the balls was significantly more effective in reducing urinary leakage than regular PFM training.

Electrical stimulation.
The aim of electrical stimulation for SUI is to strengthen the PFM, mirroring voluntary contractions. Several consensus reports have concluded that strength training is more effective than electrical stimulation to increase muscle strength for other skeletal muscles.[38,39] In most physiotherapy practices, electrical stimulation has been used for partially paralyzed muscles and to stimulate activity when the patients are not able to contract. As soon as the patient can contract voluntarily, most physical therapists would stop using electrical stimulation and continue with regular muscle training.

Surprisingly, in the area of PFM rehabilitation, there has been great interest, especially among gynecologists and general practitioners, in treating urinary incontinence with electrical stimulation. In one of the first studies in this area, Eriksen et al[40] used long-term stimulation (8 hours a day, usually during sleep, with 10 Hz) and showed significant improvement in urodynamic parameters and urinary leakage. However, the study design was uncontrolled and unblinded.

Today there are several RCTs on the effect of electrical stimulation on female SUI.[3,4] A number of different currents, apparatus, and stimulation regimens have been used (Fig. 14.4). For SUI, short-term stimulation applying 35–50 Hz has been used in most of the studies. Electrical stimulation was compared with sham or untreated control in several studies for SUI. Henalla et al,[19] Sand et al,[41] and Yamanishi et al[42] found a significant effect compared to control or sham stimulation, while Luber & Wolde Tsadik,[43] Brubaker et al,[44] and Bø et al[18] did not find significant effect. It has been concluded that more studies are needed to determine whether electrical stimulation is effective in treatment of female SUI.[3,4]

PFM training or electrical stimulation for SUI?

Hennalla et al,[19] Hofbauer et al[14] and Bø et al[18] found that PFM training was significantly better than electrical stimulation to treat SUI. Laycock & Jerwood[45] and Hahn et al[46] found no difference, and Smith[47] found that electrical stimulation was significantly better. Knight et al,[48] Hofbauer et al,[14] Gode et al,[28] and Bidmead et al[49] found no effect of adding electrical stimulation to PFM training. Many of the electrical stimulation studies are flawed, with small numbers, and RCTs with better methodologic quality should be repeated.[3,4] However, electrical stimulation has been shown to have side effects[41] and to be less tolerable to women than PFM training.[18] In addition, Bø & Talseth[50] found that voluntary PFM contraction increases urethral pressure significantly more than electrical stimulation.

There are two main concepts explaining how PFMT may work for SUI.[51]

Theory 1: Conscious PFM contraction before and during physical stress ("the knack").
Precontractions before increases in abdominal pressures have been part of PFMT in many physical therapy practices for years.[52] Miller et al[17] showed that teaching women how to contract and also to contract before coughing significantly reduced urinary leakage within a week. However, Bump et al[11] showed that only 49% of women were able to contract the PFM in a way

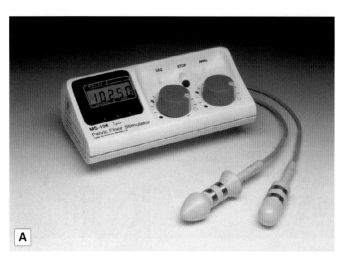

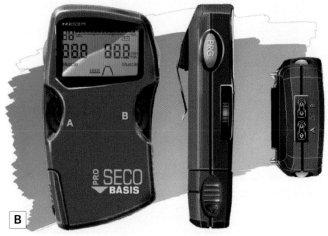

Figure 14.4 Numerous electrical stimulators are available for home use. Most of them have built-in automatic registration of adherence.

that effectively closed the urethra. Currently, we do not know the amount of strength necessary to close the urethra.

Theory 2: Strength training. The aim of strength training is to build a structural support (anatomic location of the muscles, proper attachment, tone, and hypertrophy) for the bladder and urethra. A strong structural support (stiff pelvic floor) may prevent descent of the bladder neck and urethra and close the urethra during abrupt increases in intraabdominal pressure by an automatic quick and strong PFM contraction.

In continent subjects, the PFM contraction is an automatic response without conscious voluntary contraction before activity. In addition, such precontractions are only possible before single bouts of physical exertion (for instance, sneezing). Nobody can run or dance over a longer period of time and contract the PFM voluntarily all the time. Therefore the main goal for PFMT to cure SUI is to build the muscles to reach the automatic response level.

In some studies the patients were tested both subjectively and objectively during physical activity, and had no leakage during strenuous tests after the training period.[18,23,25] The effect, therefore, most likely was due to improved automatic muscle function and not only the ability to voluntarily contract before increase in abdominal pressure.

URGE INCONTINENCE

Some authors have claimed that PFMT and electrical stimulation may be effective to treat symptoms of overactive bladder, such as urgency, frequency, and urge incontinence. In clinical practice, many patients with urge or mixed incontinence are treated with PFMT with or without biofeedback, electrical stimulation, bladder training, medication or a combination of these methods. However, based on two systematic reviews on nonpharmacologic conservative treatments for overactive bladder symptoms, there are only a few RCTs with varying quality in this area, and the results are still not convincing.[53,54]

Pelvic floor muscle training. There are two rationales for the effect of PFMT in treating urge incontinence. The most frequently cited theory is that the PFM contraction causes an inhibition of the detrusor. The patients can be taught to contract the PFM when they feel the urge to void and possibly stop the detrusor contraction. Hence, they may gain time to reach the toilet without leakage. Learning such a technique and incorporate it into daily activities can be classified as a form of "behavioral therapy."[53] Another hypothesis is that bladder overactivity is caused by fluctuations and rapid falls in urethral pressure due to PFM relaxation.[55] By regular training of the PFM, both morphologic and neuromuscular changes will occur and these

changes may reduce the neuromuscular activity causing such involuntary and frequent urethral pressure fluctuations.[55] As can be seen below, the interventions in this area are based on a combination of both theories.

Nygaard et al[56] compared the results of PFMT with and without use of an audiotape, and reported the results for the group with detrusor instability separately. Incontinence episodes per day, voids per night, and urge score were significantly reduced and there was a significant increase in PFM strength. However, pad weight gain, number of voids per day, stress score, and number of pads used per day did not change. There was no untreated control group in this study.

Burgio et al randomized 197 women aged 52–92 years with urge incontinence or mixed incontinence with predominantly urge symptoms to "behavioral treatment," oxybutynin or placebo.[57] "Behavioral treatment" consisted of 1–3 sessions of anorectal biofeedback, urge strategies (repeatedly relaxing and contracting the PFM), and home PFMT with 15 contractions, progressing to 10-second holds, three series per day for 8 weeks. The results showed that the "behavioral treatment group" significantly reduced the number of incontinence episodes compared to the other groups (80.7% versus 68.5% with oxybutynin and 39.4% with placebo). There was no significant difference in full recovery between groups but several other measured variables such as the proportion happy to continue with treatment indefinitely, proportion desiring a different form of treatment, and proportion completely satisfied with their progress were in favor of the "behavioral group." The study documented a huge placebo effect and has been criticized because of its inclusion of women with SUI, a fact that may explain some of the effect of PFMT.

Berghmans et al randomized 68 women with overactive bladder proven by ambulatory urodynamics to nine weekly sessions of "lower urinary tract exercise," vaginal electrical stimulation, combination or control.[58] The exercise program consisted of patient information, bladder training, toilet behavior, and specific PFM training to facilitate and restore the detrusor inhibition reflex. There was no significant effect of the exercise program compared to the control or any other group. The study had a small sample size and performing an intention-to-treat analysis did not improve the results for the exercise group.

Millard et al conducted an international multicenter study with 54 sites including 480 patients (75% women) with overactive bladder symptoms only.[59] The patient group was between 18 and 90 years and was randomized to tolterodine or tolterodine + PFMT. The dosage for tolterodine was 2 mg twice a day. PFMT included only written instructions to perform 15–20 contractions of 10-second holds three times a day plus performing precontractions of the PFM ("the knack") before coughing. The intervention period was 24 weeks. The results showed no additional effect of adding

PFMT to tolterodine. This study can be criticized for using a weak PFMT protocol. There was no assessment of correct contraction and several studies have shown that written instruction is not enough to ensure high adherence or improve muscle function or incontinence. Results on adherence for tolterodine were reported, but not for PFMT. Side effects of tolterodine were: dry mouth 29.6%, headache 6%, constipation 4.8%, nausea 2.7%, dry eyes 2.5%, and dizziness 2.4%.

The studies on PFMT to treat urge incontinence seem to have several flaws, and the exercise protocols are not well described. To date, the results are not convincing.

Electrical stimulation. The rationale for electrical stimulation for overactive bladder seems to be the same as for PFMT. Studies have shown that electrical stimulation can inhibit detrusor contraction and this inhibition lasts more than 1 minute after the stimulation has been given.[60] However, it is not easy to understand how this effect can be transferred to situations when the current is off. If electrical stimulation is effective for overactive bladder symptoms, there has to be a long-lasting change within the inhibitory nervous pathway to the detrusor.

There are several RCTs on electrical stimulation to treat bladder overactivity.[44,47,58,61-63] Smith randomized 38 women with detrusor instability to electrical stimulation or anticholinergic therapy (propantheline bromide) plus bladder training.[47] Electrical stimulation was given with treatment time increasing from 15 to 30, 45 and 60 minutes twice a day for 4 months and consisted of 5–25 mA, 12.5–50 Hz. Twenty-two percent were reported to be cured, 50% were improved, and 28% were failures after electrical stimulation. There were no differences between electrical stimulation and the control group. Abel randomized 22 patients with urodynamically proven urge incontinence to either maximal stimulation 20 minutes once a week for 12 weeks or sham device.[61] The results showed significant improvement in subjective evaluation for the active electrical stimulation, but no difference in leakage episodes. Brubaker et al randomized female patients with urodynamic SUI, detrusor instability or mixed incontinence to 8 weeks of 20 Hz, 0–100 mA, 20 minutes twice a day or sham device.[44] Forty-nine percent no longer had detrusor instability after the intervention.

Yamanishi et al randomized 68 men and women to 4 weeks' electrical stimulation with 10 Hz, 1 ms Pulserate, 15 minutes twice a week, for 4 weeks or sham device.[62] Bladder capacity and first and maximum desire to void significantly improved in the active group. Seven and one were cured in the active and sham groups, respectively, and 26 and nine were improved. Berghmans et al randomized 68 women with urodynamically proven bladder overactivity to "lower urinary tract exercise," vaginal functional electrical stimulation (4–10 Hz, max. level 100 mA), combination or

untreated control.[58] Significant improvement was found in the electrical stimulation group in the intention-to-treat analysis, but not in per protocol analysis. The group combining electrical stimulation and exercises did not show improvement. Wang et al randomized women with overactive bladder symptoms to PFMT, biofeedback-assisted PFMT or electrical stimulation.[63] The electrical stimulation group showed the best subjective reduction rate of symptoms.

All the RCTs on electrical stimulation to treat overactive bladder symptoms have shown significant improvement in some outcome measures. However, the researchers have used different outcome measures and different electrical stimulation equipment and parameters. It is therefore not recommended to combine results in a statistical metaanalysis. Although significantly different, the effect sizes between sham and active treatment do not seem very large and the results are not clear-cut. The electrical stimulation parameters vary between studies and it is impossible to recommend the most effective electrical parameters based on the present results. More high-quality RCTs with sufficient sample sizes are needed in this area of research. Since there are very few treatment options without side effects for this patient group, it is also important to conduct more basic research to understand how electrical stimulation works and find those who respond to treatment.

Bladder training. Bladder training is also referred to as bladder discipline, bladder drill, and bladder reeducation.[3] It describes the educational and behavioral process used to reestablish urinary control in adults. It was first described in 1966 by Jeffcote and Francis as a program of scheduled voiding.[3] Specific goals for bladder training include correcting bad habits of frequent urination, improving ability to inhibit urgency, prolonging voiding intervals, increasing bladder capacity, reducing incontinence episodes, and building patient confidence in controlling bladder function.[3]

An effective 6-week bladder training program is described in Wyman and Fantl.[64]

- Start with initial interval of 30 minutes to 1 hour between voids.
- Increase interval by 15–30 minutes per week until 2–3 hour voiding interval is achieved.
- Educate patient on distraction techniques (e.g. counting backwards from 100), relaxation techniques or PFM contractions.
- Encourage self-monitoring of voiding behavior.
- Provide positive reinforcement.
- Give other treatment options if no effect after 3 weeks.

As can be seen from the above, bladder training may or may not include PFM contraction, and technically it should therefore not be classified as PFMT. There are several RCTs comparing bladder training to untreated controls, PFMT or drug therapy. Wilson et al concluded that bladder training was an effective treatment for women with a variety of incontinence types and that it has similar effects to drug therapy in women with detrusor overactivity.[3] Burgio et al[65] and Mattiasson et al[66] confirmed that bladder training augments the effect of drug therapy.

One study showed that bladder training had similar effects on stress and urge incontinence[67] and another that it had similar effects to PFMT in women with stress, urge, and mixed incontinence.[68] Wilson et al concluded that these findings required further investigation[3] To date, there is no clear understanding of how bladder training works and it is difficult to understand how it can treat SUI if it does not include specific PFM contractions.

Adverse effects of physical therapy. Few, if any, adverse effects have been found after PFMT.[3,4,18] The only reported adverse effect is from a study by Lagro-Jansson where one woman reported pain with exercise and three had an uncomfortable feeling during the exercises.[69] In other studies no side effects have been found.[18]

Reported adverse effects after electrical stimulation have included pain, discomfort, vaginal irritations or infections, urinary tract infections, and diarrhea.[18,41,70] In a Norwegian study on 3100 women who had used electrical stimulation, 51% reported one or more side effects.[70] The most common side effects were soreness/local irritation (26%), pain (20%), and psychologic distress. Most of the cases were mild. Reported adverse effects with cones have included abdominal pain, vaginitis, and bleeding.[18]

Long-term effects of physical therapy. Several studies have reported long-term effects of PFMT.[3,4] However, usually women in the nontreatment or less effective intervention groups have gone on to other treatment after cessation of the study period. Follow-up data are therefore usually reported for either all women or for only the group with best effect. As for surgery,[7,71] there are only a few long-term studies including clinical examination.[72-74] Klarskov et al assessed only some of the women originally participating in the study.[72] Lagro-Janssen et al evaluated 88 out of 110 women with stress, urge or mixed incontinence 5 years after cessation of training and found that 67% remained satisfied with their condition.[73] Only seven of 110 had been treated with surgery. Moreover, satisfaction was closely related to compliance with training and type of incontinence, with mixed incontinent women being more likely to lose the effect. SUI women had the best long-term effect, but only 39% of them were exercising daily or "when needed."

In a 5-year follow-up, Bø and Talseth found that urinary leakage was significantly increased after cessation of organized training.[74] Three of 23 patients had been treated with surgery. Two of these women who had not been cured after the initial training were satisfied with their surgery, and had no leakage on pad test. The third woman had been cured after initial PFM training. However, after 1 year she stopped training because of personal problems connected to the death of her husband. Her incontinence problems returned and she had surgery 2 years before the 5-year follow-up. She was not satisfied with the outcome after surgery and had visible leakage on a cough test and 17 g of leakage on the pad test. Fifty-six percent of the women had a positive closure pressure during cough and 70% had no visible leakage during cough at 5-year follow-up. Seventy percent of the patients were still satisfied with the results and did not want other treatment options.

Cammu et al used a postal questionnaire and medical files to evaluate long-term effects in 52 women who had participated in an individual course of PFMT for urodynamic SUI.[75] Eighty-seven percent were suitable for analysis. Thirty-three percent had had surgery after 10 years. However, in the group which was originally successful after training only 8% had undergone surgery, whereas in the group initially dissatisfied with training, 62% had undergone surgery. Successful results were maintained after 10 years in two-thirds of the patients originally classified as successful. Bø and Kvarstein reported current status of lower urinary tract function (LUTS) from questionnaire data 15 years after cessation of organized training.[76] They found that the short-term significant effect of intensive training was no longer present. Fifty percent from both groups had interval surgery for SUI but there were no differences in reported frequency or amount of leakage between nonoperated and operated women, and women who had surgery reported more severe leakage and being more bothered by urinary incontinence during daily activities than those not operated.

The general recommendation for maintaining muscle strength is one set of 8–12 contractions twice a week.[77] The intensity of the contraction seems to be more important than frequency of training. So far, no studies have evaluated how many contractions subjects have to perform to maintain PFM strength after cessation of organized training. In the study by Bø and Talseth,[74] PFM strength was maintained 5 years after cessation of organized training with 70% exercising more than once a week. However, number and intensity of exercises varied considerably between successful women.[78] One series of 8–12 contractions could easily be incorporated into aerobic dance classes or recommended as part of women's general strength training programs. On the other hand, we do not know how a voluntary precontraction before increase in intraabdominal pressure will maintain or increase muscle strength. In the study by Cammu et al,[75] the long-term effect of PFM training appeared to be attributed to the precontraction before sudden increases in intraabdominal pressure, and not so much to regular strength training. Muscle strength was not measured in their study.

There are no long-term studies on electrical stimulation for either SUI or urge incontinence, and no studies on long-term effects of PFMT for urge incontinence.

Motivation. Several researchers have looked into factors affecting the outcome of PFM exercise for urinary incontinence.[3,4] No single factor has been shown to predict outcome and it has been concluded that many factors traditionally supposed to affect outcomes, such as age and severity of incontinence, may be less crucial than previously thought. Factors that appear to be most associated with positive outcome are thorough teaching of correct contraction, motivation, adherence to the intervention, and intensity of the program.[3,4]

Some women may find the exercises hard to conduct on a regular basis.[79] However, when analysing results of RCTs, adherence to the exercise program is generally high, and drop-out rate is low.[3,4] In a few studies, low adherence and high drop-out rates have been reported.[36,80] The physical therapist's knowledge of behavioral sciences, such as pedagogy and health psychology, and their ability to explain and motivate patients may be crucial factors in enhancing adherence and minimizing drop-outs from training. In some studies such strategies have been followed and high adherence has been achieved.[79,81] In other studies specific strategies have not been reported but emphasis has been put on creating a positive, enjoyable, and supportive training environment. Group training after thorough individual instruction may be a good concept if led by a skilled and motivating person.[18,23] (Fig. 14.5). PFMT programs with no drop-outs[82] and adherence >90%[18] are possible.

In a study by Alewijnse,[79] most women were still following advice to train 4–6 times a week 1 year after cessation of the training program. The following factors predicted adherence: positive intention to adhere, high short-term adherence levels, positive self-efficacy expectations, and frequent weekly episodes of leakage before and after initial therapy. Patients do not comply with treatment for a wide variety of reasons: long-lasting and time-consuming treatments, requirement of lifestyle changes, poor client/patient interaction, cultural and health beliefs, poor social support, inconvenience, lack of time, motivational problems, and travel time to clinics have been listed.[83]

In most countries, patients receive physical therapy on physician referral only. This means that the motivation of the general practitioner, gynecologist or urologist for PFMT and conservative treatment is extremely important. If these professions are not updated on the effect of PFMT, do not know any trained physical therapists in their area or think PFMT is boring and a big demand, then patients may not even be introduced to the option of training. PFMT can

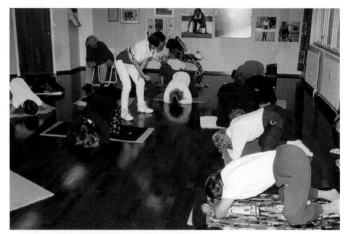

Figure 14.5 When the patients are able to contract the pelvic floor muscles correctly, it can be fun and motivating to conduct the actual training in a class. An elderly woman, not able to achieve the positions on the floor, is doing modified positions on the chair. The children at the back are not exercising! They came with their mothers to the class because they did not have a babysitter that day...

either be put forward as a "boring demanding task you need to do the rest of your life" or it can be introduced as a method that is "easy, at a low cost and with no side effects. It may take less than 10 minutes per day to build up strength if it is conducted correctly (three sets of 8–12 contractions a day), and it takes even less to maintain it." The number of physical therapists specializing in women's health and pelvic floor issues varies between countries. In order to recruit more physical therapists into the field, it may be important to include a mandatory curriculum on pelvic floor dysfunction and treatment at undergraduate education level, add courses at postgraduate level, and stimulate urologists, gynecologists, and urogynecologists to participate in teaching of physical therapists and vice versa.

FUTURE RESEARCH POSSIBILITIES

- What are the mechanisms for PFMT in treatment of SUI?
- How strong does "the knack" have to be to stop leakage during different physical tasks?
- Can responders to PFMT be described and the treatment targeted to specific groups?
- What is the effect of PFMT in the older age group (>75 years)?
- Can contraction of the PFM to inhibit detrusor contraction treat urge incontinence?
- How strong does the intentional contraction of the PFM have to be to inhibit detrusor contraction?
- How does electrical stimulation work for SUI and urge incontinence?
- How can women with UI be motivated to continue PFMT on their own?

REFERENCES

1. Kegel AH. Progressive resistance exercise in the functional restoration of the perineal muscles. Am J Obstet Gynecol 1948;56:238–249.

2. Fantl JA, Newman DK, Colling J, et al. Urinary incontinence in adults: acute and chronic management. Rockville, MD: US Department of Health and Human Services, Public Health Service, Agency for Health Care Policy and Research; 1996.

3. Wilson PD, Bø K, Nygaard I, Staskin D, Wyman J, Bourchier A. Conservative treatment in women. In: Abrams P, Cardozo L, Khoury S, Wein A, eds. Incontinence, 2nd edn. Plymouth: Health Publications Ltd; 2002: 571–624.

4. Hay-Smith E, Bø K, Berghmans L, et al. Pelvic floor muscle training fur urinary incontinence in women (Cochrane review). Oxford: Cochrane Library; 2001.

5. Abrams P, Cardozo L, Khoury S, Wein A, eds. Incontinence, 2nd edn. Plymouth, UK: Health Publications Ltd; 2002.

6. Herbison P, Plevnik S, Mantle J. Weighted vaginal cones for urinary incontinence. Oxford: Cochrane Library; 2000.

7. Smith T, Daneshgari F, Dmochowski R, et al. Surgical treatment of incontinence in women. In: Abrams P, Cardozo L, Khoury S, Wein A, eds. Incontinence, 2nd edn. Plymouth: Health Publications Ltd; 2002: 823–863.

8. Kegel AH. Stress incontinence and genital relaxation. Ciba Clin Sympos 1952;2:35–51.

9. Benvenuti F, Caputo GM, Bandinelli S, Mayer F, Biagini C, Somavilla A. Reeducative treatment of female genuine stress incontinence. Am J Phys Med 1987;66(4):155–168.

10. Bø K, Larsen S, Oseid S, Kvarstein B, Hagen R, Jørgensen J. Knowledge about and ability to correct pelvic floor muscle exercises in women with urinary stress incontinence. Neurourol Urodynam 1988;7(3):261–262.

11. Bump R, Hurt WG, Fantl JA, Wyman JF. Assessment of Kegel exercise performance after brief verbal instruction. Am J Obstet Gynecol 1991;165:322–329.

12. Bø K, Kvarstein B, Hagen R, Larsen S. Pelvic floor muscle exercise for the treatment of female stress urinary incontinence: II. Validity of vaginal pressure measurements of pelvic floor muscle strength and the necessity of supplementary methods for control of correct contraction. Neurourol Urodynam 1990;9:479–487.

13. Lagro-Janssen TLM, Debruyne FMJ, Smits AJA, Van Weel C. Controlled trial of pelvic exercises in the treatment of urinary stress incontinence in general practice. Br J Gen Pract 1991; 41:445–449.

14. Hofbauer J, Preisinger F, Nurnberger N. Der Stellenwert der Physiotherapie bei der weiblichen genuinen Stressinkontinenz. Z Urol Nephrol 1990;83:249–254.

15. Wong K, Fung B, Fung, LCW, Ma S. Pelvic floor exercises in the treatment of stress urinary incontinence in Hong Kong Chinese women. Paper presented at the ICS 27th Annual Meeting, Yokohama, Japan, 1997.

16. Henalla S, Millar D, Wallace K. Surgical versus conservative management for post-menopausal genuine stress incontinence of urine. Neurourol Urodynam 1990;9(4):436–437.

17. Miller JM, Ashton-Miller JA, DeLancey J. A pelvic muscle precontraction can reduce cough-related urine loss in selected women with mild SUI. J Am Geriatr Soc 1998;46:870–874.

18. Bø K, Talseth T, Holme I. Single blind, randomised controlled trial of pelvic floor exercises, electrical stimulation, vaginal cones, and no treatment in management of genuine stress incontinence in women. BMJ 1999;318:487–493.

19. Henalla SM, Hutchins CJ, Robinson P, MacVicar J. Non-operative methods in the treatment of female genuine stress incontinence of urine. J Obstet Gynaecol 1989;9:222–225.

20. Peschers U, Gingelmaier A, Jundt K, Leib B, Dimpfl T. Evaluation of pelvic floor muscle strength using four different techniques. Int Urogynecol J 2001;12:27–30.

21. Andersson K, Appell R, Awad S, et al. Pharmacological treatment of urinary incontinence. In: Abrams P, Cardozo L, Khoury S, Wein A, eds. Incontinence, 2nd edn. Plymouth: Health Publications Ltd; 2002: 479–511.

22. Blaivas JG, Appell RA, Fantl JA, et al. Standards of efficacy for evaluation of treatment outcomes in urinary incontinence: recommendations of the urodynamic society. Neurourol Urodynam 1997;16(145):147.

23. Bø K, Hagen RH, Kvarstein B, Jørgensen J, Larsen S. Pelvic floor muscle exercise for the treatment of female stress urinary incontinence: III. Effects of two different degrees of pelvic floor muscle exercise. Neurourol Urodynam 1990;9:489–502.

24. Glavind K, Laursen B, Jaquet A. Efficacy of biofeedback in the treatment of urinary stress incontinence. Int Urogynecol J 1998;9:151–153.

25. Mørkved S, Bø K, Fjørtoft T. Is there any additional effect of adding biofeedback to pelvic floor muscle training? A single-blind randomized controlled trial. Obstet Gynecol 2002; 100(4):730–739.

26. Dumoulin C, Lemieux M, Bourbonnais D, Morin M. Conservative management of stress urinary incontinence: a single-blind, randomized controlled trial of pelvic floor rehabilitation with or without abdominal muscle rehabilitation compared to the absence of treatment. Nerourol Urodyam 2003;22(5):543–544.

27. Glavind K, Nøhr S, Walter S. Biofeedback and physiotherapy versus physiotherapy alone in the treatment of genuine stress urinary incontinence. Int Urogynecol J 1996;7:339–343.

28. Goode P, Burgio KL, Locher JL, et al. Effect of behavioral training with or without pelvic floor electrical stimulation on stress incontinence in women. A randomized controlled trial. JAMA 2003;290(3):345–352.

29. Haskel W. Dose-response issues from a biological perspective. In: Bouchard C, Shephard RJ, Stephens T, eds. Physical activity, fitness, and health. International proceedings and consensus statement. Champaign,IL: Human Kinetics Publishers; 1994: 1030–1039.

30. Schwartz G, Beatty J. Biofeedback: theory and research. New York: Academic Press; 1977.

31. Wilson PD, Samarrai TAL, Deakin M, Kolbe E, Brown ADG. An objective assessment of physiotherapy for female genuine stress incontinence. Br J Obstet Gynaecol 1987;94:575–582.

32. Prashar S, Simons A, Bryant C, Dowell C, Moore K. Attitudes to vaginal/urethral touching and device placement in women with urinary incontinence. Int Urogynecol J 2000;11:4–8.

33. Wilson PD, Herbison P. A randomized controlled trial of pelvic floor muscle exercises to treat postnatal urinary incontinence. Int Urogynecol J 1998;9:257–264.

34. Pieber D, Zivkovic F, Tamussino K. Beckenbodengymnastik allein oder mit Vaginalkonen bei pramenopausalen Frauen mit milder und massiger Stressharninkontinenz. Gynecol Geburtshilfliche Rundsch 1994;34:32–33.

35. Cammu H, Van Nylen M. Pelvic floor exercises versus vaginal weight cones in genuine stress incontinence. Eur J Obstet Gyn Reprod Biol 1998;77:89–93.

36. Laycock J, Brown J, Cusack C, et al. Pelvic floor reeducation for stress incontinence:comparing three methods. Br J Comm Nurs 2001;6(5):230–237.

37. Arvonen T, Fianu-Jonasson A, Tyni-Lenne R. Effectiveness of two conservative modes of physical therapy in women with urinary stress incontinence. Neurourol Urodynam 2001;20:591–599.

38. Dudley GA, Harris RT. Use of electrical stimulation in strength and power training. In: Komi PV, ed. Strength and power in sport. Oxford: Blackwell Scientific Publications; 1992: 329–337.

39. Vuori I, Wilmore JH. Physical activity, fitness, and health: status and determinants. In: Bouchard C, Shephard RJ, Stephens T, eds. Physical activity, fitness and health. Consensus statement. Champaign, IL: Human Kinetics Publishers; 1993: 33–40.

40. Eriksen B, Eik-Nes SH. Long-term electrostimulation of the pelvic floor: primary therapy in female stress incontinence? Urol Int 1989;44:90–95.

41. Sand PK, Richardson DR, Staskin SE, et al. Pelvic floor stimulation in the treatment of genuine stress incontinence: a multicenter placebo-controlled trial. Am J Obstet Gynecol 1995; 173:72–79.

42. Yamanishi T, Yasuda K, Sakakibara R, Hattori T, Ito H, Murakami S. Pelvic floor electrical stimulation in the treatment of stress incontinence: an investigational study and a placebo controlled double-blind trial. J Urol 1997;158:2127–2131.

43. Luber KM, Wolde-Tsadik G. Efficacy of functional electrical stimulation in treating genuine stress incontinence: a randomized clinical trial. Neurourol Urodynam 1997;16:543–551.

44. Brubaker L, Benson JT, Bent A, Clark A, Shott S. Transvaginal electrical stimulation for female urinary incontinence. Am J Obstet Gynecol 1997;177:536–540.

45. Laycock J, Jerwood D. Does pre-modulated interferential therapy cure genuine stress incontinence? Physiotherapy 1996;79(8):553–560.

46. Hahn I, Sommar S, Fall M. A comparative study of pelvic floor training and electrical stimulation for treatment of genuine female stress urinary incontinence. Neurourol Urodynam 1991;10:545–554.

47. Smith JJ. Intravaginal stimulation randomized trial. J Urol 1996;155:127–130.

48. Knight S, Laycock J, Naylor D. Evaluation of neuromuscular electrical stimulation in the treatment of genuine stress incontinence. Physiotherapy 1998;84(2):61–71.

49. Bidmead J, Mantle J, Cardozo L, Hextall A, Boos K. Home electrical stimulation in addition to conventional pelvic floor exercises. A useful adjunct or expensive distraction? Neurourol Urodynam 2002;21(4):372–373.

50. Bø K, Talseth T. Change in urethral pressure during voluntary pelvic floor muscle contraction and vaginal electrical stimulation. Int Urogyn J 1997;8:3–7.

51. Bø K. Pelvic floor muscle training is effective in treatment of stress urinary incontinence, but how does it work? Int Urogynecol J 2004;15:76–84.

52. Mantle J. Physiotherapy for incontinence. In: Cardozo L, Staskin D, eds. Textbook of female urology and urogynecology. London: Isis Medical Media Ltd; 2001:351–358.

53. Bø K, Berghmans L. Overactive bladder and its treatments. Non-pharmacological treatments for overactive bladder: pelvic floor exercises. Urology 2000;55(Suppl 5A):7–11.

54. Berghmans L, Hendriks H, de Bie RA, et al. Conservative treatment of urge urinary incontinence in women: a systematic review of randomized clinical trials. BJU Int 2000; 85(3):254–263.

55. Mattiasson A. Characterisation of lower urinary tract disorders: a new view. Neurourol Urodynam 2001;20:601–621.

56. Nygaard IE, Kreder KJ, Lepic MM, Fountain KA, Rhomberg AT. Efficacy of pelvic floor muscle exercises in women with stress, urge, and mixed incontinence. Am J Obstet Gynecol 1996;174(120):125.

57. Burgio KL, Locher JL, Goode PS, et al. Behavioral vs drug treatment for urge urinary incontinence in older women. A randomized controlled trial. JAMA 1998;280(23):1995–2000.

58. Berghmans L, van Waalwijk van Doorn E, Nieman F, de Bie R, van den Brandt P, van Kerrebroeck P. Efficacy of physical therapeutic modalities in women with proven bladder overactivity. Eur Urol 2002;6:581–587.

59. Millard R. Clinical efficacy of tolterodine with or without a simplified pelvic floor exercise regimen. Neurourol Urodynam 2004;23:48–53.

60. Godec C, Cass AS, Ayala GF. Bladder inhibition with functional electrical stimulation. Urology 1975;6(6):663–666.

61. Abel I. Elektrostimulering og lokal østrogenterapi til behandling af urininkontinens hos postmenopausale kvinder. Denmark: Glostrup University Hospital; 1996.

62. Yamanishi T, Yasuda K, Sakakibara R, Hattori T, Suda S. Randomized, double-blind study of electrical stimulation for urinary incontinence due to detrusor overactivity. Urology 2000;55:353–357.

63. Wang A, Wang Y, Chen M. Single-blind, randomized trial of pelvic floor muscle training, biofeedback-assisted pelvic floor muscle training, and electrical stimulation in the management of overactive bladder. Urology 2004;63(1):61–66.

64. Wyman J, Fantl J. Bladder training in ambulatory care management of urinary incontinence. Urol Nurs 1991;September:11–17.

65. Burgio K, Locher J, Goode P. Combined behavioral and drug therapy for urge incontinence in older women. J Am Geriatr Soc 2000;48(4):370–374.

66. Mattiasson A, Blaakaer J, Hoye K, Wein A. Simplified bladder training augments the effectiveness of Tolterodine in patients with an overactive bladder. BJU Int 2003;91(1):54–60.

67. Fantl JA, Wyman JF, McClish DK, et al. Efficacy of bladder training in older women with urinary incontinence. JAMA 1991;265(5):609–613.

68. Elser D, Wyman J, McClish D, Robinson D, Fantl J, Bump R. The effect of bladder training, pelvic floor muscle training, or combination training on urodynamic parameters in women with urinary incontinence. Neurourol Urodynam 1999;18:427–436.

69. Lagro-Janssen A, Debruyne F, Smiths A, Van Weel C. The effects of treatment of urinary incontinence in general practice. Fam Pract 1992;9(3):284–289.

70. Indrekvam S, Hunskaar S. Side-effects, feasibility, and adherence to treatment during home-managed electrical stimulation for urinary incontinence: a Norwegian national cohort of 3198 women. Neurourol Urodynam 2002;21:546–552.

71. Black NA, Downs SH. The effectiveness of surgery for stress incontinence in women: a systematic review. Br J Urol 1996;78(497):510.

72. Klarskov P, Nielsen KK, Kromann-Andersen B, Maegaard E. Long-term results of pelvic floor training for female genuine stress incontinence. Int Urogynecol J 1991;2:132–135.

73. Lagro-Janssen T, van Weel C. Long-term effect of treatment of female incontinence in general practice. Br J Gen Pract 1998;48:1735–1738.

74. Bø K, Talseth T. Long term effect of pelvic floor muscle exercise five years after cessation of organized training. Obstet Gynecol 1996;87(2):261–265.

75. Cammu H, Van Nylen M, Amy J. A ten-year follow-up after Kegel pelvic floor muscle exercises for genuine stress incontinence. BJU Int 2000;85:655–658.

76. Bø K, Kvarstein B, Nygaard J. Lower urinary tract symptoms and pelvic floor muscle exercise adherence after 15 years. Obstet Gynecol 2005; 105:999–1005.

77. Pollock ML, Gaesser GA, Butcher JD, et al. The recommended quantity and quality of exercise for developing and maintaining cardiorespiratory and muscular fitness, and flexibility in healthy adults. Med Sci Sports Exerc 1998;30(6):975–991.

78. Bø K. Adherence to pelvic floor muscle exercise and long term effect on stress urinary incontinence. A five year follow up. Scand J Med Sci Sports 1995;5:36–39.

79. Alewijnse D. Urinary incontinence in women. Long term outcome of pelvic floor muscle exercise therapy. Maastricht: Health Research Institute for Prevention and Care/Department of Health Education and Health Promotion; 2002.

80. Ramsey IN, Thou M. A randomized, double blind, placebo controlled trial of pelvic floor exercise in the treatment of genuine stress incontinence. Neurourol Urodynam 1990;9(4):398–399.

81. Chiarelli P, Cockburn J. Promoting urinary continence in women after delivery: randomised controlled trial. BMJ 2002;324:1241.

82. Berghmans L, Frederiks C, de Bie R, et al. Efficacy of biofeedback, when included with pelvic floor muscle exercise treatment, for genuine stress incontinence. Neurourol Urodynam 1997;15:37–52.

83. Paddison K. Complying with pelvic floor exercises: a literature review. Nurs Stand 2002; 16(39):33–38.

Surgery for Urinary Incontinence

Anthony R B Smith

INTRODUCTION

This chapter covers surgery for stress incontinence, post-surgical voiding dysfunction, and refractory detrusor overactivity.

SURGERY FOR STRESS INCONTINENCE OF URINE

Surgery for stress incontinence of urine has undergone closer scrutiny than many surgical procedures over the past decade. This is partly due to the number of women who require such surgery and partly because of the wide variety of procedures performed. This section will include a critical review of the procedures.

Anterior colporrhaphy. Anterior colporrhaphy has become less popular for the treatment of stress incontinence of urine since the literature has revealed a lower chance of success and a higher chance of recurrence than with retropubic support procedures. Metaanalyses of heterogeneous studies suggest a continence rate after anterior repair of between 67.8% and 72.0%.[1,2] Randomized trials which include anterior repair in one arm and suprapubic studies in the other arm show a continence rate of 66% for anterior repair.[3] A 10-year follow-up of anterior repair reported a success rate of 38%.[4] The anterior repair is still offered as treatment for stress incontinence by some clinicians because of the relatively low morbidity associated with the procedure and also because it may be part of a prolapse repair procedure. The incidence of detrusor overactivity following the procedure is not greater than 6% and long-term voiding dysfunction following the procedure is rare.[1]

Colposuspension. Open colposuspension, which can be performed as either a primary or secondary procedure, has been shown to produce an objective cure rate of 80–90% in many series. The long-term results of Burch colposuspension have suggested that its efficacy is maintained through time, although most procedures do report recurrence. Demirci et al reported that the cure rate dropped from 87.7% in a mean follow-up of 1.5 years to 77.4% in a mean follow-up of 4.5 years.[5] Persistent voiding difficulties were reported by Viereck et al in 3.5% of a large series of women who underwent Burch colposuspension and were followed up over 3 years.[6] Shorter term voiding dysfunction occurs in 10–15% of women after colposuspension and postoperative detrusor overactivity has been described in 6.6%.[7] Genitourinary prolapse has been reported following Burch colposuspension in over 20% of women. Whilst most women are aware of the prolapse, less than 5% request further surgery.

Needle suspension. Needle suspension procedures were developed after open colposuspension in an attempt to provide a less invasive operation. Despite the early promise, such procedures have been largely abandoned due to reports of a high risk of recurrence. Glazener and Cooper performed a metaanalysis of randomized or quasi-randomized trials that included needle suspension for the treatment of stress urinary incontinence.[8] Eight trials were identified which evaluated six different types of needle suspension in 327 women compared with 407 who had other antiincontinence procedures. Although the reliability of the evidence was limited by poor quality and small trials, the authors demonstrated a 74% subjective success rate at 1-year follow-up. Needle suspension resulted in a 48% perioperative complication rate. Longer term cure rates have been generally lower than open colposuspension and Tebyani et al reported a 5% cure rate at a mean follow-up of 29 months.[9]

Laparoscopic colposuspension. Whilst there are over 50 published reports on laparoscopic colposuspension, there is still insufficient robust information to determine whether it can produce a similar cure rate to open colposuspension. The Cochrane Incontinence Review Group performed a metaanalysis of four randomized controlled trials[10-13] which demonstrated no subjective difference in outcome in up to 18 months follow-up. Objective criteria indicated an additional 9% risk of failure for laparoscopic colposuspension when compared to open colposuspension. It is widely accepted that laparoscopic surgery requires additional skills that all surgeons do not have the opportunity or desire to learn. Trials in other specialties comparing laparoscopic and open surgery have suggested that laparoscopic procedures should only be performed where such expertise is available.[14]

There is evidence to suggest that a minimum of two sutures should be used on each side when performing colposuspension.[15] Whilst some studies have demonstrated reduced postoperative morbidity following laparoscopic colposuspension, most studies have shown that operating time is longer with the laparoscopic procedure. Although studies have suggested that blood loss is reduced with the laparoscopic procedure and postoperative stay is shorter, all studies published to date suffer from insufficient numbers and short-term follow-up.

Further trial reports are awaited to determine whether laparoscopic colposuspension has a role in the treatment of stress urinary incontinence.

Slings.
Pubovaginal slings have been described since the beginning of the 20th century. While advancements have been made in sling surgery, there are many variables which influence outcome in ways that are not yet fully understood. Autologous slings (using patients' own tissues) became more popular after Aldridge described the use of rectus sheath fascia in 1942.[16] Fascia lata has also been employed, and while rectus sheath and fascia lata appear to have similar properties and are not rejected, the quality of support provided by such procedures is quite variable and there is a lack of understanding of the biologic processes which occur after insertion.

Cure rates following autologous slings range from 50%[17] to 100%.[18] Long-term follow-up of autologous sling procedures suggests that success is sustained over time.

Sling procedures have been associated with voiding dysfunction in some series but it is believed that this resulted from use of excessive tension in the sling.

Allograft slings.
The use of cadaveric materials avoids the dissection required for autologous material but in recent years concern about the risk of transmission of HIV and CJD has tempered enthusiasm for this approach. Some studies have shown higher recurrence rates than with autologous materials and this is believed to be due to tissue lysis.[19]

Xenograft slings.
Animal tissues have been used in cutaneous and soft tissue reconstruction for many years. Bovine and porcine epidermis and intestinal submucosa have been employed but there are no studies that are sufficiently robust to indicate that xenograft materials should be used instead of autologous or allograft slings. Most series reported are small and with short follow-up. Long-term evaluation is required before biocompatibility and risk can be fully assessed.

Tension-free vaginal tape (TVT).
Since the TVT procedure was first described in 1996,[20] widespread adoption of this suburethral sling procedure has occurred. The TVT procedure is based on a theory of pathophysiology of stress incontinence presented by Petros and Ulmsten.[21] TVT has been compared with open colposuspension in a multicenter randomized trial for primary treatment of stress urinary incontinence.[22] No difference in subjective and objective cure rates was found between the two procedures at 6 months follow-up. Ward and Hilton assessed cure using objective and subjective means and, although the two procedures produced a similar cure rate, the trial highlighted the variation in cure rate according to how cure was defined. When cure was assessed by pad test, 80–90% of women were cured whilst when a symptom questionnaire was used, only 30% of women were completely dry.

Although perioperative morbidity in the form of bladder injury was more common during the TVT procedure, there were no long-term sequelae from the bladder injuries reported (9% for the TVT versus 3% for colposuspension). Delayed voiding, operation time, hospital stay, and return to normal activity were all significantly longer after open colposuspension. At 2-year follow-up, objective cure rate was found to be similar. Reoperation for pelvic organ prolapse was higher in the colposuspension group, suggesting that colposuspension produces a higher risk of anatomic distortion resulting in prolapse postoperatively. Long-term objective results of the TVT procedure are now available from case series and suggest a sustained curative effect. Nilsson et al reported that at a median follow-up of 56 months, 85% of women were objectively and subjectively cured.[23]

Numerous procedures similar to the TVT have been produced by commercial organizations with little data to support their introduction. The introduction of the obturator tape also lacks long-term evidence to support its use and the purported advantage with respect to the avoidance of bladder and vessel injuries has yet to be substantiated.

Injectable agents.
Numerous injectable agents have been described over the past century, including autologous tissues such as fat and cartilage, bovine collagen, polytetrafluoroethylene (Teflon) and polydimethylxyldioxane elastomer (silicone). Each of these different agents has variable biophysical properties that influence factors such as tissue compatibility, tendency for migration, radiographic density, durability, and safety. The ideal periurethral injectable agent has not yet been identified.

Injectable agents can be introduced transurethrally, with or without endoscopic assistance, or transperineally. Most of the agents can be introduced without general or regional anesthesia and have therefore been recommended for women who wish to avoid more invasive therapy. The optimal location has not been defined to date.

Most trials of periurethral injectable agents involve few patients with short-term follow-up. In theory, injectable agents should be of more value in patients with intrinsic sphincter deficiency, although there is evidence that women with urethral hypermobility may also benefit from periurethral injection.

Collagen has been compared to carbon-coated zirconium beads and the agents were found to be equally effective at 12 months follow-up.[24] Collagen has been found to be more effective than autologous fat in women with intrinsic sphincter deficiency[25] although fat has not been found to be superior to an injection of saline periurethrally.[26] When collagen injection was compared to autologous pubovaginal slings in 50 women with stress incontinence due to ISD and urethral hypermobility at a mean of 22 months follow-up, the respective cure rates were 81% and 25%.[27] It would therefore appear that whilst periurethral injections may offer advantage in no more than 20% of women in the longer term, they are less invasive than other procedures described and may be considered of value by some women. The morbidity associated with periurethral injectable agents is low and includes urinary tract infection, allergic reactions, and particle migration for nonabsorbable agents.

Artificial urinary sphincters.

The literature related to the use of artificial urinary sphincters is difficult to evaluate since reports include patients with a heterogeneous history and range of symptoms. Most series include patients who have had numerous previous continence procedures. A 92% cure rate has been reported if the detrusor remains stable after surgery.[28] Many patients require surgical revision and some ultimately require removal. Richard reported that 17% of patients required an average of two revisions over an 8-year follow-up.[29]

POSTSURGICAL VOIDING DYSFUNCTION SURGERY

The reported incidence of voiding dysfunction due to obstruction after incontinence surgery ranges from 2.5 to 24%. Raz defined three distinct groups of patients with bladder outlet obstruction symptoms after previous continence surgery:[30]

- obstructed only: these patients produce a detrusor pressure greater than 35 cmH$_2$O without urinary flow
- poor detrusor function
- obstructed and incontinent.

There have been no randomized trials to define the optimal management for each of these groups.

Although women with voiding dysfunction may present with frequency, hesitancy, poor urinary stream, and a sensation of incomplete bladder emptying, there is often a poor correlation of such symptoms and the finding of high residual urine. Irritative symptoms are often recorded and recurrent urinary infection and incontinence may complicate the clinical picture. Diagnosis is best made by recording a careful history, including a urinary diary, and physical examination to assess the position of the anterior vaginal wall and urethra, particularly under strain, and the presence of additional pelvis masses, including a loaded rectum. Urodynamics, including uroflowmetry, cystometry and pressure flow studies, should give vital information to procure a diagnosis. Radiographic studies during cystometry (voiding cystourethrogram) may provide additional information but most clinicians would only employ this when the diagnosis is unclear using conventional studies.

Treatment

Clean intermittent self-catheterisation. Most women find clean intermittent self-catheterization (CISC) an undesirable but effective means of managing bladder emptying. The recommended frequency varies depending on the patient's voiding but ideally the catheterization volume should be kept below 400 ml to reduce the risk of urinary infection. If the patient suffers from irritative symptoms, anticholinergic drugs may be added to the regime, although inevitably natural voiding will be further inhibited.

Urethral dilation. Urethral dilation and calibration may be helpful particularly in women whose urethral caliber is reduced by either surgery or atrophy. Urethral dilation has never been carefully evaluated.

Urethrolysis. Urethrolysis may be performed vaginally or retropubically and may involve a simple separation of the paraurethral tissues or a complete surgical mobilization of the urethra. When a TVT has been inserted, the tape can be divided under the urethra or paraurethrally. All such procedures carry a risk of a return of stress incontinence postoperatively and many women prefer to perform self-catheterization rather than take such a risk.

SURGERY FOR REFRACTORY DETRUSOR OVERACTIVITY

Surgical treatment of nonneurogenic detrusor overactivity incontinence is generally reserved for patients who have failed trials of nonsurgical treatment. Such surgical treatment has not been studied in robust clinical trials and most of the evidence is from case series.

Endoscopic surgical procedures

Endoscopic bladder transection. Circumferential endoscopic incision proximal to the bladder neck, termed endoscopic bladder transection, has been employed to denervate the bladder. Although the early reports indicated that it was an effective technique, subsequent series have failed to reproduce these results and the procedure is now rarely performed.

Cystodistension. Overdistension of the bladder under regional or general anesthesia has been utilized for over 30 years to treat bladder cancer, interstitial cystitis, and detrusor overactivity. There have been no randomized controlled trials to assess the value of cystodistension and the literature on cystodistension for detrusor overactivity incontinence includes mainly small retrospective case series with short-term follow-up and subjective outcome parameters. Eighty percent substantial improvement or cure at 13 months follow-up has been reported.[31] Conversely, Delaere et al reported only 11% cure at 12 months follow-up with 21% improved.[32] Cystodistension with a balloon has been reported but in a series of 46 patients, Pengally et al noted that none of their patients' urodynamics demonstrated a stable bladder after the procedure.[33] Cystodistension is not without risk, with complications such as bladder rupture and voiding dysfunction being reported postoperatively.

Transvesical phenol injection. A 5% aqueous solution of phenol injected endoscopically into the trigone of the bladder with a view to producing a chemical denervation has been described. Whilst early reports indicated response rates between 58% and 83%,[34] further longer term follow-up studies reported much lower success rates and at 4-year follow-up, no patients were found to have a sustained response.[35] Furthermore, 1/10 women may suffer a significant complication of the phenol injection.

Open surgical procedures

Ingelman-Sundberg denervation. Surgical transsection of preganglionic pelvic nerves near the inferior surface of the bladder through a transvaginal approach was first described by Ingelman-Sundberg in 1959. This report has been followed by a number of small series with short-term follow-up. Some surgeons have employed injection of local anesthetic in the region of the trigone as an indicator of the potential value of the surgical procedure. Using this approach, a 68% cure or improved rate has been reported at a mean follow-up of 44 months.[36] No randomized blinded or placebo-controlled studies to evaluate this technique have been performed. The most frequently reported complication is voiding dysfunction.

Augmentation cystoplasty. The aim of augmentation cystoplasty is to create a high-capacity, low-pressure reservoir during the filling/storage phase of the micturition cycle. Bladder augmentation using different portions of the gastrointestinal tract has been reported in a small number of case series in nonneurogenic detrusor overactivity incontinence. In a series of 51 women published by Awad et al, only 53% of the women classified themselves as "happy" with the outcome of the surgery and 18% continued to have disabling symptoms of urinary incontinence.[37] Neurogenic detrusor overactivity series have reported more satisfactory outcomes. Augmentation of the bladder with a segment of bowel may lead to significant complications in the short and long term. The need for intermittent self-catheterization to ensure complete bladder emptying, mucous build-up, and malignant transformation are all significant complications which may contribute to the decreasing satisfaction rates with time.

Detrusor myotomy or myectomy has been reported as a form of autoaugmentation. Autoaugmentation avoids the complications related to the use of a bowel segment and is believed to produce its effect by creating a pseudo-diverticulum. Most reports of autoaugmentation include children and reports on adults involve only small case series. Ter Meulen et al reported initial improvement but deterioration in four out of five women treated with ongoing involuntary detrusor contractions, continuing on follow-up cystometry.[38]

Complications of autoaugmentation include recurrent urinary infection and urinary extravasation. A study comparing detrusor myectomy with augmentation cystoplasty in 61 patients reported similar rates of success between the two procedures but a significantly lower incidence of complications in the detrusor myectomy group (22% versus 3%).[39]

Urinary diversion. Abdominal urostomy is chosen by some women to avoid the problems created by urinary incontinence to the perineum. Alternatively, the ureters can be diverted to a segment of ileum but these techniques have not been published for the treatment of nonneurogenic detrusor overactivity.

Neuromodulation. Neuromodulation or nerve stimulation may be employed in the form of sacral nerve stimulation (SNS) or peripheral nerve stimulation (SANS). The mechanism of the action of these techniques is not understood.

SACRAL NERVE STIMULATION. Sacral nerve stimulation (SNS) involves the stimulation of the sacral nerves to modulate the neural reflexes that influence the bladder, sphincter, and pelvic floor. Since it was first reported in 1981 for bladder dysfunction, its use has been extended to include significant urgency, frequency, and idiopathic urinary retention.

Placement of stimulation electrodes is usually a two-stage procedure. In stage 1, a stimulation lead is implanted next to the dorsal root of S3 for a few weeks. If the patient's symptoms improve more than 50%, stage 2 follows, in which a permanent neural stimulator is implanted. Schmidt reported a multicenter series of 76 patients who were randomized to either implantation or a control group (in whom implantation was delayed for 6 months).[40] Of the 34 patients who were implanted, 16 were completely dry and 10 demonstrated a greater than 50% reduction in incontinence episodes. However, when the stimulators were inactivated, this group returned to their pretreatment level of incontinence.

Complications of sacral nerve stimulation include pain at the site of the stimulator implant, infection and lead migration.

PERIPHERAL NERVE STIMULATION (SANS). Following a report demonstrating that peripheral tibial nerve stimulation in monkeys inhibited detrusor overactivity, this form of neuro-modulation has been introduced in humans. Govier et al reported on the results of a multicenter study of 53 patients.[41] Following a 12-week course of stimulation, 71% of the patients had at least a 25% decrease in their day-time or night-time frequency. No adverse events were noted.

Sacral and peripheral neuromodulation have demonstrated some potential for treatment in refractory detrusor overactivity. Robust clinical trials are required to determine whether these therapies will have a long-term place.

REFERENCES

1. Jarvis GJ. Urodynamics (Ed Mundy A, Stephenson TP and Wein A), Stress incontinence, 1994, 299–326.
2. Jarvis GJ. Surgery for genuine stress incontinence. Br J Obstet Gynaecol 1994;101:371–374.
3. Jarvis GJ, Abrams P, Khoury S, Wein A. Surgical treatment for incontinence in adult women. In: Incontinence (Ed Abrams, Khoury and Wein), 1998, 637–68.
4. Demirci F, Yildirim U. Demirci E, et al. Ten-year results of Marshall Marchetti Krantz and anterior colporrhaphy procedures. Aust NZ J Obstet Gynaecol 2002;42(5):513–514.
5. Demirci F, Yucel O, Eren S, et al. Long-term results of Burch colposuspension. Gynecol Obstet Invest 2001;51(4):243–247.
6. Viereck V, Pauer HU, Bader W, et al. Introital ultrasound of the lower genital tract before and after colposuspension: a 4-year objective follow-up. Ultrasound Obstet Gynecol 2004;23(3):277–283.
7. Bidmead J, Cardozo L, McLellan A, et al. A comparison of the objective and subjective outcomes of colposuspension for stress incontinence in women. Br J Obstet Gynaecol 2001;108(4):408–413.
8. Glazener CM, Cooper K. Bladder neck needle suspension for urinary incontinence in women. Cochrane Database Syst Rev 2002(2):CD003636.
9. Tebyani N, Patel H, Yamaguchi R, et al. Percutaneous needle bladder neck suspension for the treatment of stress urinary incontinence in women: long-term results. J Urol 2000;163(5):1510–1512.
10. Carey M, Rosamilia A, Maher C, et al. Laparoscopic versus open colposuspension: a prospective multicentre randomized single-blind. Neurourol Urodynam 2000;19:389–391.
11. Fatthy H, El Hao M, Samaha I, Abdallah K. Modified Burch colposuspension: laparoscopy versus laparotomy. J Am Assoc Gynecol Laparosc 2001;8(1):99–106.
12. Su TH, Wang KG, Hsu CY, et al. Prospective comparison of laparoscopic and traditional colposuspensions in the treatment of genuine stress incontinence. Acta Obstet Gynecol Scand 1997;76(6):576–582.
13. Summitt R, Lucente VL, Karram MM, et al. Randomised comparison of laparoscopic and transabdominal Burch urethropexy

for the treatment of genuine stress incontinence. Obstet Gynecol 2000;95(4/suppl1):2S.
14. O'Dwyer T, MacIntyre I, Grant A. MRC Laparoscopic Groin Hernia Trial Group. Lancet 1999;354 (9174):185–190.
15. Persson J, Wolner-Hanssen P. Laparoscopic Burch colposuspension for stress urinary incontinence: a randomized comparison of one or two sutures on each side of the urethra. Obstet Gynecol 2000;95(1):151–155.
16. Aldridge A. Transplantation of fascia for relief of urinary stress incontinence. Am J Obstet Gynecol 1942;44:398–411.
17. Beck RP, McCormick S, Nordstrom L. The fascia lata sling procedure for treating recurrent genuine stress incontinence of urine. Obstet Gynecol 1988;72(5):699–703.
18. Hassouna ME, Ghoniem GM. Long-term outcome and quality of life after modified pubovaginal sling for intrinsic sphincteric deficiency. Urology 1999;53(2):287–291.
19. Wright EJ, Iselin CE, Carr LK, et al. Pubovaginal sling using cadaveric allograft fascia for the treatment of intrinsic sphincter deficiency. J Urol 1998;160(3 Pt 1):759–762.
20. Ulmsten U, Henriksson L, Johnson P, et al. An ambulatory surgical procedure under local anesthesia for treatment of female urinary incontinence. Int Urogynecol J Pelvic Floor Dysfunct 1996;7(2):81–85; discussion 85–86.
21. Petros PE, Ulmsten UI. An integral theory of female urinary incontinence. Experimental and clinical considerations. Acta Obstet Gynecol Scand 1990;153(suppl): 7–31.
22. Ward KL, Hilton P. A prospective multicenter randomized trial of tension-free vaginal tape and colposuspension for primary urodynamic stress incontinence: two-year follow-up. Am J Obstet Gynecol 2004;190(2):324–331.
23. Nilsson CG, Kuuva N, Falconer C, et al. Long-term results of the tension-free vaginal tape (TVT) procedure for surgical treatment of female stress urinary incontinence. Int Urogynecol J Pelvic Floor Dysfunct 2001;12(suppl 2):S5–8.
24. Lightner D, Calvosa C, Andersen R, et al. A new injectable bulking agent for treatment of stress urinary incontinence: results of a multicenter, randomized, controlled, double-blind study of Durasphere. Urology 2001;58(1):12–15.
25. Haab F, Zimmern PE, Leach GE. Urinary stress incontinence due to

intrinsic sphincteric deficiency: experience with fat and collagen periurethral injections. J Urol 1997;157(4):1283–1286.

26. Lee PE, Kung RC, Drutz HP. Periurethral autologous fat injection as treatment for female stress urinary incontinence: a randomized double-blind controlled trial. J Urol 2001;165(1):153–158.

27. Kreder KJ, Austin JC. Treatment of stress urinary incontinence in women with urethral hypermobility and intrinsic sphincter deficiency. J Urol 1996;156(6):1995–1998.

28. Webster GD, Perez LM, Khoury JM, et al. Management of type III stress urinary incontinence using artificial urinary sphincter. Urology 1992;39(6):499–503.

29. Richard F, Lefore TJM, Bitker NO, et al. Female incontinence with primary sphincter deficiency: results of artificial urinary sphincter with long term follow up. J Urol 1996; 156A(suppl):34–36.

30. Raz S. Editorial Comment. J Urol 1989;142:1038–1039.

31. Ramsden PD, Smith JC, Dunn M, et al. Distension therapy for the unstable bladder. Later results including an assessment of repeat distension. Br J Urol 1976;48:623–629.

32. Delaere KP, Debruyne FM, Michiels HG, et al. Prolonged bladder distension in the management of the unstable bladder. J Urol 1980;124(3):334–337.

33. Pengally AW, Stephenson TP and Milroy EJG. Results of prolonged bladder distension as treatment for detrusor instability. Br J Urol 1978; 50:243–245.

34. Blackford HN, Murray K, Stephenson TP et al. Results of transvesical infiltration of the pelvic plexuses with phenol in 116 patients. Br J Urol 1984;56(6):647–649.

35. Wall LL, Stanton SL. Transvesical injection of pelvic nerve plexuses in females with refractory urge incontinence. Br J Urol 1989; 63(5):465–468.

36. Westney OL, Lee JT, McGuire EJ et al. Long term results of Ingelman-Sundberg denervation procedure for urge incontinence refractory to medical therapy. J Urol 2002;168(3):1044–1047.

37. Awad SA, Al-Zahrani HM, Gajewski VB, et al. Long term results and complications of augmentation ileocystoplasty for idiopaltic urge incontinence in women. Br J Urol 1998;81(4):569–573.

38. Ter Meulen PH, Heesahkers JP, Janknegt RA. A study on the feasability of vesicomyotomy in patients with motor urge incontinence. Eur Urol 1997;32(2):166–169.

39. Leng WW, Blalock HJ, Fredriksson WH et al. Enterocystoplasty or detrusor myectomy? Comparison of indications and outcomes for bladder augmentation. J Urol 1999;161(3):758–763.

40. Schmidt RA. Sacral nerve stimulation for treatment of refractory urinary urge incontinence sacral nerve stimulation Study Group. J Urol 1999;162(2):352–357.

41. Govier FE. Percutaneous afferent neuromodulation for the refractory overactive bladder; results of a multicentre study. J Urol 2001;165(4):1193–1198.

SECTION 6

Treatment of anal incontinence

Conservative Treatment of Anal Incontinence

Christine Norton

INTRODUCTION

There are currently no comparisons of conservative versus surgical management of anal incontinence (AI) and very little guidance on how to select options for individual patients. Apart from clear cloacal injuries or defects and complete rectal prolapse, it is usual to encourage a trial of nonsurgical interventions before embarking on surgery.[1] Figure 16.1 gives an algorithm for patient management.[2] Conservative options, although described separately here, are in clinical practice often combined, and it is that combination which will often yield the best results.

PATIENT TEACHING AND EDUCATION

Patient education and teaching may have a value, even without any formal exercises or other interventions.[3,4] Many people have limited knowledge about how the bowel works and limited understanding of the implications of their symptoms. This can lead to ineffective or even counterproductive measures being taken by the patient. Several books[5,6] and websites (www.iffgd.org; www.bowelcontrol.org.uk) give useful information for patients. The patient who has insight into the condition will often be a more active participant in her own care and this is vital for most conservative options.

LIFESTYLE INTERVENTIONS

There are known associations in the epidemiologic literature between certain "lifestyle" factors and fecal incontinence (FI) (see Chapter 8). However, it is not known at present whether weight loss, smoking cessation, avoiding heavy lifting or any other measure is useful clinically for patients with FI. Nicotine is a known colonic stimulant[7] and clinically some patients with urgency seem to benefit from reducing smoking or altering the timing of smoking to avoid stimulating the urge to defecate.

DIETARY MANAGEMENT

Diet has a major influence on bowel function and stool consistency, and as such is an obvious target for manipulation in patients with FI. Usually, firmer stool is easier to control and less likely to leak. However, there have been remarkably few studies either on the relationship of diet to symptoms or on dietary interventions as treatment. It has been found that people with FI do not eat a diet which differs significantly from controls without bowel symptoms.[8] Both increasing[9] and decreasing[10] fiber content have been found useful in FI. In patients with FI associated with loose stool, one RCT has found benefit from two different sources of soluble fiber, when compared to placebo. The type of fiber and the initial baseline in the diet may be important, although this remains to be defined.

A diet and bowel diary can help the patient to identify any foods which may be associated with worsening of symptoms. Specific foods can make a huge difference to some patients, particularly those with the irritable bowel syndrome. This seems to be very individual and finding any associations is largely a matter of trial and error. Where a sensitivity or allergy is suspected, formal advice and even an exclusion diet supervised by a dietician can be helpful. If dairy products are found to worsen symptoms, care must be taken that adequate calcium intake is maintained, especially in postmenopausal women.

Reducing caffeine intake can improve frequency and urgency, although if caffeine intake is high, this should be reduced gradually to avoid headaches consequent on caffeine withdrawal. Artificial sweeteners, especially sorbitol, can also cause loose stool and can be reduced. If alcohol intake is contributing to intestinal hurry, this should be moderated.

The importance of an adequate fluid intake to promote a regular bowel habit and prevent constipation has been questioned,[11] although there is some evidence that severe restriction to the point of dehydration can promote

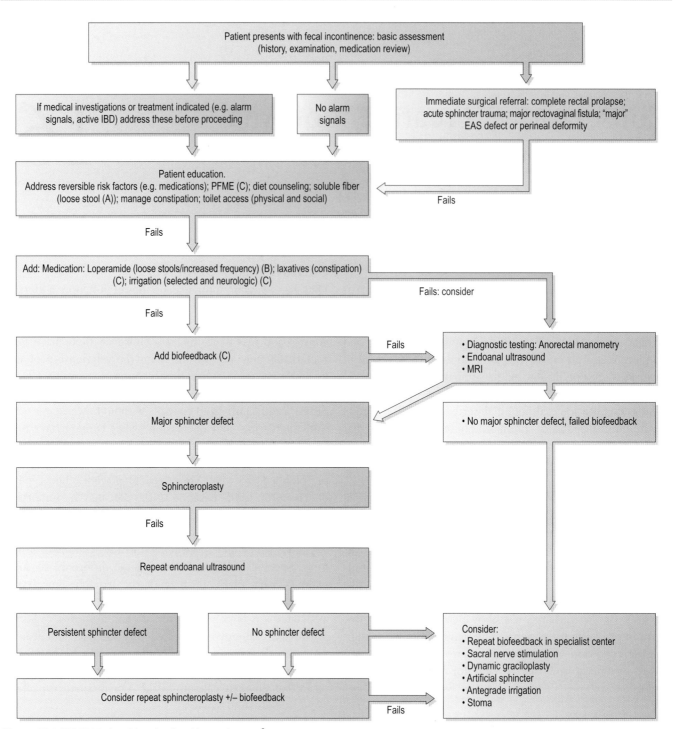

Figure 16.1 ICI 2005 algorithm for fecal incontinence.[2]

constipation.[12] As long as the patient is adequately hydrated, any extra fluid intake is more likely to influence urine than stool output.

The role of probiotics in bowel function is gaining increasing attention. These "good bacteria" have been found to be beneficial in inflammatory bowel disease and may have a more generally beneficial effect in regulating or modifying bowel function.

BOWEL HABIT AND RETRAINING

Unlike the bladder, where urine is present continuously 24 hours a day, bowel function is for most people episodic. If complete evacuation can be achieved at a predictable time, the role of the sphincters is relatively minor and the patient can be continent even with quite severely impaired sphincter function. For this reason, an attempt to regularize bowel habit and achieve complete evacuation should be made. Bowel motility is at its maximum in the morning after rising and eating or drinking and, where feasible, the patient is encouraged to make time and privacy after breakfast to attempt defecation. This can be difficult in modern lifestyles.

The patient can also be helped to achieve complete evacuation by instruction on defecation posture and pushing without straining (see Box 16.1). It can take several weeks until a regular habit is established. If the patient is actually constipated, with "overflow" type FI, achieving complete bowel evacuation is associated with reduced FI.[13] This is mostly relevant to frail or disabled people and children, and may need to be achieved by the use of laxatives and/or rectal evacuants.

Biofeedback is often used to treat adults with chronic constipation by teaching correct evacuation techniques.[14] There has been no study of its use to treat constipation-

associated FI in adults but children with constipation-associated FI can learn to relax the pelvic floor muscles during attempts to defecate. An RCT by van der Plas and colleagues[15] showed that combined treatment with biofeedback and laxatives was associated with a higher success rate at the end of training (39% vs 19%), but by follow-up 12 months later, there were no differences between groups. Other studies support these findings by showing either no difference between the laxative-only group and a biofeedback group[16] or faster acquisition of continence in the biofeedback group but no long-term difference in success rate.[17]

Patients with urgency often benefit from bowel retraining in the form of an urge resistance program akin to bladder retraining for an overactive bladder. If you have experienced urge fecal incontinence once, the natural temptation is then to rush to the toilet at the first sensation of rectal filling, in

---

Box 16.1 Patient instruction for complete evacuation

Getting into a regular habit

Most people's bowels respond best to a regular habit. Some of us are too busy to make time for our bowels. Others live a very irregular lifestyle which makes a habit difficult.

The bowel usually goes to sleep at night and wakes up in the morning. Eating, drinking, and moving around all stimulate the bowel. The most likely time for a bowel action is about 30 minutes after the first meal of the day.

This makes it important not to skip breakfast. Try to eat at least something for breakfast and take two warm drinks. Try to make 5–10 minutes of free uninterrupted time about 30 minutes later. This is not always easy if your house is busy in the morning, so you may need to plan ahead or get up a little earlier while you retrain your bowel.

Sitting properly

The way you sit on the toilet can make a big difference to ease of opening your bowels. The "natural" position (before toilets were invented) is squatting. Countries where squat (hole in the floor) toilets are still common seem to have fewer problems with constipation.

While actually squatting is not very practical, many people find that adopting a "semi-squat" position helps a lot. One of the footstools that toddlers use to reach a sink is ideal, 8–12 inches high (20–30 cm). Position this just in front of your toilet and rest your feet flat on the stool, keeping your feet and knees about 1 foot (30 cm) apart. Lean forwards, resting your elbows on your thighs. Try to relax.

Breathing

It is important not to hold your breath when trying to open your bowels. Many people are tempted to take a deep breath in and then hold their breath while trying to push. Try to avoid this. Sit on the toilet as described above, relax your shoulders and breathe normally. You may find it easiest to breathe in through your nose and out through your mouth.

If you hold your breath and push, this is STRAINING which tends to close your bottom more tightly. Also, if you hold your breath, you are limited in how long you can hold this and when you have to take the pressure off and breathe, you tend to be back to square one.

If you find that you cannot help straining and holding your breath, try breathing out gently, or humming or reciting a nursery rhyme.

Pushing without straining

The best way to open your bowels is by using your abdominal (stomach) muscles to push. Leaning forward, supporting your elbows on your thighs and breathing gently, relax your shoulders. Make your abdominal muscles bulge outwards to "make your waist wide." Now use these abdominal muscles as a pump to push backwards and downwards into your bottom. Keep up the gentle but firm pressure.

Relaxing the back passage

The final part of the jigsaw is to relax the back passage. Many people with constipation actually tighten the back passage when they are trying to open the bowels, instead of relaxing, without realizing what they are doing. This is like squeezing a tube of toothpaste while keeping the lid on!

To locate the muscles around the back passage, firstly squeeze as if you are trying to control wind. Now imagine that the muscle around the anus is a lift. Squeeze to take your lift up to the first floor. Now relax, down to the ground floor, down to the basement, down to the cellar.

Putting it all together

This is a bit like learning to ride a bike. The above instructions tell you WHAT to do but do not tell you HOW to do it. It sounds simple but coordinating everything takes practice, and you have to work it out for yourself. Some people find it easier than others.

- Sit properly
- Breathe normally
- Push from your waist downwards
- Relax the back passage

Keep this up for about 5 minutes, unless you have a bowel action sooner. If nothing happens, don't give up. Try again tomorrow. It often takes several weeks of practice until this really starts to work and a regular habit is established.

order to preempt an accident. This can become a vicious circle of hypersensitivity and vigilance, with any rectal sensation resulting in a feeling of panic and a flight to the toilet "just in case." Just as deliberate ignoring of the call to stool can result in reduced bowel frequency,[18] it is feasible that continual attempts to defecate, coupled with anxiety, could stimulate gut activity and result in even greater frequency.

Patients with urgency are given a progressive program of urge resistance, on or near the toilet to start with and then progressively holding on for longer and farther away from the toilet as confidence grows. This can take courage and perseverance but is helpful for many patients, even without formal exercises.[3] It can be accompanied by progressive rectal distension training during biofeedback sessions (see below).

EXERCISES AND BIOFEEDBACK

The mainstay of conservative management of FI in the colorectal and gastroenterology literature is "biofeedback." There have been almost no studies of exercises alone, in the manner of pelvic floor exercises for urinary incontinence. Almost all studies until very recently have utilized some method of biofeedback. Many studies have been very small and most are case series with no controls. The almost universally positive results in over 40 reports, even allowing for publication bias in favor of submitting and publishing positive reports, do suggest at least some clinical merit, with two-thirds of patients with FI deriving at least some benefit and up to half reporting symptom resolution.[19]

Three different types of biofeedback have been described.

Rectal sensitivity training.
A rectal balloon is gradually distended with air or water and the patient is asked to report first sensation of rectal filling. Once this threshold volume is determined, repeated reinflations of the balloon are performed with the objective being to teach the patient to feel the distension at progressively lower volumes.[20] The rationale is that some patients are found to have high threshold volumes and if the patient detects stool arriving sooner, there is more possibility to either find a toilet or use an anal squeeze, or both. Conversely, the same technique has also been used to teach the patient to tolerate progressively larger volumes in those with urgency and a hypersensitive rectum.[21]

Strength training.
Biofeedback techniques have been used to demonstrate anal sphincter pressures to the patient, thereby enabling teaching of anal sphincter exercises and giving feedback on performance and progress. This can be achieved by using EMG skin electrodes, manometric pressures or intraanal EMG. The patient is encouraged, by seeing or hearing the signal, to enhance squeeze strength and endurance. There is no consensus on an optimum exercise regimen for use at home between sessions, nor on the number of squeezes, the frequency of exercises or treatment duration, with different authors describing very different programs.[19] Box 16.2 gives one suggested program.[10]

Coordination training.
Some authors have described a three-balloon system for biofeedback for FI. One distension balloon is situated in the rectum; the second and third

---

Box 16.2 Patient instructions for anal sphincter exercises

Note: Length of squeeze and number of repetitions are individualized (figures in brackets), depending on what is achieved at the initial assessment.

Sit comfortably with your knees slightly apart. Now imagine that you are trying to stop yourself passing wind from the bowel. To do this, you must squeeze the muscle around the back passage. Try squeezing and lifting that muscle as tightly as you can, as if you are really worried that you are about to leak. You should be able to feel the muscle move. Your buttocks, tummy, and legs should not move much at all. You should be aware of the skin around the back passage tightening and being pulled up and away from your chair. Some people find it helpful to imagine that they are trying to pick up a penny from the chair with their anal sphincter muscles. You are now exercising your anal sphincter. You should not need to hold your breath when you tighten the muscles!

Now imagine that the sphincter muscle is a lift. When you squeeze as tightly as you can, your lift goes up to the 4th floor. But you cannot hold it there for very long, and it will not get you safely to the toilet, as it will get tired very quickly. So now squeeze more gently, take your lift only up to the 2nd floor. Feel how much longer you can hold it than at the maximum squeeze.

Practising your exercises

1. Sit, stand or lie with your knees slightly apart. Tighten and pull up the sphincter muscles as tightly as you can. Hold tightened for at least (5) seconds and then relax for at least 10 seconds to allow the muscle to recover.
   Repeat at least (5) times. This will work on the strength of your muscles.
2. Next, pull the muscles up to about half of their maximum squeeze. See how long you can hold this for. Then relax for at least 10 seconds.
   Repeat at least (5) times. This will work on the endurance, or staying power, of your muscles.
3. Pull up the muscles as quickly and tightly as you can and then relax and then pull up again, and see how many times you can do this before you get tired. Try for at least (5) quick pull-ups.
4. Do these exercises—(5) as hard as you can, (5) as long as you can and as many quick pull-ups as you can—at least (10) times every day.
5. As the muscles get stronger, you will find that you can hold for longer than 5 seconds, and that you can do more pull-ups each time without the muscle getting tired.
6. It takes time for exercise to make muscle stronger. You may need to exercise regularly for several months before the muscles gain their full strength.

smaller pressure-recording balloons are situated in the upper and lower anal canal. Rectal distension triggers the rectal–anal inhibitory reflex (see Chapter 3).

This momentary anal relaxation is a point of vulnerability for people with FI and incontinence can occur at this time. By distending the rectal balloon and showing the patient this consequent pressure drop, the aim is to teach the patient to counteract this by a voluntary anal squeeze, hard enough and for long enough for resting pressure to return to its baseline level. Some patients are performing unintentional counterproductive maneuvers when they feel the urge to defecate, such as bearing down or thinking that they are squeezing when no pressure rise is seen, and this can also be corrected.

These three methods are not mutually exclusive and many protocols combine two or three elements together. One small controlled study has suggested that the sensory training may be the most effective element.[22] Recent controlled studies have suggested that the "biofeedback" element, in what is inevitably a complex intervention involving a lot of time, attention and patient teaching and advice, may not be the most important element,[3,23] with equally good results achieved using exercises taught and monitored without biofeedback, and indeed equal results without any exercises if the same amounts of time, attention, and teaching are given.[3] However, it remains a useful adjunct in some patients and can be seen as providing a framework for consultation sessions.

ELECTRICAL STIMULATION

Attempts have been made to improve anal sphincter function by using surface electrical stimulation delivered by various methods. Older methods such as faradism were uncomfortable and interferential current was ineffective, but newer equipment is much more comfortable and well tolerated. Skin electrodes or intraanal plugs may be used, with the latter delivering current more directly to the sphincter muscles. A few case series have reported benefit, although there are very few controlled studies.[24]

One controlled study found that electrical stimulation plus biofeedback was possibly superior to biofeedback alone for 40 women with postnatal FI, but the study did not compare like methods of biofeedback in the two groups.[25] Other uncontrolled studies have reported improvement[26,27] although not all studies have been positive.[28,29] If electrical stimulation is effective, the mechanism could be via direct muscle stimulation and/or by improving sensation and responsiveness. There is one controlled study suggesting that sensitization may be the primary mechanism as stimulation at 35 Hz and at 1 Hz has equal effect.[30] The optimum stimulation parameters remain to be determined.

DRUG MANAGEMENT

Drug treatment for FI aims to modify gut motility, increase sphincter pressures or achieve complete evacuation. The evidence base is very limited[31] and as most of the medication used is off patent, it does not seem likely that large new studies will be developed.

Loperamide (Imodium) is seen as the drug of first choice in patients with FI associated with loose stool, urgency or passive loss of soft/liquid stool.[32] It has several potentially helpful modes of action, including reducing colonic motility and increasing colonic water reabsorption, thereby firming stool consistency, dampening the gastrocolic response, and raising anal sphincter pressures.[33,34] Loperamide is well tolerated by the majority of patients and is safe in doses up to 16 mg daily, although many patients obtain benefit from 2–4 mg daily or p.r.n. Onset of action is within 30–60 minutes, so it is useful on a p.r.n. basis and most patients do not seem to need to escalate the dose over time. Patients with postprandial urgency should take loperamide 30 minutes before eating. Those with early morning urgency can take a dose at night. Those who fear going out should take it before activities. Constipation seems to be the only common side-effect, which is intentional. If the capsule/tablet formulation of loperamide constipates too much, a liquid version can be used and very small doses titrated to individual needs (as low as 0.5–1 mg).

Codeine phosphate is an alternative if loperamide is not tolerated, but is associated with more side effects, the most troublesome of which is drowsiness, and development of tolerance and even dependence. Loperamide and codeine can be combined in severe diarrhea, although obviously unexplained diarrhea needs prior investigation.

A few patients with FI that cannot be controlled in any other way will deliberately choose to take enough medication to stop all spontaneous bowel evacuation and then use suppositories or an enema to empty the bowel at their own convenience and a predictable time. The only study of this was in a nursing home setting,[35] where success was good if compliance was achieved.

Other constipating drugs can have an incidental beneficial effect on FI and as urinary and fecal incontinence so often coexist, this can be harnessed; for instance, drugs with anticholinergic effects may improve both conditions. Conversely, many drugs have an unintentional effect of loosening stool and modifying a drug regimen can improve FI symptoms (e.g. oral diabetic medication, nonsteroidal antiinflammatories or antibiotics).

Patients with FI associated with incomplete evacuation may use a suppository or mini-enema to achieve more complete evacuation. Some of the bulking agents used for constipation may improve stool consistency and FI.

A more recent approach is to attempt to modify anal sphincter activity pharmacologically. Phenylephrine raises internal anal sphincter pressure in healthy volunteers and is clinically useful in patients with anal leakage secondary to formation of an ileoanal pouch, especially at night.[36,37] However, its value in patients with impaired sphincter function may be less[38] and it has not yet reached the market. Other approaches are in development and it is not known if drugs developed for the treatment of stress urinary incontinence might be helpful.

ANAL PLUG AND OTHER PRODUCTS

Many people with FI wear the absorbent pads designed for urinary or menstrual loss. Unfortunately, these are often ineffective in containing stool and do nothing to protect the skin or disguise odor. There are few satisfactory solutions to this. A few patients can tolerate a specially designed anal plug, which retains stool in the rectum, although most find it uncomfortable, or even that it stimulates defecation.[39,40] Many of the skincare products used for ostomy care are helpful as stool leakage can cause rapid skin excoriation, especially if the patient has undergone colectomy and the stool is corrosive ileal content.

IRRIGATION

Rectal irrigation is gaining acceptance as a management for FI.[41,42] Companies are now developing specific equipment designed for the purpose, although some patients use equipment designed for stoma irrigation or a bladder catheter. The patient is taught to introduce a rectal catheter into the anus, usually while seated on the toilet. Several hundred milliliters of water are introduced into the rectum, the catheter is then removed and the bowel evacuated as completely as possible. This is not effective for all patients and some do not find the procedure, or the time needed (30–60 minutes), acceptable. A surgically constructed irrigation port may be an alternative (see Chapter 17).

COMPLEX PACKAGES OF INTERVENTION

In clinical practice, many of the interventions described above are used in combination, making it very hard to tell which are the effective elements. It would not be unusual to use medication, exercises, diet, and suppositories all in the same patient. Much more research is needed to define which approaches are best targeted to which patients.

PREVENTION

Little work has been conducted to date on prevention of FI. Many groups are at high risk of FI and active case finding is important given the reluctance of many patients to discuss their symptoms (Box 16.3).

Box 16.3 Targets for secondary prevention through early recognition[2]

Patient characteristics

Dementia/cognitive impairment

Physical limitations/impaired mobility

Diseases and disorders

Urinary incontinence

Pelvic organ prolapse

Hemorrhoids, grade 3 and 4

Irritable bowel syndrome

Diarrhea

Constipation

Diabetes mellitus

CNS injury: stroke, head injury, Alzheimer's

Spinal cord injury: traumatic cord injury, spina bifida

Multiple sclerosis

Congenital anorectal anomalies: imperforate anus

Surgical interventions

Vaginal delivery with sphincter laceration

Instrumented vaginal delivery

Colectomy, with or without ileal reservoir

Internal anal sphincterotomy for anal fissure, hemorrhoids, Hirschprung's disease

Prostatectomy, especially by perineal approach

Drugs and diet

Drugs that cause diarrhea as a side effect

Foods that cause diarrhea: dairy products in lactase-deficient individuals, some fruits

Food additives that cause diarrhea or gas: artificial sweeteners

Radiologic treatment of pelvic cancer

The first vaginal delivery carries the greatest risk of new-onset FI[43] and each subsequent delivery adds to that risk.[44-47] There is a debate about elective cesarean section, especially in high-risk groups such as those with preexisting bowel disorders, but this obviously has major ramifications if recommended as a preventive measure for FI. Forceps delivery is a risk factor for FI, with the evidence on vacuum extraction being more equivocal.[2] It seems likely that avoiding episiotomy, especially midline episiotomy, except for specific indications related to fetal distress, might reduce AI via reduction of anal sphincter trauma.[2,48]

There is very limited evidence on the value of any intervention designed to reduce the incidence of FI after childbirth, either after normal delivery or that complicated by forceps or a third-degree tear. One study[49] designed to address postnatal urinary incontinence has found less FI at 1 year in women who perform pelvic floor exercises versus controls (4% vs 10%), but no study to date has directly addressed FI. It is to be hoped that in the future much greater emphasis is placed on researching ways of either reducing risk factors or preventing symptom development in those at risk by targeted interventions.

REFERENCES

1. Whitehead WE, Wald A, Norton N. Treatment options for fecal incontinence: consensus conference report. Dis Colon Rectum 2001;44:131–144.
2. Norton C, Whitehead WE, Bliss DZ, Metsola P, Tries J. Conservative and pharmacological management of faecal incontinence in adults. In: Abrams P, Khoury S, Wein A, Cardozo L, eds. Incontinence. Proceedings of the Third International Consultation on Incontinence. Plymouth: Health Books; 2005.
3. Norton C, Chelvanayagam S, Wilson-Barnett J, Redfern S, Kamm MA. Randomized controlled trial of biofeedback for fecal incontinence. Gastroenterology 2003;125:1320–1329.
4. Heymen S, Jones KR, Ringel Y, Scarlett Y, Drossman DA, Whitehead WE. Biofeedback for fecal incontinence and constipation: the role of medical management and education. Gastroenterology 2001;120(Suppl 1):A397.
5. Schuster MM, Wehmueller J. Keeping control: understanding and overcoming faecal incontinence. London: Johns Hopkins Press; 1994.
6. Norton C, Kamm MA. Bowel control: information and practical advice. Beaconsfield: Beaconsfield Publishers; 1999.
7. Rausch T, Beglinger C, Alam N, Meier R. Effect of transdermal application of nicotine on colonic transit in healthy nonsmoking volunteers. Neurogastroenterol Mot 1998;10:263–270.
8. Bliss DZ, McLaughlin J, Jung H, Savik K, Jensen L, Lowry AC. Comparison of the nutritional composition of diets of persons with fecal incontinence and that of age and gender-matched controls. J Wound Ostomy Cont Nurs 2000;27(2):90–97.
9. Bliss DZ, Jung H, Savik K, et al. Supplementation with dietary fiber improves fecal incontinence. Nurs Res 2001;50(4):203–213.
10. Norton C, Chelvanayagam S. Conservative management of faecal incontinence in adults. In: Norton C, Chelvanayagam S, eds. Bowel continence nursing. Beaconsfield: Beaconsfield Publishers; 2004: 114–131.
11. Muller-Lissner SA, Kamm MA, Scarpignato C, Wald A. Myths and misconceptions about chronic constipation. Am J Gastroenterol 2005; in press.
12. Klauser AG, Beck A, Schindlbeck NE. Low fluid intake lowers stool output in healthy male volunteers. Zeitschr Gastroenterol 1990;28:606–609.
13. Chassagne P, Jego A, Gloc P, et al. Does treatment of constipation improve faecal incontinence in institutionalized elderly patients? Age Ageing 2000;29(2):159–164.
14. Horton N. Behavioural and biofeedback therapy for evacuation disorders. In: Norton C, Chelvanayagam S, eds. Bowel continence nursing. Beaconsfield: Beaconsfield Publishers; 2004.
15. Van der Plas RN, Benninga MA, Redekop WK, Taminiau JA, Buller HA. Randomised trial of biofeedback training for encopresis. Arch Dis Child 1996;75(5):367–374.
16. Wald A, Chandra R, Gabel S, Chiponis D. Evaluation of biofeedback in childhood encopresis. J Pediatr Gastroenterol Nutr 1987;6(4):554–558.
17. Loening-Baucke V. Biofeedback treatment for chronic constipation and encopresis in childhood: long-term outcome. Pediatrics 1995;96(1 Pt 1):105–110.
18. Klauser AG, Voderholzer WA, Heinrich CA, Schindlbeck NE, Muller-Lissner SA. Behavioural modification of colonic function: can constipation be learned? Dig Dis Sci 1990; 35:1271–1275.
19. Norton C, Kamm MA. Anal sphincter biofeedback and pelvic floor exercises for faecal incontinence in adults: a systematic review. Aliment Pharmacol Therapeut 2001;15:1147–1154.
20. Chiarioni G, Bassotti G, Stranganini S, Vantini I, Whitehead WE, Stegagnini S. Sensory retraining is key to biofeedback therapy for formed stool incontinence. Am J Gastroenterol 2002; 97:109–117.
21. Norton C, Chelvanayagam S. Methodology of biofeedback for adults with fecal incontinence: a program of care. J Wound Ostomy Cont Nurs 2001;28:156–168.
22. Miner PB, Donnelly TC, Read NW. Investigation of the mode of action of biofeedback in the treatment of faecal incontinence. Dig Dis Sci 1990;35(10):1291–1298.
23. Solomon MJ, Pager CK, Rex J, Roberts R, Manning J. Randomised, controlled trial of biofeedback with anal manometry, transanal ultrasound, or pelvic floor retraining with digital guidance alone in the treatment of mild to moderate fecal incontinence. Dis Colon Rectum 2003; 46(6):703–710.
24. Hosker G, Norton C, Brazzelli M. Electrical stimulation for faecal incontinence in adults (Cochrane review). Cochrane Library Issue 2. Chichester: John Wiley Ltd; 2002.
25. Fynes MM, Marshall K, Cassidy M, et al. A prospective, randomized study comparing the effect of augmented biofeedback with sensory biofeedback alone on fecal incontinence after obstetric trauma. Dis Colon Rectum 1999;42(6):753–758.
26. Pescatori M, Pavesio R, Anastasio G, Daini S. Transanal electrostimulation for faecal incontinence: clinical, psychologic and manometric prospective study. Dis Colon Rectum 1991; 34:540–545.
27. Menard C, Trudel C, Cloutier R. Anal reeducation for postoperative fecal incontinence in congenital diseases of the rectum and anus. J Pediatr Surg 1997;32(6):867–869.
28. Scheuer M, Kuijpers HC, Bleijenberg G. Effect of electrostimulation on sphincter function in neurogenic fecal continence. Dis Colon Rectum 1994;37(6):590–593.
29. Leroi AM, Karoui S, Touchais JY, Berkelmans I, Denis P. Electrostimulation is not a clinically effective treatment of anal incontinence. Eur J Gastroenterol Hepatol 1999; 11(9):1045–1047.
30. Norton C, Gibbs A, Kamm MA. Randomised trial of electrical stimulation for faecal incontinence. Dis Colon Rectum 2005; online.
31. Cheetham M, Brazzelli M, Norton C, Glazener CM. Drug treatment for faecal incontinence in adults (Cochrane review). Cochrane Library Issue 2. Chichester: John Wiley Ltd; 2004.
32. Kamm MA. Faecal incontinence: clinical review. BMJ 1998;316:528–532.
33. Read M, Read NW, Barber DC, Duthie HL. Effects of loperamide on anal sphincter function in patients complaining of chronic diarrhoea with faecal incontinence and urgency. Dig Dis Sci 1982;27:807–814.
34. Sun WM, Read NW, Verlinden M. Effects of loperamide oxide in gastrointestinal transit time and anorectal function in patients with chronic diarrhoea and faecal incontinence. Scand J Gastroenterol 1997;32:34–38.
35. Tobin GW, Brocklehurst JC. Faecal incontinence in residential homes for the elderly: prevalence, aetiology and management. Age Ageing 1986;15:41–46.
36. Carapeti EA, Kamm MA, Evans BK, Phillips RK. Topical phenylephrine increases anal sphincter resting pressure. Br J Surg 1999;86(2):267–270.

37. Carapeti EA, Kamm MA, Phillips RK. Randomized controlled trial of topical phenylephrine in the treatment of faecal incontinence. Br J Surg 2000;87:38–42.

38. Cheetham M, Kamm MA, Phillips RK. Topical phenylephrine increases anal canal resting pressure in patients with faecal incontinence. Gut 2001;48:356–359.

39. Mortensen NJ, Smilgin Humphreys M. The anal continence plug: a disposable device for patients with anorectal incontinence. Lancet 1991;338:295–297.

40. Norton C, Kamm MA. Anal plug for faecal incontinence. Colorect Dis 2001;3:323–327.

41. Gardiner A, Marshall J, Duthie GS. Rectal irrigation for relief of functional bowel disorders. Nurs Stand 2004;19(9):39–42.

42. Briel JW, Schouten WR, Vlot EA, et al. Clinical value of colonic irrigation in patients with continence disturbances. Dis Colon Rectum 1997;40(7):802–805.

43. Zetterstrom J, Lopez A, Anzen B, Norman M, Holmstrom B, Mellgren A. Anal sphincter tears at vaginal delivery: risk factors and clinical outcome of primary repair. Obstet Gynecol 1999;94(1):21–28.

44. Fornell EU, Wingren G, Kjolhede P. Factors associated with pelvic floor dysfunction with emphasis on urinary and fecal incontinence and genital prolapse: an epidemiological study. Acta Obstet Gynecol Scand 2004;83:383–389.

45. Chen GD, Hu SW, Chen YC, Lin TL, Lin LY. Prevalence and correlations of anal incontinence and constipation in Taiwanese women. Neurourol Urodynam 2003;22(7):664–669.

46. MacLennan AH, Taylor AW, Wilson DH, Wilson D. The prevalence of pelvic floor disorders and their relationship to gender, age, parity and mode of delivery. Br J Obstet Gynaecol 2000;107(12):1460–1470.

47. Faltin D, Sangalli MR, Curtin F, Morabia A, Weil A. Prevalence of anal incontinence and other anorectal symptoms in women. Int Urogynecol J Pelvic Floor Dysfunct 2001;12(2):117–120.

48. Signorello LB, Harlow BL, Chekos AK, Repke JT. Midline episiotomy and anal incontinence: retrospective cohort study. BMJ 2000;320:86–90.

49. Glazener CM, Herbison P, Wilson PD, MacArthur C, Lang GD. Conservative management of persistent postnatal urinary and faecal incontinence: randomised controlled trial. BMJ 2001;323:593–596.

Surgical Treatment of Anal Incontinence

Noelani M Guaderrama and Charles W Nager

INTRODUCTION

Surgical treatment of anal incontinence should be considered after conservative measures have been exhausted. The efficacy of surgical treatment of anal incontinence is difficult to conclude from the medical literature. Most of the studies are retrospective case series with small numbers of patients and limited follow-up. Outcome measures are not consistent and difficult to compare. Although there are recently developed validated instruments for scoring of symptom severity and measuring quality of life, these have not been universally accepted and employed.[1,2]

ANAL SPHINCTEROPLASTY

An overlapping anal sphincter repair is the treatment of choice for patients with anal incontinence and evidence of an anal sphincter defect. This remains the general consensus despite the lack of randomized controlled trials comparing this to other surgical treatments.

The technique involves a semilunar or transverse incision anterior to the anus, approximately 1–2 cm beyond the anal verge (Fig. 17.1). Sharp dissection is performed laterally to the ischiorectal fat, posteriorly toward the anal verge, and cephalad to the rectovaginal septum to identify the two ends of the external anal sphincter muscle with intervening scar tissue. Care is taken to avoid the nerve and blood supply from branches of the pudendal nerve and artery that reach the muscle from the posterolateral directions. Most of the case series that include a description of the technique describe dividing the scar in the midline, leaving a portion of scar tissue attached to each end of the sphincter muscle.[3-10] The two ends of the external anal sphincter must be

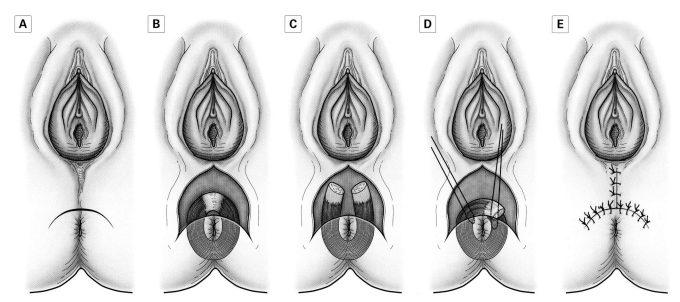

Figure 17.1   Overlapping anal sphincteroplasty. (**A**) A semilunar incision is made anterior to the anus. (**B**) The external anal sphincter with defect and intervening scar is exposed. (**C**) The scar is divided to allow for overlapping repair. (**D**) Two U-shaped sutures are placed in the overlapped ends of the sphincter. (**E**) The incision is closed in a V-Y fashion with interrupted sutures.

sufficiently mobilized to allow overlap in the midline. If the internal anal sphincter can be identified with a defect, this defect can be repaired at the same time.

Although no randomized controlled studies have been performed comparing overlapping with direct apposition (end-to-end) techniques in secondary repair, most of the case series on anal sphincteroplasty since 1984 describe an overlapping technique. Most authors describe suturing the overlapped muscle ends with mattress sutures. A variety of suture materials have been described by various authors including polyglactin,[3-5,7,11] prolene,[6,11] and polydioxanone surgical (PDS).[13] The skin edges are typically closed in a V-Y fashion. A drain may be used.

Table 17.1 shows the results of several series of overlapping anal sphincteroplasty procedures with a minimum of 30 patients.[3,4,7,8,11,12,14-25] These series involved median or mean follow-up periods from 3 to 58.5 months. Although the authors used various definitions of success, overall it is reasonable to conclude that about two-thirds of patients obtain reasonable resolution of symptoms after the procedure. When the data are specifically examined for the percentage of patients achieving "continence to solid and liquid stool," the results range from 30% to 83%. These studies illustrate the common disparity between resolution of incontinence symptoms and the sense of improvement noted by patients. In every study that reported subjective improvement, the percentage of patients who felt they were improved after anal sphincteroplasty (ranging from 69% to 85%) was higher than the percentage of patients with resolution of incontinence symptoms.

More recently, a few series have been published with long-term follow-up after overlapping anal sphincteroplasty.[10,26,27] The results from these long-term studies are summarized in Table 17.2. In 2000, Malouf et al[26] published a follow-up study on the group's original series.[16] They were able to report on 46 patients with a median follow-up of 77 months (range 60–96 months). They found that seven (15%) of the patients required further surgery for incontinence and one (2%) of the patients never had her original colostomy closed, making the outright failure rate 17%. They defined failure as the need for further continence surgery, non-closure of the colostomy or urge incontinence of at least once per 2 weeks and reported a failure rate of 50%. Four (9%) of the patients were continent to solid and liquid stool.

Halverson and Hull[10] reported on results from 49 patients with a median follow-up of 62.5 months (range 47–141 months). Eighteen patients (37%) were continent to solid and liquid stool and only 13% were completely continent. Bravo Gutierrez et al[27] reported follow-up data on a previous study from the same group.[24] They mailed the Fecal Incontinence Quality of Life Scale (FIQLS) to the 191 original patients and received responses from 130. Median follow-up was 10 years (range 7–16 years). They found that 6% were completely continent and 23% were continent to solid and liquid stool. Even with these low success rates in these long-term studies, 62–71% of patients still reported improvement from the procedure.

Many researchers have tried to identify factors that predict successful outcome after anal sphincteroplasty. The data would suggest that age, duration of symptoms, and anal manometry measurements are not predictive of success. An area of controversy is the relationship between pudendal nerve function and outcome of anal sphincteroplasty (Table 17.3). Pudendal neuropathy has correlated with poor outcome in a number of studies[5,15,19,28-30] but not in others.[8,11,16,17,24,31] Two of the studies that found no effect of pudendal neuropathy on outcome had inadequate power to detect a significant difference at the levels of success percentages seen in the studies.[11,24] Oliveira et al[18] failed to show a significant difference in outcomes between the two groups even though patients with normal pudendal nerve terminal motor latencies (PNTML) had a success rate of 73% and those with abnormal PNTML had a success rate of 38%. They argued that there may be a type II error due to a small sample size (n=55).

Table 17.3 summarizes the results of these studies and the outcome differences for patients with and without abnormal PNTML. All these studies report short-term results. Overall, patients with normal PNTML had a success rate of 69% and those with abnormal PNTML had a success rate of 49%. Therefore, the abundance of data would suggest that abnormal PNTML is a risk factor (RR=1.65; with 95% CI from 1.31 to 2.07) for a lower success rate. We conclude that abnormal preoperative PNTML studies confer a poorer prognosis, but not a contraindication, for surgery. Although the results of PNTML studies may alter prognosis, they usually do not alter plans for surgical management in a patient with a known anatomic defect. Therefore the utility of this diagnostic investigation as a preoperative test remains controversial.

When anal sphincteroplasty fails, the optimal choice for subsequent treatment is not clear. Biofeedback has been studied as an adjunct to surgery and was reported to improve continence after sphincteroplasty.[32] Surgical options for treatment of persistent or recurrent incontinence include muscle transposition procedures, artificial bowel sphincter placement, and sacral neuromodulation.

POSTANAL REPAIR

Initially described by Parks in 1975,[33] the postanal repair can be performed to treat anal incontinence in patients with an intact external anal sphincter, including those with idiopathic or neurogenic incontinence.

Table 17.1 Short-term results of overlapping anal sphincteroplasty from several series with a minimum of 30 subjects

Author, year	Number of subjects	Follow-up	Success rate	Definition of success	Subjective improvement or satisfaction	Preoperative predictors of success
Fang, 1984	76 (62 women)	Mean 35 mo. (range 2–62 mo.)	58%	Continent of solid, liquid, and gas		
Hawley, 1985	128 (80 women)	Not stated	52%	Continent of solid, liquid, and gas		
Ctercteko, 1988	44	Range 0.5–10 years	54%	Continent of solid and liquid	82% satisfied	Age Duration of symptoms
Jacobs, 1990	30	Range 7–60 months	83%	Continent of solid and liquid		1) Not manometry 2) Postop EMG: –in failures: all showed denervation –in successes: none showed denervation
Gibbs, 1993	33	Mean 43 mo. (range 4 mo. to 9.5 yrs	30%	Continent of solid and liquid	85% improved	
Londono-Schimmer, 1994	94	Median 58.5 mo. (range 12–98 mo.)	60%	Continent of solid and liquid (< or= 1/week)		Not PNTML
Engel, 1994	55	Median 15 mo. (range 6–36 mo.)	76%	Continent of solid and liquid	76% improved	Not PNTML Not age Not manometry
Sitzler, 1996	31 (27 women)	Range 1 mo. to 3 years	74%	Continent of solid and liquid		Not PNTML Not manometry
Nikiteas, 1996	42 (32 women)	Median 38 mo. (range 12–66 mo.)	60%	Continent of solid and liquid		Not PNTML Not manometry Not age
Oliveira, 1996	55	Mean 29 mo. (range 3–61 mo.)	71%	Pt graded as excellent or good		Not PNTML Not age
Young, 1998	56 (54 women)	Mean 27 mo. (range 1–77 mo.)	86%	Pt reported improved or complete continence		Not PNTML Not age
Gilliland, 1998	77	Median 24 mo. (range 2–96 mo.)	55%	Pt graded as excellent or good	69% improved	Not manometry Not age PNTML
Rasmussen, 1999	38	3 mo.	68%	Continent of solid and liquid		Age Not PNTML
Karoui, 2000	74 (68 women)	Median 35 mo. (range 9–98 mo.)	51%	Continent of solid and liquid	76% improved	
Morren, 2000	55	Median 40 mo. (range 5–137 mo.)	56%	Pt graded as excellent or good		Not PNTML
Ha, 2001	49 (46 women)	6 mo.	63%	Continent of solid and liquid	71% improved	Not PNTML Not manometry
Buie, 2001	158	Mean 43 mo. (range 6–120 mo.)	62%	Continent of solid and liquid	82% improved 83% satisfied	Preop incont type Not PNTML Not age Not manometry
Pinta, 2003	39	Median 22 mo. (range 2–99 mo.)	59%	Continent of solid and liquid		Age

Table 17.2   Long-term results of overlapping anal sphincteroplasty

Author, year	Number of subjects	Follow-up	Success rate	Definition of success	Subjective improvement or satisfaction	Preoperative predictors of success
Malouf, 2000 (follow-up study of Engel, 1994)	46	Median 77 mo (range 60–96 mo)	50%	No further surgery & incontinence with a frequency of <1/mo.	71% said they were improved	Parks score at 15 mo. The pt's rating of % improvement at 15 mo.
			9%	Continent of solid and liquid		Not PNTML Not manometry
Halverson, 2002	49	Median 62.5 mo (range 47–141 mo)	37%	Continent of solid and liquid	36% with highest score of QOL 13% complete continence	Not age Not manometry
Bravo Gutierrez, 2004 (follow-up study of Buie, 2001)	130	Median 120 mo (range 7–16 yr)	39%	No further surgery & cont to solid	62% improved 74% satisfied 6% complete continence	Age Poor early outcome predicts poor late outcome
			23%	Continent to solid and liquid		Not PNTML Not manometry

The technique starts with a curvilinear incision about 5 cm posterior to the anal verge. Dissection into the intersphincteric plane divides the internal and external sphincters. This is continued in a cephalad direction until the puborectalis is reached. The anorectum is bluntly dissected anteriorly, Waldeyer's fascia is divided, and the pararectal fat is reached. Thus, the levator ani is exposed and plicating sutures are placed, bringing the two sides together, recreating the anorectal angle and restoring the flap-valve mechanism. Parks reported an 83% success rate and postulated that the mechanism of continence relied upon an acute anorectal angle creating a flap valve. He reported that postoperative anorectal angles were more acute than preoperative angles. Subsequent studies failed to confirm these findings.

Henry and Simson[34] performed postanal repairs on 242 patients. They reported on 204 patients who were followed for an average of 46 weeks, with 58% being continent to solid and liquid stool. Other studies also reported similar short-term success rates of about 50%. Studies that examined anorectal angles failed to show a difference in angles between incontinent patients and asymptomatic controls. Furthermore, studies failed to show a change in the anorectal angle after the postanal repair.[35-38] Finally, long-term studies revealed that the success rates of the postanal repair decreased to 20–30%.[39-41]

MUSCLE TRANSPOSITION PROCEDURES

The two main categories of muscle transposition procedures are graciloplasties and gluteus maximus transpositions. There are different modifications of each of these. These procedures are generally reserved for patients who have failed an overlapping anal sphincteroplasty. They involve a range of surgical complexity and are associated with high morbidity.

Passive graciloplasty. In 1952, Pickrell first described a unilateral passive gracioplasty for the treatment of anal incontinence in four children with spina bifida.[42] He described using three incisions along the length of the middle thigh. The gracilis muscle is cut at its tendinous insertion into the tibia and is bluntly dissected and tunneled through the incisions to the perineal area. Care is taken to keep the blood and nerve supply to the gracilis intact. Then two incisions are made anteriorly and posteriorly around the anus. Four pulleys are created in the levator ani muscles laterally and in the raphae anteriorly and posteriorly. The gracilis muscle is brought through the four pulleys and the distal end is anchored to the contralateral ischial tuberosity. The end result is a muscle sling that passively increases the bulk around the anal canal. Pickrell reported that 100% of his patients achieved complete continence but these results have not been duplicated.

Two retrospective series reported on a combined 36 patients with a follow-up of about 5 years.[43,44] Corman et al reported that 50% of the patients were continent to solid and liquid stool while Faucheron et al reported 36% with the same outcome.

A variation of this procedure is the bilateral passive gracioplasty. Kumar et al[45] performed this procedure in 10 patients and reported results after an average follow-up of 24 months (range 6–40 months). They describe cutting both gracilis muscles at the insertion into the tibia, wrapping both

Table 17.3 The effect of preoperative pudendal neuropathy on surgical outcome of overlapping anal sphincteroplasty

Author, year	No. of subjects	Follow-up	Success rate with normal PNTML	Success rate with abnormal PNTML	P value	Comments
Studies that suggest preoperative pudendal neuropathy results in poor surgical outcome						
Laurberg, 1988	19	Range 9 mo. to 3 years	80% (8/10) "excellent or good results" or higher grade than preop	11% (1/9)	P<0.05	Defined abnormal as prolonged PNTML &/or increased fiber density on EMG Success= improvement
Wexner, 1991	16	Mean 10 mo. (range 3–16 mo.)	86% (12/14) "excellent or good result"	0% (0/2)	Not calculated	Only had 2 subjects with prolonged PNTML; both had daily to weekly incont. of solid stool
Simmang, 1994	10	12 mo.	100% (7/7) "cont. to solid and liquid"	33% (1/3) includes uni & bilat	Not calculated	Suggests that at least one side must be intact for good outcome
Londono-Schimmer, 1994	94	Median 58.5 mo. (range 12–98 mo.)	55% (41/74) "excellent or good results"	30% (6/20)	P<0.01	
Sangwan, 1996	15	Mean 16 mo. (range 4–32 mo.)	100% (8/8) "excellent or good results" & higher grade than preop	14% (1/6)	Not calculated	Suggests adverse effect of uni and bilat damage
Gilliland, 1998	71	Median 24 mo. (range 2–96 mo.)	63% (37/59) "excellent or good results"	17% (2/12) includes uni & bilat	P<0.01	
Studies that suggest preoperative pudendal neuropathy does not result in poor surgical outcome						
Engel, 1994	55	Median 15 mo. (range 6–36 mo.)	–	–	NS	Compared mean PNTMLs between success and failure outcome groups
Felt-Bersma, 1996	18	Mean 14 mo. (range 3–39 mo.)	–	–	NS	Numbers not included
Sitzler,1996	29	Range 1 mo. to 3 years	73% (14/19)	70% (7/10)	NS	
Nikiteas, 1996	26	Median 38 mo. (range 12–66 mo.)	67% (6/9)	53% (9/17)	NS	Only looked at bilateral neuropathy
Oliveira, 1996	55	Mean 29 mo. (range 3–61 mo.)	73% (29/40) "excellent or good results"	38%	NS	Possible type II error
Young, 1998	56	Mean 27 mo. (range 1–77 mo.)	90% (35/39)	78% (14/18)	NS	Inadequate power to detect a sig diff
Buie, 2001	158	Mean 43 mo. (range 6–120 mo.)	61% (35/57) 72%	72% (23/32)	NS	Largest study shows trend in opposite direction (abnormal PNTML with higher success rates)
Total	622		69% (232/336) (from studies with these numbers available)	49% (67/137)		RR=1.65 (95% CI: 1.31–2.07) "Abnormal PNTML increases risk of failure 1.65 times"

muscles around the anus, and suturing them to each other. They reported that 9/10 were continent to solid and semisolid stool.

Bilateral gluteus maximus transpositions.

In 1982, Hentz first described the transposition of the gluteus maximus muscles to the anal canal.[46] Two incisions are made on the buttocks in a parallel direction with the caudal part of the muscles. The lower 5 cm of the muscle is dissected from the sacrum, along with its attached fascia and periosteum and with its neurovascular bundle intact. Two incisions are made in a curvilinear shape at the lateral parts of the anus. The muscle flaps are tunneled to the anal incisions, bifurcated, and then wrapped around the anus.

Other surgeons have made modifications to this procedure with regard to the method of wrapping the anus with the ends of the muscle flap. Christiansen et al reported on seven patients undergoing the bilateral gluteus maximum transposition.[47] After a follow-up period ranging from 14 to 27 months, they reported that three of the seven had some improvement although they were still incontinent to liquid. Devesa et al performed a similar procedure on 20 patients and reported that 62% of the patients graded their results as excellent or good after a follow-up of 3 months to 9 years.[48] The wound infection rate was 35%. Two of the patients had to undergo reoperations due to anal stenosis. Pearl et al reported on seven patients who underwent bilateral gluteus maximus transposition.[49] Two of the patients (29%) were continent to solid and liquid stool. They reported a wound infection rate of 43%.

Because of high complication rates and limited success rates, this procedure is not commonly performed.

Dynamic graciloplasty.

In all the passive muscle transpositions, the patient is unable to voluntarily control contraction of the transposed muscle. The muscle slings are made up of skeletal muscle and therefore are not tonically contracted. Because of these flaws, research has aimed at creating a tonically contracted muscle sling. The concept of continuous electrical stimulation was applied to these surgical techniques. Electrical stimulation causes the conversion of type II fast-twitch, fatigue-prone muscle fibers to type I slow-twitch, fatigue-resistant muscle fibers. The continuous electrical stimulation can be controlled by an external device and deactivated for defecation to occur. Two different techniques were independently developed for muscle stimulation. Baeten et al described an intramuscular stimulation and Williams et al developed direct stimulation on the obturator nerve.[50,51]

The first part of the surgical procedure is identical to the passive unilateral graciloplasty (Fig. 17.2). Initial studies used a staged technique, where the gracilis muscle flap was created and anchored first, and then several weeks later, the electrical leads and pacemaker were implanted. This staged technique is no longer performed and the entire procedure is done at once. The distal end electrical lead is placed within the gracilis muscle and the proximal end is tunneled to a subcutaneous pocket in the lower abdominal wall. The lead wire is connected to a pulse generator. Stimulation is initiated about 3 days after implantation. An external magnetic device is used by the patient to turn off the pulse generator in order to defecate.

Table 17.4 summarizes some of the larger case series studying the efficacy and complication rates for dynamic graciloplasty.[52-57] Overall, the procedure is efficacious in

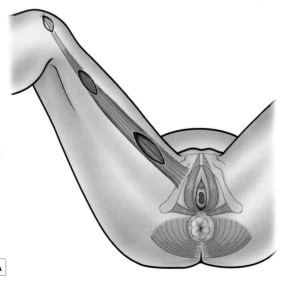

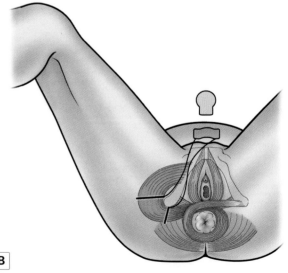

A **B**

Figure 17.2 Dynamic graciloplasty. **(A)** Three incisions are made along the medial aspect of the thigh to expose the gracilis muscle. The muscle is cut from its tendinous insertion on the tibia. **(B)** The gracilis muscle is wrapped around the anal canal and sutured to the contralateral ischial tuberosity. Two electrodes are placed on the gracilis muscle with the wires tunneled through the subcutaneous tissue to the lower abdomen. An external magnet is shown which allows for control of the electrical stimulation.

Table 17.4 Efficacy and complications of dynamic graciloplasty from several large series

Author, year	No. of subjects	Follow-up	Success rate	Definition of success	Morbidity
Baeten, 1995	52	Median 2.1 yrs (range 3 mo. to 7.4 yrs)	73%	Continent to solid and liquid	13% infection rate
Mavrantonis, 1999	37	Mean 21 mo.	46%	Continent to solid and liquid	23 device-related complications
Madoff, 1999	128	Median 24 mo.	66%	≥70% reduction in incontinent episodes for solid stool	138 complications; 32% major, 29% minor
Matzel, 2001 & Baeten, 2000 (same study)	121	Mean 23 mo. (range 1–52 mo.)	60%	≥50% reduction in incontinent episodes	211 complications in 93 patients; 89 severe events
Rongren, 2003	191	Median 261 weeks	72%	Continent to solid and liquid	138 complications

about 60% of patients (range 46–73%) in relieving incontinence to solid and liquid stool. However, the complication rate is extremely high, with morbidity events ranging from 0.14 to 2.08 per patient (average 1.12 events per patient).[58]

Artificial anal sphincter. The artificial anal sphincter is similar to the muscle transposition procedures in indications, cost, and morbidity. It involves the placement of a silastic inflatable cuff around the anus through a perineal incision or two incisions at the lateral aspects of the anus.

The original device described by Christiansen et al was a modification of the AMS 800 (American Medical Systems, Minneapolis, MN) which is an artificial urinary sphincter.[59] The device in current use is the Acticon Neosphincter also made by AMS. Both devices are similar in design and they are made up of three parts: a cuff, a pressure-regulating balloon, and a patient-activated pump. The cuff is made in variable widths and lengths and is placed as high as possible around the anal canal, preferably at the level of the anorectal junction. Some authors recommend its placement above the anococcygeal raphae posteriorly and above the transverse perinei muscle anteriorly. The cuff is connected to the pressure-regulating balloon that is placed in the retropubic space. This balloon acts as a reservoir when the cuff is deflated. The patient-activated pump is placed in the labium majus or scrotum and is used by the patient to deflate the cuff in order to defecate.

Since Christiansen's first retrospective case series in 1992, there have been several small series of artificial anal sphincter in the literature.[60-67] All these studies contain fewer than 30 patients. They report rates of continence to solid and liquid stool from 24% to 78%. The explantation rate (due to complications such as infection) ranged from 14% to 50%. In 2002, Wong et al reported 1-year follow-up results from a multicenter study including 13 sites and 112 patients.[68] They found a significant reduction in continence scores and an overall success rate of 53% (success was defined as a drop of at least 24 points in the continence scoring system). In the patients that retained the device, the success rate was 85%. The morbidity rates were high, including 384 device-related adverse events, 51 (46%) revisions, 41 (37%) explant procedures, and 38 (34%) infections.

Diversion. Diversion of the gastrointestinal tract is an option for patients with intractable fecal incontinence. This procedure can be done temporarily, such as at the same time as another distal procedure, or as a permanent solution.

Sacral neuromodulation. The technique of sacral neuromodulation is used to treat a variety of urinary conditions including urinary retention, urinary urge incontinence, and urgency/frequency. Although it is not currently FDA approved for this indication, it has also been studied for the treatment of intractable anal incontinence. The mechanism is poorly defined but involves remodulation of the sacral reflexes that effect bladder, anal canal, and pelvic floor functions. It may be indicated for the same patients in whom muscle transfer procedures or artificial anal sphincter would be considered: failed anal sphincteroplasty, incontinence with an intact anal sphincter, idiopathic and neurogenic anal incontinence. It has several advantages over the other techniques. The procedure allows for a temporary trial to test effectiveness and since it is performed distant from the anal canal, it carries reduced morbidity and infection rates.

There are two techniques available for placement. The test stimulation can be done either percutaneously with a temporary lead or as staged implant with the permanent quadripolar lead. Insulated spinal needles are placed through one of the sacral foramina (preferably S3 but sometimes S2 or S4) so that the lead lies adjacent to one of these sacral nerves. Once an appropriate test response is achieved, the lead is placed through the spinal needle and then connected to a temporary pulse generator. The test stimulation is performed for about 7–14 days and the patient keeps a bowel diary to assess response. Most authors define a positive response as at least 50% improvement in symptoms and then proceed to the permanent stimulation procedure. This involves the implantation of a permanent pulse generator and final placement of the quadripolar lead if necessary.

The first sacral neuromodulation device for the treatment of bowel dysfunction was implanted in 1995 by Matzel et al.[69] They reported on three patients who all experienced improved functional continence at 6 months. The possibility of a placebo effect was tested by Vaizey et al.[70] They studied

two patients who had been implanted with the device 9 months previously. The study involved a double-blinded crossover design and recorded incontinence episodes with a diary card. The stimulation parameters were set below the sensory threshold. They showed a dramatic change in episodes of incontinence when the stimulator was turned on as compared to when it was turned off. This study also showed that the beneficial effect of sacral neuromodulation is dependent on continued stimulation as the symptoms recurred when the stimulation was discontinued.

Table 17.5 summarizes the clinical results from various series of sacral neuromodulation.[69,71-79] Most of these series include a small number of patients for a limited amount of follow-up (all with median less than 2 years). All report a decrease in incontinent episodes or improvement in conti-

Table 17.5 Results of sacral neuromodulation in the treatment of anal incontinence

Author, year	No. of subjects	Follow-up	Success rate	Median episodes of fecal incontinence		Comments
				Pre-treatment	**Post-treatment**	
Matzel, 1995	3	6 mo	66% completely continent 100% improved continence	8 per 7d	0	Increase in resting and squeeze pressures Increase in squeeze pressure
Vaizey, 1999	9	Only percutaneous testing				Change in urge volume Change in rectal compliance
Malouf, 2000	5	Median 6 mo. (range 3–26 mo.)	100% had improvement or a significant decrease in continence scores	11 per 7d	0	No long-term change in resting, squeeze pressures, or sensory threshold **Improvement in SF-36 QOL**
Rosen, 2001	20	Median 15 mo. (range 3–26 mo.)	16 pts had permanent placement (4 failures, all with neurologic etiology)	6 per 21d	**2**	**Improvement in QOL**
Matzel, 2001	6	Range 5–66 mo.	Cleveland Clinic continence score (mean)	17 score	2.5 score	Increase in squeeze pressure No change in resting pressure
Ganio, 2001	5	Median 19 mo. (range 5–37 mo.)	100% completely continent	5.5 per 7d	0	Increase in resting pressure Improvement seen in pts with urge incontinence only No benefit in pts with complete neurologic etiology
Leroi, 2001	6	Range 3–6 mo.		3.5 per 7d	0.5	No change in resting or squeeze pressures
Ganio, 2001	16	Mean 15.5 mo. (range 3–45 mo.)		11 per 14d	0	Increase in resting pressure

Table 17.5   Results of sacral neuromodulation in the treatment of anal incontinence—cont'd

Author, year	No. of subjects	Follow-up	Success rate	Median episodes of fecal incontinence		Comments
				Pre-treatment	*Post-treatment*	
Kenefick, 2002	15	Median 24 mo. (range 3–60 mo.)	73% completely continent	11 per 7d	0	**Improvement in all subscales of SF-36 except health transition** Increase in squeeze pressure after test and permanent Increase in resting pressure after test stim (not sig. after permanent) Improvement in rectal sensation
Matzel, 2004	34	Median 23.9 mo.	37% completely continent	16.4 per 7d mean	2	ACSRS QOL showed improvement in all scales

nence score with the procedure. Many of them report a significant increase in quality-of-life measures.[72,73,78,79] Initially, these procedures were performed only in patients with intact external anal sphincters but most recent articles include patients with defects, as well as patients with neurogenic and idiopathic incontinence. Overall, these studies indicate an acceptable success rate while incurring very little morbidity. Although many of the studies examined the effect of sacral neuromodulation on parameters of anal manometry, the results are inconsistent.

Summary. After conservative treatment has been exhausted in the treatment of anal incontinence, surgical treatment options should be considered. If the patient has an identifiable defect in the sphincter muscle then an overlapping anal sphincteroplasty is the technique of choice, despite the lack of strict study protocols and long-term

efficacy. If this procedure fails or if there is no identifiable sphincter defect then a variety of other techniques are available. Muscle transposition procedures and artificial anal sphincters offer a successful outcome for the majority of patients but at high cost, high morbidity, and high complication rates. Sacral neuromodulation offers the hope of an alternative approach that may be more successful with much less morbidity.

All these recommendations come with the caveat that much of the research in this area is based on retrospective case series and there is very little evidence based on randomized controlled trials. Future studies need to incorporate validated instruments for symptom severity and quality-of-life measurements. There is a need for well-designed randomized trials to evaluate each of these surgical techniques as well as comparison between surgical and conservative management options.

REFERENCES

1. Rockwood TH, Church JM, Fleshman JW, et al. Patient and surgeon ranking of the severity of symptoms associated with fecal incontinence: the fecal incontinence severity index. Dis Colon Rectum 1999;42:1525–1532.
2. Rockwood TH, Church JM, Fleshman JW, et al. Fecal incontinence quality of life scale: quality of life instrument for patients with fecal incontinence. Dis Colon Rectum 2000;43:9–16.
3. Fang DT, Nivatvongs S, Vermeulen FD, et al. Overlapping sphincteroplasty for acquired anal incontinence. Dis Colon Rectum 1984;27:720–722.
4. Ctercteko GC, Fazio VW, Jagelman DG, et al. Anal sphincter repair: a report of 60 cases and review of the literature. Aust NZ J Surg 1988;58:703–710.
5. Wexner SD, Marchett F, Jagelman DG. The role of sphincteroplasty

for fecal incontinence reevaluated: a prospective physiologic and functional review. Dis Colon Rectum 1991;34:22–30.
6. Fleshman JW, Dreznik Z, Fry R, et al. Anal sphincter repair for obstetric injury: manometric evaluation of functional results. Dis Colon Rectum 1991;34:1061–1067.
7. Gibbs DH, Hooks VH. Overlapping sphincteroplasty for acquired anal incontinence. South Med J 1993;86:1376–1380.
8. Sitzler PJ, Thomson JPS. Overlap repair of damaged anal sphincter. Dis Colon Rectum 1996;39:1356–1360.
9. Tan M, O'Hanlon DM, Cassidy M, et al. Advantages of a posterior fourchette incision in anal sphincter repair. Dis Colon Rectum 2001;44:1624–1629.
10. Halverson AL, Hull TL. Long-term outcome of overlapping anal sphincter repair. Dis Colon Rectum 2002;45:345–348.

11. Young CJ, Mathur MN, Eyers AA, et al. Successful overlapping anal sphincter repair: relationship to patient age, neuropathy, and colostomy formation. Dis Colon Rectum 1998;41:344–349.

12. Hawley PR. Anal sphincter reconstruction. Langenbecks Arch Chir 1985;366:269–272.

13. Tjandra JJ, Han WR, Goh J, et al. Direct repair vs. overlapping sphincter repair: a randomized, controlled trial. Dis Colon Rectum 2003;46:937–943.

14. Jacobs PP, Scheuer M, Kuijpers JH, et al. Obstetric fecal incontinence. Role of pelvic floor denervation and results of delayed sphincter repair. Dis Colon Rectum 1990;33:494–497.

15. Londono-Schimmer EE, Garcia-Duperly R, Nicholls RJ, et al. Overlapping anal sphincter repair for faecal incontinence due to sphincter trauma: five year follow-up functional results. Int J Colorectal Dis 1994;9:110–113.

16. Engel AF, Kamm MA, Sultan AH, et al. Anterior anal sphincter repair in patients with obstetric trauma. Br J Surg 1994;81:1231–1234.

17. Nikiteas N, Korsgen S, Kumar D, et al. Audit of sphincter repair: factors associated with poor outcome. Dis Colon Rectum 1996;39:1164–1170.

18. Oliveira L, Pfeifer J, Wexner SD. Physiological and clinical outcome of anterior sphincteroplasty. Br J Surg 1996;83:502–505.

19. Gilliland R, Altomare DF, Moreira H, et al. Pudendal neuropathy is predictive of failure following anterior overlapping sphincteroplasty. Dis Colon Rectum 1998;41:1516–1522.

20. Rasmussen O, Puggaard L, Christiansen J. Anal sphincter repair in patients with obstetric trauma: age affects outcome. Dis Colon Rectum 1999;42:193–195.

21. Karoui S, Leroi AM, Koning E, et al. Results of sphincteroplasty in 86 patients with anal incontinence. Dis Colon Rectum 2000;43:813–820.

22. Morren GL, Hallböök O, Nyström PO, et al. Audit of anal-sphincter repair. Colorectal Dis 2001;3(1):17–22.

23. Ha HT, Fleshman JW, Smith M, et al. Manometric squeeze pressure difference parallels functional outcome after overlapping sphincter reconstruction. Dis Colon Rectum 2001;44:655–660.

24. Buie WD, Lowry AC, Rothenberger DA, et al. Clinical rather than laboratory assessment predicts continence after anterior sphincteroplasty. Dis Colon Rectum 2001;44:1255–1260.

25. Pinta T, Kylänpää-Bäck ML, Salmi T, et al. Delayed sphincter repair for obstetric ruptures: analysis of failure. Colorectal Dis 2003;5:73–78.

26. Malouf AJ, Norton CS, Engel AF, et al. Long-term results of overlapping anterior anal-sphincter repair for obstetric trauma. Lancet 2000;355:260–265.

27. Bravo Gutierrez A, Madoff RD, Lowry AC, et al. Long-term results of anterior sphincteroplasty. Dis Colon Rectum 2004;47:727–732.

28. Laurberg S, Swash M, Henry MM. Delayed external sphincter repair for obstetric tear. Br J Surg 1988;75:786–788.

29. Simmang C, Birnbaum EH, Kodner IJ, et al. Anal sphincter reconstruction in the elderly: does advancing age affect outcome? Dis Colon Rectum 1994;37:1065–1069.

30. Sangwan YP, Coller JA, Barrett RC, et al. Unilateral pudendal neuropathy: impact on outcome of anal sphincter repair. Dis Colon Rectum 1996;39:686–689.

31. Felt-Bersma RJF, Cuesta MA, Koorevaar M, et al. Anal sphincter repair improves anorectal function and endosonographic image: a prospective clinical study. Dis Colon Rectum 1996;39:878–885.

32. Jensen LL, Lowry AC. Biofeedback improves functional outcome after sphincteroplasty. Dis Colon Rectum 1997;40:197–200.

33. Parks AG. Royal Society of Medicine, Section of Proctology; Meeting 27 November 1974; President's Address. Anorectal incontinence. Proc R Soc Med 1975;68(11):681–690.

34. Henry MM, Simson JNL. Results of postanal repair: a retrospective study. Br J Surg 1985;72(Suppl):S17–S19.

35. Miller R, Bartolo DCC, Locke-Edmunds JC, et al. Prospective study of conservative and operative treatment for faecal incontinence. Br J Surg 1988;75:101–105.

36. Womack NR, Morrison JFB, Williams NS. Prospective study of the effects of postanal repair in neurogenic faecal incontinence. Br J Surg 1988;75:48–52.

37. Hunter RA, Saccone GTP, Sarre R, et al. Faecal incontinence: manometric and radiological changes following postanal repair. Aust NZ J Surg 1989;59:697–705.

38. Orrom WJ, Miller R, Cornes H, et al. Comparison of anterior sphincteroplasty and postanal repair in the treatment of idiopathic fecal incontinence. Dis Colon Rectum 1991;34:305–310.

39. Setti Carraro P, Kamm MA, Nicholls RJ. Long-term results of postanal repair for neurogenic faecal incontinence. Br J Surg 1994;81:140–144.

40. Engel AF, Baal SJ, Brummelkamp WH. Late results of postanal repair for idiopathic faecal incontinence. Eur J Surg 1994;160:637–640.

41. Matsuoka H, Mavrantonis C, Wexner SD, et al. Postanal repair for fecal incontinence: is it worthwhile? Dis Colon Rectum 2000;43:1561–1567.

42. Pickrell KL, Broadbent TR, Masters FW, et al. Construction of a rectal sphincter and restoration of anal continence by transplanting the gracilis muscle: a report of four cases in children. Ann Surg 1975;135(6):853–862.

43. Corman ML. Gracilis muscle transposition for anal incontinence: late results. Br J Surg 1985;72(Suppl):S21–S22.

44. Faucheron J, Hannoun L, Thome C, et al. Is fecal continence improved by nonstimulated gracilis muscle transposition? Dis Colon Rectum 1994;37:979–983.

45. Kumar D, Hutchinson R, Grant E. Bilateral gracilis neosphincter construction for treatment of faecal incontinence. Br J Surg 1995;82:1645–1647.

46. Hentz VR. Construction of a rectal sphincter using the origin of the gluteus maximus muscle. Plast Reconstr Surg 1982;70:82–85.

47. Christiansen J, Rønholt Hansen C, Rasmussen O. Bilateral gluteus maximus transposition for anal incontinence. Br J Surg 1995;82:903–905.

48. Devesa JM, Fernandez Madrid JM, Rodriguez Gallego B, et al. Bilateral gluteoplasty for fecal incontinence. Dis Colon Rectum 1997;40:883–888.

49. Pearl RK, Prasad ML, Nelson RL, et al. Bilateral gluteus maximus transposition for anal incontinence. Dis Colon Rectum 1991;34:478–481.

50. Baeten CG, Konsten J, Spaans F, et al. Dynamic graciloplasty for treatment of faecal incontinence. Lancet 1991;338:1163–1165.

51. Williams NS, Patel J, George BD, et al. Development of an electrically stimulated neoanal sphincter. Lancet 1991;338:1166–1169.

52. Baeten CG, Geerdes BP, Adang EM, et al. Anal dynamic graciloplasty in the treatment of intractable fecal incontinence. N Engl J Med 1995;332:1600–1605.

53. Mavrantonis C, Wexner SD. Stimulated graciloplasty for treatment of intractable fecal incontinence. Dis Colon Rectum 1999;42:497–504.

54. Madoff RD, Rosen HR, Baeten CG, et al. Safety and efficacy of dynamic muscle plasty for anal incontinence: lessons from a prospective, multicenter trial. Gastroenterology 1999;116:549–556.

55. Matzel KE, Madoff RD, LaFontaine LJ, et al. Complications of dynamic graciloplasty: incidence, management, and impact on outcome. Dis Colon Rectum 2001;44:1427–1435.

56. Baeten CG, Bailey HR, Bakka A, et al. Safety and efficacy of dynamic graciloplasty for fecal incontinence. Dis Colon Rectum 2000;43:743–751.

57. Rongren M-JGM, Uludag Ö, El Naggar K, et al. Long-term follow-up of dynamic graciloplasty for fecal incontinence. Dis Colon Rectum 2003;46:716–721.

58. Chapman AE, Geerdes B, Hewett P, et al. Systematic review of dynamic graciloplasty in the treatment of faecal incontinence. Br J Surg 2002;89:138–153.

59. Christiansen J, Sparso B. Treatment of anal incontinence by an implantable prosthetic anal sphincter. Ann Surg 1992; 215:383–386.

60. Christiansen J, Rasmussen O, Lindorff-Larsen K. Long-term results of artificial anal sphincter implantation for severe anal incontinence. Ann Surg 1999;230(1):45–48.

61. Lehur PA, Michot F, Denis P, et al. Results of artificial sphincter in severe anal incontinence: report of 14 consecutive implantations. Dis Colon Rectum 1996;39:1352–1355.

62. Wong WD, Jensen LL, Bartolo DCC, et al. Artificial anal sphincter. Dis Colon Rectum 1996;39:1345–1351.

63. O'Brien PE, Skinner S. Restoring control: the Acticon Neosphincter® artificial bowel sphincter in the treatment of anal incontinence. Dis Colon Rectum 2000;43:1213–1216.

64. Altomare DF, Dodi G, LaTorre F, et al. Multicentre retrospective analysis of the outcome of artificial anal sphincter implantation for severe faecal incontinence. Br J Surg 2001;88:1481–1486.

65. Ortiz H, Armendariz P, DeMiguel M, et al. Complications and functional outcome following artificial anal sphincter implantation. Br J Surg 2002;89:877–881.

66. Michot F, Costaglioli B, Leroi AM, et al. Artificial anal sphincter in severe fecal incontinence: outcome of prospective experience with 37 patients in one institution. Ann Surg 2003;237(1):52–56.

67. Lehur PA, Roig JV, Duinslaeger M. Artificial anal sphincter: prospective clinical and manometric evaluation. Dis Colon Rectum 2000;43:1100–1106.

68. Wong WD, Congliosi SM, Spencer MP, et al. The safety and efficacy of the artificial bowel sphincter for fecal incontinence: results from a multicenter cohort study. Dis Colon Rectum 2002;45:1139–1153.

69. Matzel KE, Stadelmaier U, Hohenfellner, et al. Electrical stimulation of sacral spinal nerves for treatment of faecal incontinence. Lancet 1995;346:1124–1127.

70. Vaizey CJ, Kamm MA, Toy AJ, et al. Double-blind crossover study of sacral nerve stimulation for fecal incontinence. Dis Colon Rectum 2000;43:298–302.

71. Vaizey CJ, Kamm MA, Turner IC, et al. Effects of short term sacral nerve stimulation on anal and rectal function in patients with anal incontinence. Gut 1999;44:407–412.

72. Malouf AJ, Vaizey CJ, Nicholls J, et al. Permanent sacral nerve stimulation for fecal incontinence. Ann Surg 2000;232(1):143–148.

73. Rosen HR, Urbarz C, Holzer B, et al. Sacral nerve stimulation as a treatment for fecal incontinence. Gastroenterology 2001;121:536–541.

74. Matzel KE, Stadelmaier U, Hohenfellner M, et al. Chronic sacral spinal nerve stimulation for fecal incontinence: long-term results with foramen and cuff electrodes. Dis Colon Rectum 2001;44:59–66.

75. Ganio E, Luc AR, Clerico G, et al. Sacral nerve stimulation for treatment of fecal incontinence: a novel approach for intractable fecal incontinence. Dis Colon Rectum 2001;44:619–631.

76. Leroi AM, Michot F, Grise P, et al. Effect of sacral nerve stimulation in patients with fecal and urinary incontinence. Dis Colon Rectum 2001;44:779–789.

77. Ganio E, Ratto C, Masin A, et al. Neuromodulation for fecal incontinence: outcome in 16 patients with definitive implant. The initial Italian sacral neurostimulation group (GINS) experience. Dis Colon Rectum 2001;44:965–970.

78. Kenefick NJ, Vaizey CJ, Cohen CG, et al. Medium-term results of permanent sacral nerve stimulation for faecal incontinence. Br J Surg 2002;89:896–901.

79. Matzel KE, Kamm MA, Stösser M, et al. Sacral spinal nerve stimulation for faecal incontinence: multicentre study. Lancet 2004;363:1270–1276.

SECTION 6 Treatment of anal incontinence

SECTION 7

Treatment of pelvic organ prolapse

Nonsurgical Management

Kari Bø

PELVIC FLOOR ANATOMY, FUNCTION, AND DYSFUNCTION

Anatomy. The pelvic floor muscles (PFM) consist of the pelvic and the urogenital diaphragm. They are located inside the pelvis and form the floor of the abdominal cavity (Fig. 18.1). The PFM consists of a muscular plate expanding from the pubic symphysis, along the front side walls of the ileum towards the coccyx (Fig. 18.2). The muscles are innervated from S2–4 and have a thickness of approximately 1 cm.[1,2]

Function and dysfunction. The PFM contract constantly, except directly before and during voiding.[3] In addition to this constant firing, there is increasing and decreasing activity according to the level of abdominal pressure. However, the PFM can also be contracted intentionally. If any of the several muscles of the pelvic floor could contract in isolation, they would all act differently due to their individual fiber direction. However, the only known voluntary function of the PFM is a mass contraction described as an inward lift and squeeze around the urethra, vagina, and anus.[4-8] Because of their location inside the pelvis, the PFM are the only muscle group in the body capable of giving structural support for the pelvic organs and the pelvic openings (urethra, vagina, and anus).

During a voluntary contraction, the PFM lift inwardly. The urethra closes and the PFM resist downward movement, thereby stabilizing the urethra.[7,9,10] However, studies from different countries have shown that >30% of women are not able to contract the PFM even after thorough individual instruction at their first consultation.[11-14] The most common error is to contract hip adductor, abdominal, and gluteal muscles instead of the PFM. In addition, straining is a common error.[11,12] Bump et al[11] showed that 25% of women were straining instead of performing the correct lift and squeeze. They also found that only 49% were able to perform a PFM contraction that effectively increased urethral pressure. Contractions of other muscle groups such as the gluteals, hip adductors, and abdominals cause co-

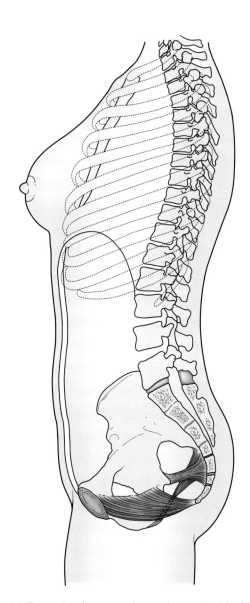

Figure 18.1 The pelvic floor muscles are located inside the pelvis and form a structural support for internal organs (reproduced with permission from Hahn I, Myrhage R. Bekkenbotten. Bygnad, funktion och traning. AnaKomp AB, 1999).

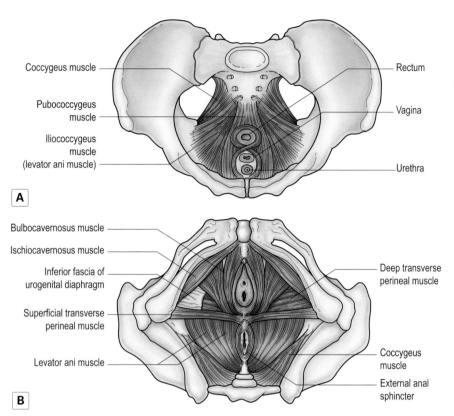

Coccygeus muscle

Pubococcygeus muscle

Iliococcygeus muscle (levator ani muscle)

Rectum

Vagina

Urethra

A

Bulbocavernosus muscle

Ischiocavernosus muscle

Inferior fascia of urogenital diaphragm

Superficial transverse perineal muscle

Levator ani muscle

Deep transverse perineal muscle

Coccygeus muscle

External anal sphincter

B

Figure 18.2 The pelvic floor muscles. (Reproduced with permission from Bø K. Pelvic floor muscle exercise for the treatment of female stress urinary incontinence. Methodological studies and clinical results. Doctoral thesis, Norwegian University of Sport and Physical Education, Oslo, Norway, 1990)

contractions of the PFM in healthy volunteers.[15-18] However, none of these other muscles can act as a structural support to the pelvic organs, prevent descent of the bladder and urethra during increases in abdominal pressure, or increase urethral closure pressure by their own isolated contractions.

Pelvic floor dysfunction can cause urinary and fecal incontinence, pelvic organ prolapse (POP) with prolapse of the anterior vaginal wall (cystocele), posterior vaginal wall (rectocele), vaginal apex (enterocele), and uterus, or pain and sexual dysfunction.[19,20]

PELVIC ORGAN PROLAPSE AND THE PELVIC FLOOR

The pathophysiology and etiologic factors causing prolapse are not yet totally understood.[21,22] Hence, rationales for appropriate methods to prevent and treat the condition are not easy to recommend. Causes and contributing factors have been classified as:

- *congenital*: bladder exstrophy, collagen defects (e.g. "benign hypermobility joint syndrome," type IV Ehlers–Danlos or Marfan's syndrome), race (white women at higher risk), and anatomy
- *childbirth* (trauma with rupture of ligaments, fascia and muscle fibers, denervation)
- *raised abdominal pressure* (chronic obstructive airway disease, straining, constipation, heavy lifting, obesity, hard physical activity)

- *menopause* (estrogen deficiency)
- *iatrogenic* (pelvic surgery, e.g. hysterectomy, colposuspension, sacrospinous fixation).[19,22,23]

POP is difficult to classify and measure. The most commonly used clinical classification is the Pelvic Organ Prolapse—Quantified (POP-Q) system. This has been tested and found to be reproducible and valid.[24] Ultrasonography and MRI can be used in lying, sitting, and standing (only ultrasonography) positions. However, more research is needed to test reproducibility and sensitivity of these imaging methods to measure location and size of the prolapse.[21,25-30]

Symptoms associated with POP include the following.

- *Urinary symptoms* (stress incontinence, frequency, urgency and urge incontinence, hesitancy, poor and prolonged urinary stream, feeling of incomplete emptying, positional changes to start or complete emptying)
- *Bowel symptoms* (difficulty in defecation, incontinence of flatus, liquid or solid stool, urgency of defecation, digitations or splinting of vagina, perineum or anus to complete defecation, feeling of incomplete evacuation)
- *Sexual symptoms* (inability to have or infrequent coitus, dyspareunia, lack of satisfaction or orgasm, incontinence during sexual activity)
- *Other local symptoms* (feeling of pressure or heaviness in the vagina, pain in the vagina or perineum, sensation of awareness of protrusion from the vagina, low back pain,

which is eased by lying down, abdominal pressure or pain, blood-stained and purulent discharge.)[22]

Hence, POP may affect activities of daily living, stop women from participating in regular physical activities, and reduce quality of life.[31]

The incidence and prevalence rates of POP are difficult to establish. Many women do not seek medical advice or treatment for the condition.[22] It is estimated that approximately 50% of all women lose some of the supportive mechanisms of the pelvic floor due to childbirth, leading to different degrees of POP. Brubaker et al[21] state that there is a variation in the literature on prevalence of POP reaching the hymen from 2% to 48% and below the hymen between 2% and 4%. The variation in prevalence may be due to differences in populations studied, age, race, parity, measurement methods, and classification systems. Samuelsson et al[32] studied 487 women 20–59 years old attending routine gynecology assessment (participation rate 76%) and found that 30.8% presented with some degree of POP. Only 2% had prolapse at introitus and none outside introitus. Symptoms were voiding and bowel difficulties (10%) and perception of heaviness (9.7%). The results showed that prevalence of POP was associated with age, parity, and PFM weakness measured with vaginal palpation.[32]

Only 10–20% of women with POP may seek help for their problem.[22] Ten percent of women may end up with prolapse surgery.[23] In the United Kingdom, 20% of the waiting list for gynecologic surgery are women with POP.[22] The incidence of posthysterectomy POP in need of surgery is 3.6% per 1000 women a year. It has been estimated that approximately 25% have relapse after prolapse surgery and that 80% of relapses become apparent within 2 years.[31]

The risk of prolapse development increases with age. Hence, as women live longer, there will be an increase in prevalence of POP in the elderly population.[22] Prolapse may be asymptomatic until the descending organ is through the introitus and therefore POP may not be recognized until an advanced condition is present.[21] In some women the prolapse advances rapidly, while others remain stable for many years. There are no published studies on the natural history of POP but most clinicians would agree that POP does not seem to regress.[21]

CONSERVATIVE TREATMENT OF PELVIC ORGAN PROLAPSE

Treatment options for POP include surgery, use of mechanical support (pessary), and pelvic floor muscle training (PFMT).[21,22] According to Brubaker et al,[21] the indications for treatment of POP are unclear. This chapter only deals with conservative treatments such as the use of mechanical support and PFMT.

Mechanical support. Mechanical support, such as pessaries, is used to restore the prolapsed organs to normal position and thereby alleviate symptoms. According to Poma,[33] several techniques to restore genital prolapse have been used since ancient times and Hippocrates recommended a pessary consisting of half a pomegranate soaked in wine. Traditionally, pessaries have been considered a choice for:

- patients unfit for surgery
- patients awaiting surgery
- patients who decline surgery.[34]

However, Cundiff and Addison[34] suggest that younger gynecologists and especially urogynecologists now consider pessaries as an alternative to surgery for POP.

A wide range of mechanical devices have been described for the treatment of prolapse, and Poma states that there are more than 120 types on the market.[33] According to Cundiff and Addison,[34] there are two broad categories of pessaries: support pessaries and space-filling pessaries. Support pessaries use a spring mechanism that rests in the posterior fornix and against the posterior aspect of the pubic symphysis while space-filling pessaries maintain their position by creating suction between the pessary and vaginal walls, by providing a diameter larger than the genital hiatus, or by both mechanisms.[34] The most recent models are made of rubber, clear plastic or soft plastic with some of them also containing metal and silicone.[33,35] Fritzinger et al[36] listed the following types of pessaries available in the US: Gelhorn pessary, donut pessary, ring pessary with and without support, cube pessary, Smith-Hodge type, Gehrung pessary, Shaatz pessary, incontinence dish and ring, Suarez and Cook continence rings, and the Introl pessary.

Several factors may affect a woman's success in using a pessary, such as hormonal status, sexual activity, prior hysterectomy, pelvic floor muscle strength, and stage and site of the prolapse.[34] However, currently, there seems to be little knowledge about what is the most effective pessary for different types and degrees of pelvic organ prolapse.

There are potential complications associated with pessary use such as vaginal wall irritation, bleeding, ulceration and pain, fistula formation and bowel herniation.[33,34] Recommendations for minimizing complications are: choosing a not too tight fitting pessary, emphasizing proper pessary care including frequent and regular monitoring with checks of vaginal mucosa erosions, regular cleansing, and use of estrogen replacement therapy. The optimum frequency of pessary removals has not yet been established. Neither has the role of local estrogens in preventing complications.[37] However, Fritzinger et al[36] recommended women to return for evaluation of vaginal tissue damage 1–2 weeks after initial insertion of the pessary, and Poma[33] suggested checks every 3–6 months after initial evaluation.

Studies have shown that 85% of gynecologists[38] and 98% of urogynecologists prescribe pessaries.[35] In a Cochrane review,[37] no RCTs were identified on which to base management by mechanical devices in women with POP. Only one retrospective study of 101 patients fitted with a pessary was found.[39] At an unspecified follow-up period, 49% were continuing with the pessary, 4% had died, 26% had discontinued usage and had surgery, and 21% had discontinued usage without surgery. In a new search for studies, one new report was found. Clemons et al[40] conducted a prospective observational study in 100 consecutive women with symptomatic POP. They were examined and fitted with either a ring or Gelhorn pessary. Successful pessary fitting was defined as a woman continuing to use a pessary 1 week after being fitted. Seventy-three were classified as successful and 27 as unsuccessful. A short vaginal length (=6 cm) and a wide vaginal introitus (four fingerbreadths) were risk factors for unsuccessful pessary fitting.[40]

In preparation for this chapter, two uncontrolled studies were found from a search on PubMed. Handa and Jones[41] followed 56 consecutive women, mean age 75 years (range 62–83 years) fitted with either ring or donut pessaries. Nineteen (33.9%) continued use for at least 1 year. By comparing baseline and follow-up examination with use of the POP-Q, they found that four women had an improvement in stage of the prolapse and no women had worsening. The authors are well aware of the limitations of the study: it was uncontrolled and unblinded, there may be variances in measurement technique, only a few women attended the follow-up visit, and there was no control of confounding factors, e.g. concomitant PFMT or lifestyle changes. The researchers suggest that there may be a therapeutic effect associated with the use of pessary, and discuss an interesting hypothesis for a possible mechanism. They refer to studies showing an association between overstretching of the pelvic floor and pudendal neuropathy, and that prolonged passive stretch impairs skeletal muscle strength. Thus, the pessary may support the pelvic organs which in turn may allow recovery from passive stretch, resulting in improved levator function.[41] This hypothesis needs to be tested in a randomized controlled study with measurement of pelvic floor muscle function.

Clemons et al[42] found that of 73 women with successful fitting, nearly all prolapse symptoms resolved from baseline to 2 months: bulge from 90% to 3% ($P<0.001$), pressure from 49% to 3% ($P<0.001$), discharge from 12% to 0% ($P<0.003$), and splinting from 14% to 0% ($P<0.001$). Among women with concurrent urinary symptoms at baseline, stress incontinence improved in 45%, urge incontinence improved in 46%, and voiding difficulty improved in 53% after 2 months. However, de novo stress incontinence occurred in 21%, de novo urge incontinence in 6%, and de novo voiding difficulty in 4%. At 2 months, 92% were satisfied with their pessary, while 8% were dissatisfied and discontinued pessary use. Dissatisfaction was associated with occult stress urinary incontinence with an odds ratio of 17.1; 95% CI, 1.9–206, $P=0.004$.

The Cochrane review group concludes that despite the common usage of pessaries, there are wide gaps in our knowledge of treatment outcomes using mechanical devices. Therefore there is a need for well-designed RCTs of a mechanical device versus control/waiting list/no active treatment, a mechanical device versus surgery, and a mechanical device versus pelvic floor muscle training and/or lifestyle interventions.[37]

Pelvic floor muscle training. In a clinical review article by Thakar and Stanton,[22] it was stated that PFMT may limit progression and alleviate mild prolapse symptoms such as low back pain and pelvic pressure. They concluded that PFMT is not useful if the prolapse extends to or beyond the vaginal introitus. Also, Davila[43] suggest that "Kegel exercises" may alleviate mild prolapse symptoms. None of the above-mentioned authors, however, refer to any studies to support their statements on PFMT for POP. One uncontrolled study has been found. Mimura et al[44] followed 32 women with rectocele >2 cm below "the expected line" at proctography. The patients had biofeedback training with a nurse every 2–3 weeks, usually for 4–5 sessions. Twenty-five women met for follow-up assessment. The results showed that complete resolution of symptoms was achieved in 12%. At follow-up 14 patients (56%) felt that their constipation had improved a little and 11 (34%) felt that it had improved a lot.

In a Cochrane review of PFMT on POP, it was concluded that there are no RCTs on the efficacy of PFMT in prevention and treatment of POP, and that high-quality RCTs in this area are needed.[31] Hence, statements on whether it is effective or not, or only effective for subgroups, e.g. prolapse with mild symptoms, are not based on evidence from research data. A survey of UK women's health physiotherapists (response rate 71%) showed that 92% assessed and treated women with POP. The most commonly used treatment was PFMT with and without biofeedback.[31] However, there were no available guidelines to follow in clinical practice.[31]

A new PubMed search for studies on PFMT and POP revealed one RCT from 2003. Piya-Anant et al[45] conducted both a cross-sectional study in 682 women and an intervention study of 654 of the same women (mean age 67 years, SD±5.6). Seventy percent were diagnosed as having POP. Thirty percent were classified as severe and 40% as mild prolapse. The women were randomly allocated to either an experimental or a control group. Women in the experimental group were taught to contract the PFM 30 times after a meal every day. Women not able to contract were asked to return to the clinic once a month until they could perform correct contractions. In addition, they were advised to eat more vegetables and fruit and to drink at least two liters of water per day to prevent constipation. There were follow-up visits every 6 months throughout the 2-year intervention period. The results showed that the intervention was only effective in the group with severe prolapse. The rate of worsening of POP was significantly greater in the control group than the PFMT group—72.2 % versus 27.8%, respectively.

To date, this seems to be the only study of PFMT and POP. The study showed improvements in a significant number of women with severe prolapse after PFMT. However, the results should be viewed with some caution. The randomization procedure was not described and there was a cointervention with change of nutrition and water intake. There was no description of methods used to evaluate PFM function, and no follow-up of the home training program, measurement of PFM strength or report of adherence to the training protocol. However, the most serious flaw is the method used to measure and classify POP. Recommended quantification systems, e.g. the POP-Q,[24] or other methods to quantify prolapse such as ultrasound or MRI[30] were not used. The evaluation methods and classification categories used are poorly described and there are no references to studies showing that the evaluation systems had been tested for reproducibility or validity. Although this study supports PFMT as a method to prevent and treat POP in severe prolapse, more high-quality RCTs are needed to confirm PFMT as an effective treatment.

Theories to support PFMT in treatment of POP.

There are two main hypotheses on how PFMT may be effective in prevention and treatment of stress urinary incontinence (SUI).[46] The same theories may apply for POP.

1. Women learn to consciously contract before and during increase in abdominal pressure, and continue to perform such contractions as a behavior modification to prevent descent.[46]

On conscious contraction of the PFM, there is a lift of the pelvic floor in a cranial and forward direction and a squeeze around the urethra, vagina, and rectum.[47,48] Ultrasonography and MRI show the lift in a cranial direction and movement of the coccyx in a forward, anterior, and cranial direction.[48,49] Mantle[50] describes a common technique termed "counterbracing," taught by physical therapists to prevent leakage during increases in abdominal pressure. The patient is taught to contract the PFM just ahead of physical stressors and to hold the contraction throughout the stress, with the rationale being that the urethra and bladder base are thus prevented from descending. In addition, the PFM contraction squeezes around the urethra and increases the urethral pressure.[11,51,52]

In 1998 Miller et al[53] named this voluntary counterbracing-type contraction the "knack." In a single-blind RCT, subjects were taught to contract before and during a cough. No additional strength training regimen was performed. A paper towel test was used at baseline and after 1 week of performing the maneuver at home. The results showed that the "knack" performed during a medium and deep cough reduced urinary leakage by 98.2% and 73.3 %, respectively. Cure rate in "real life" was not reported.

Research on basic and functional anatomy research supports the "knack" as an effective maneuver to prevent leakage. Peschers et al[54] evaluated 10 nulliparous women by perineal ultrasound and EMG during coughing with and without a voluntary PFM contraction. Bladder neck descent was significantly less when women were asked to contract the PFM before cough (4.7 mm (SD 2.9)) than when coughing without such contraction (8.1 mm (SD 2.9)). The authors concluded that the PFM voluntary contraction stabilizes the vesical neck during increases in abdominal pressure. Miller et al[26] used perineal ultrasound to compare 11 young, continent nulliparous women with 11 older, incontinent parous women when subjects coughed with and without voluntary PFM contraction. Vesical neck mobility was significantly reduced from median 5.4 mm to 2.9 mm when voluntary contraction was performed. To date, there are no studies on how much strength is necessary to prevent descent during cough and other physical exertions, and we do not know if regular counterbracing during daily activities is enough to increase muscle strength or cause morphologic changes of the PFM. There are no studies of using counterbracing /the "knack" in prevention or treatment of POP.

An interesting hypothesis but one difficult to test is whether women at risk for POP can prevent prolapse developing by performing the "knack" during every rise in abdominal pressure. Since it is possible to learn to hold a hand before the mouth before and during coughing, one would suggest that it is possible to learn to precontract the PFM before and during simple tasks such as coughing, when lifting, and performing abdominal exercises.

2. Regular strength training builds permanent muscle volume and structural support, leading to unconscious co-contractions causing prevention of descent during increased abdominal pressure.[46]

Kegel originally described PFM training as physiologic training or "tightening up" the pelvic floor, and women were asked to contract the PFM 500 times per day to strengthen the muscles.[55] Modern exercise science provides an excellent foundation for understanding PFM training in the context of strength training.

Muscle strength is defined as the "maximum force which can be exerted against an immovable object (static or isometric strength), the heaviest weight which can be lifted or lowered (dynamic strength), or the maximum torque which can be developed against a pre-set rate limiting device (isokinetic strength)."[56] Muscle strength is strongly correlated to the cross-sectional area of the muscle (muscle volume) and neural factors such as the total number of activated motor units and frequency of excitation.[57] Other determinants of muscle strength include joint angle and lever arm, the relationship between length and tension, the relationship between force and velocity (force decreases as speed increases in concentric contractions), and the metabolic component (rate at which myosin splits ATP).[56] As in other skeletal muscles, these components affect an individual's PFM strength.

The aim of a strength training regimen in regular skeletal muscles is to change muscle morphology by increasing the cross-sectional area, to improve neuromuscular function by increasing the number of activated motor neurons and their frequency of excitation, and to improve muscle "tone."[57] Connective tissue is abundant within and around all skeletal muscles including the epimysium, perimysium, and endomysium. These connective tissue sheaths provide the tensile strength and viscoelastic properties ("stiffness") of muscle and support for the loading of muscle.[58] There is evidence that physical activity and strength training can increase connective tissue mass, and that intensity of training and load bearing are major factors for effective training.[58-60]

For effective muscle strengthening in skeletal muscles in adults, exercise physiologists recommend three sets of 8–12 slow-velocity, close to maximum contractions 2–4 days a week.[61] Maximal effect may not be achieved for 5 months.[62] The PFM are regular skeletal muscles and therefore recommendations for effective PFM training should be no different from that of other skeletal muscles.

The theoretical rationale for intensive strength training (exercise) of the PFM to treat POP is that strength training may build up the structural support of the pelvis by elevating the levator plate to a permanent higher location inside the pelvis and by enhancing hypertrophy and stiffness of the PFM and connective tissue. This would facilitate a more effective automatic motor unit firing (neural adaptation), preventing descent during increase in abdominal pressure. The training may also lift the pelvic floor, and thereby the protruding organs, in a cranial direction. The pelvic openings may narrow and the pelvic organs are held in place during abdominal pressure rises.

Just as with pharmaceutical therapy, there is a dose–response relationship in all forms of exercise training.[63,64] The term "exercise dosage" includes the type of exercise, frequency, intensity, and duration of the training period.[64,65] *Type of exercise* implies correct contraction of the PFM. *Frequency* is defined as number of exercise sessions per week. *Intensity* is defined as a certain percentage of maximum

performance. For strength training, this is defined as percentage of one maximum contraction termed "one repetition maximum" (1 RM). *Duration* of the training is the length of the training period, e.g. 8 weeks or 6 months. All these factors, in addition to the extremely important adherence to the training protocol, affect the final outcome of PFMT.

Several RCTs have shown an increase in PFM strength after training to treat SUI.[66-68] However, only Bernstein et al[69] measured PFM volume before and after training. In this uncontrolled study a significant increase in muscle volume after training was shown by ultrasound. Due to the lack of a control group, more research is needed to provide conclusive evidence that muscle hypertrophies after PFM training. None of the strength training studies to date have evaluated the effect of PFM training on PFM tone or connective tissue stiffness, position of the muscles within the pelvic cavity, their cross-sectional area or neurophysiologic function. Therefore, we cannot conclude whether such changes did occur.

PFM strength training programs have proven effective in preventing leakage during prolonged provocative physical activities such as running and jumping, during which participants were not instructed to contract the PFM voluntarily during exercise[66-68] It seems unlikely, in fact, that one could continuously contract the PFM voluntarily during prolonged exercise, and thus one could postulate that morphologic changes have occurred.

Ultrasound and MRI studies have shown that parous women have a more caudal location of the pelvic floor than nulliparous women.[26,70] Difference in anatomic placement has also been shown between continent and incontinent women.[27] DeLancey et al[71] demonstrated that women with POP generated 43% less force and had more atrophy of the PFM than women without POP. One of the main theories for the effect of PFMT on SUI is that strength training increases muscle volume, neurogenic adaptation, connective tissue stiffness and strength, and shift of anatomic location of the pelvic floor to a more cranial resting position within the pelvis.[46] The only study of PFMT for POP did not measure either PFM strength or morphologic changes.

Several studies have shown that >30% of incontinent women are not able to contract the PFM correctly at their first consultation.[11,12] Assessment of ability to contract, feedback, and close follow-up are therefore mandatory in teaching PFMT.[72,73] Most women learn to contract after a few weeks of rehearsal. However, some women, and especially those bearing down or straining, may not be able to contract.[66] Bump et al[11] showed that 25% of women were straining instead of contracting. Straining is one risk factor for the development of POP and should be avoided.[21]

Since PFMT has no known side effects, has shown to be effective in RCTs and systematic reviews to treat SUI and

SECTION 7 Treatment of pelvic organ prolapse

mixed incontinence,[72] and many women present with both POP and UI, it is this author's opinion that physical therapists should continue to treat POP patients with PFMT. Basic research on pelvic floor anatomy and knowledge from exercise science suggest that PFMT is effective in prevention and treatment of POP.[46] The fact that there is no current evidence from RCTs should not prevent physical therapists trying to help women to minimize their symptoms. Since occult SUI may be a common side effect of pessary use and surgery,[21,42,74] PFMT should also be advocated in combination with pessary use and surgery. However, there is an urgent need for high-quality RCTs with appropriate training protocols to evaluate the effect of PFMT in the prevention and treatment of POP.

FURTHER RESEARCH

- RCTs to evaluate the effect of pessaries compared to no treatment.
- RCTs to compare the effect of pessaries and PFMT.
- RCTs to compare the long-term effects of surgery and pessaries.
- RCTs to compare different lifestyle interventions, such as weight reduction, avoidance of straining, and use of "the knack," with pessary use.
- RCTs to compare the effect of surgery and pessaries + PFMT.
- RCTs to compare PFMT with untreated controls.
- Anatomic and biomechanical studies to understand the mechanisms of PFMT and pessary use.

REFERENCES

1. Bernstein I, Juul N, Grønvall S, Bonde B, Klarskov P. Pelvic floor muscle thickness measured by perineal ultrasonography. Scand J Urol Nephrol 1991; 137(Suppl):131–133.

2. Mørkved S, Salvesen K, Bø K, Eik-Nes S. Pelvic floor muscle strength and thickness in continent and incontinent nulliparous women. Neurourol Urodyn 2002;21(4):358–359.

3. Fowler C, Benson J, Craggs M, Vodusek D, Yang C, Podnar S. Clinical neurophysiology. In: Abrams P, Cardozo L, Khoury S, Wein A, eds. Incontinence. Plymouth: Health Publication; 2002: 389–424.

4. Kegel AH. Stress incontinence and genital relaxation. Ciba Clin Sympos 1952;2:35–51.

5. DeLancey J. Structural aspects of urethrovesical function in the female. Neurourol Urodyn 1988;7:509–519.

6. DeLancey J. The anatomy of the pelvic floor. Curr Opin Obstet Gynecol 1994;6:313–316.

7. DeLancey J. Structural support of the urethra as it relates to stress urinary incontinence: the hammock hypothesis. Am J Obstet Gynecol 1994;170:1713–1723.

8. DeLancey J. Anatomy and physiology of urinary continence. Clin Obstet Gynecol 1990; 33(2):298–307.

9. Ashton-Miller J, Howard D, DeLancey J. The functional anatomy of the female pelvic floor and stress continence control system. Scand J Urol Nephrol 2001;207(Suppl):1–7.

10. Peschers U, Schaer G, DeLancey J, Schuessler B. Levator ani function before and after childbirth. Br J Obstet Gynaecol 1997;104:1004–1008.

11. Bump R, Hurt WG, Fantl JA, Wyman JF. Assessment of Kegel exercise performance after brief verbal instruction. Am J Obstet Gynecol 1991;165:322–329.

12. Bø K, Larsen S, Oseid S, Kvarstein B, Hagen R, Jørgensen J. Knowledge about and ability to correct pelvic floor muscle exercises in women with urinary stress incontinence. Neurourol Urodyn 1988;7(3):261–262.

13. Benvenuti F, Caputo GM, Bandinelli S, Mayer F, Biagini C, Somavilla A. Reeducative treatment of female genuine stress incontinence. Am J Phys Med 1987;66(4):155–168.

14. Hesse U, Schussler B, Frimberger J, Obernitz N, Senn E. Effectiveness of a three step pelvic floor reeducation in the treatment of stress urinary incontinence: a clinical assessment. Neurourol Urodyn 1990;9(4):397–398.

15. Bø K, Kvarstein B, Hagen R, Larsen S. Pelvic floor muscle exercise for the treatment of female stress urinary incontinence: II.Validity of vaginal pressure measurements of pelvic floor muscle strength and the necessity of supplementary methods for control of correct contraction. Neurourol Urodyn 1990;9:479–487.

16. Peschers U, Gingelmaier A, Jundt K, Leib B, Dimpfl T. Evaluation of pelvic floor muscle strength using four different techniques. Int Urogynecol J 2001;12:27–30.

17. Sapsford R, Hodges P, Richardson C, Cooper D, Markwell S, Jull G. Co-activation of the abdominal and pelvic floor muscles during voluntary exercises. Neurourol Urodyn 2001;20:31–42.

18. Neumann P, Gill V. Pelvic floor and abdominal muscle interaction: EMG activity and intra-abdominal pressure. Int Urogynecol J 2002;13:125–132.

19. Bump R, Norton P. Epidemiology and natural history of pelvic floor dysfunction. Obstet Gynecol Clin North Am 1998;25(4):723–746.

20. Abrams P, Cardozo L, Fall M, et al. The standardization of terminology of lower urinary tract function: report from the standardisation sub-committee of the International Continence Society. Neurourol Urodyn 2002;21:167–178.

21. Brubaker L, Bump R, Jacquetin B, et al. Pelvic organ prolapse. In: Abrams P, Cardozo L, Khoury S, Wein A, eds. Incontinence. Plymouth,UK: Health Publications; 2002: 243–266.

22. Thakar R, Stanton S. Management of genital prolapse. BMJ 2002;324:1258–1262.

23. Hagen S, Stark D, Maher C, Adams E. Conservative management of pelvic organ prolapse in women. Cochrane Review, Issue 2. Oxford: Cochrane Library; 2004.

24. Bump R, Mattiasson A, Bø K, et al. The standardization of terminology of female pelvic organ prolapse and pelvic floor dysfunction. Am J Obstet Gynecol 1996;175:10–17.

25. Artibani W, Anderse J, Gajewski J, Ostergaard D, Raz S, Tubaro A. Imaging and other investigations. In: Abrams P, Cardozo L, Khoury S, Wein A, eds. Incontinence. Plymouth: Health Publications; 2002: 425–478.

26. Miller J, Perucchini D, Carchidi L, DeLancey J, Ashton-Miller J. Pelvic floor muscle contraction during a cough and decreased vesical neck mobility. Obstet Gynecol 2001;97:255–260.

27. Howard D, Miller J, DeLancey J, Ashton-Miller J. Differential effects of cough,valsalva, and continence status on vesical neck movement. Obstet Gynecol 2000;95:535–540.

28. DeLancey J, Hurd W. Size of the urogenital hiatus in the levator ani muscles in normal women and women with pelvic organ prolapse. Obstet Gynecol 1998;91:364–368.

29. DeLancey J, Kearney R, Chou Q, Speights S, Binno S. The appearance of levator ani muscle abnormalities in magnetic resonance images after vaginal delivery. Obstet Gynecol 2003;101:46–53.

30. Lienemann A, Sprenger D, Janssen U, Grosch E, Pellengahr C, Anthuber C. Assessment of pelvic organ descent by use of

functional Cine-MRI: which reference line should be used? Neurourol Urodyn 2004;23:33–37.

31. Hagen S, Stark D, Cattermole D. A United Kingdom-wide survey of physiotherapy practice in the treatment of pelvic organ prolapse. Physiotherapy 2004;90:19–26.

32. Samuelsson E, Victor A, Tibblin G, Svaerdsudd K. Signs of genital prolapse in a Swedish population of women 20 to 59 years of age and possible related factors. Am J Obstet Gynecol 1999;180:299–305.

33. Poma P. Nonsurgical management of genital prolapse. A review and recommendations for clinical practice. J Reprod Med 2000;45(10):789–797.

34. Cundiff G, Addison W. Management of pelvic organ prolapse. Obstet Gynecol Clin North Am 1998;25(4):907–921.

35. Cundiff G, Weidner A, Visco A, Bump R, Addison W. A survey of pessary use by members of the American Urogynecologic Society. Obstet Gynecol 2000;95(6):931–935.

36. Fritzinger K, Newman D, Dinkin E. Use of a pessary for the management of pelvic organ prolapse. Lippincott's Prim Care Pract 1997;1(4):431–436.

37. Adams E, Hagen S, Maher C, Thomsson A. Mechanical devices for pelvic organ prolapse in women. Cochrane Review, Issue 2. Oxford: Cochrane Library; 2004.

38. Pott-Grinstein E, Newcomer J. Gynecologists' patterns of prescribing pessaries. J Reprod Med 2001;46(3):205–208.

39. Sulak P, Kuehl T, Shull B. Vaginal pessaries and their use in pelvic relaxation. Reprod Med 1993;38(12):919–923.

40. Clemons J, Aguilar V, Tillinghast T, Jackson N, Myers D. Risk factors associated with an unsuccessful pessary fitting trial in women with pelvic organ prolapse. Am J Obstet Gynecol 2004;190:345–350.

41. Handa V, Jones M. Do pessaries prevent the progression of pelvic organ prolapse? Int Urogynecol J 2002;13:349–352.

42. Clemons J, Aguilar V, Tillinghast T, Jackson N, Myers D. Patient satisfaction and changes in prolapse and urinary symptoms in women who were fitted successfully with a pessary for pelvic organ prolapse. Am J Obstet Gynecol 2004;190:1025–1029.

43. Davila GW. Vaginal prolapse. Management with nonsurgical techniques. Postgrad Med 1996;99(4):171–185.

44. Mimura T, Roy A, Storrie J, Kamm M. Treatment of impaired defecation associated with rectocele by behavioral retraining (biofeedback). Dis Colon Rectum 2000;43:1267–1272.

45. Piya-Anant M, Therasakvichya S, Leelaphatanadit C, Techatrisak K. Integrated health research program for the Thai elderly: prevalence of genital prolapse and effectiveness of pelvic floor exercise to prevent worsening of genital prolapse in elderly women. J Med Assoc Thai 2004;86(6):509–515.

46. Bø K. Pelvic floor muscle training is effective in treatment of stress urinary incontinence, but how does it work? Int Urogynecol J 2004;15:76–84.

47. DeLancey J. Functional anatomy of the female lower urinary tract and pelvic floor. In: Ciba Foundation Symposium. Neurobiology of incontinence. Chichester: John Wiley, 1990.

48. Bø K, Lilleås F, Talseth T, Hedlund H. Dynamic MRI of pelvic floor muscles in an upright sitting position. Neurourol Urodyn 2001;20:167–174.

49. Bø K, Sherburn M, Allen T. Transabdominal ultrasound measurement of pelvic floor muscle activity when activated directly or via transversus abdominis muscle contraction. Neurourol Urodyn 2003;22:582–588.

50. Mantle J. Physiotherapy for incontinence. In: Cardozo L, Staskin D, eds. Textbook of female urology and urogynecology. London: Isis Medical Media Ltd; 2001: 351–358.

51. Bø K, Talseth T. Change in urethral pressure during voluntary pelvic floor muscle contraction and vaginal electrical stimulation. Int Urogynecol J 1997;8:3–7.

52. Theofrastous J, Wyman J, Bump R, et al. Effects of pelvic floor muscle training on strength and predictors of response in the treatment of urinary incontinence. Neurourol Urodyn 2002;21:486–490.

53. Miller JM, Ashton-Miller JA, DeLancey J. A pelvic muscle precontraction can reduce cough-related urine loss in selected women with mild SUI. J Am Geriatr Soc 1998;46:870–874.

54. Peschers U, Fanger G, Schaer G, Vodusek D, DeLancey J, Schussler B. Bladder neck mobility in continent nulliparous women. Br J Obstet Gynaecol 2001;108:320–324.

55. Kegel A. The non-surgical treatment of genital relaxation. Ann West Med Surg 1948;2:213–216.

56. Frontera W, Meredith C. Strength training in the elderly. In: Harris R, Harris S, eds. Physical activity, aging and sports. Vol 1:Scientific and medical research. Albany, NY: Center for the Study of Aging; 1989: 319–331.

57. DiNubile NA. Strength training. Clin Sports Med 1991;10(1):33–62.

58. Stone M. Implications for connective tissue and bone alterations resulting from resistance exercise training. Med Sci Sports Exerc 2003;20(5):162–168.

59. Vailas A, Vailas J. Physical activity and connective tissue. In: Bouchard C, Shephard R, Stephens T, eds. Physical activity, fitness and health. International proceedings and consensus statement. Champaign,IL: Human Kinetics Publishers; 1994: 369–382.

60. Stone M. Connective tissue and bone response to strength training. In: Komi P, ed. Strength and power in sport. Oxford: Blackwell Science; 1992: 279–290.

61. Pollock ML, Gaesser GA, Butcher JD, et al. The recommended quantity and quality of exercise for developing and maintaining cardiorespiratory and muscular fitness, and flexibility in healthy adults. Med Sci Sports Exerc 1998;30(6):975–991.

62. American College of Sports Medicine Position Stand. The recommended quantity and quality of exercise for developing and maintaining cardiorespiratory and muscular fitness in healthy adults. Med Sci Sports Exerc 1990;22:265–274.

63. Haskel W. Dose–response issues from a biological perspective. In: Bouchard C, Shephard RJ, Stephens T, eds. Physical activity, fitness, and health. International proceedings and consensus statement. Champaign,IL: Human Kinetics Publishers; 1994: 1030–1039.

64. Bouchard C. Physical activity and health.introduction to the dose-response symposium. Med Sci Sports Exerc 2001;33(6):347–350.

65. Kesaniemi Y, Danforth E, Jensen M, Kopelman P, Lefebvre P, Reeder B. Dose-response issues concerning physical activity and health: an evidence-based symposium. Med Sci Sports Exerc 2001;33(6 Suppl):351–358.

66. Bø K, Hagen RH, Kvarstein B, Jørgensen J, Larsen S. Pelvic floor muscle exercise for the treatment of female stress urinary incontinence: III.Effects of two different degrees of pelvic floor muscle exercise. Neurourol Urodyn 1990;9:489–502.

67. Bø K, Talseth T, Holme I. Single blind, randomised controlled trial of pelvic floor exercises, electrical stimulation, vaginal cones, and no treatment in management of genuine stress incontinence in women. BMJ 1999;318:487–493.

68. Mørkved S, Bø K, Fjørtoft T. Is there any additional effect of adding biofeedback to pelvic floor muscle training? A single-blind randomized controlled trial. Obstet Gynecol 2002;100(4):730–739.

69. Bernstein I. The pelvic floor muscles. Copenhagen: University of Copenhagen, Department of Urology; 1997.

70. Peschers U, Schaer G, Anthuber C, DeLancey J, Schussler B. Changes in vesical neck mobility following vaginal delivery. Obstet Gynecol 1996;88:1001–1006.

71. DeLancey J, Kearney R, Umek W, Ashton-Miller J. Levator ani muscle structure and function in women with prolapse compared to women with normal support. Nerourol Urodyn 2003;22(5):542–543.

72. Hay-Smith E, Bø K, Berghmans L, Hendriks H, de Bie R, van Waalwijk van Doorn ESC. Pelvic floor muscle training for urinary incontinence in women. Cochrane Review, Issue 3. Oxford: Cochrane Library; 2001.

73. Wilson PD, Bø KH-SJ, Nygaard I, Staskin D, Wyman J, Bourcier A. Conservative treatment in women. In: Abrams P, Cardozo L, Khoury S, Wein A, eds. Incontinence. Plymouth, UK: Health Publications Ltd; 2002: 571–624.

74. Maher C, Carey M, Adams EHS. Surgical management of pelvic organ prolapse. Cochrane Review, Issue 2. Oxford: Cochrane Library; 2004.

Surgical Management: The Urogynecologist's Approach

Linda Brubaker

INTRODUCTION

Surgery for pelvic organ prolapse (POP) is common. However, there are significant geographic, cultural, and specialty-based differences in surgical practices. This chapter will review urogynecologic approaches to POP repair and provide the surgical trainee with a framework for future research in this field.

DEMOGRAPHICS OF PELVIC ORGAN PROLAPSE SURGERY REPAIR

Recent estimates from large American databases indicate that POP surgery is more common than continence surgery, with approximately 200,000 patients having POP surgery annually.[1] An often quoted epidemiologic evaluation of a large north-western Kaiser-managed healthcare population suggests that American women have an 11.1% risk of POP surgery by the age of 80, with nearly 30% undergoing more than one procedure.[2] The epidemiology of recurrent POP has also recently been studied and several risk factors highlighted.[3] Although racial differences are understudied, it appears that Caucasian women have a threefold increase in surgery compared to African-American women.

Subak et al estimated that the annual direct cost of POP surgery in the United States was approximately $1012 million.[4] These statistics are likely to underestimate the real surgical burden to society. Given the prevalence of POP surgery and the high rate of POP recurrence, there is a pressing need to apply the highest quality of scientific study to this field.

DECISION FOR SURGERY

Expert opinion is virtually unanimous in the recommendation to limit POP surgery to patients who have symptoms directly attributable to their POP. Although this seems relatively straightforward, it is not always clear which pelvic symptoms are related to POP.[5,6] Many pelvic symptoms may coexist with POP. For example, urinary incontinence, constipation and disordered defecation are relatively common comorbidities. However, these concomitant disorders may not be directly related to POP and may persist after otherwise successful anatomic POP repair. Experts suggest that the symptoms of vaginal protrusion and bulging are relatively clearly related to POP and frequently are resolved by successful POP repair.

Less commonly, a patient may present with a large "asymptomatic" anatomic defect. Most commonly, this patient has developed significant adaptive behaviors, avoiding situations that emphasize the awareness of the abnormal anatomy. On occasion, a cognitively impaired patient may deny symptoms, although a caregiver clearly relates that the patient's behavior is consistent with bothersome pelvic symptoms. In these situations, upper urinary tract safety should be ensured if POP reduction is not imminent.

It is important that the patient has sufficient bother from POP to warrant surgery and to allow successful surgery to be appreciated. A minimally symptomatic patient is unlikely to have a satisfactory risk/benefit ratio and is unlikely to tolerate even minor postoperative difficulties. The presence of other pelvic symptoms should not be so severe as to overwhelm the effects of otherwise successful surgery. A woman with relatively asymptomatic uterine prolapse and severe fecal incontinence is unlikely to perceive a significant improvement in her overall pelvic health when the uterovaginal prolapse is successfully treated but the fecal incontinence remains severe.

The goals of the surgery should be clearly explained to the patient. Pelvic anatomy and symptoms are difficult even for physicians to fully comprehend and it may be necessary to review the surgical indications and perioperative plan on more than one occasion from more than one perspective. Clinically worrisome hesitation or unrealistic expectation should prompt further preoperative discussion or permanent deferral of surgery.

Once a patient and physician have made a mutual decision to proceed with POP surgery, the specific surgical recommendations should be determined. The patient's perspective may include a lack of understanding about the prolapsing tissues. It is common for a patient to believe (or have been told by a medical professional) that "her bladder is fallen." In fact, many physicians underdiagnose apical defects, indicating to the patient that a "large cystocele" is present. Prior surgery may have been unsuccessful due to a lack of comprehensive diagnosis, including apical defects. Therefore, it may be necessary to carefully explain why the current surgical plan differs from a previous unsuccessful plan. Recurrent POP surgery is further discussed later in this chapter.

The surgeon's perspective includes a continuous assessment of the risk/benefit ratio for the individual woman. For centuries, our gynecologic forefathers have emphasized the need to individualize each surgical repair for an individual patient. This remains true, although modern surgeons do not always actively practice it. Every woman has certain risk factors for recurrent POP, although this area requires further scientific study.[7] For example, a young woman who has sustained a major childbirth-provoked POP may have markedly decreased neuromuscular integrity of the pelvic function. Once she has completed her family and desires POP surgery, the surgeon must determine the procedure (or group of procedures) that will provide the highest success rate, longest durability, and lowest rate of complications. The woman's projected lifespan and the severity of her primary presentation increase her risk for recurrent POP. A similar woman may wish for uterine preservation.

Other patients may have undergone several prior POP repairs, have discontinued vaginal coital activity, and desperately wish for a definitive resolution of POP. A different procedure is likely to be appropriate for these women.

Clearly the counseling of surgical options should be an interactive process with multiple options presented to and discussed with the patient prior to reaching a mutually agreeable decision. There are two "favorable" aspects of POP: it is rarely painful and it is generally not life threatening. These favorable features allow both surgeon and patient to carefully consider a variety of treatment options and pursue surgical intervention on a convenience schedule. It would be a highly unusual situation that would require rushing a POP patient to surgery.

PHILOSOPHY OF SURGICAL PLAN

Surgeons may have highly individualistic philosophies regarding their surgical plans. The common philosophy is that the surgeon plans to do the most effective procedure that is least morbid. However, the best procedure (or combination of procedures) with which to accomplish this goal remains unknown.

Extirpative surgery is often performed during POP procedures. In the US, the uterus is removed during almost all primary POP operations. It is estimated that approximately 7–14% of hysterectomies are done for the indication of POP. However, in various European countries, the uterus is virtually always preserved. There is no clinical trial that has addressed this most basic aspect of POP surgery. Surgical series that have been reported provide sufficient information for planning such trials and would reduce the confounding and severe biases present in all surgical case series published to date. There is no evidence that uterine preservation or removal affects the primary cure rate or risk of POP recurrence. Nieminen et al confirm that concomitant hysterectomy caused a statistically significant increase in the duration for the procedure.[8]

There are reproductive issues surrounding hysterectomy at the time of POP surgery. Most experts prefer to defer POP surgery until child bearing is complete. When a woman becomes pregnant following otherwise successful POP repair, most experts recommend cesarean delivery without labor in order to avoid further pelvic damage that increases the risk of POP recurrence.

Oophorectomy is commonly performed at the time of POP repair, although less commonly than hysterectomy. It is a well-known phenomenon that vaginal hysterectomy has a lower rate of concomitant oophorectomy than abdominal hysterectomy; even when patient age and other risk factors are similar. However, oophorectomy is relatively commonly performed in recurrent POP surgery, according to prevailing gynecologic indications for removal of otherwise healthy postmenopausal adnexae.

There are several philosophic viewpoints regarding the reconstructive aspects of POP surgery. For many years, experts recommended repairing "all defects." However, it was recognized that many asymptomatic, vaginally parous women have altered vaginal topography. Because experts cannot agree on what is normal anatomy for vaginally parous women, and because there is only a vague relationship between anatomy and function, it is difficult to recommend repair of "all defects." More than two-thirds of parous women have objective evidence of POP on clinical examination. The majority of these defects are asymptomatic and fewer than 15% of them will require surgical intervention. The policy of "repair all defects" may in fact induce more dysfunction than it resolves. For example, surgical treatment of an asymptomatic posterior wall that is present at the hymen may cause significant new-onset dyspareunia.

Some POP surgery (and some concomitant continence surgery) may predispose to de novo or worsening of other POP. The specific risks for these events are only poorly understood. A small case series suggested that POP occurred in approximately 15% of women who had a Burch urethropexy.[9] Clinicians have used this report to suggest that concomitant culdeplasty was indicated at the time of Burch urethropexy. Since the publication of this report, no randomized surgical trial has addressed the risk of de novo POP at the time of Burch urethropexy.

Multiple case series have suggested vulnerabilities in various POP procedures. The sacrospinous ligament suspension is a commonly performed procedure that appears to have a relatively high rate of persistent or de novo anterior wall support defects. The combination of a needle urethropexy and sacrospinous ligament suspension has been shown to predispose to the early development of prolapse of the upper anterior vaginal segment and failure of bladder neck support.[10] Case series have highlighted the posterior vaginal support defects that may occur after sacrocolpopexy.[11]

The selection of the optimal POP procedure includes an assessment of the site-specific risks of POP recurrence for that individual woman. In a woman with a predominantly anterior support defect, a procedure that is more effective for this segment may be considered. Likewise, a predominant posterior defect may be optimally treated with a procedure that does not further challenge posterior support.

The selection of concomitant procedure may also affect the decision for a specific procedure or the components of a combined procedure complex. The effect of concomitant continence procedures will be further discussed later in this chapter.

TECHNICAL ASPECTS OF RECONSTRUCTIVE SURGERY

It is assumed that readers of this book have basic surgical knowledge and are aware of the importance of meticulous surgical technique, including respect for tissue planes, hemostasis, and surgical efficiency. Given the patient positioning and duration of many POP procedures, the surgical team should be cognisant of the risks of nerve injury and be diligent in their ongoing efforts to minimize long-term neural sequelae.

Most POP patients are positioned on the operating table with the intention to complete the repair through either a transvaginal or a transabdominal route. A minority of surgeons plan to use both routes during the same procedure in selected patients.

Selecting the optimal route for surgery is an important cornerstone of surgical planning. However, these are extraordinarily difficult studies to plan and complete.

Figure 19a.1 demonstrates the preoperative view of a stage IV uterovaginal POP that was successfully repaired with a transvaginal route. Figure 19a.2 demonstrates the preoperative physical findings in a woman with three prior vaginal POP repairs who was ultimately successfully treated with sacrocolpopexy. Clearly, different patients require different surgical approaches. Four randomized surgical trials have attempted to address this important area. Two

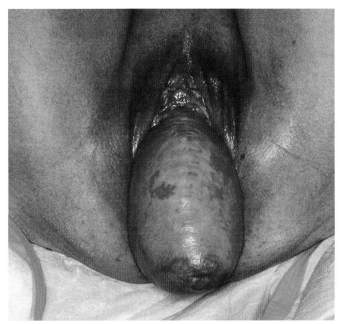

Figure 19a.1 Preoperative view of a stage IV uterovaginal POP that was successfully repaired with a transvaginal approach.

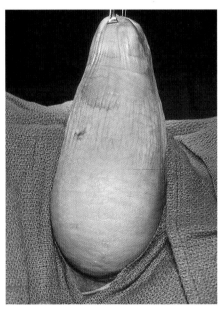

Figure 19a.2 Preoperative physical findings in a woman with stage IV POP and three prior vaginal POP repairs who was ultimately successfully treated with sacrocolpopexy.

of these trials are reported in sufficient detail to allow evaluation of their results.

Benson et al reported the first randomized surgical trial addressing the optimal route for surgery.[12] These researchers reported that abdominal surgery was significantly more likely than vaginal surgery to result in an optimal outcome (mean follow-up 2.5 years). An interim analysis revealed a clinically significant disparity between the groups and the authors felt obliged to stop the trial after 124 women were randomized over 26.5 months. The final sample of 80 women who were treated included a significant proportion of "abdominal" participants who also had vaginal procedures (anterior colporrhaphy 30% and posterior colporrhaphy 50%). The specific primary prolapse procedures performed included bilateral sacrospinous suspension, vaginal paravaginal repair, Pereyra needle urethropexy, sacrocolpopexy, retropubic paravaginal repair, and Burch colposuspension. Thus, the route of surgery was also related to specific procedures, as is common clinically.

Women in the vaginal group with recurrent POP experienced their recurrence significantly earlier than women in the abdominal group. However, women randomized to the abdominal group had significantly more complications and significantly longer operation times and hospital costs than women in the vaginal group.

The recently published study by Maher et al corroborates the Benson findings of anatomic superiority of abdominal sacrocolpopexy at a mean follow-up of 24 months.[13] However, unilateral vaginal sacrospinous suspension had an overall equal efficacy when complications and patient-centered outcomes were included in the outcome assessment.

These two important studies compare a group of POP procedures as well as the route of POP surgery. The reoperation rates for prolapse or incontinence were similar, with the vaginal approach being quicker, less expensive, and associated with a quicker return to activities of daily living. However, the vaginal approach was associated with a significantly higher rate of combined recurrent anterior and apical prolapse. This difference in objective evaluation was offset by an increased rate of posterior compartment prolapse following the sacral colpopexy, resulting in an overall similar objective outcome between the two groups.

These studies support the superiority of the abdominal route procedures compared with the vaginal route procedures as measured by the durable restoration of anatomy and lower urinary tract and vaginal function. However, this anatomic superiority may be offset by the increased morbidity of the abdominal route. Clearly, additional large clinical trials will be needed to determine the optimal approach for primary and recurrent POP surgery.

RISKS OF RECURRENT PROLAPSE

There are no long-term studies with objective outcomes to assess the durability of any POP procedure. However, there are several case series that highlight disturbingly high rates of recurrence in short-term follow-up.

Brubaker reported an unacceptably high rate of anterior wall support defects in a sacrocolpopexy series with only apical and posterior mesh placement.[14] Currently, experts recommend fixation of both anterior and posterior material at the time of sacrocolpopexy. It is well known that simple fixation of sacrocolpopexy materials to the apex only results in unacceptably high POP recurrence rates.

Weber at al reported an unacceptable high rate of anterior wall support defects in a randomized trial of three techniques for anterior wall support defect repair.[15] There were no significant differences between the groups at a mean follow-up of nearly 2 years with only 30%, 46%, and 42% experiencing satisfactory or optimal anatomic results.

Kenton et al reported a case series of defect-specific rectocele repairs in which certain functional abnormalities (manual assistance with defecation) recurred within 1 year in approximately half of the patients, despite anatomic resolution of their posterior wall anatomic defects.[16]

Most experts believe that suspension of the apex is the cornerstone of prolapse repairs, regardless of the route of surgery. Ineffective apical suspension is often misdiagnosed as "large cystoceles" or "enterocele." If the preoperative diagnosis is not accurate, it is unlikely that the surgical plan will be appropriate.

There is limited demographic information on the risk of recurrent surgery. Clearly, an estimate of repeat surgery will underestimate the number of women who actually have persistence or recurrence of their pelvic floor disorders. The risks factors for recurrent POP are generated predominantly by expert opinion and epidemiologic studies. Risks include unsuccessful prior surgery and unusually extreme forces on the repair sites.

There is a known risk of persistent, recurrent or de novo POP after POP surgery. In 1943 Victor Bonney reported that fixed vaginal retroversion predisposes to anterior segment prolapse. It is well known that sacrospinous ligament suspension is associated with anterior wall anatomic defects.[10, 17-19]

The prevalence of cystocele from 1 to 5 years after sacrospinous vault suspension has been reported to be 16–18%,[20] 36%,[10] and 92%.[19] The combination of marked retroversion of the vaginal apex resulting from the sacrospinous suspension and the marked anterior deflection of the anterior segment resulting from the needle bladder neck suspension and paravaginal repair increases the stress on the upper anterior vaginal wall, leading to much earlier and more severe recurrent anterior segment prolapse.

TECHNIQUES FOR REPAIR OF RECURRENT PROLAPSE

When faced with a patient who has POP persistence or recurrence, especially within a short period of time, the surgeon must set aside ego and arrogance. Surgeons have a tendency to overemphasize another surgeon's lack of skill as a cause of the unsuccessful surgical outcome, deflecting the role of patient selection and the procedure. It is important to consider the capabilities and surgical habits of the prior surgeon, and to review the surgical record for important clues such as material mismatching or unusual intraoper-

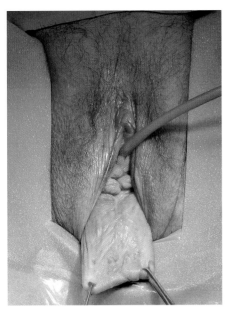

Figure 19a.3 Preoperative physical findings in a patient with multiple prior procedures whose vagina is now extremely thin and shortened.

ative findings. Figure 19a.3 demonstrates the preoperative physical findings in a patient with multiple prior procedures whose vagina is now extremely thin and shortened. Materials issues will be further discussed in the next section. It is not common to have an outstanding surgical success when performing the exact same operation that was previously unsuccessful. Alternative technique and materials are typically justified. Less commonly used techniques such as vaginal closure (colpocleisis) may be offered to select women. Figure 19a.4 demonstrates the postoperative appearance of a vaginal closure with extensive perineorrhaphy.

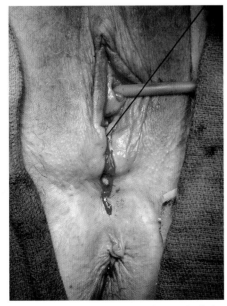

Figure 19a.4 Postoperative appearance of a vaginal closure with extensive perineorrhaphy.

ADJUNCTIVE MATERIALS FOR RECONSTRUCTION

Surgeons rely on adjunctive materials for two purposes during POP surgery.[21] The first is for a bridging purpose, such as during sacrocolpopexy where the adjunctive material actually forms a bridge and must remain in situ for the foreseeable future. It is inappropriate to use dissolving materials when constructing a bridge that needs to be permanent. The ideal permanent material does not yet exist.[22] Interested readers are referred to published literature for a more thorough understanding of the issues in this rapidly evolving area. Although permanent materials offer durability and strength, this favorable aspect must be weighed against the irreducible problems with foreign materials (of any kind) in the human body. A variety of case reports highlight the low but persistent rate of permanent materials problems in POP surgery. There are many permanent meshes available for the surgeon to use as bridging materials. The surgeon should be familiar with the properties of the material and be able to deal with foreign body complications should they arise.

The other form of adjunctive material is intended to provide additional structure to weakened native tissues, such as within the surgical planes necessary for anterior and posterior vaginal wall repair. Case series and case reports have documented inappropriate surgical use of many materials rates resorption[23] and surgical removal,[24] among other problems.[25] The recent International Consultation on Incontinence Committee on Pelvic Organ Prolapse completed a comprehensive review of this topic. There are two randomized trials to determine the role of polyglactin mesh in reducing the high anatomic recurrence rate in the anterior wall.[15,26] However, the findings of these two studies conflict. This expert review found no evidence to support the use of biologic or permanent synthetic grafts for transvaginal POP repair.

Therefore, until there is evidence of efficacy, as well as safety, the use of such adjunctive materials for the purpose of transvaginal tissue reinforcement should occur within the setting of a clinical trial. Several ongoing trials are under way and are likely to be completed following publication of this book. Interested readers are encouraged to continually assess this surgical recommendation, as there is a great deal of ongoing work in this area.

COMBINING POP AND CONTINENCE PROCEDURES

At least one-third of women who have POP surgery have concomitant continence procedures. This is an area of significant scientific uncertainty that deserves much more attention. This area is also troubled by a resolvable nomenclature problem.

Women with POP may have the full spectrum of lower urinary tract problems, including incontinence and/or retention. Using an arbitrarily set cut-off of 100 cc, FitzGerald et al demonstrated that it is uncommon to detect high postvoid residuals when women have less than stage II POP.[27] Women with stage III or IV POP may carry a high residual but this is nearly always resolved with POP repair.[28] There is a small group of women who need POP surgery who have had prior continence surgery and this group is at increased risk for unsuccessful repeat continence procedure and postoperative voiding dysfunction.

When preoperative stress urinary incontinence (SUI) is present, the surgeon typically wishes to add a concomitant procedure. Although the optimal continence procedure is not clear, a recently completed NIH clinical trial may provide some data following the publication of this book. A large variety of small case series report that a wide variety of continence procedures are "safe and effective" when combined with POP surgery. These case series have multiple significant limitations and do not effectively address this major issue in POP surgery.[29] Bump et al reported that the needle suspension procedures predisposed to recurrent prolapse when combined with sacrospinous ligament suspensions.[10] Colombo reported differential continence rates following needle suspension or posterior urethral ligament plication, although both procedures are known to have lower success rates than gold standard continence procedures such as urethropexys and slings.[30] This group also reported differential anatomic restoration rates in the anterior wall following Burch urethropexy versus anterior colporrhaphy.[31]

It is well known that stress incontinence can become apparent following POP repair.[32] The discussion of this topic is severely hampered by differences in nomenclature. Researchers and clinicians use terms such as "a potential" and "occult incontinence" in inconsistent ways. Some clinicians use these terms as descriptors of the vulnerability of all stress-continent women with POP; that is to say, they all have a risk (of unknown magnitude) of developing SUI after their POP surgery. Other clinician researchers reserve the terms for otherwise continent women who have the urodynamic finding of stress incontinence during testing. It is not clear whether this must occur with or without prolapse reduction. Most experts believe that POP reduction in a severe manner can unmask SUI in virtually all women, and is likely an artifact. The optimal method for prolapse reduction is not known, nor are urodynamic techniques for this standardized. Moreover, it is not clear what urodynamic terms should be used to describe a POP patient who does not leak at maximum capacity without reduction, but demonstrates urodynamic stress incontinence only during reduction. Most urodynamicists use the same term

"urodynamic stress incontinence," although the need to reduce the POP is not included in such standardized terminology. Therefore, clinician researchers are urged to fully describe their terms and methods in this somewhat unclear area of POP surgery.

When there is no preoperative SUI (stress-continent woman with POP), the surgeon is faced with one of three choices. The surgeon can:

1. always add a continence procedure (causing de novo symptoms in some women who do not necessarily benefit from the procedure)
2. never add a continence procedure (and probably need to reoperate on a portion of women for SUI later)
3. attempt to predict postoperative continence status, usually using a urodynamic technique.

As appealing as option 3 is, there is no standardized technique for prediction of postoperative continence status, even using high-quality urodynamic tests. Ongoing clinical trials are under way to address this important area of POP surgery.[33]

When two surgeons from different disciplines cooperate on a patient, it is extremely important to have collegial communications regarding the perioperative care of the patient. Should difficulties arise (urinary retention, recurrent POP, etc.) a unified approach to the resolution of these symptoms is critically important. It is inappropriate to bounce a patient back and forth between noncommuni-cating surgeons, especially when the surgical result is suboptimal.

The most commonly performed procedures for POP include sacrocolpopexy, sacrospinous ligament suspension, anterior colporrhaphy, and posterior colporrhaphy. All these have been the subject of randomized surgical trials. The ICI Committee on POP surgery has concluded that sacrospinous-based vaginal procedures have a higher anterior and apical anatomic recurrence rate than sacrocolpopexy-based abdominal repairs. Overall outcomes (which include quality of life) indicate that abdominal surgery and vaginal surgery are relatively equivalent. Abdominal surgery has a higher morbidity, at least in the short term.

There is no evidence that any transvaginal repair of the anterior vaginal wall is superior to any other. Similarly, there is no evidence that any transvaginal apical procedure is more effective than any other.

Experts suggest that POP may be prevented in some women by enhancing surgical efforts to suspend the vaginal cuff following hysterectomy by any route. There is no randomized trial that supports this recommendation; however, the risk/benefit ratio of careful cuff suspension is in the patient's favor.

DETERMINING SURGICAL OUTCOMES

The outcome of surgery is typically assessed clinically. This form of clinical assessment is vulnerable to overestimation of the surgical efficacy. Patients with suboptimal outcomes often do not return to their primary surgeon. Surgeon's bias is a well-known phenomenon that may be enhanced by the patient's desire to please her surgeon. It is preferable to have some form of standardized objective outcome measures that are obtained by someone other than the surgeon. These assessments should include anatomic, functional, and patient-oriented outcome measures. All experienced surgeons have met with postoperative patients who were happy despite a significant anatomic defect while in the next examination room was a patient with perfect postoperative anatomy who was dismally unhappy. All pelvic surgeons should make a concerted effort to understand and meet the patient's individual goals and expectations for her surgical outcome.[34]

CONCLUSION

In summary, there are many surgical approaches for POP repair. Several methods appear superior, at least given the amount of surgical research completed to date. Careful patient selection, thoughtful procedure selection, optimal technical performance, and an honest postoperative assessment allow surgeons to improve their skills in the surgical treatment of POP.

REFERENCES

1. Boyles S, Weber A, Meyn L. Procedures for pelvic organ prolapse in the United States, 1979–1997. Am J Obstet Gynecol 2003;188(1):108–115.
2. Olsen AL, et al. Epidemiology of surgically managed pelvic organ prolapse and urinary incontinence. Obstet Gynecol 1997;89(4):501–506.
3. Clark AL, et al. Epidemiologic evaluation of reoperation for surgically treated pelvic organ prolapse and urinary incontinence. Am J Obstet Gynecol 2003;189(5):1261–1267.
4. Subak LL, et al. Cost of pelvic organ prolapse surgery in the United States. Obstet Gynecol 2001;98(4):646–651.
5. Swift SE, Tate SB, Nicholas J. Correlation of symptoms with degree of pelvic organ support in a general population of women: what is pelvic organ prolapse? Am J Obstet Gynecol 2003;189(2):372–377; discussion 377–379.
6. Ellerkmann RM, et al. Correlation of symptoms with location and severity of pelvic organ prolapse. Am J Obstet Gynecol 2001;185:1332–1338.
7. Bump RC, Norton PA. Epidemiology and natural history of pelvic floor dysfunction. Obstet Gynecol ClinNorth Am 1998;25(4):723–746.
8. Nieminen K, Heinonen PK. Sacrospinous ligament fixation for massive genital prolapse in women aged over 80 years. Br J Obstet Gynaecol 2001;108(8):817–821.
9. Wiskind AK, Creighton SM, Stanton SL. The incidence of genital prolapse after the Burch colposuspension. Am J Obstet Gynecol 1992;167(2):399–404; discussion 404–405.
10. Bump RC, et al. Randomized prospective comparison of needle colposuspension versus endopelvic fascia plication for potential stress incontinence prophylaxis in women undergoing vaginal reconstruction for stage III or IV pelvic organ prolapse. The Continence Program for Women Research Group. Am J Obstet Gynecol 1996;175(2):326–333; discussion 333–335.
11. Baessler K, Schuessler B. Abdominal sacrocolpopexy and anatomy and function of the posterior compartment. Obstet Gynecol 2001;97(5 Pt 1): 678–684.
12. Benson JT, Lucente V, McClellan E. Vaginal versus abdominal reconstructive surgery for the treatment of pelvic support defects: a prospective randomized study with long-term outcome evaluation. Am J Obstet Gynecol 1996;175(6):1418–1421; discussion 1421–1422.
13. Maher CF, et al. Abdominal sacral colpopexy or vaginal sacrospinous colpopexy for vaginal vault prolaspe: a prospective randomized study. Am J Obstet Gynecol 2004;190:20–26.

14. Brubaker L. Sacrocolpopexy and the anterior compartment: support and function. Am J Obstet Gynecol 1995;173(6):1690–1695; discussion 1695–1696.
15. Weber AM, et al. Anterior colporrhaphy: a randomized trial of three surgical techniques. Am J Obstet Gynecol 2001;185(6):1299–1304; discussion 1304–1306.
16. Kenton K, Shott S, Brubaker L. Outcome after rectovaginal fascia reattachment for rectocele repair. Am J Obstet Gynecol 1999;181(6):1360–1363; discussion 1363–1364.
17. Shull BL, et al. Preoperative and postoperative analysis of site-specific pelvic support defects in 81 women treated with sacrospinous ligament suspension and pelvic reconstruction. Am J Obstet Gynecol 1992;166(6 Pt 1):1764–1768; discussion 1768–1771.
18. Shull BL, et al. Bilateral attachment of the vaginal cuff to iliococcygeus fascia: an effective method of cuff suspension. Am J Obstet Gynecol 1993;168(6 Pt 1):1669–1674; discussion 1674–1677.
19. Holley RL, et al. Recurrent pelvic support defects after sacrospinous ligament fixation for vaginal vault prolapse. J Am Coll Surg 1995;180:444–448.
20. Morley GW, DeLancey JO. Sacrospinous ligament fixation for eversion of the vagina. Am J Obstet Gynecol 1988;158(4):872–881.
21. Birch C, Fynes MM. The role of synthetic and biological prostheses in reconstructive pelvic floor surgery. Curr Opin Obstet Gynecol 2002;14(5):527–535.
22. Iglesia CB, Fenner DE, Brubaker L. The use of mesh in gynecologic surgery. Int Urogynecol J 1997;8(2):105–115.
23. Fitzgerald MP, Mollenhauer J, Brubaker L. Donor fascia in urogynaecological procedures: a canine model. BJU Int 2001;87(7):682–689.
24. Julian TM. The efficacy of Marlex mesh in the repair of severe, recurrent vaginal prolapse of the anterior midvaginal wall. Am J Obstet Gynecol 1996;175(6):1472–1475.
25. Cosson M, et al. Rejection of stapled prosthetic mesh after laparoscopic sacropexy. Int Urogynecol J Pelvic Floor Dysfunct 1999;10(5):349–350.
26. Sand PK, et al. Prospective randomized trial of polyglactin 910 mesh to prevent recurrence of cystoceles and rectoceles. Am J Obstet Gynecol 2001;184(7):1357–1362; discussion 1362–1364.
27. FitzGerald MP, Jaffar J, Brubaker L. Risk factors for an elevated postvoid residual urine volume in women with symptoms of urinary urgency, frequency and urge incontinence. Int Urogynecol J 2001;12:237–240.
28. Fitzgerald MP, Kulkarni N, Fenner D. Postoperative resolution of

urinary retention in patients with advanced pelvic organ prolapse. Am J Obstet Gynecol 2000;183(6):1361–1363; discussion 1363–1364.

29. Cheng-Yu L, Shih-Cheng H, Der-Ji S. Abnormal clinical and urodynamic findings in women with severe genitourinary prolapse. Kaohsiung J Med Sci 2002;18:593–597.

30. Colombo M, et al. Surgery for genitourinary prolapse and stress incontinence: a randomized trial of posterior pubourethral ligament plication and Pereyra suspension. Am J Obstet Gynecol 1997;176(2):337–343.

31. Colombo M. et al. Randomised comparison of Burch colposuspension versus anterior colporrhaphy in women with stress urinary incontinence and anterior vaginal wall prolapse. Br J Obstet Gynaecol 2000;107(4):544–551.

32. Rosenzweig BA, Pushkin S, Blumenfeld D. Prevalence of abnormal urodynamic test results in continent women with severe genitourinary prolapse. Obstet Gynecol 1992;79:539–543.

33. Brubaker L, et al. A randomized trial of colpopexy and urinary reduction efforts (CARE): design and methods. Controlled Clinical Trials 2003;24(5):629–642.

34. Elkadry EA, Kenton KS, FitzGerald MP, Shott S, Brubaker L. Patient-selected goals: a new perspective on surgical outcome. American Journal of Obstetrics & Gynecology 2003;189(6):1551–1557.

SECTION 7 Treatment of pelvic organ prolapse

Surgical Management: The Urologist's Approach

Jason P Gilleran and Philippe E Zimmern

INTRODUCTION

With an aging population of women who wish to maintain a good quality of life, the demand for repair of pelvic organ prolapse (POP) is increasing. The prevalence of POP has been quoted at 20–50% in a screened population,[1,2] with a lifetime risk of surgery for prolapse estimated around 11%.[3] Based on the Medicare reimbursement schedule and measured in 1997 US dollars, the direct cost of surgical repair alone for POP has been estimated at over $1 billion.[4]

Surgical management of POP by the urologist has historically been limited to surgery for stress urinary incontinence (SUI) and cystocele repair. However, since it is not uncommon for women to undergo multiple prolapse repairs at the time of SUI repair,[5] the urologist's role in treating this condition is rapidly evolving. Although some women will choose conservative management, a large number will be bothered enough to pursue surgical repair.[6]

The ultimate goal of POP repair is to restore anatomy and function of the vagina and pelvic organs. This chapter will focus primarily on the surgical techniques for prolapse repair available to the pelvic floor reconstructive surgeon, with a review of their unique complications, results, and long-term outcome (when available). A significant portion of this chapter will discuss prolapse of the anterior vaginal wall, as these are the techniques most familiar to urologists. However, since vaginal apex and posterior compartment prolapses can coexist with anterior vaginal wall herniation, discussion of these repair techniques will be provided as well.

ANTERIOR COMPARTMENT REPAIR

The most common anterior vaginal compartment prolapse is the cystocele. Assessment of the degree of prolapse can be based on a variety of systems, the two most popular being the Baden-Walker halfway system and the pelvic organ prolapse quantified (POP-Q) grading system.[7,8] The severity of prolapse is important, as effective management of mild-to-moderate prolapse differs from that of severe prolapse.

Once the decision is made to repair a symptomatic cystocele, the choice of surgical technique is influenced by several factors, which are summarized in Box 19b.1. The options for cystocele repair are presented in Table 19b.1, stratified by degree of cystocele and approach (transvaginal versus abdominal). For each procedure discussed, we will present sequentially the goal, technique with risks and complications, and results in table form.

Vaginal repair: general comments. There are several operative steps common to all vaginal repairs. The patient is placed in the dorsal lithotomy position, with the legs placed in Allen stirrups or candy canes, and care taken to pad all pressure points. TED hose and/or pneumatic compression devices are commonly considered to prevent venous thrombosis.

After full vaginal and lower abdominal preparation, either a Lone Star (Lone Star Medical Products Inc., Stafford, TX)

Box 19b.1 Factors contributing to options for surgical management of pelvic prolapse

- Degree or stage of herniation
- Location of defect (lateral vs central)
- Prior vaginal or pelvic repairs
- Associated or unmasked stress incontinence
- Associated voiding dysfunction
- Sexual function
- Level of activity
- Upper tract status
- Hormonal status
- Presence or absence of uterus
- Medical comorbidities
- Patient expectations
- Risk factors for recurrence (obesity, chronic pulmonary disease, chronic constipation)

Table 19b.1   Options for cystocele repair based on degree of prolapse and approach

Mild-to-moderate cystocele		Severe cystocele	
Vaginal approach	Abdominal approach	Vaginal approach	Abdominal approach
Vaginal wall repairs Four-corner suspension Anterior vaginal wall suspension	Burch colposuspension	Graft interposition (allograft, xenograft, synthetic)	Mesh sacrocolpopexy
	Paravaginal repair	Anterior vaginal wall suspension	Laparoscopic sacrocolpopexy
	Laparoscopic colposuspension	Anterior colporrhaphy	

or Turner-Warwick retractor, weighted speculum, and occasionally a headlight are used to optimize exposure (Fig. 19b.1A). The bladder is drained continuously throughout the procedure with a urethral catheter. Alternatively, a suprapubic tube may be placed using a Lowsley retractor or a percutaneous suprapubic catheter set. The location of the bladder neck on the anterior vaginal wall can be marked at the level of the catheter balloon. Injection of normal saline, or a 1% lidocaine + epinephrine solution, into the anterior vaginal wall may facilitate dissection of the plane between the vaginal mucosa and the bladder wall. An estrogen cream- or antibiotic-soaked vaginal pack can be placed postoperatively to encourage hemostasis. The pack and catheter are usually removed within 24 hours, although a urethral catheter may be left longer in cases of inadvertent bladder injury or if there is a concern for prolonged urinary retention.

Low-grade cystocele

Bladder neck/base suspension procedures. The goal of these procedures is placement of suspension sutures to support the anterior vaginal wall which will in turn stabilize the bladder neck and base. By correcting the anterior vaginal wall laxity, each technique corrects urethral hypermobility whether there is associated stress incontinence or not. Historically, all these types of procedures derive from the Pereyra and Raz bladder neck suspension techniques, and thus share common features.

FOUR-CORNER (RAZ) SUSPENSION

Technique. In the initial series described by Raz, an inverted U-shaped incision was made in the anterior vaginal wall with the apex of the U at the midpoint between the bladder neck and urethral meatus.[9] The dissection begins distally at the level of the bladder neck and extends laterally towards the undersurface of the pubic bone. The retropubic space is entered to allow for passage of the suspension sutures. On each side, two sets of nonabsorbable sutures are passed through the vaginal wall 2–3 times in a helical fashion, excluding epithelium. The distal sutures are passed at the bladder neck and proximal urethra incorporating the ure-

thropelvic ligament, while sutures at the base of the incision incorporate the underlying pubocervical fascia.

Then, through a small suprapubic incision, the sutures are transferred retropubically and above the rectus fascia using a double-pronged suture carrier. During passage of the carrier, perforation of the anterior bladder wall may occur, often not associated with any evidence of gross hematuria. Therefore, cystoscopy is done to exclude bladder injury and to visualize the bladder neck support upon lifting the sutures. Following closure of the vaginal incision, the suspension sutures are first tied independently, then to each other on each side, then lastly to each other across the midline.

MODIFIED PROCEDURES: 1. The concept of broad-based suture anchoring for improved support of the vaginal wall in the four-corner suspension was introduced by Zimmern and Leach.[10] This modification incorporated findings by Bruskewitz et al, who demonstrated decreased suture pull-through using looped sutures over a greater cross-sectional area in a rabbit model.[11]

Technique. The inverted-U shaped incision of the four-corner suspension is modified into two parallel, longitudinal incisions, which begin on each side of the bladder neck. The retropubic space is entered and nonabsorbable sutures are passed helically beneath the vaginal wall at the level of the bladder neck distally, omitting the urethropelvic ligament. Proximally, the cardinal ligament complex (if the uterus is still present) or the vaginal cuff is incorporated in the sutures. The four sets of sutures are then transferred through the retropubic space with a ligature carrier. The distal sutures are anchored to the rectus fascia or pubic bone,[12] while the proximal sutures are secured to the rectus fascia, with all sutures tied with minimal tension.

MODIFIED PROCEDURES: 2. The six-corner suspension is a further modification reported by Raz which uses a similar incision and dissection to the four-corner suspension but in this case, three sets of sutures are passed on each side: one at the midurethra (incorporating the urethropelvic ligament), one at the bladder neck, and one at the level of the cardinal

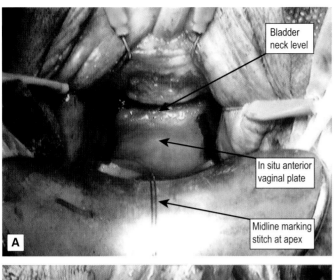

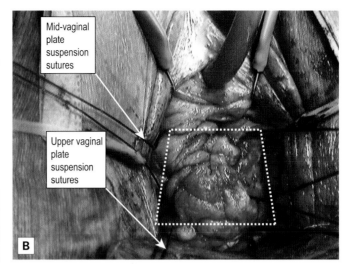

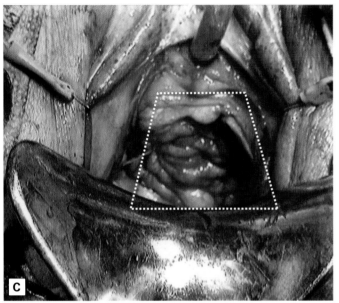

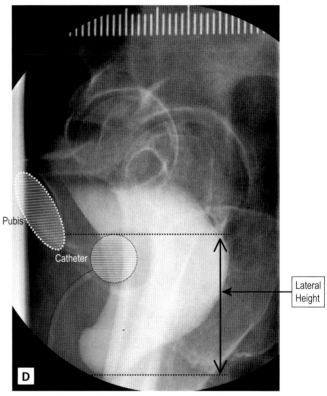

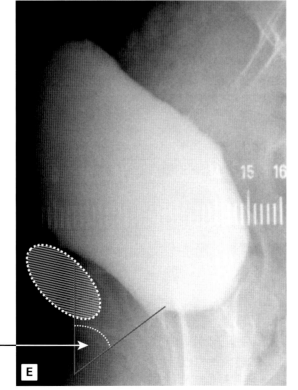

Figure 19b.1 Anterior vaginal wall suspension (AVWS).
(**A**) Cystocele coming towards introitus at rest. Exposure is facilitated by a Lone Star™ retractor and a weighted speculum. The level of the bladder neck is marked transversely, and two oblique incision lines delineate the lateral edges of the in situ anterior vaginal wall plate. (**B**) On each side, two sets of permanent suspension sutures (labeled) have been passed helically in the vaginal wall to support a broad segment of the vaginal plate. These sutures will then be transferred suprapubically under finger-tip guidance with a ligature carrier. (**C**) After tying the four suspension sutures with minimal tension, the anterior vaginal wall plate (still in dashed outline) appears well supported. Support of the anterior vaginal wall will return the bladder neck and bladder base to their normal anatomic position. (**D**) Preoperative standing, voiding cystourethrogram (VCUG) with lateral view during straining. Bladder base is seen to descend 5 cm below the symphysis pubis (dashed line represents lower edge of pubis). The angle of the urethra is noted over the catheter, and is approximately 60° with respect to the vertical. (**E**) Postoperative straining, lateral view VCUG in same patient 6 months following AVWS. The symphysis pubis is outlined. The urethral support and bladder base have returned to normal.

199

ligaments. The most proximal suture incorporates the cardinal and uterosacral ligaments, which are thought to be the strongest anchoring points. The sutures are then transferred retropubically in an identical fashion, tied at the level of the rectus fascia first, then tied to each other over a 1 cm fascial bridge.[13]

ANTERIOR VAGINAL WALL SUSPENSION. Experience with and principles learned from the techniques described above led to the development of the anterior vaginal wall suspension (AVWS). The AVWS incorporates suture placement over a broad area of vaginal wall to prevent suture pull-through, and tightens the vaginal wall hammock by excising vaginal flaps laterally to eliminate potential for recurrence of midline cystocele.

Technique. The vaginal cuff (after hysterectomy) or anterior cervical crease is tagged with three stay sutures (one midline and two 1.5 cm lateral on each side). Two longitudinal incisions are made in the anterior vaginal wall from just lateral to the bladder neck to each lateral marking suture. This leaves an in situ trapezoidal vaginal plate beneath the bladder neck and bladder base to be used for support. The plate dimensions, on average, are 2.5–3 cm in width distally, 3–4 cm in width proximally, and 4–8 cm in vaginal length. The vaginal flaps lateral to the incisions are dissected off the underlying bladder wall using low-current electrocautery to minimize blood loss. These flaps correspond to the site of the lateral defect and can be excised according to the degree of redundancy.

The in situ vaginal plate is divided into four quadrants with a marking pen. No. 1 polypropylene sutures are passed helically beneath the vaginal mucosa to incorporate a broad segment of vaginal wall in each quadrant and then are tagged separately (Fig. 19b.1B). Alternatively, a single set on each side may be sufficient if the vaginal plate is short in length. A 3 cm transverse incision is then made one fingertip above the pubis on the midline. The tendinous insertion of the rectus fascia on the back of the symphysis pubis is exposed, and the wound is packed with antibiotic gauze.

Returning to the vaginal incisions, the endopelvic fascia is perforated and the retropubic space is entered on each side using blunt dissection. Sharp dissection using Metzenbaum scissors may be necessary if scar tissue is encountered from prior repair. Once the retropubic space is free and with the bladder fully drained, a double-pronged ligature carrier is then passed under fingertip guidance from the suprapubic incision down into the vagina. If four sets of sutures are used, the carrier is passed twice on each side. After IV indigo carmine is administered, cystoscopy documents that no bladder or ureteral injury has occurred. The vaginal incisions are closed with running absorbable sutures (Fig. 19b.1C). Each suspension suture is clamped at least 2 cm above the fascia with a rubber-shod right angle clamp, and tied under no tension. Excessive tension is avoided by vaginal examination, which confirms a flat plate anteriorly with a posterior slant at the apex.[14] Respecting the configuration of the anterior and upper vagina may avoid secondary vault prolapse or enterocele.

Results. Results of bladder suspension procedures are summarized in Table 19b.2. Due to evolution of technique, long-term data greater than 10 years are not yet available. Results differ with regard to anatomic outcome, continence status, and outcome measure (supine physical exam or standing voiding cystourethrogram). Most studies have used

Table 19b.2	Results of anterior suspension repairs for cystocele					
Author (yr)	n	Type of suspension	Mean follow-up (mos)	Recurrence definition	Recurrent cystocele
Raz (1989)[9]	107	Four-corner	24	Physical exam (B-W ≥grade 2)	2%
Juma (1995)[14]	10	AVWS	30	PE (not defined)	10%
Dmochowski (1997)[10]	47	Four-corner	37	PE (3rd party, ≥grade 2), and VCUG (bladder descent below pubic bone)	40% (grade 1) 17% (grade 2)
Bai (2002)[21]	42	Six-corner	12	PE (POP-Q <stage II)	30%
Costantini (2002)[19]	37	Four-corner	62	PE (B-W ≥grade 2)	0% (preoperative grade 1,2) 39% (preoperative grade 3)

AVWS: Anterior Vaginal Wall Suspension, B-W: Baden-Walker Halfway Classification System, PE: Physical Exam, VCUG: Voiding Cystourethrogram, POP-Q: Pelvic Organ Prolapse Quantification, NR: Not Reported

a cystocele of Baden-Walker grade 2 (prolapse at the introitus with straining) or higher to define recurrence, though physical examination by the author alone may be biased, as reflected in one study noting a lower rate of success using an independent examiner.[10]

In one study by Showalter et al, the lateral height of 52 patients with grade 1–2 cystocele was measured before and after AVWS, noting statistically significant improvement in lateral height on video cystourethrogram (VCUG) 3–6 months postoperatively.[15] Representative pre- and postoperative VCUG images are provided in Figures 19b.1D,E. However, both physical examination and imaging modalities suffer from the lack of a standardized and reproducible technique for straining.[10]

Beyond the assessment of anatomic repair, issues regarding voiding function, sexual function, patient satisfaction, and overall quality of life (QOL) were seldom addressed in these studies. Based on a mailed questionnaire, Lemack et al reported the number of women sexually active following AVWS to be equal to those active preoperatively. They noted a 20% rate of postoperative dyspareunia but this was decreased from a preoperative rate of 29%.[16] In regard to patient satisfaction, at 37 months mean follow-up Dmochowski et al reported 33/47 (70%) of women who stated they would be willing to undergo the same procedure again.[10]

Complications. The most frequent complications encountered during bladder suspension procedures, namely bleeding and bladder injury, are related to retropubic dissection and needle passage. The reported transfusion rate following transvaginal suspension is estimated at 3%.[17] Unrecognized suture passage through the bladder or urethra, or secondary migration can result in stone formation over the exposed suture and/or recurrent UTI. During cystoscopy, careful inspection with a 70° lens may avoid this complication.

Voiding dysfunction following bladder suspension, either de novo urgency and/or bladder outlet obstruction, may occur in 5% of cases.[17]

Persistent suprapubic pain is uncommon and can be due to sutures tied too tight over the rectus fascia or entrapment of the genitofemoral nerve following passage of the carrier too far lateral. In such cases, osteitis pubis should be considered, particularly in cases using bone anchors. The exact incidence of osteitis pubis is difficult to determine due to a lack of consensus about its definition.[18] Plain films may be suggestive but often bone scan or MRI is necessary to confirm the diagnosis.

Secondary vault and/or posterior compartment prolapse has been reported at less than 10% in two series.[10,19] Extrusion of suture through the vaginal wall, quoted at less than 2%, is a minor complication, often asymptomatic and usually requiring only local excision.[19,20]

Abdominal and laparoscopic repair

BURCH COLPOSUSPENSION

Goal. First described by Burch in 1961 as a modification of the Marshall-Marchetti-Kranz (MMK), the goal of this procedure is to suspend the bladder neck and urethra by several interrupted sutures secured to Cooper's ligament bilaterally, thus restoring support to the distal anterior vaginal wall. Although historically regarded as an anti-incontinence procedure, the Burch has been described as a means of repairing a low-grade cystocele as well.

Technique. The colposuspension is commonly performed through a short Pfannenstiel incision, often as an adjunctive procedure to an abdominal hysterectomy or a mesh sacrocolpopexy. After the retropubic space is entered, the bladder neck is identified by the Foley catheter balloon. A finger or lubricated sponge clamp is placed in the vagina to tent up the lateral wall. Usually 2–3 nonabsorbable or delayed-absorbable sutures are placed in the vaginal submucosa on each side, lateral to the proximal urethra and bladder neck. Cystoscopy confirms no injury to the urethra, bladder neck or ureters. Each suture is transfixed through Cooper's ligament before being tied. Elevation of the vaginal wall to the level of Cooper's ligament was portrayed in Burch's original drawings, but this resulted in an overcorrected urethra and provoked secondary voiding difficulties. To provide support without overcorrection, it is now common to leave a suture bridge between the vaginal wall and the ligament (Fig. 19b.2).

Results. The Burch procedure is traditionally employed for the surgical repair of stress incontinence, but may be an option as an isolated procedure for mild-to-moderate (grade 1–2) cystocele, particularly in the patient with a short anterior vaginal wall.[22] However, the Burch procedure may be performed in conjunction with other prolapse repairs,

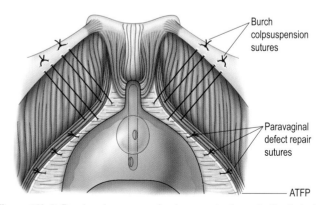

Figure 19b.2 Burch colposuspension/paravaginal repair. Cephalad view of pelvis showing final support of bladder base and urethra after placement of sutures in Cooper's ligament (Burch colposuspension) and in ATFP (paravaginal defect repair). (Modified with permission from Miklos JR, Kohli N. Urology 2000;56:64–69.[37])

such as anterior colporrhaphy or paravaginal repair.[23] Results are summarized in Table 19b.3, which includes type and number of adjunctive prolapse procedures, as well as outcomes on continence.

LAPAROSCOPIC COLPOSUSPENSION. The retropubic approach of the Burch lends itself to laparoscopic application of the open technique while avoiding the morbidity of an abdominal incision.

Technique. A three-port approach is commonly used via either a transperitoneal or extraperitoneal route. The retropubic space of Retzius is first dissected free on each side. As with the open procedure, nonabsorbable sutures are passed through the vaginal wall at the level of the bladder neck and proximal urethra. Once bladder or ureteral injury is excluded by cystoscopy, the sutures are fixed to Cooper's ligament and tied intra- or extracorporeally with a knot pusher. To avoid excessive tension on the bladder neck, elevation of the urethrovesical axis can be monitored through the vagina during laparoscopic tying. Several techniques for this have been published, including Q-tip test[21] and measuring the distance between the bladder neck and superior symphysis pubis.[24]

RESULTS. There is scant information regarding anatomic outcome following laparoscopic Burch procedure, as most series focus on continence alone. Although short-term data have shown comparable outcomes to that of the abdominal approach, long-term data on continence have not been as promising.[24-26] McDougall et al noted that following laparoscopic Burch, only 30% of 58 patients were completely continent at a mean follow-up of 45 months.[25] Complication rates, however, have not been reported to be significantly different from open repair.[27]

Complications. Bleeding from pelvic veins during retropubic dissection or vaginal suture placement can lead to transfusion, with a rate of 5% quoted in a large literature review.[17] Proponents of the laparoscopic approach argue that the pneumoperitoneum tamponades venous bleeding, leading to decreased blood loss.[28] Decreased bleeding during laparoscopy, however, may be detrimental to retropubic scar formation and may explain the lower continence rates reported after laparoscopic Burch.

Overcorrection of the urethrovesical junction following Burch colposuspension may lead to bladder outlet obstruction with urinary retention or de novo urge incontinence. Rates of postoperative urinary retention are similar to those of transvaginal suspension procedures at 4–5%, while de novo urgency or detrusor overactivity after Burch procedure has been reported to occur in 11–17% of patients.[17,29]

Alteration of the anterior vaginal axis may expose the apical and posterior compartments to rises in abdominal pressure, thus predisposing to vault prolapse, enterocele or rectocele. Secondary pelvic organ prolapse following isolated Burch urethropexy has been estimated at 18–33%.[29,30] Although posterior compartment defects (rectocele, enterocele) are initially the most common, secondary anterior compartment defects have been reported in longer follow-up series.[30]

PARAVAGINAL REPAIR

Goal. The goal of the paravaginal repair is to attach the lateral vaginal wall to the arcus tendineus fascia pelvis (ATFP) to correct a lateral defect.[33] The procedure is most often performed abdominally, though vaginal techniques have been reported.[34,35]

Technique. The abdominal approach is similar to that described for the open Burch colposuspension. The ATFP,

Author (yr)	n	Mean follow-up (mo/yr)	Adjunctive procedures	Recurrence definition	Recurrent cystocele
Sekine (1999)[23]	14	40 mo	AC (6)	No change on bead-chain cystogram at 3 months	29% (Burch + AC) 50% (Burch only)
Colombo (2000)[31]	35	14.2 yr, RCT	USLF (35), Culdoplasty (17)	PE (B-W ≥grade 2)	34%
Lovatsis (2001)[22]	189	2.3 yr	USLF (57), SCP (1)	PE (B-W grade 0)	36% (at 5 years)
Cugudda (2002)[32]	14	53 mo	AC (4)	PE ("no vaginal prolapse")	11%

Table 19b.3 Anatomic and functional results of Burch colposuspension for cystocele repair

USLF: Uterosacral Ligament Fixation, PE: Physical Exam, AC: Anterior Colporrhaphy, B-W: Baden-Walker Halfway Classification System, NR: Not Reported, RCT: Randomized, Controlled Trial

or "white line," is identified along the medial border of the obturator internus muscle, extending from the posterior pubic symphysis to the ischial spine on each side. Elevation of the anterior vagina by the surgeon's finger may help identify a discrete lateral detachment. A series of 4–6 interrupted, nonabsorbable sutures are passed through the lateral vaginal wall to suspend it to the ATFP, starting distally in the posterior pubourethral ligament and ending near the ischial spine (see Fig. 19b.2).[33] The original series described the middle suture on each side passing through Cooper's ligament for additional support.

When performed using the vaginal approach, a midline anterior vaginal wall incision is made from the bladder neck to the vaginal apex. The dissection is carried out laterally until the retropubic space is reached, then extended along the inferior ramus of the pubis.[33] A fiberoptic light source is helpful for visualization of the retropubic space. The obturator internus muscle is identified as well as the condensation of the ATFP. A long, straight needle passer is used to place a series of nonabsorbable sutures in the ATFP, extending from just anterior to the ischial spine to the pubic bone. Each suture incorporates the ATFP and fascia of the obturator internus muscle and is left untied prior to passage through the lateral periurethral fascia and vaginal wall. Following cystoscopy as described previously, the sutures are tied sequentially from distal to proximal, and the vaginal incision is closed with running, absorbable sutures.

The laparoscopic paravaginal repair has been described using a transperitoneal approach, and parallels that of the open technique. Once the space of Retzius is entered and bluntly dissected to expose the ATFP, the vaginal wall is secured to the white line bilaterally using 2–4 nonabsorbable sutures or mesh.[36] If a colposuspension is being performed for SUI, the paravaginal repair is completed first to avoid overelevation of the Burch sutures at the bladder neck.[37]

Results. The anatomic outcomes following paravaginal repair using different approaches are summarized in Table 19b.4. Despite limited follow-up of a small number of patients, most series report low recurrence rates for cystocele. However, definitions of recurrence are vague or poorly explained in many series, using only supine physical examination for evaluation. Adjunctive procedures for concomitant SUI are common, as the paravaginal repair alone has not demonstrated long-term, durable success for incontinence in one randomized trial.[35,38]

Complications. As with the Burch colposuspension, bleeding requiring transfusion has been reported at between 0% and 16%,[33-35] with lower rates for the laparoscopic approach. Reported blood loss in series using the vaginal approach may be slightly higher, though this has not been examined in comparison to the abdominal approach.[35,39]

The bladder and ureters are susceptible to injury or obstruction during passage of vaginal wall sutures at or proximal to the bladder neck. This is relatively rare, as one large series of 171 laparoscopic paravaginal repairs noted a 2.3% bladder injury rate with no cases of ureteral compromise.[37] Although not performed in the original series,[33] cystoscopy has been described in later reports to help recognize any urinary tract injury intraoperatively.[40]

Table 19b.4 Anatomic and functional results of paravaginal repair

Author (yr)	n	Approach	Mean follow-up (mos)	Adjunctive procedures	Recurrence definition	Recurrent cystocele
Shull (1989)[33]	149	Abdominal	NR	AC (7), "abdominal cystocele repair" (5)*	PE (no change from preop B-W exam)	5%
Bruce (1999)[42]	52	Abdominal	61	Rectus muscle sling (27)	PE (lateral defect cystocele)	8%
Shull (1994)[41]	62	Transvaginal	20	AC (62)	PE (B-W ≥grade 2)	8%
Scotti (1998)[35]	40	Transvaginal	39	Burch (35) SCP (27) AC (27)	PE (No bulge or minimal descent, NY)	9%
Young (2001)[34]	100	Transvaginal	11	AC (100)	PE (B-W <grade 1)	2% 22% (midline)
Mallipeddi (2001)[39]	45	Transvaginal	20	AC/PC (45), SSLF (12)	PE (B-W ≥grade 1)	3%
Washington (2003)[36]	12	Laparoscopic	12	Culdoplasty (12)	ΔBA on POP-Q	18%

PE: Physical Exam, AC: Anterior Colporrhaphy, PC: Posterior Colporrhaphy, POP-Q: Pelvic Organ Prolapse Quantification, BW: Baden-Walker Halfway Classification System, SCP: Sacrocolpopexy, NY: New York Classification System (similar to POP-Q), NR: Not Reported, SSLF: Sacrospinous Ligament Fixation, ΔBA: Change in Point of Greatest Descent on Anterior Vaginal Wall, *Done for Concurrent Midline Defects

Secondary prolapse, particularly a midline cystocele defect, is a concern as the focus of support is laterally, rather than in the midline. Not surprisingly, a 22% midline cystocele recurrence was noted in one study. Concomitant transvaginal midline plication was mentioned in several reports.[35,39,41] Development of apical or posterior compartment prolapse following paravaginal repair is estimated at between 2% and 11% in larger studies.[33,35]

High-grade cystocele

ANTERIOR COLPORRHAPHY

Goal. The procedures listed thus far have addressed early-grade cystoceles generally due to lateral defects bilaterally. Closure of the central defect through which the bladder base is herniating is the goal of the Kelly type plication, which is the most practiced form of anterior colporrhaphy (AC). Although generally indicated for large cystocele repair, a limited colporrhaphy, particularly at the bladder neck, has been used as a primary repair for stress incontinence.

Technique. A midline anterior vaginal wall incision is made, starting at the bladder neck and extending to the vaginal apex in the posthysterectomy patient. Two lateral flaps are elevated off the bladder wall to expose the midline defect beneath the bladder base. If the hernia is easily reducible, it is repaired with a series of interrupted, Lembert or purse-string absorbable suture(s) to plicate the pubocervical fascia over the midline (Fig. 19b.3).[43] Some authors have not found this to be a discrete fascial layer, but rather a fibromuscular layer of the vaginal wall itself.[32,44] In larger hernias, in older patients with weak tissues or in patients undergoing simultaneous lateral defect repair, identification of this tissue and satisfactory midline plication may be challenging.

Cystoscopy is recommended, as direct injury or overplication of the trigone can obstruct one or both ureters. In addition to visualizing bilateral ureteral efflux, the bladder neck and urethra should be carefully examined to exclude significant distortion, which may result in bladder outlet obstruction. Depending on the degree of known or expected sexual activity, redundant vaginal mucosa is excised before the midline vaginal incision is closed with running absorbable sutures.

Variations of this technique include the "goalpost" technique, during which two parallel, longitudinal incisions are made on each side of the midurethra to 1 cm proximal to the bladder neck (the posts).[45] Then, a crossbar incision is created by connecting the proximal ends of the posts, followed by a midline incision from the midpoint of the crossbar to the vaginal cuff or anterior cervix (Fig. 19b.4). This incision allows for a combined bladder neck suspension (lateral support) and anterior colporrhaphy (midline support). The parallel incisions create a short distal vaginal plate, which is suspended as previously described for the four-corner suspension and acts as a support for the bladder

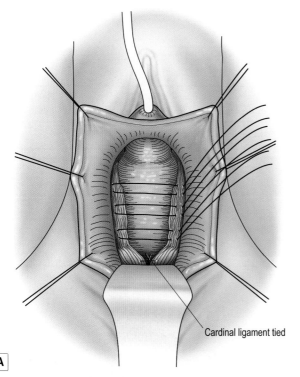

Cardinal ligament tied

A

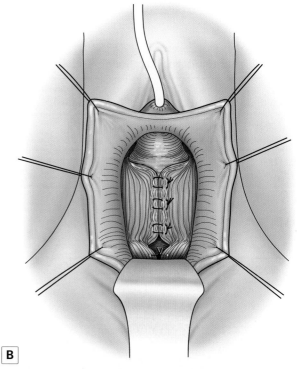

B

Figure 19b.3 Anterior Colporrhaphy. After reduction of the cystocele superiorly, sutures are placed to close the central herniation **(A)** by reapproximating the pubocervical fascia over the midline **(B)**. (Reproduced with permission from Raz S, et al. J Urol 1991;146:988–992.[46])

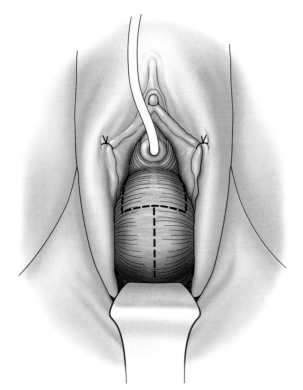

Figure 19b.4 Goalpost incision for large cystocele. Anterior vaginal wall incision ("goalpost") for combined bladder neck suspension and anterior colporrhaphy in repair of large cystocele with urethral hypermobility. (Reproduced with permission from Safir M, et al. J Urol 1999;161:587–594.[45])

tems, the anterior colporrhaphy appears to yield a moderate rate of cystocele recurrence, ranging from 3–43% (Table 19b.5). Nonetheless, most series examine small populations retrospectively and rarely extend beyond 2 years. One randomized controlled trial has shown AC to be superior to the Burch procedure for repair of the grade 2–3 cystocele.[31] Adjunctive antiincontinence procedures are common in several reports, although one study suggests that cystocele recurrence rates may be higher when a concomitant bladder neck suspension is performed, compared to AC alone.[44]

Complications. Ureteral injury, via kinking of the intramural ureters medially or direct ligation, is rare and recognizable by performing an intraoperative cystoscopy to confirm ureteral patency. If ureteral obstruction or injury is suspected, the plicated fascia should be reopened and bilateral efflux confirmed by cystoscopy. On occasion, ureteral stents may be necessary to complete the operation safely.

Tight plication of the cystocele too far distally runs the risk of obstructing the bladder neck, leading to voiding dysfunction and possibly urinary retention requiring prolonged catheterization, which has been reported in 2–3% of cases.[46,47] Ischemic necrosis of these tissues may result in the rare but distressing complication of vesicovaginal, ureterovaginal or urethrovaginal fistula.

Vaginal narrowing following tight anterior plication can significantly compromise sexual function postoperatively. To ensure adequate vaginal caliber at completion of the case, the introitus should accommodate three fingerbreadths, estimated at 10–12 cm in diameter, which is considered adequate for intercourse.[48]

Secondary complications include midline cystocele recurrence and stress incontinence. In the case of an

neck and proximal urethra. The midline posterior incision allows access to the pubocervical fascia for midline plication to support the bladder base.

Results. Based on physical examination alone, often performed by the authors themselves and using different staging sys-

Table 19b.5   Outcomes for anterior colporrhaphy

Author (yr)	n	Mean follow-up (mo/yr)	Adjunctive surgery	Recurrence definition	Recurrent cystocele
Raz (1991)[46]	46	34 mo	Four-corner suspension (46)	PE (B-W grade ≥2)	7%
Kohli (1996)[44]	27	13 mo	AC alone	PE (B-W grade ≥1)	7%
	40	13 mo	AC + BNS	32%	
Cross (1997)[43]	36	20 mo	Pubovaginal sling	PE (B-W grade ≥1)	8%
Colombo (2000)[31]	33	13.9 yr, RCT	AC vs Burch; USLF, PC	PE (grade 2-3 cystocele)	3%
Sand (2001)[50]	70	12 mo, RCT	AC alone vs AC + mesh	PE (B-W ≥grade 2)	43%
Weber (2001)[47]	33	23 mo, RCT	AC alone vs AC + mesh	PE (POP-Q ≥stage II)	30%
Cugudda (2002)[32]	18	53 mo	Burch (5)	VCUG (not defined)	17%
deTayrac (2002)[51]	28	36 mo	None	PE (not defined)	7%

B-W: Baden-Walker Halfway Classification System, BNS: Bladder Neck Suspension, RCT: Randomized, Controlled Trial, USLF: Uterosacral Ligament Fixation, PC: Posterior Colporrhaphy, NR: Not Reported

unrecognized lateral defect preoperatively, the midline plication may, in fact, aggravate the lateral detachment and cause a secondary cystocele recurrence.[42] Occult stress incontinence may be unmasked in 8–22% of patients following repair of a high-grade cystocele.[49]

NONSYNTHETIC GRAFT INTERPOSITION

Goal. The high recurrence rate seen after primary repair for large cystocele has prompted a search for tissue interposition. Cadaveric dermis or fascia lata, as well as graft materials from nonhuman species (xenograft), have been used for large cystocele repair, alone or in combination with pubovaginal sling.

Technique. The approach is similar to the anterior colporrhaphy, using a midline vaginal incision from the midurethra to the apex or anterior cervix. The bladder and urethra are dissected off the anterior vaginal wall and mobilized to perforate the endopelvic fascia on each side and enter the retropubic space.[52] A single 6 × 8 cm patch of graft material can be configured into a T-shape, using the narrow distal portion to support the bladder neck and urethra, while the "cross" of the T is used to support the bladder base. Graft size may vary depending on patient anatomy and surgeon preference. The corners of the graft are folded on them-

selves to prevent suture pull-through, and the sling portion is secured with bone anchors attached to nonabsorbable sutures.[53] The base of the patch is secured to the medial edge of the levator muscles bilaterally with absorbable sutures[53] or to the ATFP with interrupted delayed-absorbable sutures to correct the cystocele.[54] The midline vaginal incision is closed after cystoscopy with indigo carmine is performed to exclude urinary tract injury.

Results. The vast majority of the published data on grafts for cystocele repair originate from case series, with relatively short follow-up. The success of the tissue interposition is partially credited to surrounding tissue ingrowth which further stabilizes the repair, and early reports show promise (Table 19b.6). However, these results are confounded by varying surgical techniques, graft material used, and definitions of failure. Long-term data on the durability of cadaveric or xenograft tissue have yet to be generated.

SYNTHETIC REPAIR. The advantages of synthetic material (mesh) over other grafts include decreased cost and elimination of the concern for viral or proteinaceous particle transmission. However, as with any nonautologous tissue, the risk of infection or erosion is higher, and the impact of the use of synthetics on voiding, defecatory or sexual function

Table 19b.6	Outcomes of cystocele repair with nonautologous (graft, synthetic) material				
Author	**n**	**Material**	**Mean follow-up (mos)**	**Recurrence definition**	**Recurrence rate**
Julian (1996)[55]	12	Marlex mesh	24	PE (B-W ≥grade 2); two examiners	0%
Safir (1999)[45]	112	Polyglycolic acid*	21	PE (B-W >grade 2)	8%
Sand (2001)[50]	73	Polyglycolic acid*	12, RCT	PE (B-W >grade 2)	22%
Weber (2001)[47]	35	Polyglycolic acid*	23.3, RCT	PE (point Aa at stage 0 or I)	58%
Groutz (2001)[56]	21	Cadaveric fascia lata	20.1	PE ("recurrent prolapse")	0%
Kobashi(2002)[53]	172	Cadaveric fascia lata	12.4	PE (B-W ≥grade 1)	12.9%
Chung (2002)[57]	19	Cadaveric dermal allograft	28	PE or fluorourodynamics	11%
Powell (2004)[58]	58	Cadaveric fascia lata	24.7	PE (POP-Q ≥stage II)	19%
Gomelsky (2004)[54]	70	Porcine dermal xenograft (Pelvicol)	24	PE (B-W ≥grade 2)	8.6% (grade 2) 4.3% (grade 3)
Leboeuf (2004)[59]	19	Porcine dermal xenograft (Pelvicol)	15	PE (B-W ≥ grade 2), SEAPI test	15%

PE: Physical Exam, B-W: Baden-Walker Halfway Classification System, POP-Q: Pelvic Organ Prolapse Quantification, RCT: Randomized, Controlled Trial, *Absorbable (Vicryl) mesh

has not yet been studied. A "tension-free" technique has been advocated by some to minimize the risk of erosion or secondary enterocele.[60]

Recent data have emerged on mesh selection based on ultrastructural properties, with fewer complications noted for type I meshes (e.g. Marlex, Prolene), which are macro-porous (>75 μ pore width) and allow bacteria as well as macrophages into the spaces.[61,62] Multifilamentous mesh contains interstices <10 μ wide, which may harbor bacteria, restrict macrophage entrance, and lead to higher infection rates.

While reports of synthetic material in the vaginal repair of cystocele are emerging, much remains unknown regarding long-term outcomes. In light of the scarcity of data that exists at this time regarding the safety and efficacy of synthetic materials, one must proceed with caution in the use of mesh for vaginal repair of cystocele outside the setting of a controlled, randomized trial.[63]

Lastly, two recent randomized trials, looking at the role of an absorbable mesh in cystocele repair, deserve specific mention. Weber et al randomized 109 patients to AC with or without absorbable Vicryl mesh, and found no statistically significant improvement in recurrence rate (defined as point Aa or Ba at stage II (−1 cm or lower) unchanged or worse from preoperative staging) or symptom resolution between the two groups at 23 months follow-up.[47] However, at 1 year follow-up, Sand et al found a significant decrease in cystocele recurrence (defined as descent to the midvaginal plane or hymenal ring) in 160 women randomized to AC with polyglactin mesh versus those who underwent AC alone.[50] However, this difference in outcomes may be related to a stricter definition of recurrence followed in the former study.

VAGINAL VAULT PROLAPSE REPAIR

Vaginal vault prolapse (VVP) may present in conjunction with uterine prolapse or years following hysterectomy as a vaginal mass or bulge, often asymptomatic. In the presence of a coexisting anterior or posterior compartment prolapse, there may be associated voiding or defecatory dysfunction. The indications for surgical intervention are dictated mainly by patient symptomatology, severity, and degree of sexual activity, though some women may choose a nonoperative approach, such as pessary placement, when it is effective.

The vaginal approach is usually the first option considered, as it is associated with decreased morbidity and faster recovery. This is particularly relevant in the older woman (>65 years), who is more likely to present with this condition. Vaginal mucosal ulceration associated with long-standing, high-grade vault prolapse mandates a vaginal approach, and local estrogen therapy should be administered

for 4–6 weeks preoperatively to improve tissue quality. Abdominal repair may be offered as a primary procedure in younger patients, those with a foreshortened vagina or as a secondary procedure in those who have failed prior vaginal repair.[64] The desire for uterine preservation in the younger woman, and uterine size or other pathology in those undergoing hysterectomy, may also influence the surgical approach.

Vaginal repair. All vaginal repair procedures address apical prolapse by plication of or fixation to surrounding structures to restore normal vaginal axis, position, and function. Historically, the McCall culdoplasty was the first technique described for repair of vault prolapse, and it is still in use today.

MCCALL (MAYO) CULDOPLASY
Goal. In the initial series, this technique was described as an adjunct to the vaginal hysterectomy to obliterate the pouch of Douglas by a series of continuous sutures to correct an enterocele, and support the vaginal apex.[65] It is most commonly used today to prevent enterocele formation after vaginal hysterectomy.

Technique. A midline vaginal incision is made from the apex posteriorly. The enterocele sac is identified and inverted. With the patient in Trendelenburg position, a nonabsorbable suture is passed 2 cm above the cut edge of one of the uterosacral ligaments, which can be tagged at the time of hysterectomy. This same suture is passed several times through the redundant enterocele sac, then through the contralateral uterosacral ligament. An additional 2–3 interrupted sutures are passed in similar fashion and held without tying. Between these sutures, a series of through-and-through absorbable sutures including the uterosacral ligaments and vaginal wall are placed, with the highest suture at the vaginal apex to preserve vaginal length. The upper third of the vagina is ultimately supported in a presacral position over the levator plate.

Results. A large series from the Mayo Clinic of 693 patients operated on for vault prolapse with a minimum 5-year follow-up showed durable success with good support throughout the vagina in 89% and secondary anterior or posterior prolapse requiring repair in 6%.[66]

Complications. The risk of ureteral obstruction or injury with this procedure is not mentioned in the original series but is a concern, particularly with placement of the highest suture in the vaginal apex. Comiter et al reported one ureteric obstruction in 104 patients who underwent transvaginal culdosuspension using a similar technique.[67]

SACROSPINOUS LIGAMENT FIXATION

Goal. The goal of the sacrospinous ligament fixation (SSLF), first described by Richter in 1968,[68] is to use the sacrospinous ligament, which extends from the sacrum to the ischial spine, as an anchoring point to suspend the vaginal apex.

Technique. If a hysterectomy or other prolapse repair is required, this is performed first. The posterior vaginal wall is incised in the midline over the entire prolapse segment. Blunt and sharp dissection is used to perforate the right prerectal fascia for a right-handed surgeon in a unilateral repair. The sacrospinous ligament is palpated as a cord-like structure within the body of the coccygeus muscle. Access to the ligament may require a headlight or fiberoptic lighted-tip suction catheter, and/or Breisky-Navratil retractors to retract the peritoneal contents superiorly and the rectum medially.[69]

The challenge of suture passage into the ligament deep in the pelvis has led to the development of special instruments, some of which rely on direct vision of the area, including the Miya hook and the Deschamps ligature carrier. The Capio device is a laparoscopic instrument that relies on finger guidance for suture passage.[70] In all cases, 1–2 nonabsorbable sutures are passed from top down into the ligament two fingerbreadths medial to the ischial spine.[71] Important structures to avoid include the sciatic nerve and pudendal nerves and vessels, which are found superolateral and posterior to the sacrospinous ligament (Fig. 19b.5).

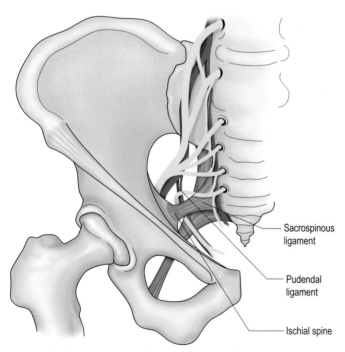

Figure 19b.5 Sacrospinous ligament fixation. Illustration demonstrating the sacrospinous ligament and surrounding vascular and neural structures at risk for injury during suture placement in the sacrospinous ligament fixation procedure. (Reproduced with permission from Cespedes RD. Urology 2000;56:70–75.[71])

The sutures are then passed through the vaginal submucosa and tied outside the vagina prior to excision of redundant vaginal wall and closure. If the knot cannot be safely tied outside the vagina, slow-absorbable sutures may be used. The distance between the vaginal wall and the ligament often precludes tying these fixation sutures without tension. Ideally, the vaginal apex is tied flush to the ligament but if vaginal length does not allow for tying without tension, a suture bridge is left. Interposition of a local vaginal strip to avoid this problem has been reported.[72] Bilateral fixation has been reported but is technically challenging due to the risk of excessive tension on the vaginal cuff,[71] and in one prospective study was able to be completed in only 26/40 (65%) of patients with uterine or vault prolapse.[73]

Results. Results from several series with varying lengths of follow-up are summarized in Table 19b.7. In most published reports, vault prolapse was associated with prior hysterectomy and tended to be high grade with multiple associated prolapse defects. Recurrence rates are based on physical examination alone with differing definitions. In one prospective randomized trial, the SSLF matched the mesh sacro-colpopexy results for repair of vault prolapse, although the appearance of secondary prolapse in other compartments was slightly higher for the SSLF.[74]

Complications. Vascular injury, particularly to the inferior gluteal and pudendal vessels which are located superior and behind the ligament, may lead to transfusion, with rates ranging from 0.6% to 16%.[75-78] In one study, mean blood loss with the SSLF procedure was reported to be higher than for sacrocolpopexy or uterosacral ligament fixation.[79]

Neural injury or entrapment following SSLF should be suspected if a patient complains of gluteal pain or numbness postoperatively. The incidence is not uniformly reported but has been estimated to occur in 2–7% of procedures.[71,79] In the majority of cases, symptoms are transient and can be managed conservatively.

The occurrence of secondary cystocele after SSLF has been reported in up to 20% of cases. This may be due to excessive posterior deviation of the vaginal axis, opening the anterior vaginal wall to rises in intraabdominal pressures. Following SSLF in 122 women, Nieminen et al noted recurrent prolapse in 26 (21%), 10 of which were symptomatic, with the most common prolapse being cystocele in 14 (11%).[80] Of these, six patients (5%) were reoperated for prolapse. However, one retrospective review of a large cohort of patients suggested that SSLF by itself is not associated with an increased risk of de novo cystocele compared to those who underwent other prolapse repairs without SSLF or anterior repair.[81]

With regard to sexual function, the majority of the data rely on a small subset of patients, as women undergoing

Labels on figure:
Sacrospinous ligament
Pudendal ligament
Ischial spine

Table 19b.7   Results for sacrospinous ligament fixation for vaginal vault prolapse

Author (Yr)	n	Mean F/U (mos)	Adjunctive Procedures	Definition of Recurrence	Recurrence (%)
Richter (1981)[84]	81	NR	None	PE ("ideal results"—no other prolapse)	36%
Morley (1988)[76]	100	8, 4.3 Yr*	AC (7), PC (30), AC + PC (30)	PE (objective), postal questionnaire (subjective)	4%
Cespedes (2000)[71]	28	17	AC (28), rectocele (28), enterocele (28), PVS (25)	PE (B-W grade 1)	4%
Giberti (2001)[85]	12	16	AC (8), PC (9), enterocele (1)	PE (not defined)	8%
Nieminen (2001)[77]	25	33	AC (23), PC (16)	PE (B-W ≥grade 2)	11%
Cruikshank (2003)[75]	173 221	43	AC (15) AC (43), PC(22), PVS(75)	PE (mild, moderate, severe) at rest PE (B-W at rest + Valsalva, no grade defined)	12.7% 5%
	301		AC (75), PC (61), PVS (76), PVR (78)	PE (ICS)	1%
Maher (2004)[74]	48	22, RCT	PC (44), enterocele repair (28)	PE (B-W ≥grade 1)	31%
Silva-Filho (2004)[78]	158	64	None	PE (B-W <grade 2)	2.5% vault 11% total

AC: Anterior Colporrhaphy, PC: Posterior Colporrhaphy, PVS: Pubovaginal Sling, PVR: Paravaginal Repair, PE: Physical Exam, B-W: Baden-Walker Halfway Classification System, ICS: International Continence Society Classification, RCT: Randomized, Controlled Trial, *Objective Follow-Up 8 Months, Questionnaire Follow-Up 4.3 years

repair of vault prolapse tend to be older and less active sexually. The quoted incidence of new-onset dyspareunia ranges from 2.4% to 9%.[80,82] Total vaginal length has not been shown to be significantly decreased after SSLF, although there is evidence that vaginal length after mesh sacrocolpopexy is better maintained.[83] Nevertheless, the relationship between vaginal length and sexual function has not yet been clarified.[48]

UTEROSACRAL LIGAMENT FIXATION

Goal. This procedure uses the same principle as the SSLF to suspend the vaginal vault at a fixed point, in this case the uterosacral ligament, which is located medial and cephalad to the ischial spine and sacrospinous ligament.

Technique. A midline vaginal incision over the entire vaginal wall overlying the prolapsed segment is made after stay sutures are placed in the vaginal cuff. The uterosacral ligaments can be identified in a retroperitoneal position on each side of the rectum. After dissection of the enterocele sac, a No.1 nonabsorbable suture is passed through a thin portion of the peritoneum and uterosacral ligament on each side.[69] Visible movement of the proximal portion of the ligament assures secure and accurate placement of the suture. One end of each suture is passed anteriorly through peritoneum, pubocervical fascia, and vaginal epithelium, while the free end is passed through peritoneum, rectovaginal fascia, and

vaginal epithelium posteriorly with a Mayo needle. These can be left untied until all other repairs are completed. After tying the fixation sutures, cystoscopy is performed to exclude bladder injury and/or ureteral ligation. The vaginal wall is then closed with running, absorbable sutures.

Results. Cure rates for this procedure range from 67% to 90%.[69] Amundsen et al reported a mean improvement in vaginal cuff position by 7.3 cm (point C on the POP-Q system from −1.7 to −9.0 cm), with a 6% recurrence of stage II vault prolapse and 12% rectocele rate at 28 months. Shull et al followed 289 patients and found a 13% and 5% grade 1 and 2 vault prolapse recurrence, respectively.[86] Follow-up was short, however, with a mean of 12 months in those who did not recur and 25 months in those who did. Comiter et al reported an overall recurrence rate of 4% at 17.3 months follow-up.[67]

Complications. The ureters traverse the pelvis very close to the lowest, or cervical, portion of the ligaments and are at risk for injury or ligation during suture passage. This has been reported in 1.5–11% of cases[79,86,87] and must be excluded by cystoscopy as previously described. Any concern should prompt removal of one or both suspensory sutures with reevaluation or retrograde ureterogram. More extensive injuries may require ureteroneocystostomy. As the suspension suture is placed more proximally towards the sacrum, the risk of ureteral injury is lower, though this carries the drawback of decreased ligament strength.[87]

As with the sacrospinous fixation, one should be wary of hemorrhage from pelvic vessels, although the reported transfusion rate is low, ranging between 0% and 3%.[67,69,86]

Sexual function following this procedure has not been studied extensively, though the limited data suggest adequate preservation of function. Amundsen et al did note a decrease in total vaginal length by, on average, 0.9 cm following uterosacral fixation but found no cases of new-onset dyspareunia in a subset of sexually active women.[69]

LEVATOR MYORRHAPHY

Goal. The principle behind this method is to recreate the anatomy of the upper vagina resting over the levator muscle complex (Fig. 19b.6A). This technique rebuilds a strong levator plate, which acts as a broad base of support for the vaginal vault, and closes the midline defect to prevent subsequent enterocele formation.

Technique. A betadine-soaked gauze is inserted in the rectum and isolated from the rest of the field. After infiltration with saline, a midline vaginal incision is begun at the vaginal apex and extended over the vaginal bulge towards the introitus. Lateral vaginal flaps are elevated from the underlying enterocele sac and rectocele as identified by the preplaced rectal pack (Fig. 19b.6B).

Starting 3 cm above the junction of the levator and rectum, the levator muscle is reapproximated over the midline using large absorbable sutures.[88] The most distal

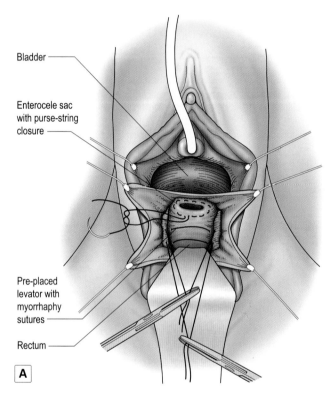

Bladder

Enterocele sac with purse-string closure

Pre-placed levator with myorrhaphy sutures

Rectum

A

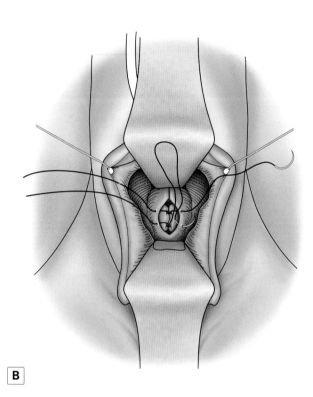

B

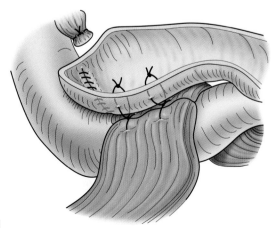

C

Figure 19b.6 High-midline levator myorrhaphy (HMLM) repair. (**A**) The enterocele sac is closed prior to placing the extraperitoneal levator myorrhaphy sutures. (**B**) Before closing the vaginal apex, the HMLM sutures are transfixed from inside-out to secure the vault to the repaired levator plate. (**C**) Sagittal view demonstrating final position and posterior angulation of the vagina after levator myorrhaphy. *Continued*

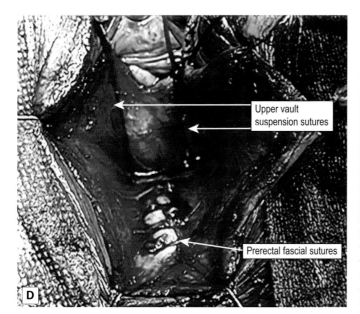

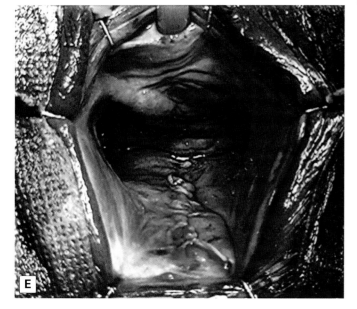

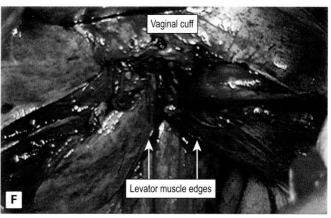

Figure 19b.6, cont'd (**D**) Extraperitoneal HMLM showing upper vault suspension procedures at vaginal apex (above), and after vaginal wall closure following a traditional posterior colporrhaphy repair (below). (**E**) Final view of repaired posterior vaginal wall after closure of vaginal mucosa. (**F**) Intraoperative pelvic view of high-midline levator myorrhaphy, with edges of levator muscles identified after midline reapproximation.

suture is placed first, proceeding proximally and posteriorly along the levator plate (Fig. 19b.6C). These are tied in sequence from distal to proximal; these sutures can be placed intraperitoneally before closure of the enterocele sac or, if the sac is dissected and not entered, they can be placed extraperitoneally (Fig. 19b.6D). Formal repair of the enterocele is discussed later in this chapter. After closure of the sac and tying of the sutures, cystoscopy is performed to verify ureteral patency.[88] Cystoscopy is recommended also for the extraperitoneal technique of levator myorrhaphy although it is recognized that the risk of ureteral injury is very much lower.

After completion of the posterior repair and perineorrhaphy when indicated, each high levator myorrhaphy suture is transfixed from inside out through the uppermost portion of the posterior vaginal wall using a free Mayo needle (Fig. 19b.6D,E). This maneuver will anchor the vagina vault to the rebuilt levator plate underneath it by direct tissue apposition. These sutures are left on stay clamps. Redundant vaginal flaps are excised according to degree of patient sexual activity and the vaginal incision is closed from the apex down with a running absorbable suture (Fig. 19b.6F). Then the levator myorrhaphy sutures are tied down on each side of the apex (vaginal apices) and the vagina is packed with an antibiotic-soaked gauze.

Results. The first 5-year data on this technique were presented in 1994 on a series of 22 patients for traction enterocele or vault prolapse, with a mean follow-up of 29 months.[89] No recurrent enterocele was observed. In a single-center review of 47 women who underwent levator myorrhaphy for vaginal vault prolapse, Lemack et al noted recurrent prolapse requiring reoperation in five (11%) patients at a mean follow-up of 27.9 months.[90] By telephone interview, 17/23 (74%) reported extreme satisfaction (>90%) with the procedure. Four of these patients (9%) had undergone at least one prior reconstructive surgery for vault prolapse. Cespedes et al followed 136 patients with grade 2–4 vault prolapse and reported recurrent grade 1 vault prolapse in five patients, resulting in a cure rate of 96% at a mean follow-up of 29 months.[91]

Complications. As with any prolapse repair, hemorrhage and ureteral injury can occur. Ureteral injuries were noted in 7/120 patients (5.8%) over a 10-year period, with five being recognized intraoperatively and managed with removal of one suture.[88] Complications unique to the levator myorrhaphy include rectal injury, pain with defecation, and sexual dysfunction. In a telephone interview of 36 patients, 14 reported themselves to be sexually active, with 11 of these (79%) reporting no discomfort during intercourse.[90]

COLPOCLEISIS

Goal. The techniques thus far described are reconstructive, designed to restore the original anatomy and position of the vagina. Elderly patients who are no longer sexually active and may not tolerate prolonged anesthesia for a reconstructive repair may be offered an obliterative procedure. The Le Fort colpocleisis is designed to correct high-grade prolapse through vaginal closure (Fig. 19b.7).[92]

Technique. With the patient in high lithotomy position, a superficial circumscribing incision is made through the vaginal mucosa at the base of the prolapse at a level adjacent to the hymenal ring.[93] The edges of the mucosa are grasped with Allis clamps and stripped off the underlying fascia using blunt and sharp dissection. Once hemostasis is obtained, the anterior and posterior fascias are approximated with absorbable sutures. To reduce the entire protruding mass, these sutures are passed through the endopelvic fascia (which may be difficult to identify), either in a sequential purse-string fashion or following an interrupted anteroposterior direction.

Results. Success rates for colpocleisis in regard to prolapse correction range from 97% to 100% at short-term follow-up.[92-95] The patient population undergoing colpocleisis for vaginal eversion are often elderly and long-term data are unavailable as many patients are lost to follow-up or die during the follow-up period.

Abdominal repair

ABDOMINAL MESH SACROCOLPOPEXY

Goal. The mesh sacrocolpopexy (MSC) is designed to correct vault prolapse but may be performed in conjunction with repair of a high-grade cystocele or a posterior compartment defect (enterocele or rectocele). The MSC can be chosen as a primary procedure or performed in women who have failed prior vault suspension procedures or other prolapse compartment repairs.

Technique. The patient is placed in low lithotomy position to allow vaginal and cystoscopic access. After the bowel contents are packed away to expose the pelvis, the posterior peritoneum is incised over the right ureter lateral to the sacral promontory and medial to the common iliac vessels. The ureter is isolated and can be placed on a vessel loop for identification. A broad peritoneal flap is raised up from the level of the promontory down to the vaginal cuff to facilitate closure over the mesh at the end of the procedure. A lubri-

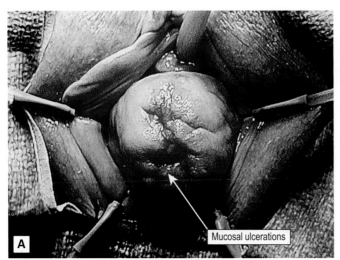
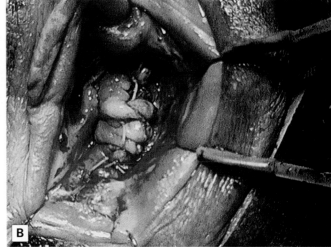

Figure 19b.7 Colpocleisis. (**A**) Complete vaginal vault prolapse with vaginal wall ulcerations (labeled) in a posthysterectomy 94-year-old woman. (**B**) Following excision of vaginal wall lining, the completed colpocleisis shows reduction of prolapse with foreshortened vagina.

SECTION 7 Treatment of pelvic organ prolapse

cated sponge clamp or vaginal dilator is helpful to elevate and mobilize the vaginal cuff during dissection of the rectum off the posterior vaginal wall.

To correct an associated high-grade cystocele, the vesicovaginal space must be entered.[96,97] This is quite possibly the most critical part of the procedure, as any perforation of the bladder or vagina may preclude mesh placement or predispose the patient to secondary infection or erosion. The plane between the vagina and bladder may be difficult to identify after a previous repair, such as an anterior colporrhaphy. The dissection of the bladder base from the anterior vaginal wall must be carried down to, but not beyond, the level of the interureteric ridge. After indigo carmine is administered intravenously, cystoscopy is performed to exclude bladder or ureteral injury.

Next, the sacral promontory is exposed, with care taken to avoid the middle sacral artery and the iliac vessels, and 1–2 nonabsorbable sutures are placed through the anterior common vertebral ligament. These pre-placed sutures will be secured at the upper edge of the mesh once it has been secured to the vagina.

A rectangular segment of Mersilene or Marlex mesh is soaked in antibiotic solution and measured to a length that will reach the promontory without tension (Fig.19b.8A). The mesh is generally secured with interrupted sutures that are passed shallow through the outer layer of the vaginal wall. In one series, the rate of erosion was higher with full-thickness suture passage in the vaginal wall.[98] Closure of the peritoneum over the mesh is paramount to avoid complications from direct contact between bowel and mesh (Fig. 19b.8B).[99]

When the uterus is still present, the choice of using mesh may be limited by the risk of vaginal erosion when securing a synthetic material to a freshly closed vaginal cuff after the hysterectomy. Uterine preservation in the younger patient who still wants to bear children can be accomplished by hysteropexy using an anterior and posterior limb of mesh secured to the vaginal wall and passed through each broad ligament of the uterus.[100] Leaving a cervical stump to which to secure the mesh is another option to minimize the risk of mesh infection. However, both techniques require the patient to continue lifelong surveillance for potential future cervical or uterine malignancies.

RESULTS. Abdominal sacrocolpopexy has proven to be a durable repair in several studies, with a success rate of 78–100%.[101] LeFranc et al reviewed 85 cases over a median length of 10.5 years and found only two patients with vault prolapse recurrence.[102] Fox et al quoted a 27% postoperative vault prolapse incidence in 29 women who underwent MSC, although all were designated as grade I by International Continence Society (ICS) standard.[103] Two studies, one randomized comparing MSC to sacrospinous fixation, reported higher success rates with the MSC.[74,104]

In the situation of uterine preservation, recurrent prolapse following sacrohysteropexy has been reported at between 0% and 7%.[100,105,106] However, these results were reported from small series, with 3–30 patients, with only one having a mean follow-up of >16 months.

Although the mesh sacrocolpopexy can be combined with antiincontinence procedures, most commonly a Burch colposuspension, there does appear to be a slightly higher rate of postoperative incontinence and posterior vaginal prolapse after combined interventions.[99,107] This observation suggests the MSC may provide enough support to the anterior vaginal wall, and additional bladder neck suspension procedures may abnormally alter the vaginal axis.

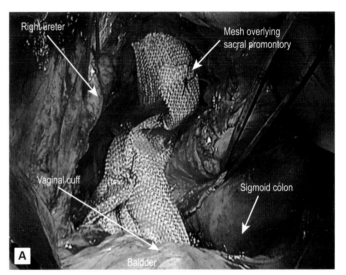

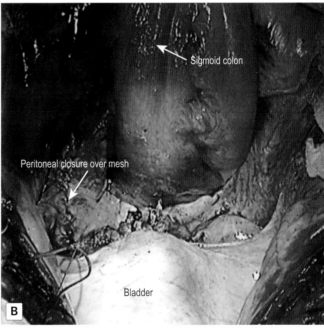

Figure 19b.8 Intraoperative views of completed mesh sacrocolpopexy. (**A**) Marlex mesh secured to sacral promontory and vaginal cuff with sigmoid colon retracted laterally by the forceps (labeled). (**B**) Closure of peritoneum over Marlex mesh, with the sigmoid colon now returned to its normal position.

LAPAROSCOPIC SACROCOLPOPEXY

Technique. The steps of open sacrocolpopexy have been reproduced by laparoscopy. A four-port approach is most commonly used, with a 10 mm umbilical port, two 5 mm ports lateral to the rectus abdominis muscles and 3 cm medial from the anterior superior iliac spine, and a 10 mm port in the suprapubic position.[108] If a hysterectomy is performed in the same setting, the uterus can be delivered through an extended abdominal or vaginal incision.

The vesicovaginal and rectovaginal spaces can be dissected to receive a Y-shaped piece of Marlex or Mersilene mesh with a single arm extending to the presacral ligament. The mesh can be secured to the presacral ligament with staples or a tacker, as suture passage in the promontory with laparoscopic instruments may be challenging.[109] If the uterus is being preserved, the mesh can be passed between the uterus and bladder. Similar to the open approach, the peritoneum is closed over the entire mesh to protect the enteric contents from the mesh.

Results. As the laparoscopic experience for prolapse repair is still limited, there are few long-term data duplicating the durable outcomes seen with the abdominal MSC. Success rates in series with short-term follow-up have been comparable to open repair, ranging from 84% to 94%.[99,108,109] Antiphon et al noted higher failure rates in all categories of prolapse when a single anterior mesh was used, as opposed to dual anterior–posterior meshes.[99]

Complications. Vaginal erosion is a concern in any procedure using mesh, but particularly with the MSC due to the large surface area of material secured to the vaginal wall. The reported incidence is 5–9%, though the presentation can vary from a small, asymptomatic vaginal opening to infection, abscess or fistula formation.[110,111] Management depends on extent of erosion, and in mild cases observation or local debridement and closure may be sufficient. Removal of all or part of the material may be necessary if there is evidence of infection. Despite removal of the mesh, prolapse recurrence is not inevitable, as the resulting scar tissue may be adequate for sustained support.[112]

If the MSC is being done concomitantly with an abdominal hysterectomy, the likelihood of mesh erosion has been found to be higher in two series.[113,114] Other studies have not shown concurrent hysterectomy to be associated with a higher risk of vaginal erosion.[98,115]

Complications arising from the sacral component of the procedure include hemorrhage from the presacral vessels, which can be particularly troublesome. In intractable cases, it can be managed by coagulation, suture ligation or thumbtacks.[103] The vascular anatomy of the sacral promontory is highly variable, and the pneumoperitoneum during laparoscopic sacrocolpopexy may conceal low-pressure venous bleeding, which could go unrecognized following release of the intraabdominal gas. Spondylodiscitis, an infective and/or inflammatory process resulting from direct extension of mesh violating the lumbosacral disc space, can lead to sacral abscess. Although a rare and dreaded complication, spondylodiscitis can generally be prevented by superficial passage of the suture(s) in the anterior longitudinal ligament alone.[109]

POSTERIOR COMPARTMENT REPAIR
Enterocele

Indications. Prolapse of the peritoneal contents may feature the peritoneum alone (peritoneocele), small intestine (enterocele) or small intestine with omentum. They may be found as an isolated prolapse or in conjunction with rectocele or vaginal vault descent. Reduction and repair of an enterocele is indicated in symptomatic cases, particularly as part of a vault prolapse repair. However, many peritoneoceles/ enteroceles are asymptomatic and may be observed, and the question of whether or not to close a deep pouch of Douglas preventively at the time of a hysterectomy has yet to be answered.

VAGINAL REPAIR

Goal. The goal of transvaginal repair of an enterocele is to isolate the peritoneocele, free and reduce the bowel contents, close the hernia, and prevent its recurrence. In patients who have undergone multiple prior abdominal surgeries, the abdominal approach may be preferred due to the risk of adhesions that may be encountered transvaginally.

Technique. If multiple areas of prolapse are being addressed, the enterocele is repaired first, followed by anterior, then posterior wall repair.[88] Visualization of light from a cystoscope can help differentiate cystocele from enterocele in high-grade prolapse.[116] Broad-spectrum antibiotic coverage is administered preoperatively due to the potential for bowel injury.

For isolated enteroceles, an apical midline vaginal incision is made and the sac is dissected from the vaginal wall as previously described. Once the sac is opened, laparotomy pads are used to pack away enteric contents. Closure of the cul-de-sac is usually done with 1–2 nonabsorbable purse-string sutures to include prerectal fascia posteriorly, parietal peritoneum laterally, and the posterior peritoneal surface of the bladder anteriorly. After removal of the packs, the purse-string suture is then cinched down snugly under direct vision to avoid bowel entrapment. Cystoscopy with IV indigo carmine confirms ureteral integrity.

Results. Most series report on prevention of posthysterectomy prolapse or recurrence of de novo enterocele following culdoplasty. Cruikshank randomized 100 women at the time of vaginal hysterectomy to one of three surgical methods of posterior/apical closure: a Moschowitz-type operation (purse-string suture bringing the uterosacral–cardinal complex together in the midline), a McCall culdoplasty (plication of the complex and elevation of redundant vaginal apex), or closure of the peritoneum only.[117] At 3 years follow-up, they found that the McCall culdoplasty was superior to the other two methods described in preventing postoperative enterocele.

Tulikangas et al followed 54 women at a mean of 16 months and reported 16 grade II apical prolapse recurrences (28%).[118] The functional outcomes did not differ between those with grade I and II prolapses. Raz et al followed 81 women at a mean follow-up of 15.7 months and reported an overall success rate, defined as no recurrence of enterocele, in 86%.[119]

ABDOMINAL REPAIR

Technique. Two main techniques for obliteration of the cul-de-sac following abdominal hysterectomy exist. The Halban, or Nichols, procedure uses a series of interrupted, non-absorbable sutures to approximate the vaginal cuff to the prerectal fascia and taenia of the rectosigmoid, thus obliterating the pouch of Douglas. Each suture is passed, tagged, and then tied sequentially at the end.

The Moschowitz technique involves multiple purse-string sutures which incorporate the vaginal cuff, uterosacral–cardinal ligament complex, perivesical, and prerectal fascia and close the pouch of Douglas from the bottom up. This technique is more prone to ureteric injury, thus prompting the need for a cystoscopy procedure with IV indigo carmine at completion of the repair.

Results. Few reports exist on isolated abdominal repair of enteroceles, as this condition will often be addressed at the time of vaginal vault fixation or other pelvic organ prolapse repair. Cronje et al analyzed 130 women with enteroceles repaired by a variety of techniques, including a Moschowitz repair with suspension of the vault to the sacrum in 13 patients.[120] Follow-up in this series was 7.4 months but they reported no recurrences (defined as grade II or more vaginal vault prolapse) over this short time period. Scarpero et al performed a concomitant Halban culdoplasty at the time of Marlex mesh sacrocolpopexy in 20 women with enterocele, cystocele, and vaginal vault prolapse.[121] All these patients showed good support of the vaginal vault with no recurrent enterocele at a mean follow-up of 11.3 months. Brieger et al treated 45 cases of pulsion enterocele via combination abdominoperineal approach, using Mersilene mesh in completing a simultaneous sacrocolpopexy, and reported a 92.5% success rate at a short follow-up of 6 months.[122]

LAPAROSCOPIC REPAIR

Technique. Adapting the concepts of open or vaginal enterocele repair to the laparoscopic approach has been described. The enterocele sac is dissected, then excised with monopolar electrocautery or harmonic scalpel. Next, the pubocervical and rectovaginal fascias are identified and reapproximated with interrupted nonabsorbable sutures.[123,124]

Results. Long-term data on outcomes following laparoscopic enterocele repair are lacking but the preliminary results appear promising. Recently, Cook et al reported a 93% success rate based on objective assessment using the POP-Q system in 45 women after 3 years follow-up, with a 4.4% incidence of major complications.[123] Cadeddu et al reported on three women repaired laparoscopically using a Moschowitz technique with no recurrences at a follow-up of 10.5 months.[125]

Complications. The primary complication is a ureteric injury. Other complications, such as bleeding from ovarian vessels or bladder/bowel perforation during dissection, are rare.

Rectocele.
Rectocele is defined as a herniation of the rectum through the posterior vaginal wall, though not all posterior wall defects are rectoceles. A posterior vaginal wall defect may allow protrusion of small bowel, rectum or both. Management of the asymptomatic rectocele remains controversial, although defecatory dysfunction (constipation, anal incontinence, or both) will often prompt a patient to seek intervention.

Vaginal repair

POSTERIOR COLPORRHAPHY

Goal. The goal of the posterior colporrhaphy is to close the posterior wall herniation by reapproximation of the medial edge of the levator muscles over the midline.

Technique. With the patient in dorsal lithotomy position, two Allis clamps are placed at the 5 and 7 o'clock positions on the introitus, exposing the perineal body. Saline hydrodissection may be used to identify the proper plane between the vagina and rectum. A triangular incision with the apex pointing downward is made, excising a segment of perineal skin at the mucocutaneous junction, with a second, inverted triangular incision made to further expose the prerectal space. Otherwise, a midline incision is made in the posterior vaginal wall, extending to the posterior edge of the vaginal cuff. Vaginal flaps are developed on each side to separate the vaginal wall from the rectum, identifying in the process the proximal defect in the levator hiatus and the attenuated prerectal fascia. This dissection is done as close as possible to the vaginal wall to avoid rectal injury.

The prerectal fascia may be plicated with a series of interrupted absorbable sutures.[126] With a narrow right-angle retractor retracting the rectum downward for protection, the most proximal suture is passed first incorporating the medial edge of the levator muscles. Several absorbable sutures are placed sequentially moving distally towards the perineal body, and are left on stay clamps to be tied at the end or are tied progressively. It is important to avoid overtightening the mid or upper vagina or creating a transversal ridge across the posterior vaginal wall which could result in dyspareunia. Before closing the vaginal incision, excision of redundant vaginal flaps may be necessary but must take into account the patient's age and degree of sexual activity.

Results. Long-term success of the posterior colporrhaphy has been reported, with reported anatomic cure rates of 76–96%,[50,127,128] as summarized in Table 19b.8. In 25 women followed up to 5.1 years, Lopez et al found one clinical recurrence of rectocele and five recurrences by dynamic defecography.[127] In the study, rectocele was diagnosed as an outpocketing of the anterior rectal and posterior vaginal wall into the lumen of the vagina, ranging in size from 1.5 to 4 cm.

Of these, only one patient underwent repeat posterior colporrhaphy. Thus, defecography may be limited in its role of defining clinically relevant prolapse, as Shorvon et al demonstrated the prevalence of occult rectoceles in 47 asymptomatic volunteers undergoing defecography.[129]

SITE-SPECIFIC REPAIR

Goal. The concern for postoperative dyspareunia due to vaginal narrowing after posterior colporrhaphy has led to the concept of the site-specific repair, which involves closing isolated defects in the rectovaginal fascia.

Technique. A midline posterior vaginal wall incision is made over the bulging rectocele, and the vaginal mucosa is dissected off the underlying rectovaginal septum. The surgeon's finger is placed in the rectum to delineate the defects. Identification of the fascial defect(s) relies on both palpation and visualization of the shiny, white rectovaginal fascia against the ruddy rectal muscularis layer.[130] Allis clamps may be placed on the fascial edges to reapproximate the defect, while the finger in the rectum carefully reduces the rectocele to avoid bowel injury. The fascial tear is closed with interrupted delayed-absorbable sutures[131,132] or reattached to the perineal body with longitudinal, interrupted sutures.[133] If there is no tension on the vaginal closure, a short strip of redundant flap may be excised on each

Table 19b.8	Clinical outcomes from recent rectocele repair series						
Author (yr)	n	Mean follow-up (mo/yr)	Definition of recurrence	Recurrence rate	New-onset dyspareunia	Symptom imprvmt
Posterior colporrhaphy						
Kahn (1997)[128]	244	42.5 mo	PE (presence of "large" rectocele)	24%	16%	62%
Lopez (2001)[127]	24	5.1 yr	PE (not defined) Defecography*	4% 21%	33%	91%
Maher (2004)[139]	38	24 mo	Point Bp ≥stage II	21%	4%	89%
Site-specific repair						
Cundiff (1998)[132]	43	12 mo (median)	PE (no change or worsening in POP-Q stage)	18%	19%	87% (60/69)
Kenton (1999)[133]	46	12 mo	PE (POP-Q Ap point at −1 or greater)	23%	7%	43–92%
Porter (1999)[134]	125	18 mo	PE (B-W >grade 2)	18% (16/89)	12%	35–74%
Graft interposition						
Sand (2001)[50]	80	12 mo	PE (B-W ≥grade 2)	8% (6/73)	NR	NR
Kohli (2002)[135]	43	13 mo	PE (POP-Q Ap point ≥-0.5)	2% (2/30)	0%	NR

PE: Physical Exam, POP-Q: Pelvic Organ Prolapse Quantification, B-W: Baden-Walker Halfway Classification System, NR: Not Reported,
* Outpocketing of the Anterior Rectal and Posterior Vaginal Wall into the Lumen of the Vagina

side. The edges are then reapproximated with a running absorbable suture.

Results. The definition of objective success, which has been reported at 82–86% (see Table 19b.8) has not been limited to anatomic repair, as several series have examined the change in bowel symptoms and sexual function from baseline just as closely as anatomic success.[132-134] Although the literature on site-specific repair suggests it to be superior to the posterior colporrhaphy in alleviating the symptoms associated with a rectocele, clinical evaluation of rectovaginal fascial defects was found to be in concordance with surgical findings in only 59.4% of cases.[130]

GRAFT INTERPOSITION

Goal. Reconstruction of the posterior pelvic floor under no tension and without narrowing the vagina may prove challenging in some cases with a standard posterior plication or site-specific repair. The strength of the repair can be augmented with the use of nonautologous material, either graft (e.g. cadaveric dermis) or synthetic (mesh).

Technique. The vaginal incision and dissection of the rectovaginal space are identical to those of the previously described procedures. The size of the material needed varies based on surgeon preference and individual anatomy, but a 4×7 or 2×6 cm piece has been described. In one report using dermal graft, this material was reconstituted in normal saline for 20 minutes and then secured to the edges of the levator muscles bilaterally with interrupted permanent sutures.[135] The graft may also be sutured distally and proximally to prevent migration. A synthetic mesh can similarly be secured with permanent or delayed-absorbable sutures.

Results. Experience with graft interposition is limited to small patient populations with short follow-up, although in one randomized prospective trial, Sand et al showed that addition of an absorbable (Vicryl) mesh did not affect the likelihood of rectocele recurrence at 1-year follow-up.[50] They reported an overall success rate, defined as no rectocele beyond the hymenal ring, of 90% in 132 subjects. Kohli et al followed 30 patients for 12.9 months after dermal graft augmentation and found a 93% surgical cure rate, defined as an Ap measurement of −0.5 or greater using the POP-Q score.[135] No graft-related complications were reported in this series.

Abdominal repair

Goal. A large rectocele associated with loss of the perineal body and vaginal vault prolapse may be reconstructed through an abdominal approach, similar to the sacrocolpopexy previously described.

Technique. Placement of a synthetic mesh to the posterior vagina for support may be extended to reach the perineal body and repair a rectocele in the same setting. The incision, exposure, and dissection are identical to the abdominal mesh SCP. The dissection between the vagina and rectum is carried distally until the perineal body is reached, at which point the mesh is secured directly to the perineal body. If the superficial perineal muscles are separated, they may be reapproximated by a vaginal route (perineorrhaphy) prior to mesh placement in select cases.[136]

Results. There are scant reports on the outcome of rectocele repair with this technique. One anecdotal series followed 19 patients and found stage 0 or I prolapse in 84% and improvement of point Ap and Bp in 18 patients.[136] However, the follow-up was at a mean of 8 weeks, with only five patients followed beyond 3 months.

Complications. Narrowing or shortening of the vagina has been reported in between 6% and 33% of patients (see Table 19b.8).[90,127,128] Worsening of sexual function was reported to be 19% in one study.[134] Improvement in sexual function ranges from 10% to 92%, the disparity due to differences in follow-up and the small number of sexually active women in most series. Careful excision of redundant vaginal flaps may help prevent vaginal narrowing or leaving uneven ridges in the closure. When a perineorrhaphy is associated, a high labial ridge can cause introital dyspareunia.

Preoperative bowel function is highly variable and does not correlate with severity of prolapse.[137] Furthermore, improvement of some bowel symptoms after rectocele repair has not been shown, despite anatomic repair. Resolution of constipation ranges from 10% to 40%,[128,133] though one study noted 11% and 23% of patients reporting increased and de novo constipation, respectively.[134] Lopez et al reported an improvement in rectal emptying symptoms in 91% of 24 patients at extended follow-up of 5.1 years.[127] Improvement in manual evacuation ranges from 36% to 63%. Fecal incontinence has been reported to improve in 35–57% of cases, while 3–13% reported de novo incontinence.[132,134]

Rectal injury can result in rectovaginal fistula, which has been reported previously in up to 5% of patients.[126] Bowel wall injury may be difficult to recognize in the absence of a rectal examination intraoperatively or a packed rectum with povidone-iodine gauze. Sutures through the rectal wall must be recognized and released.[138]

CONCLUSION

The surgical repair of pelvic organ prolapse must be tailored to the individual, addressing the many aspects of this complex disease. Degree and location of the defect, tissue quality, risk factors, and patient goals must be taken into account to insure a satisfactory result. However, long-term data on success are sparse, and the same risk factors that led to the development of the prolapse initially may contribute to recurrence of the condition. Surgical correction of POP is challenging, requiring a thorough understanding of the underlying pathophysiology and of the currently available repair procedures with their advantages, limitations, risks, and complications. The ultimate goal of each technique is to reconstruct the pelvic anatomy and prolapsed organs, and restore their normal function.

REFERENCES

1. Versi E, et al. Urogenital prolapse and atrophy at menopause: a prevalence study. Int Urogynecol J Pelvic Floor Dysfunct 2001;2:107–110.
2. Handa V, et al. Progression and remission of pelvic organ prolapse: a longitudinal study of menopausal women. Am J Obstet Gynecol 2004;190:27–32.
3. Subak LL, et al. Cost of pelvic organ prolapse surgery in the United States. Obstet Gynecol 2001;98(4):646–651.
4. Olsen AL, et al. Epidemiology of surgically managed pelvic organ prolapse and urinary incontinence. Obstet Gynecol 1997;89(4):501–506.
5. Ng C, Rackley R, Appell R. Incidence of concomitant procedures for pelvic organ prolapse and reconstruction in women who undergo surgery for stress urinary incontinence. Urology 2001;57:911–913.
6. Heit M, et al. Predicting treatment choice for patients with pelvic organ prolapse. Obstet Gynecol 2003;101:1279–1284.
7. Baden WF, Walker TA. Genesis of the vaginal profile: a correlated classification of vaginal relaxation. Clin Obstet Gynecol 1972;15:1048–1054.
8. Bump RC, et al. The standardization of terminology of female pelvic organ prolapse and pelvic floor dysfunction. Am J Obstet Gynecol 1996;175:10–17.
9. Raz S, Klutke G, Golomb J. Four-corner bladder and urethral suspension for moderate cystocele. J Urol 1989;142:712–715.
10. Dmochowski R, et al. Role of the four-corner bladder neck suspension to correct stress incontinence with mild to moderate cystocele. Urology 1996;49: 5–40.
11. Bruskewitz R, et al. Bladder neck suspension material investigated in a rabbit model. J Urol 1989;142:1361–1363.
12. Appell R. In situ vaginal wall sling. Urology 2000;56:499–503.
13. Raz S, Stothers L, Chopra A. Raz techniques for anterior vaginal wall repair. In: Raz S, ed. Female urology. Philadelphia: WB Saunders; 1996:344–366.
14. Juma S. Anterior vaginal suspension for vaginal vault prolapse. Tech Urol 1995;1(3):150–156.
15. Showalter P, et al. Standing cystourethrogram: an outcome measure after anti-incontinence procedures and cystocele repair in women. Urology 2001;58:33–37.
16. Lemack GE, Zimmern PE. Sexual function after vaginal surgery for stress incontinence: results of a mailed questionnaire. Urology 2000;56:223–227.
17. Leach GE, et al. Female stress urinary incontinence clinical guidelines panel summary report on surgical management of female stress urinary incontinence. J Urol 1997;158:875–880.
18. Winters JC, Scarpero HM, Appell RA. The use of bone anchors in urology. Urology, 2000;56 (Suppl 6A):15–22.
19. Costantini E, et al. Four-corner colposuspension: clinical and functional results. Int Urogynecol J Pelvic Floor Dysfunct 2003;14:113–118.
20. Kaplan SA, et al. Prospective analysis of 373 consecutive women with stress urinary incontinence treated with a vaginal wall sling: the Columbia-Cornell University experience. J Urol 2000;164:1623–1627.
21. Bai SW, et al. The effectiveness of modified six-corner suspension in patients with paravaginal defect and stress urinary incontinence. Int Urogynecol J Pelvic Floor Dysfunct 2002;13:303–307.
22. Lovatsis D, Drutz HP. Is transabdominal repair of mild to moderate cystocele necessary for correction of prolapse during a modified Burch procedure? Int Urogynecol J Pelvic Floor Dysfunct 2001;12:193–198.
23. Sekine H, et al. Burch bladder neck suspension for cystocele repair: the necessity of combined vaginal procedures for severe cases. Int J Urol 1999;6:1–6.
24. Huang WC, Yang JM. Anatomic comparison between laparoscopic and open Burch colposuspension for primary stress urinary incontinence. Urology 2004;63:676–681.
25. McDougall EM, et al. Laparoscopic bladder neck suspension fails the test of time. J Urol 1999;162: 2078–2081.
26. Moehrer B, et al. Laparoscopic colposuspension for urinary incontinence in women. Cochrane Review. Oxford: Update Software; 2002.
27. Walter AJ, et al. Laparoscopic versus open Burch retropubic urethropexy: comparison of morbidity and costs when performed with concurrent vaginal prolapse repairs. Am J Obstet Gynecol 2002;186: 723–728.
28. Cheon WC, Mak J, Liu JYS. Prospective randomized controlled trial comparing laparoscopic and open colposuspension. Hong Kong Med J 2003;9:10–14.
29. Langer R, et al. Long-term (10–15 years) follow-up after Burch colposuspension for urinary stress incontinence. Int Urogynecol J Pelvic Floor Dysfunct 2001;12: 323–327.
30. Kwon CH, et al. The development of pelvic organ prolapse following isolated Burch retropubic urethropexy. Int Urogynecol J Pelvic Floor Dysfunct 2003;14: 321–325.
31. Colombo M, et al. Randomised comparison of Burch colposuspension versus anterior colporrhaphy in women with stress urinary incontinence and anterior vaginal wall prolapse. Br J Obstet Gynaecol 2000;107: 554–551.
32. Cugudda A, et al. Long term results of Burch colposuspension and anterior colpoperineorrhaphy in the treatment of stress urinary incontinence and cystocele. Ann Urol 2002;36(3):176–181.
33. Shull BL, Baden WF. A six-year experience with paravaginal defect repair for stress urinary incontinence. Am J Obstet Gynecol 1989;160:1432–1440.
34. Young SB, Daman JJ, Bony LG. Vaginal paravaginal repair: one-year outcomes. Am J Obstet Gynecol 2001;185:1360–1367.
35. Scotti RJ, et al. Paravaginal repair of lateral vaginal wall defects by fixation to the ischial periosteum and obturator membrane. Am J Obstet Gynecol 1998;179: 1436–1445.
36. Washington JL, Somers KO. Laparoscopic paravaginal repair: a new technique using mesh and staples. J Soc Laparoendosc Surg 2003;7:301–303.
37. Miklos JR, Kohli N. Laparoscopic paravaginal repair plus Burch colposuspension: review and descriptive technique. Urology 2000;56 (Suppl 6A): 64–69.
38. Colombo M, et al. A randomized comparison of Burch

colposuspension and abdominal paravaginal defect repair for female stress urinary incontinence. Am J Obstet Gynecol 1996;175(1): 78–84.

39. Malipeddi PK, et al. Anatomic and functional outcome of vaginal paravaginal repair in the correction of anterior vaginal wall prolapse. Int Urogynecol J Pelvic Floor Dysfunct 2001;12: 83–88.

40. Richardson AC, Edmonds P, Williams N. Treatment of stress urinary incontinence due to paravaginal fascial defect. Obstet Gynecol 1981;57:357–362.

41. Shull BL, Benn SJ, Kuehl TJ. Surgical management of prolapse of the anterior vaginal segment: an analysis of support defects, operative morbidity, and anatomic outcome. Am J Obstet Gynecol 1994;171:1429–1439.

42. Bruce RG, Rizk ES, Galloway NT. Paravaginal defect repair in the treatment of female stress urinary incontinence and cystocele. Urology 1999;54:647–651.

43. Cross C, Cespedes R, McGuire E. Treatment results using pubovaginal slings in patients with large cystoceles and stress incontinence. J Urol 1997;158: 431–434.

44. Kohli N, et al. Incidence of recurrent cystocele after anterior colporrhaphy with and without concomitant transvaginal needle suspension. Am J Obstet Gynecol 1996;175:1476–1482.

45. Safir M, et al. 4-Defect repair of grade 4 cystocele. J Urol 1999;161:587–594.

46. Raz S, et al. Repair of severe anterior vaginal wall prolapse (grade IV cystourethrocele). J Urol 1991;146: 988–992.

47. Weber A, et al. Anterior colporrhaphy: a randomized trial of three surgical techniques. Am J Obstet Gynecol 2001;185:1299–1306.

48. Weber A, Walters M, Piedmonte M. Sexual function and vaginal anatomy in women before and after surgery for pelvic organ prolapse and urinary incontinence. Am J Obstet Gynecol 2000;182:1610–1615.

49. Barnes NM, et al. Pubovaginal sling and pelvic prolapse repair in women with occult stress urinary incontinence: effect on postoperative emptying and voiding symptoms. Urology 2002;59:856–860.

50. Sand PK, et al. Prospective randomized trial of polyglactin 910 mesh to prevent recurrence of cystoceles and rectoceles. Am J Obstet Gynecol 2001;184:1357–1364.

51. de Tayrac R, Salet-Lizee D, Villet R. Comparison of anterior colporrhaphy versus Bologna procedure in women with genuine stress incontinence. Int Urogynecol J Pelvic Floor Dysfunct 2002;13: 36–39.

52. Kobashi, KC, Mee SL, Leach GE. A new technique for cystocele repair and transvaginal sling: the cadaveric prolapse repair and sling (CaPS). Urology 2000;56 (Suppl 6A): 9–14.

53. Kobashi KC, et al. Continued multicenter followup of the cadaveric prolapse repair with sling. J Urol 2002;168: 2063–2068.

54. Gomelsky A, Rudy DC, Dmochowski RR. Porcine dermis interposition graft for repair of high grade anterior compartment defects with or without concomitant pelvic organ prolapse procedures. J Urol 2004;171:1581–1584.

55. Julian TM. The efficacy of Marlex mesh in the repair of severe, recurrent vaginal prolapse of the anterior midvaginal wall. Am J Obstet Gynecol 1996;175(6):1472–1475.

56. Groutz A, et al. Use of cadaveric solvent-dehydrated fascia lata for cystocele repair— preliminary results. Urology 2001;58:179–183.

57. Chung SY, et al. Technique of combined pubovaginal sling and cystocele repair using a single piece of cadaveric dermal graft. Urology 2002;59:538–541.

58. Powell CR, Simsiman AJ, Menefee SA. Anterior vaginal wall hammock with fascia lata for the correction of stage 2 or greater anterior vaginal wall compartment relaxation. J Urol 2004;171:264–267.

59. Leboeuf L, et al. Grade 4 cystocele repair using four-defect repair and porcine xenograft acellular matrix (Pelvicol): outcome measures using SEAPI. Urology 2004;64:282–286.

60. Migliari R, et al. Tension-free vaginal mesh repair for anterior vaginal wall prolapse. Eur Urol 2000;38: 151–155.

61. Amid PK, et al. Biomaterials for "tension-free" hernioplasties and principles of their applications. Minerva Chir 1995;50(9): 821–826.

62. Cervigni M, Natale F. The use of synthetics in the treatment of pelvic organ prolapse. Curr Opin Urol 2001;11: 429–435.

63. Maher C, et al. Surgical management of pelvic organ prolapse in women. Cochrane Review, Issue 4. Oxford: Update Software; 2004.

64. Cespedes RD. Diagnosis and treatment of vaginal vault prolapse conditions. Urology 2002;60(1):8–15.

65. McCall ML. Posterior culdeplasty: surgical correction of enterocele during vaginal hysterectomy; a preliminary report. Obstet Gynecol 1957;10(6):595–602.

66. Sze E, Karram M. Transvaginal repair of vault prolapse: a review. Obstet Gynecol 1997;89:466–475.

67. Comiter CV, Vasavada SP, Raz S. Transvaginal culdosuspension: technique and results. Urology 1999;54: 819–822.

68. Richter K. [The surgical anatomy of the vaginae fixatio sacrospinalis vaginalis. A contribution to the surgical treatment of vaginal blind pouch prolapse] [German]. Geburtshilfe Frauenheilkd 1968;28(4):321–327.

69. Amundsen CL, Flynn BJ, Webster GD. Anatomical correction of vaginal vault prolapse by uterosacral ligament fixation in women who also require a pubovaginal sling. J Urol 2003;169: 1770–1774.

70. Ginsberg DA. Vaginal vault prolapse: evaluation and repair. Curr Urol Rep 2003;4: 404–408.

71. Cespedes RD. Anterior approach bilateral sacrospinous ligament fixation for vaginal vault prolapse. Urology 2000;56 (Suppl 6A): 70–75.

72. Alsultan H, et al. [Sacral colpopexy by the abdominal route: possible!] J Gynecol Obstet Biol Reprod 1995;24(4): 452–453.

73. Pohl JF, Frattarelli JL. Bilateral transvaginal sacrospinous colpopexy: preliminary experience. Am J Obstet Gynecol 1997;177: 1356–1362.

74. Maher CF, et al. Abdominal sacral colpopexy or vaginal sacrospinous colpopexy for vaginal vault prolapse: a prospective randomized study. Am J Obstet Gynecol 2004;190: 20–26.

75. Cruikshank SH, Muniz M. Outcomes study: a comparison of cure rates in 695 patients undergoing sacrospinous ligament fixation alone and with other site-specific procedures. A 16-year study. Am J Obstet Gynecol 2003;188: 1509–1515.

76. Morley GW, DeLancey J. Sacrospinous ligament fixation for eversion of the vagina. Am J Obstet Gynecol 1988;158:872–881.

77. Nieminen K, Heinonen PK. Sacrospinous ligament fixation for massive genital prolapse in women aged over 80 years. Br J Obstet Gynaecol 2001;108: 817–821.

78. Silva-Filho AL, et al. Sacrospinous fixation for treatment of vault prolapse and at the time of vaginal hysterectomy for marked uterovaginal prolapse. J Pelvic Med Surg 2004;10(4): 213–218.

79. Young SB, et al. A survey of the complications of vaginal prolapse surgery performed by members of the Society of Gynecologic Surgeons. Int Urogynecol J Pelvic Floor Dysfunct 2004;15: 165–170.

80. Nieminen, K, Huhtala H, Heinonen PK. Anatomic and functional assessment and risk factors of recurrent prolapse after vaginal sacrospinous fixation. Acta Obstet Gynecol Scand 2003;82: 471–478.

81. Smilen SW, et al. The risk of cystocele after sacrospinous ligament fixation. Am J Obstet Gynecol 1998;179:1465–1472.

82. Goldberg RP, et al. Anterior or posterior sacrospinous vaginal vault fixation: long-term anatomic and functional evaluation. Obstet Gynecol 2001;98(2):199–204.

83. Brubaker L, Bump R, Jacquetin B, et al. Pelvic organ prolapse. In: Abrams P, Cardozo L, Khoury S, Wein A, eds. Incontinence. Second International Consultation on Incontinence. Plymouth, UK: Plymbridge Distributors; 2002: 245–265.

84. Richter K, Albrich W. Long-term results following fixation of the vagina on the sacrospinal ligament by the vaginal route. Am J Obstet Gynecol 1981;141: 811–816.

85. Giberti C. Transvaginal sacrospinous colpopexy by palpation—a

new minimally invasive procedure using an anchoring system. Urology 2001;57: 666–669.

86. Shull BL, et al. A transvaginal approach to repair of apical and other associated sites of pelvic organ prolapse with uterosacral ligaments. Am J Obstet Gynecol 2000;183: 1365–1374.

87. Barber MD, et al. Bilateral uterosacral ligament vaginal vault suspension with site-specific endopelvic fascia defect repair for treatment of pelvic organ prolapse. Am J Obstet Gynecol 2000;183: 1402–1411.

88. Lemack GE, Zimmern PE, Blander DS. The levator myorrhaphy repair for vaginal vault prolapse. Urology 2000;56 (Suppl 6A): 50–54.

89. Zimmern PE, et al. Five years experience with transvaginal repair of vaginal vault prolapse and prevention of enterocele recurrence by high, midline levator myorraphy. J Urol 1994;151(5): 421A.

90. Lemack GE, et al. Vaginal vault fixation and prevention of enterocele recurrence by high midline levator myorraphy: physical examination and questionnaire-based follow up. Eur Urol 2001;40: 648–651.

91. Cespedes RD, Kraus S. Extraperitoneal levator myorrhaphy for moderate grade vault prolapse: experience in 136 cases. J Urol 2002;167(4): 76.

92. Glavind K, Kempf L. Colpectomy or Le Fort colpocleisis—a good option in selected elderly patients. Int Urogynecol J Pelvic Floor Dysfunct 2004;16(1):48–51.

93. DeLancey JO. Morley GW. Total colpocleisis for vaginal eversion. Am J Obstet Gynecol 1997;176(6):1228–1232.

94. Fitzgerald MP, Brubaker L. Colpocleisis and urinary incontinence. Am J Obstet Gynecol 2003;189: 1241–1244.

95. Von Pechmann WS, et al. Total colpocleisis with high levator plication for the treatment of advanced pelvic organ prolapse. Am J Obstet Gynecol 2003;189:121–126.

96. Marinkovic SP, Stanton SL. Triple compartment prolapse: sacrocolpopexy with anterior and posterior mesh extensions. Br J Obstet Gynaecol 2003;110: 323–326.

97. Von Theobald P, Labbe E. La triple operation perineal avec protheses. J Gynecol Obstet Biol Reprod 2003;32:562–570.

98. Visco AG, et al. Vaginal mesh erosion after abdominal sacral colpopexy. Am J Obstet Gynecol 2001;184: 297–302.

99. Antiphon P, et al. Laparoscopic promontory sacral colpopexy: is the posterior, recto-vaginal, mesh mandatory? Eur Urol 2004;45: 665–661.

100. Barranger E, Fritel X, Pigne A. Abdominal sacrohysteropexy in young women with uterovaginal prolapse: long-term follow-up. Am J Obstet Gynecol 2003;189:1245–1250.

101. Nygaard I, et al. Abdominal sacrocolpopexy: a comprehensive review. Obstet Gynecol 2004;104(4):805–823.

102. Le Franc JP, et al. Longterm followup of posthysterectomy vaginal vault prolapse abdominal repair: a report of 85 cases. J Am Coll Surg 2002;195: 352–358.

103. Fox SD, Stanton SL. Vault prolapse and rectocele: assessment of repair using sacrocolpopexy with mesh interposition. Br J Obstet Gynaecol 2000;107: 1371–1375.

104. Hardiman PJ, Drutz HP. Sacrospinous vault suspension and abdominal colposacropexy: success rates and complications. Am J Obstet Gynecol 1996;175: 612–616.

105. Leron E, Stanton SL. Sacrohysteropexy with synthetic mesh for the management of uterovaginal prolapse. Br J Obstet Gynaecol 2001;108(6): 629–633.

106. Addison W, Timmons M. Abdominal approach to vaginal eversion. Clin Obstet Gynecol 1993;36: 995–1004.

107. Cosson M, et al. Long-term results of the Burch procedure combined with abdominal sacrolcolpopexy for treatment of vault prolapse. Int Urogynecol J Pelvic Floor Dysfunct 2003;14: 104–107.

108. Cosson M, et al. Laparoscopic sacrocolpopexy, hysterectomy, and Burch colposuspension: feasibility and short-term complications of 77 procedures. J Soc Laparoendosc Surg 2002;6:115–119.

109. Wattiez A, Mashiach R, Donoso M. Laparoscopic repair of vaginal vault prolapse. Curr Opin Obstet Gynecol 2003;15: 315–319.

110. Cosson M, et al. [Laparoscopic sacral colpopexy: short-term results and complications in 83 patients.] J Gynecol Obstet Biol Reprod 2003;29(7):644–649.

111. Hart SR, Weiser EB. Abdominal sacral colpopexy mesh erosion resulting in a sinus tract formation and sacral abscess. Obstet Gynecol 2004;103(5 Pt 2):1037–1040.

112. Lindeque BG, Nel WS. Sacrocolpopexy—a report on 262 consecutive operations. S Afr Med J 2002;92 (12): 982–985.

113. Mattox T, Stanford E, Varner E. Infected abdominal sacrocolpopexies: diagnosis and treatment. Int Urogynecol J Pelvic Floor Dysfunct 2004;15 (5): 319–323.

114. Culligan P, et al. Long-term success of abdominal sacral colpopexy using synthetic mesh. Am J Obstet Gynecol 2002;187: 1473–1482.

115. Brizzolara S, Pillai-Allen A. Risk of mesh erosion with sacral colpopexy and concurrent hysterectomy. Obstet Gynecol 2003;102: 306–310.

116. Vasavada SP, Comiter CV, Raz S. Cystoscopic light test to aid in the differentiation of high-grade pelvic organ prolapse. Urology 1999;54: 1085–1087.

117. Cruikshank SH, Kovac SR. Randomized comparison of three surgical methods used at the time of vaginal hysterectomy to prevent posterior enterocele. Am J Obstet Gynecol 1999;180(4):159–165.

118. Tulikangas PK, Piedmonte MR, Weber AM. Functional and anatomic follow-up of enterocele repairs. Obstet Gynecol 2001;98: 265–268.

119. Raz S, Nitti V, Bregg K. Transvaginal repair of enterocele. J Urol 1993;149: 724–730.

120. Cronje HS, De Beer J, Bam R. The pathophysiology of an enterocele and its management. J Obstet Gynaecol 2004;24(4): 408–413.

121. Scarpero H, Cespedes RD, Winters J. Transabdominal approach to repair of vaginal vault prolapse. Tech Urol 2001;7(2):139–145.

122. Brieger GM. Abdominoperineal repair of pulsion enterocele. J Obstet Gynaecol Res 1996;22(2): 151–156.

123. Cook JR, Seman EI, O'Shea RT. Laparoscopic treatment of enterocele: a 3-year evaluation. Aust NZ J Obstet Gynaecol 2004;44: 107–110.

124. Paraiso MF, Falcone T, Walters MD. Laparoscopic surgery for enterocele, vaginal apex prolapse and rectocele. Int Urogynecol J Pelvic Floor Dysfunct 1999;10: 223–229.

125. Cadeddu JA, et al. Laparoscopic repair of enterocele. J Endourol 1996;10(4): 367–369.

126. Rovner ES, Ginsberg DA. Posterior vaginal wall prolapse: transvaginal repair of pelvic floor relaxation, rectocele, and perineal laxity. Tech Urol 2001;7(2): 161–168.

127. Lopez A, et al. Durability of success after rectocele repair. Int Urogynecol J Pelvic Floor Dysfunct 2001;12: 97–103.

128. Kahn MA, Stanton SL. Posterior colporrhaphy: its effects on bowel and sexual function. Br J Obstet Gynaecol 1997;104: 82–86.

129. Shorvon PJ, et al. Defecography in normal volunteers: results and implications. Gut 1989;30(12): 1737–1749.

130. Burrows LJ, et al. The accuracy of clinical evaluation of posterior vaginal wall defects. Int Urogynecol J Pelvic Floor Dysfunct 2003;14: 160–163.

131. Lukacz ES, Luber KM. Rectocele repair: when and how? Curr Urol Rep 2002;3: 418–422.

132. Cundiff GW, et al. An anatomic and functional assessment of the discrete defect rectocele repair. Am J Obstet Gynecol 1998;179(6): 1451–1457.

133. Kenton K, Shott S, Brubaker L. Outcome after rectovaginal fascia reattachment for rectocele repair. Am J Obstet Gynecol 1999;181(6): 1360–1363.

134. Porter WE, et al. The anatomic and functional outcomes of defect-specific rectocele repairs. Am J Obstet Gynecol 1999;181(6): 1353–1358.

135. Kohli N, Miklos J. Dermal graft-augmented rectocele repair. Int Urogynecol J Pelvic Floor Dysfunct 2002;14: 146–149.

SECTION 7 Treatment of pelvic organ prolapse

136. Cundiff GW, et al. Abdominal sacral colpoperineopexy: a new approach for correction of posterior compartment defects and perineal descent associated with vaginal vault prolapse. Am J Obstet Gynecol 1997;177(6): 1345–1353.

137. Weber AM, et al. Posterior vaginal prolapse and bowel function. Am J Obstet Gynecol 1998;179: 1446–1450.

138. Nichols DH. Posterior colporrhaphy and perineorrhaphy: separate and distinct operations. Am J Obstet Gynecol 1991;164: 714–721.

139. Maher CF, et al. Midline rectovaginal fascial plication for repair of rectocele and obstructed defecation. Obstet Gynecol 2004;104(4):685–689.

SECTION 7 Treatment of pelvic organ prolapse

SECTION 8

Fistula

Vesicovaginal Fistula: Vaginal Approach

Matthew Rutman, Donna Deng, Larissa Rodriguez and Shlomo Raz

INTRODUCTION

A vesicovaginal fistula is an abnormal communication between the bladder and vagina, which results in continuous urine leakage through the vagina. It is one of the most significant and devastating morbidities in female urology and urogynecology. Vesicovaginal fistulae have been recognized and described since ancient times but successful repair was not documented until James Marion Sims' first paper in 1852.[1] His transvaginal repair included the use of silver wire suture, and many principles described are still applicable today. Subsequent advances included the first "layered" repair by Mackenrodt[2] and the interposed labial fat graft of Martius[3] in the late 1920s.

The most common cause of vesicovaginal fistula in developing countries remains birth trauma. This is secondary to prolonged and obstructed labor, which leads to pressure necrosis of the anterior vaginal wall and the underlying bladder neck and urethra. This is in stark contrast to developed countries where the large majority of fistulae are the result of complications of gynecologic and other pelvic surgery. Regardless of the cause, surgical repair remains the gold standard and primary treatment of vesicovaginal fistula.

ETIOLOGY

In the United States and other industrialized nations, vesicovaginal fistulae occur as a result of surgical trauma, with the most common cause being abdominal or vaginal hysterectomy. Inadvertent suture placement into the bladder during vaginal cuff closure results in tissue necrosis and subsequent fistula formation. Excessive blunt dissection of the bladder can result in ischemia or an unrecognized tear in the posterior bladder wall, with resultant fistula formation. Overall, around 75% of vesicovaginal fistulae are reported to occur after hysterectomy for benign disease.[4] The overall incidence of vesicovaginal fistula after hysterectomy is approximately 0.5–1%.[5] Vesicovaginal fistulae have also been documented after anterior colporrhaphy, sling procedures for stress incontinence, cystocele repair, colposuspension procedures, and urethral or bladder diverticulectomy. Overall, approximately 90% of vesicovaginal fistulae in North America are caused by gynecologic procedures. The remaining 10% are caused by radiation, advanced local malignancy (cervical, vaginal, and endometrial), inflammatory bowel disease, foreign bodies, and infectious processes of the urinary tract such as tuberculosis.

PREVENTION

Recognizing that the majority of vesicovaginal fistulae are iatrogenic, it is paramount that the surgeon takes critical steps to prevent their occurrence. Risk factors for fistula development include prior cesarean section, endometriosis, and previous cervical conization and radiation treatment.[6] During abdominal hysterectomy, the bladder is most often injured during the dissection of the posterior bladder wall from the anterior surface of the uterus at the level of the vaginal cuff. Placement of an indwelling Foley catheter and meticulous sharp dissection can diminish inadvertent injury. Iatrogenic injuries can be nearly impossible to avoid secondary to difficult reoperations and dense adhesions that obliterate surgical planes. Every attempt should be made to diagnose and repair the injury intraoperatively. Filling the Foley catheter with methylene blue to check for leakage is simple but effective. If a bladder injury is identified, it should be repaired with a two-layered closure after adequate exposure is provided. A drain should then be placed. Intraoperative discovery and repair of a bladder injury will mandate keeping the catheter in for longer than the usual 1–2 days post hysterectomy. An interposition flap can provide additional coverage.

EVALUATION

Symptoms and signs. Most commonly, patients will present with continuous urinary drainage (day and night) from the vagina after gynecologic/pelvic surgery. Any patient who presents with urinary incontinence early after pelvic surgery should be evaluated for a vesicovaginal fistula. The fistula may manifest itself immediately postoperatively but often becomes clinically apparent days to weeks later. Vesicovaginal fistulae tend to present earlier than ureterovaginal fistulae. Ten percent of patients with vesicovaginal fistula have an associated ureterovaginal fistula.[7] Patients in the early postoperative course may present with fevers, ileus, abdominal pain, hematuria, and lower urinary tract symptoms.

Fistulae related to a past history of radiation therapy may present anywhere from 6 months to 20 years after treatment.[8] The fluid draining from the vagina could be urine, lymph, peritoneal fluid, fallopian tube fluid or vaginal secretions. The differential diagnosis of vesicovaginal fistula includes urethrovaginal fistula, ureterovaginal fistula, ectopic ureter, peritoneal fluid drainage, and vaginal cuff infection.

Diagnosis. To confirm that urine is leaking from the vagina, the fluid can be sent for creatinine. Elevated levels, relative to serum, will establish the diagnosis of a communication between the urinary tract and the vagina. Physical examination is the most critical element in the evaluation of a woman with a suspected fistula. The depth, diameter, mobility, and mucosa of the vagina must all be evaluated. Concomitant prolapse, urethral hypermobility, and incontinence should be assessed. Vaginal examination with a speculum can isolate the point of leakage. The most common location for vesicovaginal fistula after hysterectomy is at the level of the vaginal cuff. Pooling of urine at the vaginal apex and in the fornices is often seen. The surrounding vaginal mucosa may appear erythematous and edematous, making it difficult to identify the opening. Placing a Foley catheter into the bladder can assist if the balloon is visualized.

If all the above measures fail to identify a fistula, dye tests can be performed for confirmation. Methylene blue can be instilled through the Foley catheter and the vagina inspected for leakage of blue fluid. Having the patient ambulate with a vaginal pack in place will often stain the packing blue. If a vesicovaginal fistula is still not identified, the patient should be given oral phenazopyridine, which stains the urine orange. The vagina is then packed and orange staining confirms a fistula. A negative methylene blue instillation with a positive phenazopyridine test strongly suggests a ureterovaginal fistula.

All patients with a urinary fistula should undergo cystoscopy and upper tract evaluation. Cystoscopy should identify the location and size of the fistula, and its relationship to the ureteral orifices. It is important to ascertain that there is adequate bladder capacity and to rule out a foreign body as the source of the fistula. Careful surveillance for multiple fistulae is imperative. For patients that have a radiation- or malignancy-associated fistula, biopsy of the site

is mandatory prior to repair. Upper tract evaluation can be done with either intravenous pyelography (IVU) or retrograde pyelography. Ureteral involvement can be demonstrated by hydronephrosis or extravasation on IVU, although the ipsilateral kidney can appear normal with prompt drainage.

Retrograde pyelography remains the most sensitive test to evaluate for ureteral involvement in the presence or absence of a vesicovaginal fistula. Voiding cystourethrogram (VCUG) can also help identify the presence and location of a fistula. Coexisting vesicoureteral reflux, urethral diverticulum, stress incontinence, and cystocele can also be identified, which may alter the surgical plan. Furthermore, VCUG can help elucidate fistulae involving the rectum or uterus. Vaginoscopy can assist in identifying the vaginal communication.

TREATMENT
Conservative management. Small vesicovaginal fistulae may close spontaneously with continuous Foley catheter drainage in up to 10% of cases. By the time patients have sought consultation with a specialist, this has usually been attempted. Three weeks of drainage is a reasonable option if the fistula is discovered early in the postoperative period. Mature fistula tracts are unlikely to resolve with this technique. Prolonged catheter drainage requires coverage with antibiotics.

Another conservative treatment includes fulgurating the lining of the fistula tract. However, this should not be attempted with large fistulous tracts. In fistulae less than 3 mm, Stovsky reported closure in 11 of 17 patients with fulguration and 2 weeks of catheter drainage.[9] Recent reports have shown success with fibrin therapy to treat small vesicovaginal fistulae.[10] Most conservative measures ultimately fail in the attempt to cure vesicovaginal fistulae. Formal surgical repair remains the gold standard. For larger, complex, and radiation-induced fistulae, there is only a minor role for conservative treatment.

Preoperative considerations. Prior to formal repair of a vesicovaginal fistula, multiple factors must be considered. This will optimize the chances of a successful first repair. Traditionally, most authors advocated waiting 3–6 months prior to surgical repair in order to allow the fistula to completely mature.[11,12] This allowed maximal healing during the posthysterectomy inflammatory stage. Women with vesicovaginal fistulae experience enormous physical, social, and psychologic stress during this time period, which greatly hinders their quality of life. Many contemporary authors have reported excellent results with early repair, avoiding the great patient distress throughout the waiting period.[13,14]

Typically, early transvaginal repair is performed 2–3 weeks after the time of injury. This technique is most commonly performed in women with fistulae that form after abdominal hysterectomy. Patients with vaginal cuff infections or pelvic abscesses are not candidates for early repair and must be treated with long-term antibiotics prior to any repair attempt. Patients with previously failed repairs and radiation fistulae are not candidates for early intervention, and should wait at least several months prior to formal repair.

The most appropriate approach to formal surgical repair of vesicovaginal fistula is the one most familiar to the surgeon. Choosing between an abdominal and vaginal approach will depend on the surgeon's experience, training, and comfort level. The highest success rates are associated with the first operation, regardless of the approach. Traditionally, location of the fistula dictated the surgical approach. Supratrigonal fistulae were repaired transabdominally and infratrigonal and bladder neck fistulae were repaired vaginally. With good surgical technique and tissue interposition, even complex high vesicovaginal fistulae can be repaired utilizing a transvaginal approach. The advantage of the abdominal approach is the ability to perform simultaneous procedures for coexisting intraabdominal pathology. These include augmentation cystoplasty, ureteral reimplantation, and repair of bowel fistulae. The vaginal approach avoids an abdominal incision with possible bladder bivalving. It is associated with decreased morbidity, shorter hospital stay, and quicker patient convalescence. We utilize the transvaginal approach for the overwhelming majority of vesicovaginal fistulae. Therefore, this will be the focus of the chapter.

Regardless of the approach chosen, many principles are integral in fistula repair. Excellent exposure with watertight, tension-free closure utilizing multiple, nonoverlapping suture lines provide an approximately 90% chance of cure on the first attempt. Continuous catheter drainage postoperatively is mandatory. If any question exists, interpositional grafts will optimize the chance for cure.

Preoperative preparation includes antibiotics to clear any associated infection and provide a sterile environment for repair. Routine urine culture should document absence of infection beforehand. Broad-spectrum intravenous antibiotics are provided in the preoperative area. Estrogen-containing vaginal cream is used in the postmenopausal or posthysterectomy patient to improve the quality of the vaginal tissues.

Traditional repair of vesicovaginal fistula included excision of the tract to provide clean and vascular edges, which was thought to increase chances for cure. Raz and associates have demonstrated excellent results and no adverse outcomes without excising the fistulous tract.[15,16] Excising the fistula enlarges the tract and potentially causes iatrogenic bleeding, requiring hemostatic measures that may inhibit healing. In addition, excising fistulous tracts located near the ureteral orifices may require ureteral reimplantation.

Prior to any surgical repair, the surgeon should be familiar with several techniques for interposition of tissue. Although these grafts are often necessary in large, complex, postradiation, and failed primary repairs, it is difficult to accurately predict which fistulae will require the additional layer of coverage to avoid a tenuous repair.

Preoperative evaluation should always attempt to identify those patients who have stress urinary incontinence. Simultaneous sling procedure or bladder neck suspension can be performed to avoid the need for a second procedure. Concomitant repair for stress incontinence has been shown to cause no increase in fistula recurrence rate.[17] It is also important to consider the sexual function of the patient and ensure preservation of vaginal depth in the sexually active patient. This can require rotational flaps in patients with large fistulae and vaginal stenosis. Local estrogen replacement should be considered in patients with vaginal atrophy.

Transvaginal operative technique. We routinely repair vesicovaginal fistulae through a vaginal approach and will describe the basic technique for this procedure. This avoids the morbidity of a laparotomy and is performed on an outpatient basis.

Step 1: Patient preparation. The patient is placed in the low lithotomy position and prepped in standard fashion. A headlight provides excellent visualization for the primary surgeon. Cystoscopy with ureteral catheterization is done in cases where the fistula is located in proximity to the ureteral orifices. A curved Lowsley retractor is used to assist in placement of a 16 F suprapubic catheter through a small suprapubic incision. A relaxing incision (posterolateral episiotomy) may be necessary to aid in exposure in cases with a narrow vagina. The labia are sutured apart and a ring retractor is placed for optimal exposure. A urethral Foley catheter is placed as well, to ensure maximal urinary drainage. An Allis clamp is used to elevate the anterior vaginal wall and a posterior weighted speculum is positioned.

Step 2: Isolation of fistula. The fistulous tract is then identified and catheterized with an 8 or 10 F Foley catheter which aids in retraction throughout dissection (Fig. 20.1). Metal sounds may aid in dilating the tract prior to catheter placement. An inverted J incision is made, with care taken to circumscribe the fistulous tract (Fig. 20.2). The long end of the J should extend to the apex of the vagina, which will facilitate advancement and rotation of a posterior flap later in the procedure. Fistulae located high in the vaginal cuff may require an inverted incision, with the base of the flap facing the urethral meatus.

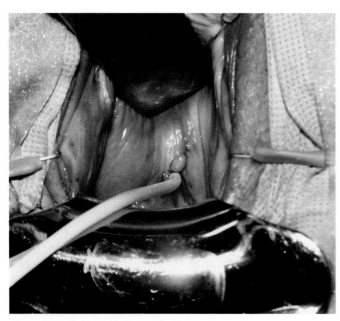

Figure 20.1 Catheterization of fistulous tract.

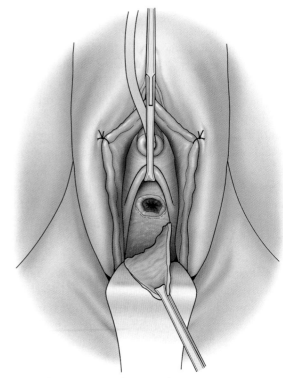

Figure 20.3 Development of vaginal flaps.

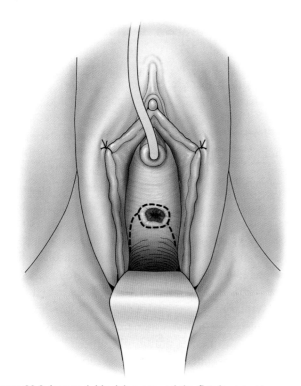

Figure 20.2 Inverted J incision around the fistulous tract.

Step 3: Creation of flaps. Anterior and posterior based vaginal flaps are dissected on each side of the fistulous tract, starting with healthy tissue away from the fistula (Fig. 20.3). This allows a natural plane of dissection and helps prevent enlargement of the fistulous tract or inadvertent bladder perforation. The ring of vaginal tissue at the opening of the fistula is left intact. The flaps should be developed at least 2–4 cm away from the fistulous tract, exposing the under-

lying perivesical fascia. The flaps are now retracted with the hooks of the ring retractor.

Step 4: Closure of fistula. The standard vesicovaginal fistula repair is done in three layers. The first layer closes the epithelialized edges of the fistula tract and a few mm of the surrounding tissue (including bladder wall) with interrupted 3-0 absorbable sutures (Vicryl or Dexon) in a transverse fashion (Fig. 20.4). The fistula catheter is removed and the sutures are tied, closing the fistulous tract. The second layer of the repair incorporates the perivesical fascia and deep muscular bladder wall using the same suture material (Fig. 20.5). The sutures are placed at least 1 cm from the prior suture line and secured tension free. The suture should be placed in a line 90° from the first suture layer to minimize overlapping suture lines. The bladder is filled with indigo carmine diluted in saline and the integrity of the repair is tested.

Step 5: Completion of operation. In a standard vesicovaginal fistula repair (without tissue interposition) the procedure is now completed. The previously raised posterior flap is now rotated beyond the fistula closure site by at least 3 cm (Fig. 20.6). Excess vaginal flap tissue is excised. This is closed using a running, locking absorbable 2-0 suture (Vicryl or Dexon). This covers the tract with healthy vaginal tissue and provides a third layer of closure with no overlapping of suture lines. An antibiotic-

SECTION 8 Fistula

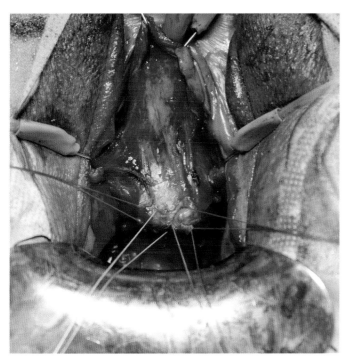

Figure 20.4 First layer of repair: transverse closure of fistulous tract without excision.

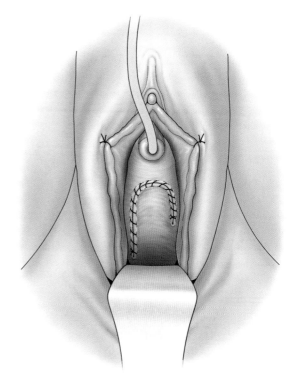

Figure 20.6 Third layer of repair: vaginal flap advancement.

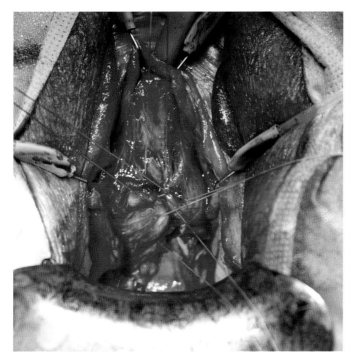

Figure 20.5 Second layer of repair: imbricates first layer with perivesical fascia.

impregnated vaginal pack is placed and the urethral and suprapubic catheters are left to dependent drainage.

The majority of cases of uncomplicated vesicovaginal fistula require only a three-layer tension-free repair. Complicating factors which mandate additional protection include prior radiation, failed prior surgery, and poor tissue quality. These conditions require tissue interposition and will be described below.

Transabdominal technique. This approach is outside the objectives of this chapter and is briefly described for discussion purposes only.

In our hands, the abdominal approach is utilized only in select patients requiring concomitant abdominal procedures such as augmentation cystoplasty or ureteral reimplantation. Preoperative bowel preparation is necessary in cases where augmentation is anticipated. The patient is placed supine with the legs in modified lithotomy for intraoperative vaginal access. The abdomen and vagina are prepped in standard fashion and a suprapubic tube is placed with a Lowsley retractor. A lower midline or Pfannenstiel incision is made, and the space of Retzius is exposed. An extra-peritoneal approach can be used, although an intraperitoneal approach assists in optimizing exposure and allows an omental flap to be positioned.

A Foley catheter is inserted into the bladder. Identification of the fistula may be aided by intravesical instillation of methylene blue. The dome of the bladder is elevated and dissection is performed between the base of the bladder and vagina toward the fistulous tract. The bladder is dissected completely free from the vagina with margins of at least 3 cm, and the fistulous tract is identified. The bladder is open only in the area of the fistula, without excising the fistula or bivalving the bladder. The bladder and vaginal defects are then each repaired in two layers using interrupted, absorbable sutures. Interposition with omentum, perivesical fat or peritoneum provides an additional layer of coverage. The abdominal wound is then closed and the suprapubic and Foley catheters are left to drainage.

Other techniques. Other authors advocate the O'Conor technique, a transvesical approach with bivalving of the bladder.[11] An anterior cystotomy is made in the sagittal plane and extended posteriorly to the fistula. The bladder is mobilized completely from the vagina and the fistula is excised. The openings in the bladder and vagina are closed separately in two layers with interrupted 2-0 absorbable sutures. An omental flap is placed between the bladder and vagina and the wound is closed.

The Latzko operation, described in 1942, uses a partial colpocleisis to treat vesicovaginal fistula.[18] The operation consists of denudement of the vaginal wall around the fistula without excising the fistulous tract. A separate layered closure is then performed including the bladder, vesico-vaginal fistula, and vagina. A potential drawback to this procedure is vaginal shortening. However, success rates of 93% and 95% have been reported in two series of 43 and 20 patients, respectively, with no significant patient-reported vaginal shortening or sexual dysfunction.[19,20] The technique is still performed by many gynecologists today due to its technical ease and minimal morbidity.

Transurethral suture cystorrhaphy without fistula tract excision has recently been described as a minimally invasive alternative for smaller fistulae (5–8 mm) located away from the ureteral orifices. The technique requires fulguration of the tract and surrounding bladder mucosa prior to combined transurethral/abdominal endoscopic suture placement. A minimum 2–3 week period of bladder drainage is necessary. Eight of 11 patients (73%) treated with this technique were cured.[21]

Vesicovaginal fistula repair has been described laparo-scopically since the recent explosion of minimally invasive surgery.[22] The approach was first described in 1994 and has undergone various modifications, including use of an endostapler, omental interposition, and layered closure.[23]

COMPLEX FISTULAE

Complex vesicovaginal fistulae include those fistulae asso-ciated with malignancy or prior radiation, recurrent fistulae, fistulae of large size (greater than 3 cm), fistulae involving the bladder neck and trigone, and those associated with poor tissue quality or difficult closure. In these cases it is manda-tory to modify the standard transvaginal vesicovaginal fistula repair. Multiple techniques of tissue interposition exist, providing an additional layer of closure and enhancing the quality of the reconstructive repair.

Radiation fistulae. Radiation-induced vesicovaginal fistulae represent a unique subset requiring special consid-eration. The site of fistula formation is typically in the trigone region. Since the trigone is in a relatively fixed position, radiation effects are more likely to occur. Radiation fistulae have been reported in 1–5% of patients treated for cervical or uterine carcinoma. The fistulae typically present in a delayed fashion, possibly up to 15–20 years later.[15] Fistulae occurring after radiation should always be biopsied to rule out recurrence of the primary malignancy.

Radiation-induced fistulae occur secondary to oblitera-tive endarteritis in the irradiated field.[24] The microvascular injury compromises healing and the tissues surrounding the fistula are also affected by the endarteritis, complicating an already difficult repair. Video urodynamics and cystoscopy allow assessment of bladder capacity and compliance. If there is adequate capacity and compliance, transvaginal repair is performed with certain modifications. Tissue inter-position with a Martius graft or omental flap is critical, as is prolonged postoperative catheter drainage. If the bladder has small capacity and poor compliance, augmentation cystoplasty is required and an abdominal approach is taken. Careful inspection of the bowel is necessary to ensure usage of a nonirradiated segment for the augmentation. Tissue interposition and prolonged catheter drainage are necessary steps, regardless of the approach, when repairing radiation-induced vesicovaginal fistulae.

Martius graft. The Martius graft (fibrofatty labial flap) was first described in 1928.[3] This technique is commonly used in perineal reconstructive surgery and has great utility in vesicovaginal fistula, rectovaginal fistula, urethral recon-struction, and urethrovaginal fistula. It has high reported success rates in complex fistula repair[25] and is the most convenient source of interposition in transvaginal vesico-vaginal repair. We use a Martius flap in all cases unless the fistula is located high in the vaginal vault (post hysterec-tomy). In these cases, the peritoneum is our preferred source of tissue interposition.

The Martius graft is a long band of adipose tissue from the labia majora. It has excellent strength (contains end fibers of round ligament) and vascularity. The blood supply is threefold. Branches of the external pudendal artery supply the graft superiorly and anteriorly. Obturator branches enter the graft at its lateral border. The inferior labial artery and vein supply the graft inferiorly. The graft may be mobilized superiorly or inferiorly depending on the desired location of transfer.

The first two layers of the fistula are closed as described earlier. The vaginal flaps are left intact and the labial retraction suture is removed. A vertical incision is then made over the labia majora and the subcutaneous tissues are dissected laterally to the lateral border of the dissection, the labiocrural fold. The flap is then dissected posteriorly to Colles' fascia and medially to the labia minora/bulbocavernosus muscle. The main vascular supply is at the base and the entire thickness of the fat pad is carefully encircled by a Penrose drain. The superior and anterior segment of the graft is clamped, transected, and suture-ligated. The remaining dissection is completed and the flap is now freed, except at its base (Fig. 20.7). A tunnel is then created between the vaginal wall and the perivaginal tissues. The graft is then passed from the labial area to the vaginal area (through the tunnel) with the aid of a hemostat (Fig. 20.8). The Martius graft is then placed over the fistula site and secured tension free with interrupted absorbable sutures. The vaginal flap is now advanced and closed as previously described, providing a fourth layer of closure. A light pressure dressing may be applied and ice packs are routine.

Eilber et al reported a 97% cure rate with transvaginal repair using Martius graft interposition in 34 patients with complex fistulae.[26]

Peritoneal flap.
We utilize a peritoneal flap in the repair of high fistulae located at the vaginal vault, which are seen most commonly after hysterectomy. Extending a Martius graft to this location may result in inadvertent vaginal shortening. A peritoneal flap is an easily available, well-vascularized tissue that can be harvested without a second incision.

The fistula repair begins as described in the first three steps of the transvaginal technique. The fistula is now circumscribed and vaginal flaps are prepared. A catheter in the fistula can help in dissection of the flaps. Sharp dissection is used to expose the peritoneum and preperitoneal fat. The fistulous tract is then closed in two layers, as previously described. The preperitoneal fat and peritoneum are now advanced to cover the fistula repair and secured to the perivesical fascia with tension-free interrupted sutures (Fig. 20.9). The vaginal flap is then advanced and closed.

Raz et al reported a 91% success rate in their initial experience using a peritoneal flap in 11 patients with vesicovaginal fistula.[27] Eilber et al reported a 96% cure rate using a peritoneal flap in 83 patients who underwent complex fistula repair.[26] It has high success rates, minimal morbidity, and equal outcomes to a Martius graft, without a second incision.

Omental interposition.
Omental interposition is primarily used in the abdominal approach for fistula repair, although it can be accessed transvaginally in women who have had previous procedures. Understanding the blood supply to the omentum is critical prior to mobilization in vesicovaginal fistula repair. Vascular supply to the omentum is derived from the right gastroepiploic artery (branch off the gastroduodenal artery) and the left gastroepiploic artery (branch off the splenic artery). The right and left omental arteries take origin from their respective gastroepiploic branches and unite at the inferior aspect of the stomach in a U-shaped fashion. Variably, there is a middle omental artery which bisects the U into two sections. Omental flaps are typically based on the right gastroepiploic artery, as it is the dominant supply in the majority of cases.

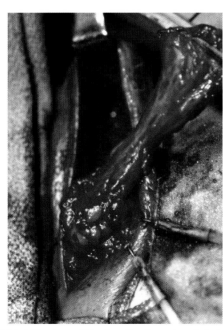

Figure 20.7 Mobilization of Martius flap based on inferior pedicle.

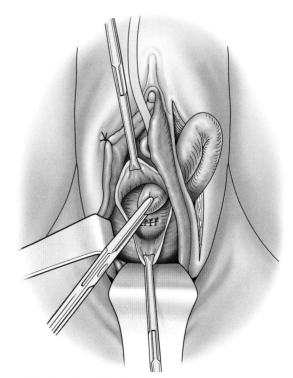

Figure 20.8 Transfer of Martius flap to cover fistula repair.

The omentum can be quite redundant in certain cases and reach down into the pelvis with minimal to no mobilization. If the omentum only requires minimal mobilization, an L-shaped incision below the transverse colon (based on the right omental artery) may be all that is required. Additional length can be obtained by dissecting the omentum off its attachments to the transverse colon. In cases requiring major mobilization, the left short gastric arteries are taken down, the transverse colon attachments are dissected off, and an incision is made down the center of the omentum. These techniques all result in an omental graft which can be placed between the bladder and vagina for an additional layer of protection.

Full-thickness labial flap. In select complex cases with loss of vaginal wall, insufficient vaginal epithelium may preclude primary vaginal closure. A full-thickness labial flap can be rotated to substitute for the missing vaginal wall. The fistula is closed as previously described, and the vascularized flap is rotated to provide full-thickness skin coverage.

After closure of the fistula, a U-shaped incision is made over the labia including the lateral labial skin and underlying tissue. The base of the flap is at the level of the posterior fourchette. The flap is dissected from the fascia overlying the pubic bone and then rotated to cover the repair. Interrupted absorbable sutures are used to secure the edges in place.[28] Small series have reported excellent results. Carr and Webster reported excellent outcomes in four patients.[29] Postoperative complications include sensory deficit at the harvest site and poor cosmetic result, in addition to wound infection and flap sloughing.

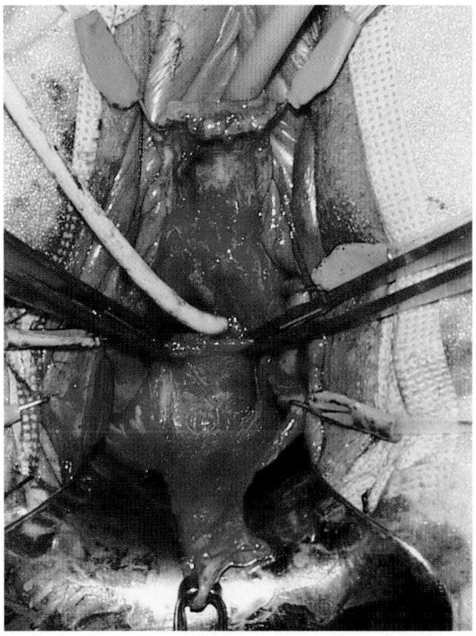

Gluteal skin flap. Gluteal skin flaps are used predominantly in patients with postradiation fistulae or severe vaginal wall atrophy with no other available and viable skin source. The first two layers of the fistula are closed and the vaginal flaps raised as described earlier. A longitudinal incision is made in the vaginal wall toward the midportion of the labia majora. This is then extended in a semicircular fashion in the gluteal skin. The skin is then undermined and the flap is rotated and advanced into the vaginal canal to cover the fistula. The flap is secured with interrupted, absorbable sutures and the vaginal flaps are secured to the skin flap edges.[30] Complications include wound infection, sloughing of the flap, and injury to the anal sphincter.[31] Meticulous surgical technique is mandatory to avoid the latter complication.

Myocutaneous gracilis flap. The gracilis muscle-based myocutaneous flap has been frequently described in association with repair of the postradiation vesicovaginal fistula in patients with vaginal atrophy or absence. The gracilis muscle is a long slender muscle which extends from the inferior pubic symphysis to the medial condyle of the femur. It is an accessory muscle used for thigh adduction and knee flexion and can be sacrificed with no loss of function. It sits between the adductor magnus medially and the adductor longus laterally. Its blood supply is derived from the medial femoral circumflex artery, a branch of the deep femoral artery.

The flap is harvested with a tennis racquet incision on the medial aspect of the thigh over the gracilis muscle. It begins around 10 cm below the pubic tubercle and extends 20 cm toward the knee (Fig. 20.10). The skin and underlying muscle are mobilized, with care taken to preserve the vascular supply. The gracilis is transected at its distal insertion. A tunnel is then created underneath the medial aspect of the

Figure 20.9 Peritoneal flap advancement.

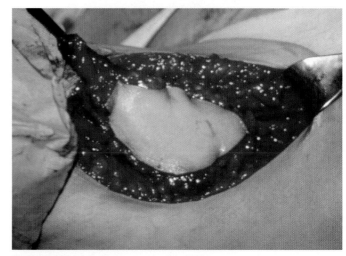

Figure 20.10 Gracilis myocutaneous flap.

SECTION 8 Fistula

thigh and labia, and the flap is transferred to the vaginal area for additional coverage of the fistula tract and reconstruction of the vaginal canal. This can result in considerable cosmetic scarring but there is no functional defect.

INTRAOPERATIVE COMPLICATIONS

Bleeding and ureteral injury represent the two major potential intraoperative complications. Hemostasis is critical during the vaginal flap dissection and can be controlled with fine absorbable sutures. Electrocautery should be avoided. Anything short of perfect hemostasis can lead to hematoma formation with possible disruption of the fistula repair.

Ureteral catheterization is recommended for fistulae close to the trigone because of the higher risk of iatrogenic ureteral injury. Fistulae located elsewhere do not usually require this maneuver. If there is any concern about ureteral injury, perform cystoscopy after intravenous indigo carmine is administered. Ureteral catheterization can also be performed.

POSTOPERATIVE MANAGEMENT (TRANSVAGINAL REPAIR)

The vagina is packed with an antibiotic-impregnated gauze which is left for several hours. Surgery is mostly performed on an outpatient basis. The suprapubic and Foley catheters (joined to a Y-connector) are left to dependent drainage for a minimum of 2–3 weeks. Anticholinergics are given to minimize bladder spasm and augment patient comfort. An oral quinolone or cephalosporin is continued until the Foley catheter is removed. Patients are instructed to resume normal activity except for strenuous exercise. In addition, sexual intercourse is prohibited for 12 weeks. The urethral catheter is removed 2–3 weeks after surgery and a suprapubic cystogram is performed. If the cystogram demonstrates no extravasation, the suprapubic catheter is removed.

OUTCOMES

Many factors must be considered when assessing patient outcomes. Cure rate, morbidity, and patient satisfaction are critical factors in determining patient success and the ideal approach. There have been no prospective, randomized studies comparing vaginal and abdominal approaches in vesicovaginal fistula repair. Many series have shown success rates of 90–100% with both approaches.[15,32-34] The best approach remains the one with which the surgeon has the most expertise.

POSTOPERATIVE COMPLICATIONS

Early complications such as vaginal bleeding, bladder spasms, and vaginal infection must be treated aggressively and immediately to avoid fistula recurrence. Secondary vaginal bleeding is treated with repacking and bedrest. Prophylactic anticholinergics should minimize bladder spasms. B and O suppositories can be used if required. Perioperative antibiotics continued in the postoperative period are important in preventing vaginal infections.

The most important delayed complication is fistula recurrence. Others include vaginal shortening and stenosis, and unrecognized ureteral injury. Tension-free, multi-layered closure, with tissue interposition as needed, results in a greater than 95% success rate. If the fistula recurs, a second vaginal repair may be performed with a Martius graft or peritoneal flap. A waiting period of at least 3 months after previous repair allows for resolution of postoperative inflammation. Care must be taken to not perform excessive resection of the vaginal wall, as this can result in significant shortening and stenosis. In these cases secondary vaginoplasty is required. Unrecognized ureteral injury presents more commonly as an obstruction than a leak. An antegrade approach with percutaneous nephrostomy is preferred to a retrograde procedure due to the possible disruption of the repair via a transurethral approach.

CONCLUSION

Vesicovaginal fistula remains a significant source of morbidity in the female after gynecologic and pelvic surgery. Transvaginal surgical repair is an outpatient procedure associated with high success rates, minimal morbidity, and quick convalescence times. It remains our preferred method of repair in all but the select few cases requiring concomitant abdominal surgery.

REFERENCES

1. Sims JM. On the treatment of vesico-vaginal fistula. Am J Med Sci 1852;23:59–82.
2. Mackenrodt A Die operative Heiling grosser Blasencheindenfisteln. Zentralbl Gynakol 1894;8:180–184.
3. Martius H. Uber die Behandlung von Blasenscheidenfisteln, insbesondere met Hilfe einer Lappenplastik. Geburtshilfe Gynakol 1932;103:22–34.
4. Lee RA, Symmonds RE, Williams TH. Current status of genitourinary fistula. Obstet Gynecol 1998;72:313–319.
5. Drutz HP, Mainprize TC. Unrecognized small vesicovaginal fistula as a cause of persistent urinary incontinence. Am J Obstet Gynecol 1988;158:237.

6. Kursh ED, Morse RM, Resnick MI, et al. Prevention of the development of a vesicovaginal fistula. Surg Gynecol Obstet 1988;166(5):409–412.

7. Symmonds RE. Incontinence: vesical and urethral fistulas. Obstet Gynecol 1984;27:499–514.

8. Graham JB. Vaginal fistulae following radiotherapy. Surg Gynecol Obstet 1965;120:1019–1030.

9. Stovsky MD, Ignaroff JM, Blum MD, et al. Use of electrocoagulation in the treatment of vesicovaginal fistulas. J Urol 1994;152:1443–1444.

10. Morita T, Tokue A. Successful endoscopic closure of radiation induced vesico-vaginal fistula with fibrin glue and bovine collagen. J Urol 1999;162:1689.

11. O'Conor VJ. Review of experience with vesico-vaginal fistula repair. J Urol 1980;123(3):367–369.

12. Wein AJ, Malloy TR, Carpiniello VL, et al. Repair of vesico-vaginal fistula by a suprapubic transvesical approach. Surg Gynecol Obstet 1980;150:57–60.

13. Blaivis JG, Heritz DM, Romanzi LJ. Early versus late repair of vesicovaginal fistulas: vaginal and abdominal approaches. J Urol 1995;153(4):1110–1112.

14. Raz S, Little NA, Juma S. Female urology. In: Walsh PC, Retik AB, Stamey TA, eds. Campbell's urology, 6th edn. Philadelphia: WB Saunders; 1992.

15. Zimmern PE, Hadley HR, Staskin DR, Raz S. Genitourinary fistulae: vaginal approach for repair of vesicovaginal fistulae. Urol Clin North Am 1985;12(2):361–367.

16. Leach GE, Raz S. Vaginal flap technique: a method of transvaginal vesicovaginal fistula repair. In: Raz S, ed. Female urology. Philadelphia: WB Saunders; 1992.

17. Arrowsmith SD. Genitourinary reconstruction in obstetric fistulas. J Urol 1994;152(1): 403–406.

18. Latzko W. Postoperative vesicovaginal fistulas: genesis and therapy. Am J Surg 1942;58: 211–228.

19. Tancer ML. The post-total hysterectomy (vault) vesicovaginal fistula. J Urol 1980;123: 839–840.

20. D'Amico AM, Lloyd KL. Latzko repair of vesicovaginal fistula. J Urol 1999;161(4S):202.

21. Mckay HA. Vesicovaginal fistula repair: transurethral suture cystorrhaphy as a minimally invasive alternative. J Endourol 2004;18(5):487–490.

22. Ou C, Huang U, Tsuang M, Rowbotham R. Laparoscopic repair of vesicovaginal fistula. J Laparoendoscopic Adv Surg Tech 2004;14(1):17–20.

23. Nezhat CH, Nezhat F, Nezhat C, et al. Laparoscopic repair of vesicovaginal fistula: a case report. Obstet Gynecol 1994;83:899–901.

24. Perez Ca, Grigsby PW, Lockett MA, et al. Radiation therapy morbidity in carcinoma of the uterine cervix: dosimetric and clinical correlation. Int J Radiat Oncol Biol Phys 1999;44:855–866.

25. Margolis T, Elkins TE, Seffah J, et al. Full-thickness Martius grafts to preserve vaginal depth as an adjunct in the repair of large obstetric fistulas. Obstet Gynecol 1994;84(1):148–152.

26. Eilber KS, Kavaler E, Rodriguez LV, et al. Ten-year experience with transvaginal vesicovaginal fistula repair using tissue interposition. J Urol 2003;169:1033–1036.

27. Raz S, Bregg KJ, Nitti VW, et al. Transvaginal repair of vesicovaginal fistula using a peritoneal flap. J Urol 1993;150:56.

28. Raz S. Atlas of transvaginal surgery. Philadelphia: WB Saunders; 2002.

29. Carr LK, Webster GD. Full-thickness cutaneous Martius flaps: a useful technique in female reconstructive urology. Urology 1996;48:461–463.

30. Stothers L, Chopra A, Raz S. Vesicovaginal fistula. In: Raz S, ed. Female urology, 2nd edn. Philadelphia: WB Saunders; 1996.

31. Wang Y, Hadley HR. The use of rotated vascularized pedicle flaps for complex transvaginal procedures. J Urol 1993;149:590–592.

32. Langkilde NC, Pless TK, Lundbeck F, et al. Surgical repair of vesicovaginal fistulae: a ten-year retrospective study. Scand J Urol Nephrol 1999;33:100–103.

33. Diaz CE, Calatrava GS, Caldentey GM, et al. Surgical repair of vesico-vaginal fistulae with abdominal-transvesical approach. Comments on this technique with long-term results. Arch Esp Urol 1997;50:55–60.

34. Frohmuller H, Hofmockel G. Transvaginal closure of vesicovaginal fistulas. Urologe A 1998;37:102.

Vesicovaginal and Rectovaginal Fistula Repair

Christopher R Chapple and Richard Turner-Warwick

Whatever may be the cause of this distressing affection, it is a matter of serious importance to both surgeon and patient that it be rendered susceptible of cure. (Sims 1852)[1]

INTRODUCTION

Van Roonhuyse (1672) is credited with being amongst the first to carry out surgical repair of a fistula,[2] by denuding the fistula edge and then closing the defect using sharpened goose quills wrapped in red waxed silk. Joubert (1834) emphasized the importance of avoiding tension during closure and attempted the use of labial skin flaps;[3] Gosset described a surgical cure in 1834[4] and Hayward in 1839.[5] Nevertheless, Sims (1852) is widely recognized as having pioneered the modern era of fistula repair with his masterly description of a technique.[1] His repair was carried out with the patient in the prone position and emphasized the importance of good exposure (the Sims speculum), tension-free approximation of the wound edges with nonreactive silver sutures, and continuous bladder drainage after closure.

Fistulae involving the vagina in undeveloped societies are most commonly associated with obstetric trauma and as such have from ancient times represented an important cause of severe morbidity and mortality in young women. In our society, urinary–vaginal fistulae, occurring most commonly between bladder and vagina and sometimes involving the ureter, are usually associated with gynecologic surgery and occasionally complicate the management of gynecologic malignancy. Fistulous communications between the bladder or urethra and adjacent structures are a cause of great distress to the patient. Few patients are more anxious to be cured of their affliction or are more grateful when this has been accomplished. The vast majority of such fistulae occur in women and result from gynecologic or obstetric trauma, most commonly urinary vaginal fistulae involving the bladder, ureter and rarely the urethra. Vesicointestinal communications usually occur as a complication of inflammatory or malignant bowel disease, with the exception of the rare case of the radiation-damaged "frozen pelvis" following treatment of gynecologic malignancy. Urethrorectal and urethrocutaneous fistulae are the only groups which occur most commonly in men.

The subdivision of fistulae into "simple" and "complex" introduces further nomenclature. At first sight this might be considered to unnecessarily complicate matters but it serves a useful purpose in defining the appropriate surgical repair. Simple fistulae can usually be resolved by a simple closure in layers. More complex cases with associated tissue devascularization, previous failed surgical repair attempts or irradiation, extensive tissue loss or persistence of a focus of infection or malignancy may require the use of adjunctive procedures. Fistulae arising from many etiologies, whether traumatic, surgical, inflammatory, neoplastic or radiation induced, are invariably amenable to surgical repair.

DIAGNOSIS

The classic symptom of a urinary–vaginal fistula is continuous diurnal involuntary incontinence following a hysterectomy or other pelvic operation. Nevertheless, in situations where there is a small fistula, the symptomatology may be far less florid and comprises no more than a watery vaginal discharge accompanied by normal voiding.

Definition of the precise anatomic abnormality is necessary prior to taking a decision on the appropriate management of a fistula. All patients should have an intravenous urogram to assess the number of ureters and look for the presence of dilation or extravasation from a ureter which would be suggestive of its involvement in the fistula. A voiding cystourethrogram may demonstrate the presence of a fistula (Fig. 21.1) and will document any associated vesicoureteric reflux, bladder base prolapse, and stress incontinence which may either relate to the patient's symptomatology or could be usefully corrected at the time of surgical repair of the fistula.

The combined use of imaging modalities and a careful examination under anesthetic are an essential part of the

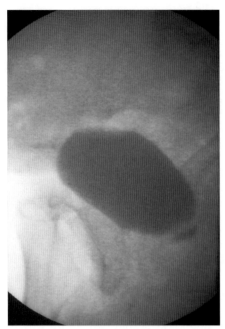

Figure 21.1 A voiding cystourethrogram may demonstrate the presence of a fistula.

management of fistulae, since in many cases more than one structure, e.g. both the bladder and ureter, is involved in the fistula. A careful cystoscopy, vaginoscopy, and examination under anesthetic (EUA) are essential in all cases and will often demonstrate small fistulae not seen on other investigation.

The majority of vesicovaginal fistulae are easy to identify. Fistulae that are associated with thin-walled bladders, in the midline above the trigone, may be large enough to feel with the tip of a finger in the vagina. Conversely, a long-established "pinhole" fistula in the base of the bladder is not associated with "tell-tale" hyperemia around its margins and it may be difficult to identify endoscopically. If the appearance is equivocal it may be helpful to distend the bladder with irrigation fluid with the patient in the lithotomy position and to observe the anterior vaginal wall for a jet or a drip leakage, using a speculum in the vagina and a fiberlight sucker. Alternatively, endoscopic examination of both the bladder and the vagina with a cystoscope, with gentle probing of suspicious areas with a guidewire, can also be extremely helpful since catheterization of a fistula which might not be easy to spot can suddenly make the situation much clearer. It is important to remember that there may be more than one fistulous track, especially after the failure of a previous repair procedure.

A biopsy should be taken from the edges of the fistula in all cases where there is any history of pelvic malignancy. If ureteric damage is suspected, ascending bulb ureterograms can be carried out and this can be followed by the insertion of double pigtail "JJ stents." In addition, the demonstration of associated functional abnormalities and the presence of

malignant disease are all important contributory factors which need to be considered and investigated prior to undertaking reparative surgery. In principle, any vesicovaginal fistula is amenable to surgical repair. Fistula occurring in association with current malignancy following therapy for a gynecologic malignancy may still be suitable for surgical intervention as excisional surgery may be curative.

Where doubt remains as to the exact diagnosis even at the time of an EUA, the synchronous use of the "three-sponge test" can provide helpful additional information (Fig. 21.2), as can insufflation of the vagina which in the presence of a fistula produces a stream of air bubbles which can be seen at cystoscopy. The "three-sponge" test simply involves the placement of three separate and suitably sized gauze sponges to gently fill the vagina, one above the other. A colored fluid such as aqueous methylene blue is then introduced into the bladder with a catheter and the three sponges are removed after about 20 minutes. Remember to remove the urethral catheter after filling the bladder, to avoid masking a urethrovaginal fistula.

- If only the lowermost sponge is colored it suggests that the leakage has come down the urethra, indicating either a low urethral fistula or simply urethral incontinence backtracking into the introitus.
- If both the lower sponges are unstained and the top sponge is wet with unstained urine, it generally indicates a ureterovaginal fistula.
- If only the upper sponge is stained, it suggests a vesicovaginal fistula. Very occasionally dye staining of the uppermost sponge can result from reflux of the dye from the bladder into the ureter and its leakage from a ureterovaginal fistula.

CONSERVATIVE MANAGEMENT

What are the indications for surgery versus conservative treatment? In a proportion of patients with small "simple" vesicovaginal and ureterovaginal fistulae, conservative therapy may result in resolution of the fistula. In such patients the use of continuous drainage with a urethral catheter or internal splintage with a double pigtail stent, respectively, needs to be considered. Nevertheless it must be borne in mind that there is a low incidence of such spontaneous closure in many series; indeed, Marshall reported only one case in a series of 92 patients.[6]

A number of adjunct measures can be used in addition to drainage.

- Local or systemic estrogen therapy[7]
- Antibiotic prophylaxis[8]
- Cystoscopic fulguration of the fistula[9]
- Corticosteroid therapy[10]

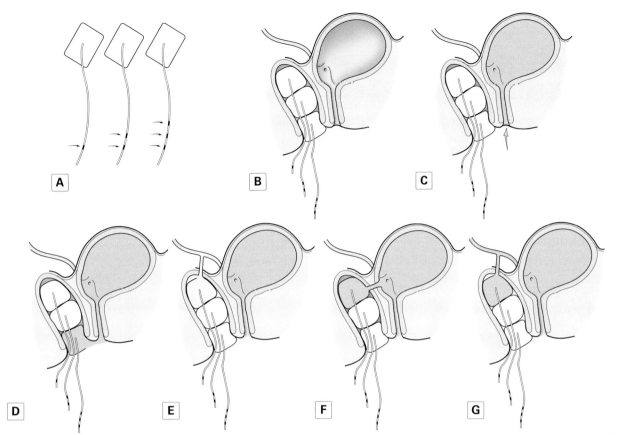

Figure 21.2 Three-swab test showing the importance of identifying individual swabs and the way in which this can localize a site of leakage. Note bottom right a false positive due to reflux up the ureter and leakage from a ureterovaginal fistula.

Both estrogen therapy in the postmenopausal patient and antibiotic prophylaxis are likely to help by improving the quality of the tissues and would certainly aid subsequent surgery. Cauterization of the fistula was described as of limited benefit, except in small fistulae, by Sims, a sentiment reiterated by O'Conor who reported success with six patients.[9] It seems unlikely that corticosteroid therapy has much to recommend it since, although it will reduce edema, it will also impair healing.

With all nonsurgical management, it must be remembered that the majority of fistulae will fail to heal and this needs to be balanced against the near certainty of a surgical cure, particularly if there is an iatrogenic etiology.

TIMING OF SURGERY

It is an essential requirement prior to surgery to have accurate knowledge of the patient's vaginal and urinary tract bacteriology, so that any pathogens can be eradicated by appropriate antimicrobial therapy; antibiotic prophylaxis should be used routinely.

It is difficult to generalize about the appropriate timing of surgical intervention for every case, since this will depend upon the systemic and local factors influencing the healing potential of the local tissues in the individual case. In the otherwise uncomplicated simple postoperative fistula, it is invariably possible to resolve the problem by early exploration within a few weeks, before the processes of inflammation and repair render surgery difficult. The majority of evidence suggests that if this window of opportunity is missed, it is wise to defer surgery for at least 3 months,[6,11] as it would be inappropriate to carry out a surgical procedure which would potentially be rendered more complex and extensive and where morbidity is likely to be higher. In more complex fistulae where tissue healing is dependent on the interposition of a pedicled flap of vascularized tissue such as omentum, this timing is less critical to healing but surgery carried out at an inappropriate time may be rendered far more difficult. Although some workers have advocated repair between 3 and 12 weeks,[12,13] it must be remembered that these cases were all repaired by the use of interposed flaps of peritoneum or omentum. It is salutary that in a reported series of 11 "early" repairs of vesicovaginal fistula, 10 cases were successfully operated on before 3 weeks had elapsed after injury but the remaining case repaired by simple layer closure at 35 days recurred on the fifth postoperative day.[14]

CHOICE OF APPROACH

The decision as to the best surgical approach for an individual case will of course be considerably biased by an individual surgeon's preference and training. It will also depend upon the etiology, position, and size of the vesical fistula and the concurrence of associated ureteric or urethral damage. Adequate surgical access to the fistula itself and to allow associated procedures such as urethral repair, ureteric reimplantation or the interposition of pedicle flaps is essential to a successful repair. These requirements should be the most important factor in determining the optimal surgical approach.

Specific patient positioning. The options for the open surgical repair for the vesicovaginal fistula are as follows.

Vaginal approach. The positioning for vaginal approach can either be with the patient in the standard lithotomy position or in the modified Sims position (see Fig. 21.3). A perineal approach provides limited access but avoids the morbidity associated with any abdominal procedure. It is ideally suited to closure of the low simple fistula and can be combined with the use of an interposed pedicled flap of labial/scrotal tissue or gracilis muscle, for more complex fistulae.

Abdominal approach. The abdominal approach is more invasive for the patient but is indicated for the repair of high or complex fistulae, and lends itself to the concomitant interposition of a pedicled omental flap in the repair. The most logical approach is to have available the expertise to utilize all of the available procedures as most appropriate,[15,16] preparing the patient for a synchronous perineo-abdominal procedure at the outset of an operation; thereby facilitating the progression of one to the other as necessary.[11]

Laparoscopy. Recent case reports have documented the use of laparoscopic techniques but they are still being perfected and cannot be considered to be mainstream therapy at this time.

REPAIR TECHNIQUE

The plethora of reports in the literature bears witness not only to the variation in success of the different surgical methods in the hands of individual surgeons, but to the diversity of different procedures available. Any surgical repair will succeed provided that it removes any predisposing etiologic cause for a fistula and reconstitutes a defect by the approximation of clean, well-vascularized tissue. These criteria are easily achieved in simple fistulae by the trimming and tension-free approximation of adjacent wound edges. In more complex cases where the fistulous defect is large or fibrosis resulting from infection, surgery or irradiation compromises tissue healing, the interposition of a pedicled flap of well-vascularized tissue markedly increases the chances of a successful repair. In these cases it must be remembered that if the tension-free apposition of an epithelial defect is not possible, the migration of epithelial cells will occur over an interposed vascularized pedicled flap and therefore it is perfectly acceptable to leave defects provided that they are adequately covered by the flap.

Specific equipment and materials. Appropriate instrumentation can greatly improve access for a fistula repair. A ring retractor is recommended along with a variety of fixed and malleable copper blades which are available for ring retraction.

- Self-retaining retractor for vaginal surgery, e.g. Parkes anal retractor
- Curved needle holders (Turner-Warwick)
- Additional targeted lighting, delivered with the aid of either a fiberlight sucker or an appropriate headlamp
- Cystoscope and Albarran catheterization bridge, 30° telescope
- Ureteric catheters × 3
- 16 F silicone Foley catheters × 2
- Standard operating instruments dictated by the surgeon's preference

Basic principles. Absorbable suture materials should be used. Interrupted sutures ensure the best possible vascularization of the tissue between tissue bites but this advantage can be compromised by inflammatory reaction at the site of knots and a rational compromise is the use of interrupted short runs. The routine use of effective prophylactic postoperative antibiotic cover is important.

Adequate postoperative drainage of the bladder via urethral and suprapubic catheters is recommended since if one of these blocks, the other would hopefully be patent, thereby protecting the bladder repair. This should be maintained postoperatively until it has served its intended function, which depends upon the surgeon's judgment. As a rule of thumb, if there is any doubt it is generally better to maintain catheter drainage a little longer rather than removing it too early, based on the principle that "there is no such thing as brave surgeons, just brave patients."

Tissue interposition support. The principles of the layer closure of a fistula are well established. The adjuvant use of an additional supporting tissue is a generally advisable routine after a layer closure whenever this is easily available. However, when the healing potential of the tissue around a fistula is compromised for any reason, such as diabetes, infection, infestation, the failure of previous repairs or irradiation, the reliability of a simple layer closure procedure diminishes and the failure rate rapidly escalates unless a definitive well-vascularized transposition graft is interposed.

A number of techniques have been described in the literature. These include the use of peritoneal interposition, first described by Bardescu in 1900,[17,18] the use of island myocutaneous and fasciocutaneous flaps,[19,20] bladder mucosa[21] and the use of omentum, which was first reported by Walters in 1935[22] and popularized in the last three decades.[23,24]

Flaps of local peritoneum. The transposition of a flap of pelvic peritoneum was described more than 100 years ago. This is sometimes useful as a simple adjuvant support of the layer closure of a "simple" fistula but its vascularization is not particularly good and it is quite inadequate when positive support is required as a result of significant local pathology that is likely to compromise healing. This is in addition to the fact that it is itself commonly compromised by this local tissue abnormality.

Pedicled flaps of skeletal muscle. Skeletal muscle had some inherent limitations as a supporting tissue.

- Its "resting" vascularization is minimal and is only maximally augmented during muscular exercise.
- It is relatively poorly adapted to resist infection; thus it can disintegrate when repositioned into the severely infected surroundings of some complex fistulae.
- It is not specially adapted to resolve inflammation so that it can contribute little to the local tissue healing when this is severely impaired.
- Inactivity of a muscle eventually results in disuse atrophy and it is largely replaced by fibrous tissue unless it is regularly exercised.

However, a muscle flap that is adequately vascularized is most useful when the reconstructive requirement is a sizeable bulk of viable interposition tissue in the situation that is not grossly infected.

Martius labial rotation flap. A Martius flap provides useful vagino-urethral interposition support after a vaginal-approach layer closure of a fistula and it was originally developed for this purpose. Its particular advantage is that it is locally available during a perineal approach without a synchronous abdominal approach.

It is a simple fat pad, which provides a thin but reasonably well-vascularized tissue bulk. It has no special healing qualities so it is by no means comparable with the omentum.

Omental support. The use of omentum should be the first-line choice. It is readily available and easy to mobilize, readily reaching down to the perineum in most cases, has a good blood and lymphatic supply, and sufficient bulk to fill dead space without producing marked fibrosis during healing, which may compromise lower urinary tract function and render subsequent surgery more difficult. In contrast, peritoneum, whilst being readily available, does not possess these other properties and is likely to have been involved in local pathology or in the irradiated field. Bladder mucosal grafts can be used in a manner analogous to the techniques using vaginal mucosa but carry the same potential disadvantages as suggested for peritoneum. Other flap procedures are an important part of the armamentarium but require particular expertise.

The omentum should always be separated from its attachment to the transverse colon and mesocolon since postoperative distension of the bowel may otherwise dislodge its attachment to the subsequent repair. The lower margin of the omental apron will reach the perineum without additional mobilization in 30% of cases. In the remaining cases some degree of mobilization of the omentum by division of part of its vascular pedicle is necessary. Whilst Kiricuta suggested that the omentum should be mobilized on the left gastroepiploic pedicle,[23] Turner-Warwick has raised the important technical point that the gastroepiploic arch becomes increasingly small towards its left extremity and that the omental flap should be based on the right gastroepiploic pedicle for a more reliable blood supply.[24] In approximately 30% of cases, sufficient elongation is achieved by division of the left gastroepiploic pedicle and those of the direct left lateral vessels to the omentum. In the remaining cases, full mobilization is required on the right gastroepiploic vessel right over to its gastroduodenal origin to prevent undue traction on individual short gastric vessels which might result in shearing and postoperative hemorrhage. Careful ligation of individual short gastric vessels is necessary using an absorbable suture. The resultant slender pedicle of this flap is protected by relocating it behind the mobilized descending colon.

Mobilization of the omentum from the stomach does result in a mild ileus and it is therefore sensible to institute gastric suction for a few days postoperatively (insertion of a gastrostomy tube is a humane alternative to a nasogastric tube, particularly as the stomach is suitably exposed).

VAGINAL REPAIR OF VESICOVAGINAL FISTULA

Exposure. The patient is placed on the operating table in a slightly head-down position, hips flexed to 30°, and legs widely abducted. The use of either the lithotomy or prone position has the disadvantage that should vaginal repair prove troublesome, then progression to a synchronous abdominal approach is difficult or impossible. Optimal exposure of the fistula is achieved by the use of either a weighted

Auvard posterior vaginal retractor, used in conjunction with temporary lateral stay sutures to the labia minora attached laterally under tension to the towels, or alternatively, a ring retractor. In the presence of a narrowed introitus, exposure can be improved by a posterolateral relaxing incision prior to insertion of the retractor.

Technique (Fig. 21.3).

Ureteric catheters facilitate the identification of the ureteric orifices and the extravesical location of the terminal ureteric segments while repairing bladder base fistulae. The vaginal orifice of the fistula is identified. Two stay sutures are inserted into the vaginal wall anterolateral to it and directional traction on these, anchored in relation to the appropriate guide-knobs of the perineal ring retractor, effectively draws the fistula down to the introitus. The traction on these stay sutures is generally preferable to the alternative procedure of traction on a balloon catheter passed through the fistula because this has to be removed before layer closure of the bladder can be achieved.

A third stay suture is inserted into the vaginal wall in the midline above the fistula to stabilize its retraction. If laxity of the anterior vaginal wall does not allow this to be drawn down effectively to the introitus, it can be usefully retracted posteriorly using the guide-locating notch in the distal margin of the posterior vaginal blade of the ring retractors with appropriate tension anchorage at the ring margin.

The margin of the fistula is circumcised (Fig. 21.4). The excision of the perifistula scarring is facilitated by traction on additionally inserted stay sutures. The layer between the vaginal wall and the bladder wall is developed.

The bladder wall is closed with an interrupted 4/0 polyglycolic acid (PGA) suture, the knots being tied on the lumen until the last two or three sutures are inserted. A Martius interposition flap is raised and tunneled through to the fistula closure site. The vaginal wall is closed: the Martius labial incision is occluded with 3/0 PGA dead space-encircling sutures.

A suprapubic catheter and a urethral catheter are positioned with the synchronous pull-in procedure. When the prone position is used for a vaginal repair, the suprapubic catheter is inserted with the patient in the supine position before she is turned over.

Closure.

It is important that the tissues used in the closure should be well vascularized and wherever possible, suture lines which are in contact should be offset or placed at 180° to each other. Absorbable sutures of interrupted 3/0 Dexon or Vicryl are used. In the first layer the bladder wall is closed vertically (Fig. 21.5A), then the perivesical tissues are

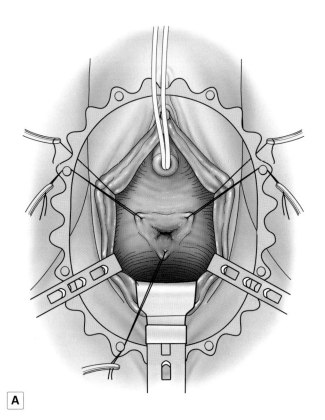

A

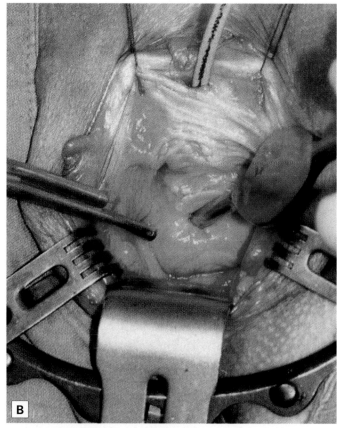

B

Figure 21.3 Ureteric catheters facilitate the identification of the ureteric orifices and the extravesical location of the terminal ureteric segments while repairing bladder base fistulae. The vaginal orifice of the fistula is identified.

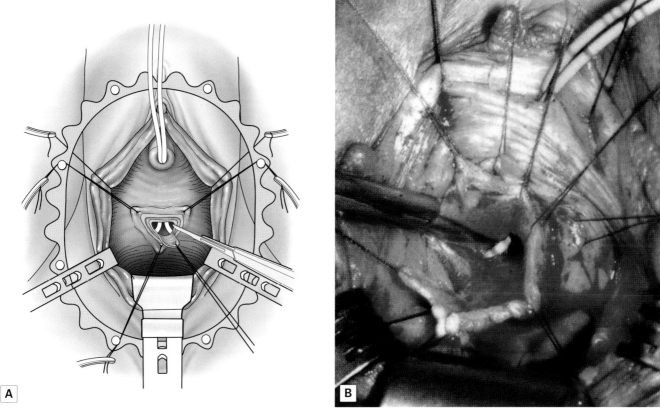

Figure 21.4 The margin of the fistula is circumcised. The excision of the perifistula scarring is facilitated by traction on additionally inserted stay sutures.

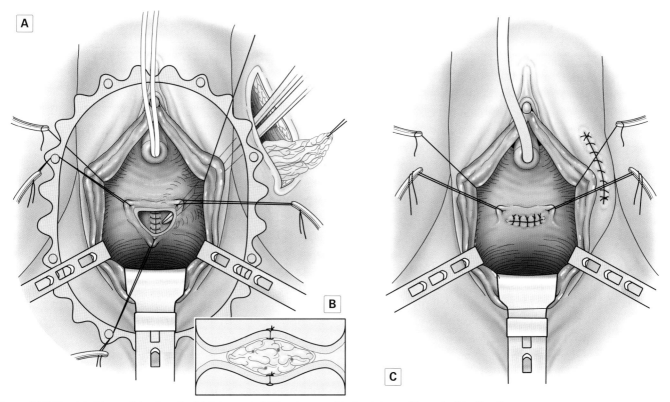

Figure 21.5 The bladder wall is closed with interrupted 4/0 sutures, with the interposition of a Martius flap.

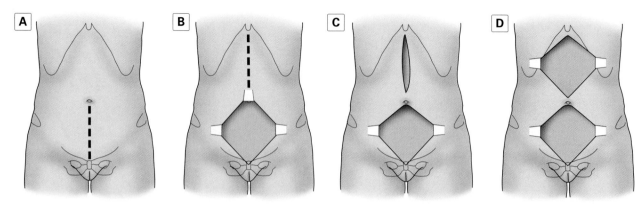

Figure 21.6 The "suprapubic cross" incision.

closed transversely (Fig. 21.5C). An alternative approach is to excise a rim of vaginal epithelium from around the fistula, allowing repair by colpocleisis using a double- or triple-layer closure of the subcutaneous tissues.[17] A modification is that reported by Twombly and Marshall[26] who suggested preservation of a flap of the vaginal epithelium which is used as the first layer closure of the defect (Fig. 21.6). These techniques do produce some shortening of the vagina but are reported to produce little interference with sexual activity.[25,27] They are most suitable for the postmenopausal patient, particularly if there is a deep vagina and a vault fistula, and can in experienced hands be applicable to a wide range of different fistulae.[28]

Postoperative care. It is important to provide a post-operative milieu that promotes satisfactory healing of the surgical anastomotic repair. Careful review of urine bacteriology should be undertaken. The urinary tract should be drained continuously under low pressure. The synchronous use of both urethral and suprapubic drainage of adequate caliber (18 F) reduces the likelihood that blockage of a catheter will result in a build-up of pressure that will disrupt the surgical repair. Catheters should be left on free drainage for at least 10 days and the integrity of the surgical repair confirmed at this juncture by the use of contrast studies. If there is any contrast leakage, the catheters should be left on drainage for a further week and radiologic reevaluation repeated at that point.

Vaginal repair of the complex fistula. In some cases the local vaginal tissues are damaged to the extent that a simple layered closure of the vagina is felt to be potentially precarious. Such a situation may result from tissue loss or tissue fibrosis produced by infection or previous surgery. In this situation it is necessary to augment the operation by the interposition of a vascularized flap between the two layers of the repair, filling dead space and bringing in a much-needed

blood and lymphatic supply. Many of these fistulae can be repaired using a vaginal procedure.

A number of techniques have been described for the mobilization and deployment of adjacent soft tissue structures. These include the transposition of the medial fibers of the levator ani;[29] use of a gracilis muscle flap[30-32] or a gracilis myocutaneous flap,[33] and the use of a pedicle flap of vulval fat and bulbocavernosus muscle.[34] Whilst procedures utilizing the gracilis are invaluable for the repair of extensive defects, the majority of cases can be satisfactorily resolved by the use of a Martius flap[34] and hence this procedure will be described in detail here.

A vertical incision is made in either labia majora, allowing a posteriorly based, pedicled, vascularized flap of labial tissue to be raised. The size of the flap is determined by the size of the fistula and can be increased by anterior extension of the incision into the mons (see Fig. 21.5A). The flap is mobilized, taking care not to damage the blood supply from the inferior hemorrhoidal vessels which enter anteriorly. Next, a tunnel is made beneath a vulval skin bridge to the site of fistula closure (see Fig. 21.5A). The labial flap is secured in position as part of the final layer closure (see Fig. 21.5B).

A problem encountered occasionally is that of a urethrovaginal fistula. The majority of those patients with a distal urethrovaginal fistula are continent and asymptomatic provided that the bladder neck mechanism is competent.[35] Vaginal repair of such a fistula is easily carried out. If there is an associated urethral mucosal defect, it can be replaced by a suitable flap of adjacent vaginal mucosa supported by a Martius flap. Alternatively, a modification of the Martius procedure can be used whereby the urethral repair is facilitated by a suitably positioned skin island left on the labial pedicle.[36] If the fistula is more proximal and a more extensive repair of urethra is likely to be necessary or if it is associated with a vesicovaginal fistula, then a combined transvesical and abdominal approach is preferable.

TRANSABDOMINAL FISTULA REPAIR

A combined transperitoneal transvesical approach to a vesicovaginal fistula is to be preferred over the conventional anterior transvesical approach first described by Trendelenburg in 1890[37] and subsequently modified[38] to a synchronous perineo-abdominal approach (PAPA). When operating via an abdominal approach, it is also sensible to have the patient in the perineo-abdominal position so that manipulation of the vagina can be easily carried out and progression to a perineo-abdominal approach facilitated.

Irrespective of whether the intended approach for a fistula repair is vaginal or abdominal, the perineum and abdomen are prepared and draped in a single sterile operating field for a synchronous procedure. When appropriate, mild additional flexion of the hips can be used for a vaginal approach in the PAPA position because this is easily flattened in the event of transfer to a synchronous abdominal approach.

During a definitive abdominal approach, the synchronous vaginal access provided by the single sterile perineo-abdominal operating field of the PAPA position has particular advantages for vesicovaginal fistula repair. However, care must be taken to avoid the complication of the anterior compartment syndrome that can result from calf pressure supports, such as the Lloyd Davies, during prolonged operations.

- It enables a finger in the vagina to guide the separation of the fused vesicovaginal tissue layers around the fistula.
- Bleeding that develops low in the abdominoperineal interposition tunnel is often controllable by vaginal finger pressure until definitive hemostasis is secured.
- It facilitates urethral catheterization and manipulation.
- Synchronous peroperative endoscopic examination and instrumentation procedures are occasionally helpful.

Technically, in terms of access and versatility, the supravesical abdominal approach provides superior access for the repair of many vesicovaginal fistulae; it is suitable for all such fistulae in all locations, down to and including the bladder neck and the proximal urethra. However, a vaginal-approach repair is a less extensive surgical procedure so this is naturally preferable when the circumstances are ideally appropriate for it.

The incision.
A midline abdominal wall incision is essential to provide appropriate access for the mobilization of the full length of the vascular omental pedicle from the stomach. This is necessary in about a third of the cases in which omental interposition is required for the reliable repair of a complex vesicovaginal fistula. The need for such an extensive mobilization of the omentum cannot be predicted preoperatively. A common clinical problem is that many of the patients who require the repair of a vesicovaginal fistula have just had a Pfannenstiel incision approach hysterectomy with a horizontal skin incision. An additional vertical midline skin incision for an omental fistula repair results in a scar that is a lasting reminder of the complication, and is best avoided.

The "suprapubic cross" incision (see Fig. 21.6). The "suprapubic cross" incision was specifically developed to enable the great majority of Pfannenstiel-approach hysterectomy fistula repairs to be completed through the original skin incision. After a slight lateral extension of this horizontal skin incision, the upper and lower skin and subcutaneous tissue flaps are separated from the rectus fascia, upwards and downwards, sufficiently to enable a midline abdominal wall incision to be made up to the level of the umbilicus and leaving the original horizontal Pfannenstiel rectus sheath closure intact. Suture reinforcement of the margins of the previous horizontal sheath closure transsected by the midline incision is generally advisable.

In the event that an upper abdominal access is required to mobilize the vascular pedicle of a short apron omentum (30–40% of cases), this can be achieved by a short additional midline epigastric skin incision and a supraumbilical extension of the midline incision in the abdominal wall, which is in continuity under the wide skin bridge between these two incisions. Thus an additional midline skin incision is avoided in the majority of patients who require a postoperative fistula repair procedure without compromising the option of an extension for full mobilization of the omental pedicle when this is necessary to ensure success.

Increasing the midline incisional access to the retropubic space. A distal prepubic extension of the midline incision into the prepubic aponeurosis, and its reflection off the surface of the pubic bone, results in a remarkably effective increase in the exposure of the retropubic space. The access to the lower recesses of the retropubic space can be further increased by a partial resection of the pubic bone but this additional exposure is rarely necessary in the female.

Operative procedure for transabdominal vesicovaginal fistula repair (Fig. 21.7).
The transperitoneal supravesical approach provides the best exposure for the abdominal repair of a vesicovaginal fistula. The traditional anterior transvesical approach for the closure of vesicovaginal fistulae, originally described by Trendelenburg, provides a very limited exposure through which only a simple layer closure of a fistula can be achieved; this is no longer advocated for this purpose. To take advantage of the special features of this approach, a perineo-abdominal

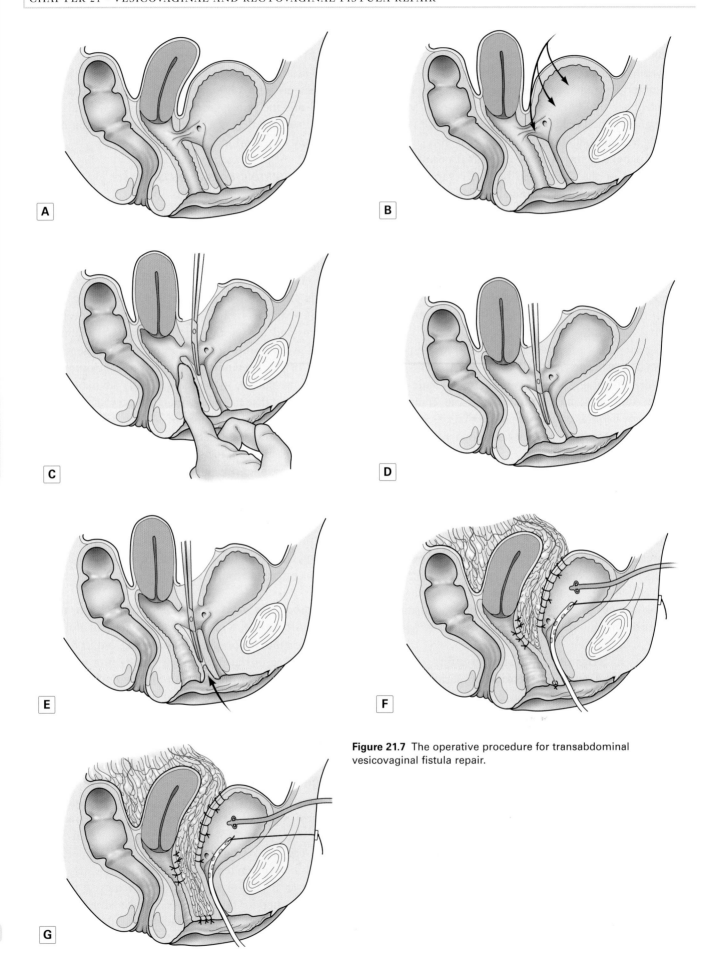

Figure 21.7 The operative procedure for transabdominal vesicovaginal fistula repair.

operating position is essential to provide synchronous perineal access. The patient is placed on the operating table in the perineo-abdominal position with an appropriate degree of head-down tilt to reduce venous pressure bleeding in the pelvis.

A midline abdominal incision is essential to enable the full length of the right gastroepiploic pedicle of the omentum to be mobilized to support the fistula repair in the event of necessity. For a simple posthysterectomy fistula, the initial lower midline incision may be achieved by the lower element of the suprapubic cross incision so that, when omental interposition support is required, it can usually be achieved using a simple horizontal Pfannenstiel-type skin incision without an epigastric extension.

The suprapubic cross incision is retracted with an abdominal ring retractor. The bladder and the vaginal vault are elevated up into the wound by suspension stay sutures retained over the margin of the ring retractor.

The elevated bladder is opened by a laterally curved vertical incision to facilitate its eventual closure. The bladder incision is extended down into the fistula itself and its lateral margins are retracted by elevating stay sutures to expose the bladder base widely.

The ureteric orifices are identified. Ureteric catheters are passed up to the kidney on either side and the distal ends exteriorized through the urethra into the sterile perineal-approach access of the PAPA position. These catheters can be passed endoscopically during the preliminary examination but they are equally easy to pass during the operation. When the bladder is open and the ureteric orifices are obscured by inflammatory changes of the bladder base, they are more easily identified by observing the almost immediate efflux of clear urine generated by the intravenous injection of a diuretic rather than by waiting for the relatively delayed excretion of an intravenous colored dye such as indigo carmine.

The separation of the fused layers of the bladder and the vagina at the margin of the fistula is greatly facilitated by scissor-tip dissection guided by the tip of the surgeon's finger in the vagina. Even when the adhesion is dense and extensive, it is remarkably easy to define it by this sharp scissor-tip cutting at a level about 3 mm from the fingertip, the thickness of the vaginal wall. This is simply estimated by finger sensation until the natural intervening tissue plane opens up.

The margins of the vaginal opening of the fistula are excised and it is closed by interrupted short runs of 3/0 PGA sutures. A suprapubic catheter and a urethral catheter are inserted. The curved incision in the bladder is easily closed by simple rotation of its inherent flap using interrupted runs of 3/0 PGA sutures.

The space for omental interposition support of the suture line can be created either by simple lateral development of the space between the bladder base closure and the vaginal closure from above, or by the synchronous development of an abdominoperineal tunnel, three fingerbreadths wide, that opens distally at the margin of the introitus behind the urethral meatus. Separation of the vaginal vault from the bladder is facilitated by an orientating finger placed within the vagina. A three fingerbreadths space is completed in the plane between bladder and vagina; it is important to create enough "space" to allow the adequate tension-free positioning of a suitable bulk of omentum. In difficult cases, and in particular those where previous surgery has been attempted, the abdominal dissection can be combined with a subsequent perineal dissection to produce an abdominoperineal tunnel, thereby allowing linear deployment of the omentum along the whole length of the vagina.[39] Although many simple fistulae can be satisfactorily closed via this approach with a layer closure as described above, an extra advantage can be gained by the addition of an interposed omental pedicled flap in the closure.[22] This surgical technique is applicable to a wide variety of fistulae and provides a virtually guaranteed closure of most fistulae.[40]

At the end of the procedure a colposuspension may be carried out where necessary to reposition the proximal urethra and bladder neck, ensuring the optimal transmission of intraabdominal pressure and thereby avoiding the development of stress incontinence.[41]

The mobilized omentum is introduced into the interpositional space. An abdominal omental interposition is anchored at the upper margin of the interposition space, an abdominoperineal tunnel interposition is fixed by including the distal margin of the apron with the sutures closing the introital incision at its lower end.

Tips and tricks for supravesical repair of vesicovaginal fistulae

- A guiding finger in the vagina greatly facilitates the separation of the back of the bladder and the urethra from the vaginal wall at the margins of the fistula.
- Bleeding deep in the pelvis is often controllable by simple vaginal finger pressure while definitive hemostasis is being secured.
- The exposure of the bladder base, the lateral paravesical space, and the retrovesical/vaginal plane enables the ureter to be mobilized and reimplanted into the bladder by a reflux-preventing procedure when this is indicated, most commonly as a result of its involvement in the margin of the fistula.
- When a vesical fistula extends down to or through the bladder neck, a definitive synchronous perineo-abdominal reconstruction of the sphincter mechanism can be achieved using a prevaginal abdominoperineal tunnel. The separation of the urethra from the vagina is continued down to a periintroital incision to create a

prevaginal abdominoperineal tunnel, 3–4 fingerbreadths wide, to accept a really effective bulk of omentum.

- Omental interposition can be achieved using the supravesical abdominal approach alone, creating an intervening space for it by a downward and lateral extension of the separation of the bladder base and the urethra from the anterior wall of the vagina. The failure of an omental interposition repair should be a very unusual event; it is important to avoid three potential surgical shortcomings:
  1. inadequate size of the abdominoperineal interposition tunnel, because this results in an insufficiency of the lateral tissue overlap. The omentum should not be used as a simple "plug"
  2. failure to mobilize a sufficient bulk of omentum to fill the appropriately sized interposition tunnel
  3. impairment of the vascularity of the mobilized omentum resulting from an inappropriate mobilization procedure or poor vascular surgical technique.

- Use of a laterally curved incision in the posterior wall of the bladder. If a vertical midline incision in the bladder is used to achieve a supravesical approach to a vesicovaginal fistula, it can be difficult, and sometimes impossible, to achieve side-to-side closure when the bladder wall and the lateral paravesical pelvic tissues are indurated, as they often are as a result of previous surgery, inflammatory fibrosis, and especially after irradiation. It is generally advisable to curve the incision in the posterior wall of the bladder laterally because this creates an eccentric laterally based flap of the bladder wall that enables closure to be achieved by its simple rotation.

Operative procedure for vesicovagino-rectal fistula repair (Fig. 21.8). The procedure is an extended development of the abdominoperineal closure of a complex vesicovaginal fistula by omental interposition. A simple loop ileostomy preliminary bowel diversion is preferred to a traditional loop colostomy because it is easier for the surgeon to make, for the patient to manage, and for the surgeon to close.

With the patient in the perineo-abdominal progression position, the fistula is opened from above, separating the rectum from the back of the bladder. The stenotic vault of an irradiated vagina is excised. After its separation from the

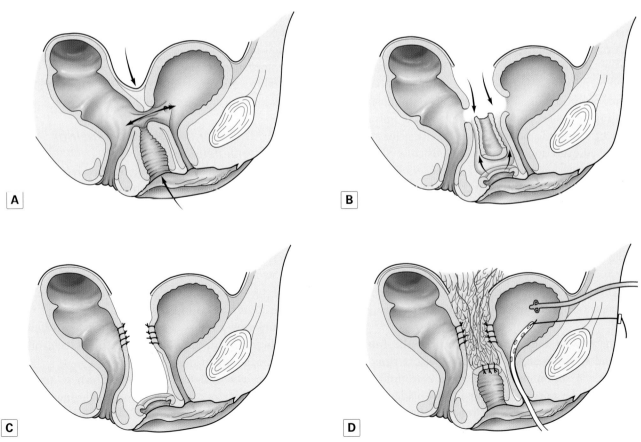

Figure 21.8 The operative procedure for vesicovagino-rectal fistula repair.

rectal wall posteriorly and the vesicourethral wall anteriorly, the vaginal wall is circumcised transvaginally at the upper limit of its preservable viability and caliber. Suprapubic and suture-retained urethral catheters are positioned. The rectal and bladder walls are closed.

The omental apron is mobilized to fill the sizeable gap between the bladder and the rectum, and its distal margin is included in the vaginal closure sutures.

If a bowel substitution vaginoplasty is indicated, it can be done as either an immediate or a deferred procedure.

POSTOPERATIVE CARE

The patient has an occlusive wound dressing applied and is left with a suprapubic and urethral catheter. All patients are continued on full antibiotic prophylaxis for 10 days at which time a cystogram is performed. Provided there is no leak from the bladder, the urethral catheter is removed and the suprapubic catheter clamped. If the patient is able to void without significant problems, the suprapubic catheter is then removed. The patient is advised to avoid excessive activity for 4–6 weeks and then to gradually mobilize towards normal by 2–3 months.

FROM SURGEON TO SURGEON

Helpful tips have been included wherever possible as the techniques have been described. In my experience, with a combination of self-retracting instruments, adequate exposure and good lighting, it is possible to close the majority of fistulae. Basic surgical principles of excising avascular tissue, avoiding dead space, producing tension-free anastomoses, draining urine, and, where appropriate, diverting the urinary stream all combine to ensure a successful outcome.

To emphasize the most clinically difficult situation, the so-called "frozen pelvis" that occasionally results from pelvic irradiation is an extensive fibrosis of interstitial tissue that largely fills the pelvis (Fig. 21.9). In my experience, the repair of complex vesicovaginal fistulae is most satisfactorily tackled via the abdominoperineal approach with omental interposition as described above.[40] Certain additional points are, however, worthy of comment. If radiotherapy is implicated in the etiology of the fistula, the wall of the bladder is usually rendered more rigid and inflexible than is normally the case. In this situation, an oblique incision in the wall of the bladder is often preferable to one in the midline as this facilitates subsequent bladder closure by the rotation of a broad-based bladder flap.

In those patients with radiation-induced fibrosis and necrosis, the surgical procedure must be considered to consist of two separate stages. It is first necessary to *excise* all macroscopically abnormal tissue. These cases are usually associated with extensive irradiation changes in the bladder, the ureters, and the rectum. Often, after treatment of cervical carcinoma, there is a fistulating radionecrotic cavity in the vaginal vault area. Traditionally, such a "frozen pelvis" was treated by a double abdominal-surface urostomy and colostomy diversion but this does not relieve the unfortunate patient of an offensive purulent discharge from a radionecrotic cavity, the avascular walls of which are incapable of generating the proliferative granulation tissue required for its occlusive healing. The surgical resolution of a "frozen pelvis" used to be widely regarded as an inoperable situation; however, after a subtotal exenteration that leaves the potentially resurrectable elements in situ (the bladder base, the lower vagina, and the anorectal mechanism), a functional reconstruction of some or all of these is often possible, especially if a sufficiency of transposable omentum is available, combined if necessary with a vaginoplasty to help fill "dead space." If residual malignancy is suspected this can be confirmed by frozen section but unless extensive, apart from biasing the surgeon towards a more radical excision, should not preclude a reconstructive procedure. The second stage of this operation involves a *functional restoration* of the integrity of the rectum, bladder, and vagina as far as this is feasible, filling the dead space within the inevitably ischemic pelvis with omentum and/or a cecolovaginoplasty.[41]

If there is an extensive defect then it may not be possible to obtain satisfactory apposition of the edges of the bladder wall without compromising its functional capacity. Closure of the bladder defect can be carried out with the additional use of an augmentation cystoplasty. Alternatively, the bladder defect can be left and the omentum used to patch it; animal studies have clearly demonstrated that the defect is covered within 2–3 weeks by new transitional epithelium with the subsequent formation of new smooth muscle layer within the omentoplasty in continuity with the margins of the detrusor muscle at the edges of the defect.[42,43] Clinical experience over the last 25 years has confirmed the efficacy of this technique in the clinical setting.[24,44,45]

In any fistula case it is advisable to obtain support from a colleague with expertise in this area since the closure of apparently simple vesicovaginal fistulae should be regarded as a specialist procedure. Often the surgeon who creates a fistula is not the one best qualified to undertake its repair, although the temptation to attempt this may be great. From the patient, medical, and medicolegal viewpoints, it is important that a postoperative fistula is repaired both expeditiously and successfully at the first attempt. The difficulty of a fistula repair can escalate when the situation becomes complex but this should rarely be the result of a previous surgical failure.

SECTION 8 Fistula

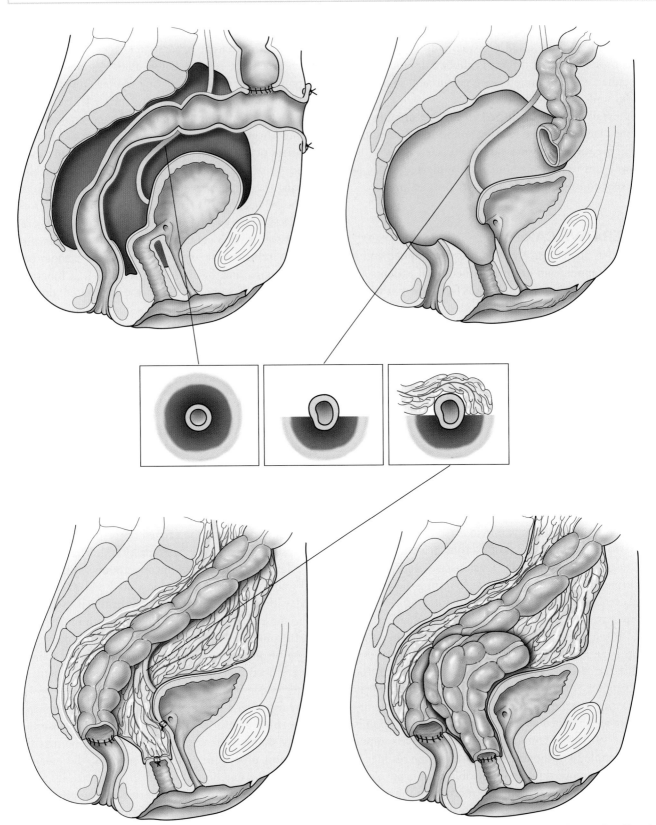

Figure 21.9 The so-called "frozen pelvis" that occasionally results from pelvic irradiation with the development of extensive fibrotic interstitial tissue that encases the pelvic organs. (Adapted from figures designed and drawn by Richard Turner-Warwick and Paul Richardson.)

REFERENCES

1. Sims JM. On the treatment of vesicovaginal fistula. Am J Med Sci 1852;23:59–83.

2. Van Roonhuyse, 1672, cited in Zacharin RF. Grafting as a principle in the surgical management of vesico-vaginal and recto-vaginal fistulae. Aust NZ J Obstet Gynaecol 1980;20:10–17.

3. Joubert AJ. Gaz Hop (Paris) 1834;8:405,437.

4. Gosset M. Calculus in the bladder: vesicovaginal fistula: advantages of the gilt wire suture (letter to the editor). Lancet 1834;345–346.

5. Hayward G. Massachussetts General Hospital. Cited in reference 9.

6. Marshall VF. Vesicovaginal fistulas on one urological service. J Urol 1979;121:25–29.

7. Collins CG, Pent D, Jones FB. Results of early repair of vesicovaginal fistula with preliminary cortisone treatment. Am J Obstet Gynecol 1960;80:1005.

8. Lawson J. The management of genitourinary fistulae. Clin Obstet Gynecol North Am 1978; 5:209–236.

9. O'Conor VJ. Review of experience with vesicovaginal fistula repair. Trans Am Assoc Genitourinary Surg 1979;71:120–122.

10. Jonas U, Petri E. Genitourinary fistulae. In: Stanton SL, ed. Clinical gynecologic urology. St Louis: CV Mosby; 1984.

11. Turner-Warwick RT. Repair of urinary vaginal fistulae. In: Rob C, Smith R, eds. Operative surgery, 3rd edn. London: Butterworths; 1977.

12. Persky L, Herman G, Guerrier K. Non-delay in vesicovaginal fistula repair. Urology 1979;13:273–275.

13. Badenoch DF, Tiptaft RC, Thakar DR, Fowler CG, Blandy JP. Early repair of accidental injury to the ureter or bladder following gynecologic surgery. Br J Urol 1987;59:516–518.

14. Cruikshank SH. Early closure of posthysterectomy vesicovaginal fistulas. South Med J 1988;81:1525–1528.

15. Roen PR. Combined vaginal and transvesical approach in successful repair of vesicovaginal fistula. Arch Surg 1960;80:628–633.

16. Weyrauch HW, Rous SN. Transvesical-transvaginal approach for surgical repair of vesicovaginal fistulae. Surg Gynecol Obstet 1966;123:121–125.

17. Bardescu N. Ein neues verfahren fur die operation der tiefen blasen-uterus-scheidenfisteln. Centralbl f Gynak 1900;24:170.

18. Eisen M, Jurkovic K, Altwein JE, Schreiter F, Hohenfellner R. Management of vesicovaginal fistulas with peritoneal flap interposition. J Urol 1974;112:195–198.

19. Robertson CN, Riefkohl R, Webster GN. Use of the rectus abdominis muscle in urological reconstructive procedures. J Urol 1986;135:963–965.

20. McCraw JB, Arnold PG. Atlas of muscle and myocutaneous flaps. Norfolk, VA: Hampton Press; 1986.

21. Coleman JW, Albanese C, Marion D, et al. Experimental use of free grafts of bladder mucosa in canine bladders: successful closure of recurrent vesicovaginal fistula utilising bladder mucosa. Urology 1985;25:515–517.

22. Walters W. Transperitoneal repair of a vesico-vaginal fistula. Proc Mayo Clin 1935;375–377.

23. Kiricuta I, Goldstein AMB. Epiplooplastia vezicala, metoda de tratament curativ al fistulelor vezico-vaginale. Obstetrica si Ginecologia Buceresti 1956;2:163.

24. Turner-Warwick RT, Wynne EJC, Handley-Ashken M. The use of the omental pedicle graft in the repair and reconstruction of the urinary tract. Br J Surg 1967;54:849–853.

25. Latzko W. Post-operative vesicovaginal fistulas. Am J Surg 1942;58:211–228.

26. Twombly GH, Marshall VF. Repair of vesico-vaginal fistula caused by radiation. Surg Gynecol Obstet 1946;83:348.

27. Rader ES. Post-hysterectomy vesicovaginal fistula: treatment by partial colpocleisis. J Urol 1975;112: 811–812.

28. Blaikley JB. Colpocleisis for difficult vaginal fistulae of bladder and rectum. Proc Roy Soc Med 1965;58:581–586.

29. Douglass M. Operative treatment of urinary incontinence. Am J. Obstet Gynecol 1936;31:268–279.

30. Garlock JH. The cure of an intractable vesico-vaginal fistula by the use of a pedicled muscle flap. Surg Gynecol Obstet 1928;47:255–260.

31. Ingleman-Sundberg A. Surgical treatment of carcinoma of the cervix (ed Meigs J.V.) London: Heinemann; 1954.

32. Hamlin RHJ, Nicholson EC. Reconstruction of urethra totally destroyed in labour. BMJ 1969;2:147–150.

33. McCraw JB, Massey FM, Shanklin KD, Horton CE. Vaginal reconstruction with gracilis myocutaneous flaps. Plast Reconstr Surg 1976;58:176–183.

34. Martius H. Die Operative Wiederherstellung der volkommen fehlenden Harnrohre und der Schliessmuskels derselben. Zentbl Gynak 1928;52:480–486.

35. Spence HM, Duckett JW. Diverticulum of the female urethra: clinical aspects and presentation of a simple operative technique for cure. J Urol 1970;104:432–437.

36. Turner-Warwick RT. The use of pedicle grafts in the repair of urinary tract fistulae. Br J Urol 1972;44:644–656.

37. Zacharin RF. Grafting as a principle in the surgical management of vesico-vaginal and recto-vaginal fistulae. Aust NZ J Obstet Gynaecol 1980;20:10–17.

38. O'Conor VJ, Sokol JK, Bulkley GJ, Nanninga JB. Suprapubic closure of vesicovaginal fistula. JUrol 1973;109:51–54.

39. Turner-Warwick RT. Urinary fistula in the female In: Harrison E, et al, eds. Campbell's urology. Philadelphia: WB Saunders; 1979.

40. Chapple CR, Turner-Warwick RT. Traumatic lower urinary tract fistulae—abdominoperineal repair with pedicled omental interposition. J Urol 1990;143:328A.

41. Turner-Warwick RT. The omental repair of complex urinary fistulae. In: Gingell C, Abrams P, eds. Controversies and innovations in urological surgery. London: Springer Verlag; 1988.

42. Goldstein MB, Dearden LC. Histology of omentoplasty of the urinary bladder in the rabbit. Invest Urol 1966;3:460–469.

43. Helmbrecht LJ, Goldstein AMB, Morrow JW. The use of pedicled omentum in the repair of large vesicovaginal fistulas. Invest Urol 1975;13:104–107.

44. Kiricuta I, Goldstein AMB. The repair of extensive vesicovaginal fistulas with pedicled omentum. J Urol 1972;108:724–727.

45. Chapple CR, Turner-Warwick RT. Surgical salvage of radiation induced fibrosis: the "frozen pelvis". J Urol 1990;143:349A.

Urethral Diverticula, Urethrovesical Fistulae

Christopher R Chapple

URETHRAL DIVERTICULA

Female urethral diverticula are estimated to occur in between 1% and 6% of all adult females and are usually diagnosed after the age of 20, the majority of the cases being in the fourth decade of life. Whilst the majority of urethral diverticula are undiagnosed as they prove to be asymptomatic, they may be complicated by infection, stones or, rarely, malignancy and by virtue of their size, may produce obstruction to the bladder outlet. Diverticula most commonly present with symptoms relating to their size, with discomfort or with episodes of repeated inflammation and infection. If a diverticulum is asymptomatic and causing the patient no concern then there is no indication for its further treatment. The presenting symptoms can be summarized as the three Ds: **d**ysuria, postvoid **d**ribbling, and **d**yspareunia (Box 22.1).

Although it has been suggested that diverticula are congenital in origin, there is no evidence to support this view as they are rarely found in children. However, this does not preclude the fact that an early diverticulum or weakness might have been present but undiagnosed. It is tempting to attribute the development of diverticula to the trauma of childbirth and whilst diverticula often present in women following childbirth, it has been shown that urethral diverticula are just as likely to arise in nulliparous patients. A strong possibility is that repeated infection and obstruction of the periurethral glands results in the formation of a cyst which eventually ruptures and drains back into the urethral lumen.[2] Another possibility is that some cases may be due to embryologic remnants, e.g. Gartner's duct or vestigial wolffian ducts, which may act as a precursor to the diverticulum formation. Indeed, diverticula in the pediatric population have been attributed to a number of congenital anomalies including an ectopic ureter draining into a Gartner's duct cyst and a forme fruste of urethral duplication.[3-5]

There are a number of possibilities in terms of differential diagnosis (Box 22.2).

Urethral diverticula invariably communicate with the urethral lumen and by virtue of their position, protrude through and stretch the periurethral smooth muscle (bearing in mind the favored hypothesis that they are based on obstructed periurethral glands). The periurethral glands are tubuloalveolar structures that predominate in the distal two-thirds of the urethra and, not surprisingly, up to 90% of diverticula open into the mid or distal urethra. Therefore, infection of the periurethral glands seems to be the most generally accepted common etiologic factor in most cases. Reinfection, inflammation, and recurrent obstruction of the neck of the cavity are theorized to result in patient symptoms and enlargement of the diverticulum. This proposed

---

Box 22.1 Presenting features of urethral diverticula[1]

Frequency/dysuria (56%)

Recurrent infection (40%)

Tender mass (35%)

Stress incontinence (32%)

Postmicturition dribble (27%)

Dyspareunia (16%)

Stones (1–10%)

Discharge of pus per urethra (12%)

Retention (4%)

Malignancy (rare—adenoca 80%)

Box 22.2 Differential diagnosis

Diverticulum

Vaginal wall cyst

Injectable

Skene's gland abscess

Ectopic ureterocele

(Carcinoma)

pathophysiology appears to adequately explain the anatomic location and configuration of most urethral diverticula. However, it should be noted that Daneshgari and colleagues have recently reported noncommunicating urethral diverticula diagnosed by MRI.[6] Whether this lesion represents a forme fruste of urethral diverticula or simply an obstructed communication with the urethral lumen is unclear.

Occasionally diverticula, by virtue of their size, extend proximally and beneath the bladder neck and trigonal area (Fig. 22.1). A urethral diverticulum is often an isolated cyst-like appendage with a single discrete connection to the urethral lumen. However, complicated anatomic patterns may exist and in certain cases the urethral diverticulum may extend partially ("saddlebag" urethral diverticulum) or circumferentially about the urethra.[7]

The diagnosis of urethral diverticula (UD) can be made with a combination of a thorough history, physical examination, appropriate urine studies, including urine culture and analysis, endoscopic examination of the bladder and urethra, urodynamics, and selective radiologic imaging.

During physical examination the anterior vaginal wall should be carefully palpated for masses and tenderness. The location, size, and consistency of any suspected UD should be recorded. Most UD are located ventrally over the middle and proximal portions of the urethra corresponding to the area of the anterior vaginal wall 2–3 cm inside the introitus. However, UD may also be located anterior to the urethra or extend partially or completely around the urethral lumen. These particular configurations may have significant implications when undertaking surgical excision and reconstruction.

A preoperative classification has been described based on the location, size, configuration, communication with the urethral lumen, and continence status (Table 22.1).[1]

A number of diagnostic techniques have been reported (Box 22.3).

Recent work in this area has clearly demonstrated that a postvoiding sagittal MRI scan (Fig. 22.2) is the most accurate way of finding their size and position. Urethroscopy, whilst often performed, usually fails to be helpful, particularly if the diverticulum is collapsed as the internal communication between the diverticulum and the urethra is often not visible.

Urodynamics is important in the preoperative assessment of patients to document the presence or absence of stress urinary incontinence prior to excision of a diverticulum. Approximately 50% of women with UD will demonstrate SUI on urodynamic evaluation[1,4] (Table 22.2).

A videourodynamic study combines both an anatomic assessment and a pressure study and will be helpful in differentiating true stress incontinence from pseudoincontinence related to emptying of a urethral diverticulum with physical activity (Fig. 22.3).

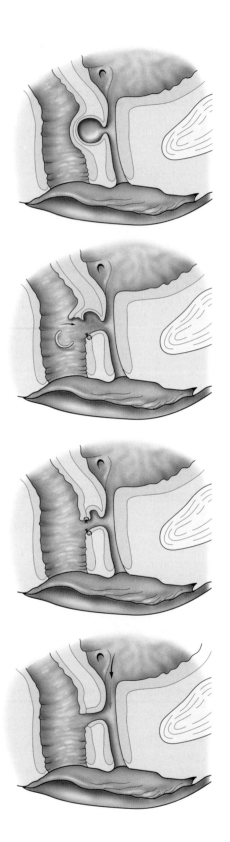

Figure 22.1 A diverticulum usually extends through all layers of the urethra, therefore marsupialization may lead to fistula. A diverticulum stretches through all layers of the urethra and surgery on it will tend to weaken the urethral sphincter.

Table 22.1   Preoperative classification of female urethral diverticula (L/N/S, C3) in 60 women

Location (L)	Number (N)	Size (S)	Configuration (C1)	Communication (C2)	Continence (C3)
Proximal, beneath the bladder neck (8)*	Single (54)	0.2 x 0.2 cm	Multiloculated (21)	Proximal urethra (15)	Completely continent (34)
Proximal urethra (7)	Multiple (6)	to	Single (39)	Midurethra (35)	Stress incontinence (26)
Midurethra (36)					
Distal urethra (9)		5.0 x 4.5 cm	Saddle shaped (13)	Distal urethra (10)	
* Number of women					

Box 22.3   Diagnostic techniques

Invasive

Urethroscopy

Double balloon urethrography[9]

VCUG[10]

Noninvasive

Postvoid IVU[11]

Transvaginal US[12]

MRI sagittal postvoid[13]

Table 22.2   Urodynamic findings in 55 women with urethral diverticula

Findings	n	Percentage
Abnormal	33	60
Stress incontinence alone	18	32.5
Stress incontinence with detrusor instability	8	14.5
Detrusor instability alone	5	9
Sensory urgency	1	2
Myogenic decompensation	1	2
Normal	22	40

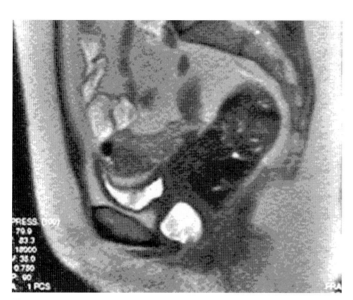

Figure 22.2 A postvoiding sagittal MRI scan is the most accurate method of diagnosis.

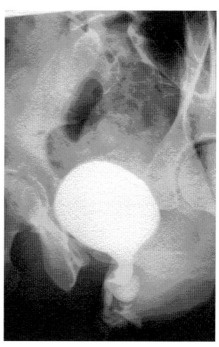

Figure 22.3 Diverticulum visible during a voiding cystogram during videourodynamics.

For patients undergoing surgery for UD with coexistent symptomatic stress urinary incontinence demonstrated on physical examination and urodynamically (USI), or those found to have an open bladder neck on preoperative evaluation, concomitant antiincontinence surgery can be offered. Multiple authors have described successful concomitant repair of urethral diverticula and stress incontinence in the same operative setting.[1,14-16] A small number of patients may have evidence of bladder outlet obstruction due to the obstructive effects of the diverticulum It should be noted that SUI may coexist with obstruction.[17] It is my practice to treat the diverticulum in the first instance where necessary by surgical excision and then reassess the appropriateness of sling insertion. I place a Martius flap in the majority of cases and this not only prevents the formation of a fistula and adds bulk which helps to alleviate stress incontinence but also facilitates subsequent surgery by preventing excessive fibrosis.

In my view, a diverticulum should only be treated if it is symptomatic and conservative measures have failed. Symptomatic patients, including those with dysuria, refractory bothersome postvoid dribbling, recurrent UTIs, dyspareunia and pelvic pain in whom the symptoms can be attributed to the UD, may be offered surgical excision. A number of surgical options have been described (Box 22.4).

Having identified a diverticulum which is asymptomatic, the treatment of choice is excision of the diverticulum. I have not found endoscopic incision to be necessary but rather would allow an infected diverticulum to settle with antibiotic therapy. Simple marsupialization of a diverticulum is one of the commonest causes of development of a urethrovaginal fistula. My standard management of these patients is to excise the diverticulum via a vaginal approach using the prone position (Fig. 22.4). This is a technique similar to that reported by Leach.[18]

The most definitive treatment of a diverticulum is to carry out a full excision with a full opening of the urethra but this does carry with it morbidity, even in experienced hands. After discussion of this, the majority of patients will

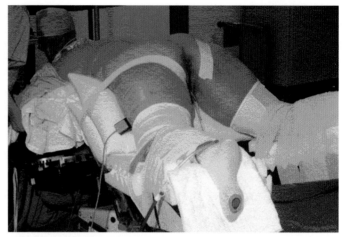

Figure 22.4 Excision of the diverticulum via a vaginal approach using the prone position.

opt for simple diverticulectomy with insertion of a Martius flap (Figs 22.5–7).

Using this surgical technique, urethrovaginal fistula formation is exceedingly rare. However, prior to surgery all patients should be warned that there is a risk of incontinence, either because it is unmasked as a consequence of removing the swollen diverticula in a patient who already had a tendency to stress incontinence or because it results from damage to the urethral sphincter mechanism during removal of the diverticulum. The patient should therefore be aware that a secondary procedure, in particular a sling procedure, may be necessary at a later date and certainly this is facilitated by the positioning of the Martius flap at the time of the diverticulectomy.

I carry out the urethral repair with 5/0 Monocril. Antibiotics are continued for at least 5 days postoperatively. The vaginal packing is removed at 24 hours and when ready, the patient is discharged home with urethral and suprapubic catheters. Antispasmodics are used liberally to reduce bladder spasms. Careful adherence to the principles of transvaginal urethral diverticulectomy should minimize postoperative complications but they may arise (Box 22.5).

Vaginal scarring or narrowing, dyspareunia, etc. Urethrovaginal fistula is a devastating complication of urethral diverticulectomy and deserves special mention. It is extremely uncommon for these to occur if a Martius flap is utilized de novo. This should be combined with meticulous attention to surgical technique, good hemostasis, avoidance of infection, preservation of a well-vascularized anterior vaginal wall flap, and multilayered closure. A fistula located beyond the sphincteric mechanism may not be associated with symptoms other than a split urinary stream. Conversely, a proximal fistula located at the bladder neck or at the

---

Box 22.4   Surgical options

Palliative

Endoscopic incision

Curative

Marsupialization

Excision

Excision and Young Dees reconstruction

254

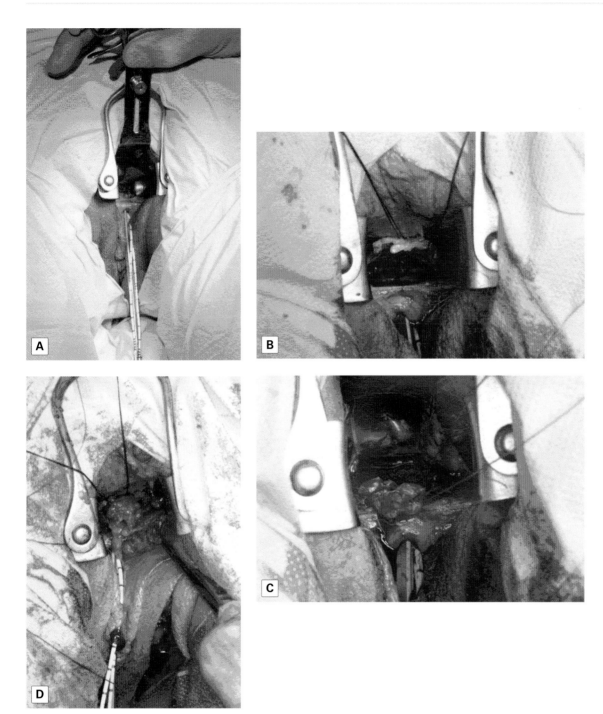

Figure 22.5 (**A**) Position and exposure with a self-retaining retractor. (**B**) Raising the anterior vaginal flap. (**C**) Excising the diverticulum. (**D**) Martius flap inlaid.

midurethra in patients with an incompetent bladder neck will likely result in considerable symptomatic urinary leakage. These patients should undergo repair with the use of an adjuvant tissue flap such as a Martius flap to provide a well-vascularized additional tissue layer.

Some patients will have persistence or recurrence of their preoperative symptoms postoperatively. The finding of a UD

following a presumably successful urethral diverticulectomy may occur as a result of a new UD or alternatively as a result of recurrence. Recurrence of UD may be due to incomplete removal of the UD, inadequate closure of the urethra or residual dead space, or other technical factors. Repeat urethral diverticulectomy surgery can always be carried out if necessary.

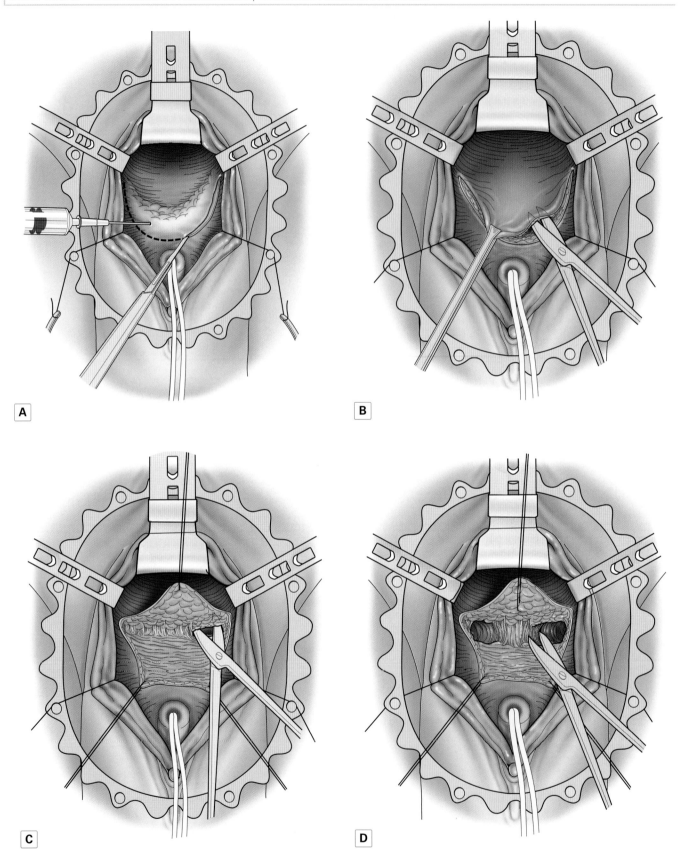

A

B

C

D

Figure 22.6 Surgery in the prone position, showing infiltration with lidocaine and adrenaline, raising the anterior vaginal flap, and the excellent view and access to the diverticulum seen with this patient positioning. *Continued*

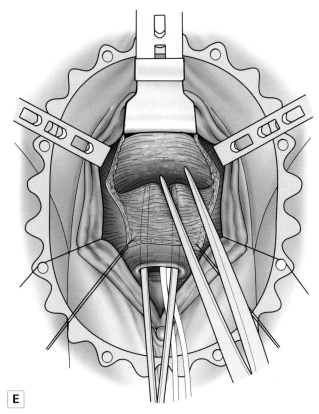

E

Figure 22.6, cont'd

URETHROVAGINAL FISTULAE AND URETHRAL SPHINCTER DEFICIENCY

Urethrovaginal fistulae are happily uncommon but invariably associated with a defect in the posterior section of the urethral sphincter mechanism. Patients present with the consequence of a fistula, namely incontinence, and any repair of these fistulae will also require definitive repair of the sphincter in order to restore continence. Urethrovaginal

Box 22.5   Complications of transvaginal urethral diverticulectomy, with % range of reported incidence[19]

Urinary incontinence (1.7–16.1%)

Urethrovaginal fistula (0.9–8.3%)

Urethral stricture (0–5.2%)

Recurrent UD (1–25%)

Recurrent UTI (0–31.3%)

Other:

- Hypospadias/distal urethral necrosis

- Bladder or ureteral injury

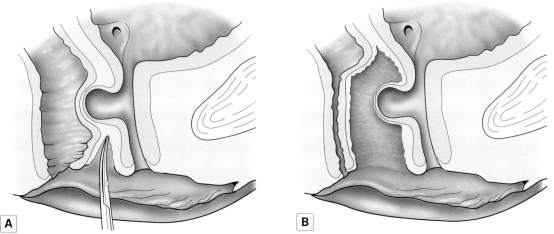

A   **B**

Figure 22.7 Plane of dissection for a diverticulum and the advantage of a full opening of the urethra to facilitate complete excision.

Continued

SECTION 8 Fistula

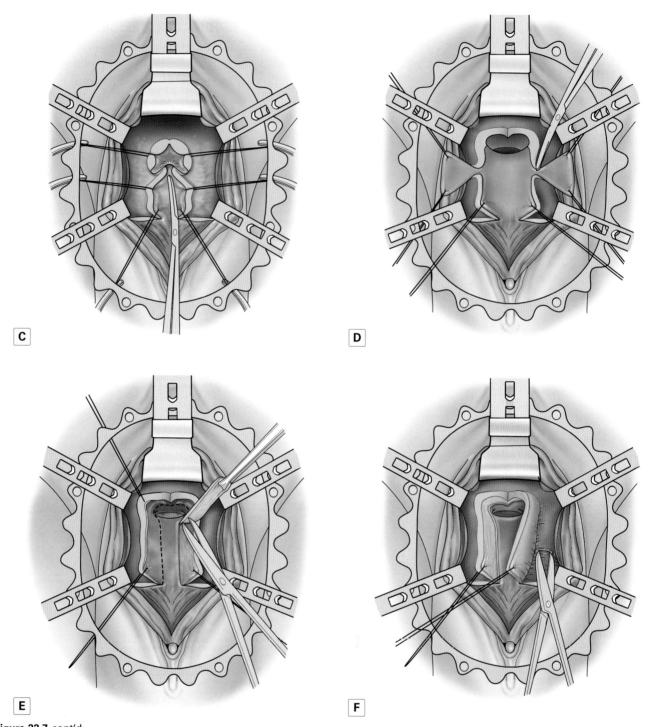

C

D

E

F

Figure 22.7, cont'd

fistulae may occur as the consequence of prolonged labor or complicated vaginal delivery where there is damage to the urethra or following surgery, particularly excision of the urethral diverticulum or surgery to the anterior vaginal wall. Urethral damage consequent upon pelvic fracture injuries is extremely rare.

Management of a urethrovaginal fistula therefore requires urethral reconstruction with careful attention to reconstructing the integrity of the urethral sphincter mechanism using a Young-Dees urethral tailoring procedure (Fig. 22.8). Such surgery should be carried out by those familiar with the principles and practice of urethral reconstruction.

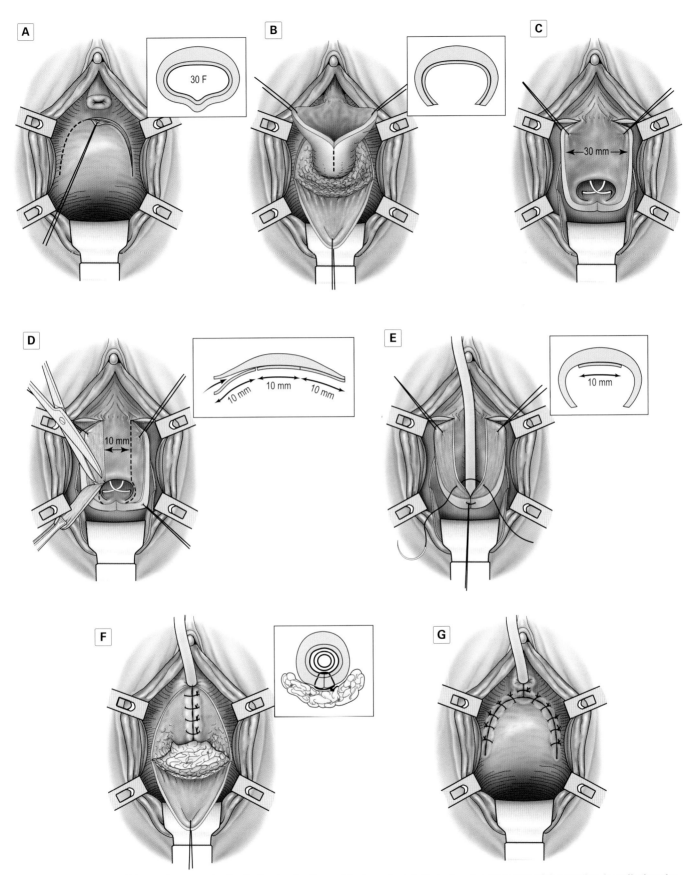

Figure 22.8 Principle of Young Dees urethral tailoring (reduction sphincteroplasty). Reducing the diameter of the urethra by tailoring the urethral roof strip, removing the damaged ventral urethra and basing the reconstruction on the intact and more robust dorsal component of the sphincter. (Adapted from figures designed and drawn by Richard Turner-Warwick and Paul Richardson.)

REFERENCES

1. Ganabathi K, Leach GE, Zimmern PE, Dmochowski R. Experience with the management of urethral diverticulum in 63 women. J Urol 1994;152 (5 Pt 1):1445–1452.

2. Young GPH, Wahle GR, Raz S. Female urethral diverticulum. In: Raz S, ed. Female urology. Philadelphia: WB Saunders; 1996: 477–489.

3. Boyd S, Raz S. Ectopic ureter presenting in midline urethral diverticulum. Urology 1993;41(6):571–574.

4. Silk MR, Lebowitz JM. Anterior urethral diverticulum. J Urol 1969;101:66–67.

5. Vanhoutte JJ. Ureteral ectopia into a Wolffian duct remnant presenting as a urethral diverticulum in two girls. Am J Roentgenol Radium Ther Nuclear Med 1970;110(3):540–545.

6. Daneshgari F, Zimmern PE, Jacomides L. Magnetic resonance imaging detection of symptomatic noncommunicating intraurethral wall diverticula in women. J Urol 1999;161(4): 1259–1261.

7. Rovner ES, Wein AJ. Diagnosis and reconstruction of the dorsal or circumferential urethral diverticulum. J Urol 2003;170(1):82–86.

8. Leach GE, Sirls LT, Ganabathi K, Zimmern PE. L N S C3: a proposed classification system for female urethral diverticula. Neurourol Urodynam 1993;12(6): 523–531.

9. Davis HJ, Cian LG. Positive pressure urethrography: a new diagnostic method. J Urol 1952;68:611–616.

10. Reid RE, Gill B, Laor E, Tolia BM, Freed SZ. Role of urodynamics in management of urethral diverticulum in females. Urology 1986;28(4):342–346.

11. Goldfarb S, Mieza M, Leiter E. Postvoid film of intravenous pyelogram in diagnosis of urethral diverticulum. Urology 1981;17(4):390–392.

12. Baert L, Willemen P, Oyen R. Endovaginal sonography: new diagnostic approach for urethral diverticula. J Urol 1992;147(2):464–466.

13. Blander DS, Rovner ES, Schnall MD et al. Endoluminal magnetic resonance imaging in the evaluation of urethral diverticula in women. Urology 2001;57(4):660–665.

14. Bass JS, Leach GE. Surgical treatment of concomitant urethral diverticulum and stress urinary incontinence. Urol Clin North Am 1991;18:365–373.

15. Faerber GJ. Urethral diverticulectomy and pubovaginal sling for simultaneous treatment of urethral diverticulum and intrinsic sphincter deficiency. Techn Urol 1998;4(4):192–197.

16. Swierzewski SJ III, McGuire EJ. Pubovaginal sling for treatment of female stress urinary incontinence complicated by urethral diverticulum. J Urol 1993;149(5):1012–1014.

17. Bradley CS, Rovner ES. Urodynamically defined stress urinary incontinence and bladder outlet obstruction can coexist in women. J Urol 2004;171:757–761.

18. Leach GE, Schmidbauer H, Hadley HR et al. Surgical treatment of female urethral diverticulum. Semin Urol 1986;4:33–42.

19. Dmochowski R. Surgery for vesicovaginal fistula, urethrovaginal fistula, and urethral diverticulum. In: Walsh PC, Retik AB, Vaughan ED Jr, Wein AJ, eds. Campbell's urology, 8th edn. Philadelphia: WB Saunders; 2002:1214.

SECTION 9

Intraoperative injury

Intraoperative Injury: Prevention and Immediate Management

Christina J Poon and Philippe E Zimmern

INTRODUCTION

Although rates of intraoperative injury during incontinence and pelvic prolapse surgery are generally very low, when permanent complications are the result of such injuries, the potential gain in quality of life that typically results from these surgeries can be severely reduced. If intraoperative injuries go unrecognized, as is the case in up to 70% of iatrogenic genitourinary injuries in some series,[1,2] the range of sequelae varies from bothersome (e.g. recurrent urinary tract infections due to a calcified bladder suture) to life threatening (e.g. urosepsis or obstructive uropathy due to ureteric ligation). Even if injuries are recognized, operative management can lengthen anesthetic time and place excessive surgical stress on an elderly patient with lower physiologic reserve. Because incontinence and pelvic prolapse are themselves not life-threatening conditions, surgical complications, when they occur, are not easily accepted by the patient. Accordingly, it is imperative that the surgeon obtains adequate informed consent preoperatively and, intraoperatively anticipates, recognizes and appropriately manages injuries in order to avoid permanent complications.

This chapter will focus on prevention, diagnosis, and immediate management of intraoperative injuries occurring in abdominal and vaginal reconstructive urogynecologic procedures. Injuries will be discussed in detail according to anatomic site: bladder, urethra, ureter, and bowel.

PREOPERATIVE PREPARATION: GENERAL MEASURES

As with any surgery, preparation involves attention to optimization of the patient's general medical condition and instituting measures to prevent specific complications such as infection, bleeding, and deep vein thrombosis. As surgeries for pelvic floor conditions are elective procedures, there is always the luxury of time to perform preoperative evaluations when indicated. In patients with cardiovascular or respiratory conditions, specialist consultation (e.g. cardiology, pneumology, anesthesiology) may be required.

Advanced age, in itself, is not an absolute contraindication to elective pelvic reconstructive surgery and, indeed, it has been shown that octogenarians tolerate these procedures as well as younger patients, in addition to obtaining similar long-term results.[3]

Infection prophylaxis involves methods to reduce bacterial counts preoperatively and administration of antibiotics perioperatively. Antibiotic prophylaxis to provide coverage for skin organisms (e.g. first-generation cephalosporins) is recommended in all cases, with the addition of antibiotics effective against uropathogens if possible entry into the urinary tract is anticipated or if an indwelling bladder catheter has been in place. A negative urine culture should be documented preoperatively in all patients. Vaginal douches and bowel enemas the day prior to surgery lower bacterial counts. Optimization of vaginal skin quality in postmenopausal women using local hormone replacement for at least 6 weeks preoperatively may enhance vaginal wound healing and minimize the risk of infection postoperatively.

Preoperative preparation to minimize the risk of bleeding involves a thorough history to ascertain any bleeding diathesis. Anticoagulants and antiplatelet agents should be discontinued at the appropriate time preoperatively. Significant bleeding during either abdominal or vaginal approaches is unusual (<1%) and cross-matching for blood transfusion should not be routine practice unless a difficult dissection is anticipated.

With the risk of deep vein thrombosis (DVT) following gynecologic surgery for benign disease as high as 29%,[4] routine prophylaxis should be practiced. Various methods including preoperative and postoperative subcutaneous heparin, graded compression stockings, and pneumatic calf compressors are available. At the authors' institution, compression stockings and calf compressors are used intraoperatively and continued postoperatively until the patient is ambulatory.

Although the dorsal lithotomy position is commonly used in both abdominal and vaginal approaches to surgery, and the associated risk of complications due to positioning factors alone is very small, attention to proper positioning minimizes this risk. DVT prophylaxis is particularly prudent when a case entails prolonged dorsal lithotomy positioning. Musculoskeletal conditions may make the dorsal lithotomy position impossible, as in patients with significant scoliosis and other spine conditions or in those with severe lower extremity contractures (e.g. related to neurologic disease). Preoperative orthopedic consultation may be appropriate in some cases. On initial positioning, care is taken to avoid hyperflexion/extension of the thighs over the hips and to pad potential pressure points to avoid nerve injuries from compression and/or stretching as well as soft tissue ischemic injury (Table 23.1). The use of pneumatic stirrups (e.g. Allen) allows adjustment of position to low lithotomy whenever possible during the course of a case. The operative table should be lined with foam/egg-crate or gel padding in prolonged cases or for those involving neurogenic patients.

To optimize positioning and surgical exposure, the need for appropriate retractors, drapes, lighting, and instruments must be anticipated. Whether a transabdominal or transvaginal approach is used, both sites should be prepped. In vaginal cases, one must anticipate the possibility of having to convert to an abdominal approach if, for example, there is an unintentional bladder injury that cannot be repaired transvaginally. Optimization of vaginal exposure involves the use of self-retaining retractors (e.g. Turner-Warwick, Lone-Star) as well as hand-held retractors (e.g. narrow malleable or Deaver), an appropriate length weighted vaginal speculum and, occasionally, retraction sutures on the labia majora. The Trendelenburg position can improve visualization of the anterior vaginal wall, which is especially important in cases of prior surgery resulting in urethral hyperelevation. Trendelenburg positioning also shifts bowels cephalad which is useful in both abdominal and vaginal surgeries, particularly when passing sutures or graft materials through the retropubic space. Use of a headlight may be critical when deep in the pelvis or vagina.

INTRAOPERATIVE BLEEDING

Hemorrhage and transfusion rates specific to reconstructive pelvic surgery are in the range of 1–5%.[5] Lambrou et al reported a hemorrhage rate of 1% and transfusion rate of 16% in 100 consecutive pelvic reconstructive procedures of varying types using abdominal and vaginal approaches.[6] Although these numbers probably overestimate the incidence of significant bleeding, due to the retrospective nature of the study, significant bleeding in pelvic reconstructive surgery may be greater than in general gynecologic procedures due to a number of factors unique to this type of surgery, including the number of procedures performed per case (which, in turn, is associated with longer operative times) and more extensive dissection often required after multiple prior procedures. In addition, older individuals may not tolerate blood loss as well as younger patients undergoing general gynecologic procedures, resulting in a lower threshold for transfusion.

There are certain procedures and sites of dissection that are associated with a greater potential for significant bleeding. The retropubic space is entered in both abdominal

Table 23.1 Potential complications during dorsal lithotomy positioning	
Injury	**Description**
Obturator nerve	Acute flexion of the thigh against the groin, especially in obese patients, can compress the obturator nerve after it exits the obturator foramen and begins to divide in the upper thigh. The resulting deficit is weakness or paralysis of the adductors of the thigh
Femoral nerve	Occurs by compression of the femoral nerve against the pubic ramus. This results in an abnormal gait
Saphenous nerve	Compression of the knee against the knee brace of the stirrup injures the saphenous nerve. The resulting deficit is loss of sensation in the medial aspect of the leg
Peroneal nerve	Pressure on the lateral aspect of the knee compresses the peroneal nerve between the fibular neck and supporting leg brace. This results in instability of the foot and foot drop
Sciatic nerve	Pressure on nerve against the sciatic notch during hip flexion or stretching of the nerve by flexing the hip with the knee extended. Results in weak knee flexion or variable loss of common peroneal or tibial nerve function
Anterior fascial compartment syndrome	Occurs due to muscle necrosis after prolonged leg suspension

and vaginal procedures such as retropubic bladder neck suspensions and pubovaginal sling procedures. The rich perivesical venous plexus can be a source of considerable bleeding which may continue postoperatively if satisfactory or complete hemostasis is not achieved at the time of surgery. Specific attention must be paid to avoiding the dorsal vein of the clitoris by limiting dissection to either side of the midline. Accessory or aberrant obturator vessels are present in up to 80% of individuals and these vessels, or the obturator artery itself, may send branches over Cooper's ligament in 10% of individuals. These vessels need to be identified when positioning retractors or placing sutures through Cooper's ligament.[7]

Although some degree of bleeding associated with defatting of the perivaginal fascia during a retropubic dissection may help identify the bladder neck and bladder edges more effectively, a more extensive dissection may result in a large retropubic hematoma which could become infected, producing a serious complication when synthetic materials are used. The risk of infection is higher in combined abdominal–vaginal procedures where contamination of the retropubic space from the vagina is more likely. Particular attention needs to be paid to hemostasis during laparoscopic procedures after which there can be delayed bleeding once the hemostatic effect of the pneumoperitoneum is released. During vaginal surgeries, the risk of significant bleeding, which can be sudden and massive, increases once the endopelvic fascia has been perforated and the retropubic space is developed. It is the authors' preference to use blunt finger dissection instead of blind sharp dissection with Metzenbaum scissors when developing the endopelvic fascia, as this minimizes the risk of excessive bleeding. However, using either technique, vaginal surgeons must be prepared for brisk bleeding and consider adhering to the following principles.

1. Complete all possible steps of the repair procedure *before* entering the retropubic space. For example, during the anterior vaginal wall suspension, lateral vaginal flaps are dissected, suspension sutures are placed and left on stay clamps, and the suprapubic incision is made before entry into the retropubic space to transfer the suspension sutures suprapubically. Similarly, for a urethrolysis procedure, the suprapubic tube, Martius fat pad (when indicated), and urethral dissection are performed before entering the periurethral space to liberate the urethra and bladder neck.
2. All suture transfers are completed efficiently and followed by rapid closure of the vaginal incision and packing of the vagina. Bleeding is usually self-limiting as the hematoma forms. Placement of a Foley catheter within gauze packing in the vagina and inflating the balloon until adequate tamponade is achieved may

optimize hemostasis.[8] The pack should remain undisturbed for 24–48 hours. Use of a Foley catheter has also been described for control of bleeding during the tension-free vaginal tape (TVT) procedure by inserting the catheter along the trocar insertion path and inflating the balloon in the retropubic space.[9]

There are three procedures that mandate special attention, as bleeding can be massive and hemostasis very difficult to secure. The first is the abdominal mesh sacrocolpopexy. Massive bleeding is rare (1.2–2.6%) but can occur with disruption of the presacral veins. Modification of the technique by securing the mesh to the sacral promontory rather than lower sacral levels reduces this risk.[10] If presacral vessels prevent suture placement, they often can be mobilized laterally with cautious dissection and very small vessels may be cauterized. If catastrophic bleeding does occur, a method using stainless steel thumbtacks has been described (Fig. 23.1).[11] Bone anchor use has been reported to minimize the dissection and avoid triggering major bleeding.

Another vault fixation technique associated with the risk of potentially life-threatening hemorrhage is the sacrospinous ligament fixation. Similarly, the risk of severe bleeding is rare but deaths due to bleeding have occurred, as indicated in one publication in which the authors state that they are "aware of several unpublished cases in which fatalities have occurred."[12] Although it is commonly believed that the vessels at risk adjacent and posterior to the sacrospinous ligament are of pudendal origin,[13] the inferior gluteal artery is most likely to be injured based on anatomic

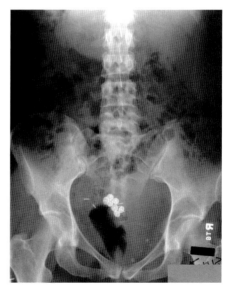

Figure 23.1 Severe bleeding during mesh sacrocolpopexy. Massive bleeding during placement of mesh sacrocolpopexy sutures into the anterior spinous ligament at lower sacral segments could not be controlled with ligature and cautery, requiring placement of multiple sterile thumbtacks for tamponade, as seen radiographically.

studies.[12] Placement of sutures posterior to the ligament and/or placement of retractors beyond the ligament superiorly or inferiorly can injure the superior gluteal artery or its branches. Bleeding may be controlled by packing the operative field tightly with several laparotomy sponges for 20–30 minutes and, if necessary, packing the perirectal space and taking the patient from the operating room for stabilization, with plans to return later to identify the bleeding site and control the vessels with surgical clips. Alternatively, selective arterial embolization may be performed.[14]

The third procedure in which massive hemorrhage can occur is the TVT midurethral sling. Although rates of significant bleeding with TVT from the 1455-patient Finnish registry[15] (>200 cc blood loss 1.9%, major vessel injury 0.07%, retropubic hematoma 1.9%) are comparable to rates reported for more conventional techniques (<1–10%),[5,16-18] massive hemorrhage requiring a 10-unit transfusion has been reported,[19] as well as two cases of external iliac vein injury.[20,21] Fatalities have been reported from secondary bleeding. Patients are now observed for 24 hours and not sent home immediately (two died of unrecognized internal bleeding secondarily).[22] The transobturator approach to tape placement has shown no statistically significant differences in bleeding risk[23,24] but theoretically should not produce catastrophic bleeding by avoiding iliac or retropubic vessels during trocar passage.

Urethral bleeding may occur during dissection between the anterior vaginal wall and periurethral fascia. Any sign of bleeding usually indicates that the dissection is proceeding in the wrong plane and that redirection is required to limit bleeding and avoid urethral injury. Hydrodissection, particularly when there has been prior surgery, may facilitate identification of the correct plane. Usually, reapposition of the periurethral fascia with a fine absorbable suture will obtain hemostasis more effectively than cautery.

BLADDER INJURY

Because pelvic reconstructive surgery involves dissection in close proximity to the urinary tract, often in patients with prior surgery, unintentional urinary tract injuries, particularly cystotomy, may occur at higher rates than in general gynecologic procedures. In a series of various pelvic reconstructive surgeries, cystotomies occurred in 6% of cases.[25] This is in contrast to a rate of 0.4% in a series of 5517 procedures for general nonradical major gynecologic procedures.[2] The risk of bladder injury is increased by any condition that can produce adhesions in the pelvis; this includes not only prior surgical procedures but also endometriosis, pelvic inflammatory disease, diverticulitis, infection, and prior radiation. Distortion of the retropubic space and pelvis may occur as a result of uterine myomas or ovarian cysts.

Injuries may result from bladder incision, excision, crushing, avulsion/tearing or involvement in a ligature. Perforation due to retropubic needle or trocar passage is the most common type of bladder injury and occurs in transvaginal sling and suspension procedures performed for incontinence. Using some basic principles described herein, most injuries can be prevented and so long as the injury is recognized and appropriately managed, unnecessary morbidity and permanent complications will be avoided. Unrecognized injuries can result in infectious complications, urinary tract fistulae, and bladder calculus formation. However, even when recognized, an extensive bladder repair may necessitate deferring the originally planned procedure to a later date, for fear of secondary urinary leakage.

A simple preventive maneuver that should be practiced, regardless of the specific surgical procedure, is placement of a urethral Foley catheter at the start of the case to ensure bladder decompression. The catheter should be kept on continuous rather than intermittent drainage in order to keep the bladder away from dissection at all times. A Foley catheter also facilitates identification of the bladder neck and urethra by palpation of the balloon in both abdominal and transvaginal procedures, in addition to monitoring for hematuria resulting from a bladder injury. It should be noted, however, that even if decompressed, the bladder can still be distorted by old adhesions; for example, prior low abdominal incisions may produce adhesions sufficient to elevate the dome of the bladder or even predispose to ventral bladder hernia, making it susceptible to incisional injury.

Bladder injury during retropubic needle or trocar passage requires specific mention with the recent popularity of the TVT procedure. The predecessor techniques utilizing retropubic needle passage, such as the Pereyra and Raz transvaginal bladder neck suspensions, were associated with bladder perforation rates of <1%.[26,27] In large series, the TVT procedure has been associated with bladder perforation rates of 0.8–3.8%[15,28] although some have shown much higher rates of up to 24%.[29,30] Fingertip guidance of retropubic passage of the needle ligature carrier was first described in the modified Pereyra bladder neck suspension and has been used in subsequent transvaginal suspensions. This maneuver is particularly important in cases of prior surgery after which retropubic scar can distort the normal anatomy and position. The technique involves initial development of the retropubic space and endopelvic fascia (usually bluntly with a finger), after which the needle tip is advanced from the suprapubic site on the finger at all times while closely approximating the posterior aspect of the pubis. Blunt dissection prior to needle passage frees up the scar tissue and helps ensure the bladder is mobilized medially out of the path of the needle. The SPARC polypropylene tensionless midurethral sling is purported to have the advantage of improved control of the trocar compared to the TVT as the trocar is passed from "top to bottom" using the same principle of fingertip guidance.[31]

One must remember that the technique of "fingertip guidance" does not imply development of the retropubic space, which is *not* routinely performed, and theoretically adds an additional element of injury prevention. Similarly, techniques to facilitate controlled passage from "bottom to top" of the TVT trocar have been proposed in order to achieve a similar safety margin.[32] The obturator approach to tape placement should, in theory, avoid bladder injury and many have suggested that cystoscopy is not mandatory; however, bladder injury during transobturator insertion of TVT has still been reported.[33]

Bladder injury is usually detected by the presence of bloody urine draining from the catheter or urine leaking into the operative field, although in some cases these signs may not be observed. Although routine intraoperative cystoscopy, first proposed by Stamey,[34] should detect all injuries and add little morbidity and time to surgery, its routine use is debated.[35,36] Proper technique for cystoscopy includes adequate distension of the bladder and use of both 30° and 70° lenses to prevent any mucosal folding from obscuring an injury (Fig. 23.2). Suprapubic pressure may facilitate visualization of the anterolateral and distal anterior bladder walls. Alternatively, a flexible cystoscope can be used. Location, size, and proximity of injury to the ureteric orifices should be observed. If cystoscopy appears normal but a bladder injury is still suspected, distending the bladder to a volume of 400–600 cc with indigo carmine or methylene blue

solution may allow for identification of dye draining through the vagina or suprapubically.

In most instances, the intended reconstructive procedure can proceed after surgical repair of the injury site or with extended postoperative bladder drainage alone. In fact, most relatively small bladder punctures (e.g. by retropubic needles, trocars, sutures, tapes) will heal without extending catheter drainage beyond 1–2 days after surgery. In a small series of cases of cystotomies occurring during transvaginal surgery for incontinence, immediate bladder closure and continuation of the planned procedure was carried out without an increased risk of vesicovaginal fistula formation.[37] When a needle ligature carrier, trocar, nonabsorbable suture or synthetic graft material enters the bladder, it should simply be removed and repositioned more laterally. Failing to recognize intrusion of a foreign body into the bladder may result in infection, stone formation, and urinary symptoms.[38] More extensive cystotomies occurring during transvaginal procedures will require formal closure; this should be performed transvaginally unless the trigone and/or ureters are involved in which case an abdominal approach is used. If the injury is very large, urine contamination precludes placement of synthetic material or if the repair extends the duration of procedure excessively from an anesthetic standpoint, the originally proposed reconstructive procedure will need to be deferred. Injuries occurring during abdominal procedures are repaired through the same incision.

Bladder repair, whether transvaginal or transabdominal, follows the same fundamental principles. The injury must

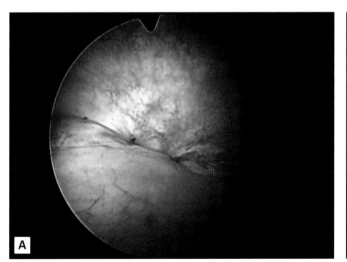
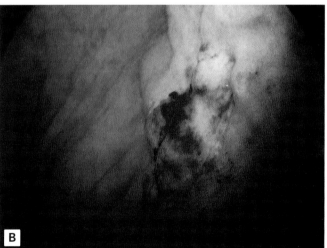

Figure 23.2 Bladder injuries identified on cystoscopy. (**A**) Cystoscopy after Burch bladder neck suspension. A transfixing posterior bladder wall suture is seen from the abdominal hysterectomy preceding the Burch procedure. The abdomen was reexplored and the suture-ligature around the uterine pedicle was removed. It is likely that in the absence of cystoscopy, this uneventful hysterectomy would have been complicated by a vesicovaginal fistula. (**B**) During a midline cystocele repair in a patient who previously underwent a paravaginal repair, dense retropubic scarring rendered transfer of suspension sutures difficult, resulting in an anterolateral bladder wall injury. Of note, there was no gross hematuria. Evaluation with a fully distended bladder and 70° cystoscope revealed a discrete site injury due to a transfixing suture. The sutures were repositioned more laterally.

first be staged for size, location, number of perforations, viability of tissue, and ureteric involvement. If ureteric injury is suspected, then intravenous indigo carmine should be administered to assess cystoscopically for blue efflux. The repair itself must be tension free and water tight. This is achieved by adequate mobilization of the bladder prior to closure, ensuring viability of the bladder tissue involved (debriding when necessary), closing with absorbable suture in multiple layers, and, in some cases, placement of pedicled interposition or advancement flaps of well-vascularized tissue (e.g. Martius labial graft, omentum, peritoneum).[39]

Transabdominal repair of a bladder laceration requires a conventional two-layer closure. If the injury is located near the trigone, then ureteric involvement needs to be assessed. This can usually be adequately performed by direct visualization through a large cystotomy, otherwise the cystotomy may need to be extended to allow better visualization. When the laceration is large or located near the vaginal cuff, interposition tissue should be placed. Omentum[40] or peritoneum[41] (including preperitoneum) can be mobilized and anchored with interrupted sutures to cover the bladder closure. A large-bore suprapubic catheter is placed through a separate cystotomy and secured to the bladder adventitia with fine absorbable suture prior to closure of the bladder injury. An extravesical closed suction drain is left in place for a short period postoperatively to monitor for any urine leakage.

For transvaginal repairs, the first step is placement of a small (approximately 10 F) Foley catheter into the bladder via the cystotomy in order to provide traction and exposure. A guidewire may facilitate passage of the catheter and is left in place to prevent loss of the tract if the Foley catheter is lost inadvertently. A suprapubic catheter is placed using a Lowsley retractor[42] as the bladder may not be easily distended to allow for a suprapubic punch catheter placement. Margins of the cystotomy are identified and tagged with fine suture or grasped with Allis clamps to better assess the extent of injury (Fig. 23.3). Debridement of devitalized tissue is rarely required. To facilitate a tension-free closure, the adjacent bladder wall is mobilized from the vaginal tissue. The closure is then performed in two layers. For the first mucosal layer, 5-0 absorbable suture is run from the two extremities of the cystotomy toward the middle. Water-tightness is checked at this point by distending the bladder with fluid and, if the closure is adequate, the second layer is closed using interrupted 3-0 absorbable suture in a direction at right angles to the first to prevent overlapping suture lines. Interposition tissue (e.g. fascia or Martius fat graft) may be positioned between the repair and the vaginal wall closure in cases of large injuries, extensive prior surgery or pelvic radiation. As the final step, cystoscopy with intravenous administration of indigo carmine is performed to ensure ureteric patency.

Postoperative care is as important as a good repair. The goal is to minimize tension on the repair to facilitate healing. This requires a period of uninterrupted catheter drainage (urethral and intraoperatively placed suprapubic) with infection and bladder spasm prophylaxis with antibiotics and antimuscarinic medications or belladonna and opioid suppositories. Duration of catheterization varies according to risk factors for poor healing: drainage for 5–7 days is adequate in uncomplicated cases but after extensive injuries or with a history of pelvic irradiation, a longer course is required (10–14 days). Prior to catheter removal, healing can be confirmed with a lateral-view cystogram. Adherence to these principles minimizes the risk of secondary vesico-vaginal fistula.

URETERIC INJURY

Ureteric injury is reported to occur at a higher rate in pelvic reconstructive procedures for prolapse and incontinence compared to general urogynecologic procedures. Rates of 1.7–4.9% have been reported in reconstructive procedures,[6,35,36,43] compared to 0.03–2% for benign gynecologic conditions.[44-48] Rates of ureteral injury during specific techniques, such as uterosacral vaginal vault suspension and Burch bladder neck suspension, vary widely depending on the series, with reported rates of 1–11%[49,50] and 0–10%[35,51] respectively. The anterior colporrhaphy, not traditionally thought to place the lower urinary tract at high risk, has been associated with a 2% risk of ureteric injury.[43] Although ureteric injuries are relatively much less common compared to bladder injuries, sequelae, particularly in cases of delayed diagnosis, are potentially much more severe and include obstructive nephropathy with kidney loss, fistula formation, and urosepsis. Intraoperative detection and repair of injuries reduces morbidity significantly.[52-54]

The most common mechanisms of ureteral injury include ligation and angulation/kinking by a suture.[55,56] Less common are laceration, transection (Fig. 23.4), excision, and devascularization (e.g. cautery injury resulting in delayed necrosis). Although several risk factors for ureteric injury have been proposed,[57] including excessive scarring due to prior surgeries, endometriosis or pelvic inflammatory disease and excessively distorted anatomy due to large cystocele, uterus or adnexal mass, some reported series of pelvic reconstructive procedures have failed to identify any parameters predicting those at risk.[35] Indeed, it has been suggested that it is in those procedures considered "routine" or "technically uncomplicated" that injuries are more likely to be unsuspected and unrecognized.[35,43,48] For this reason, the utmost vigilance is required in all cases regardless of the absence or presence of obvious risk factors.

A sound knowledge of normal ureteral anatomy as well as possible congenital or acquired variations in anatomy

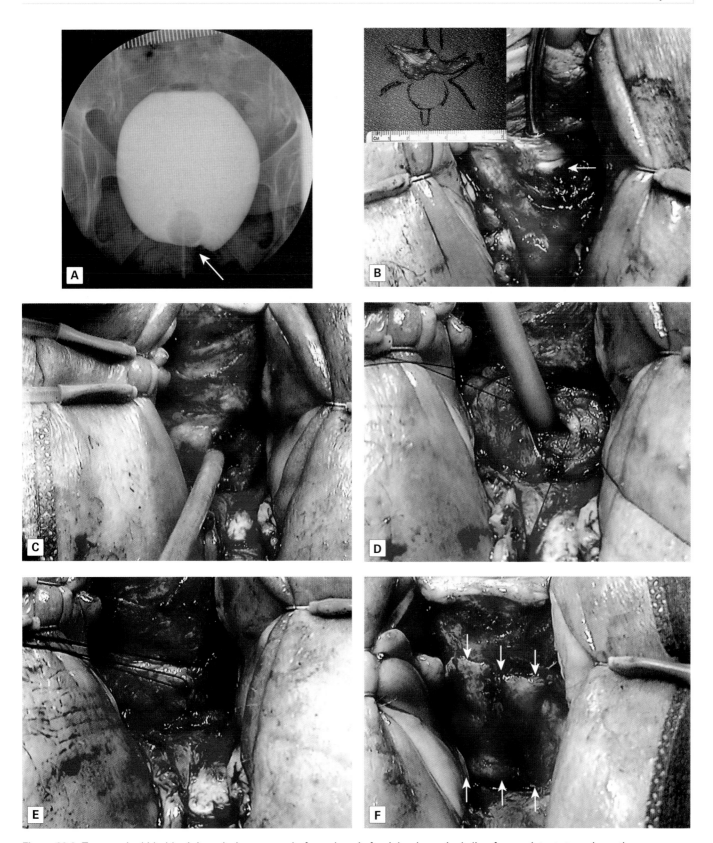

Figure 23.3 Transvaginal bladder injury during removal of a cadaveric fascial pubovaginal sling for persistent stress incontinence. (**A**) Anteroposterior view from a standing VCUG showing a filling defect indenting the left bladder neck (*arrow*). (**B**) The sling material was traced left of the bladder neck and after removal, a left-sided cystotomy was observed. [*inset excised sling specimen*] (**C**) A Foley catheter was inserted through the bladder defect to provide traction and occlusion of the injury for bladder filling required during suprapubic tube placement. (**D**) First layer closure: sutures were placed at the extremities of the defect and run towards the middle. (**E**) Second layer closure: interrupted perivesical Lembert sutures were placed at right angles to the first layer. (**F**) Completion of the planned autologous fascia sling procedure covering the defect repair.

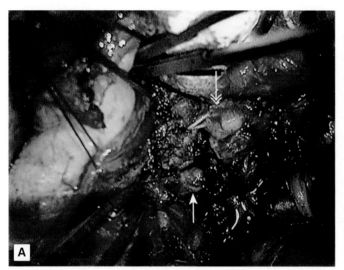
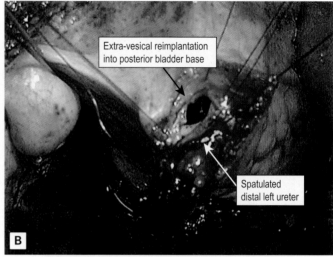

Figure 23.4 Ureteric transection. Intraoperative consultation for suspected ureteric injury during a difficult abdominal hysterectomy for a very enlarged fibroid uterus. At cystoscopy no ureteric efflux or peristalsis of the left ureteric orifice was observed. Retrograde passage of a catheter met with resistance at 2 cm proximal to the ureterovesical junction. (**A**) The proximal ureter was identified at the level of the iliac vessels and traced distally to the site of transection (*single arrowhead, distal ureter; double arrowhead, proximal ureter*). (**B**) Given the close proximity of the bladder, an extravesical Lich-Gregoir ureteric reimplantation was performed.

will allow the surgeon to identify the ureter at predictable locations intraoperatively, usually without formal dissection. Although the use of preoperative imaging has been suggested as a means of identifying preexisting ureteral abnormalities, this strategy has not shown a significant reduction in intraoperative injury in routine hysterectomy.[58,59] Still, preoperative imaging may be advisable when adverse surgical conditions are anticipated; examples include pelvic masses, pelvic inflammatory disease, prior ureteral injury, previous irradiation, known solitary kidney or renal anomalies.[60] Additionally, ureteric stent placement at the time of surgery can help.

Anatomic studies have determined the proximity of the ureter to specific anatomic landmarks and distortion produced by certain surgical procedures (Fig. 23.5). Two of the most common sites of ureteric injury are at the infundibulopelvic ligament/ovarian fossa, between the posterior peritoneum and the hypogastric vessels (medial umbilical ligament), and dorsal to the uterine artery and lateral to the cervix at the base of the broad ligament. The ureter is also at risk of injury along the lateral pelvic side wall above the uterosacral ligaments and through the tunnel in the cardinal ligament where the ureter turns medially anterior to the vaginal fornix to enter the bladder. During anterior colporrhaphy, the ureter is located at a mean of 0.9 cm from anterior colporrhaphy plication sutures and a mean of 1.0 cm from the infundibulopelvic ligament when the tube and ovary are removed.[47] Cadaveric dissection has shown the mean distance from the ureter to uterosacral ligament to be 0.9, 2.3, and 4.1 cm in the cervical, intermediate, and sacral portions of the uterosacral ligament respectively.[61] Based on computed tomography studies, the ureter is located on average 2.3 cm lateral to the cervix except in 12% of examinations in which the distance was 0.5 cm or less.[62]

While prevention of an unintentional ureteric injury is the ultimate goal, a far greater error than the injury itself is failure to recognize it. Higgins is frequently quoted as stating this in 1967: "The venial sin is the injury of the ureter, but the mortal sin is the failure of recognition."[56] Although 30 years later, a 1997 educational bulletin of the American College of Obstetricians and Gynecologists continued to advise that "both ureters and bladder should be inspected to confirm their integrity" at the conclusion of gynecologic surgery,[63] specific recommendations are not provided and there is no apparent consensus among surgeons.

Intraoperative methods to identify injuries include direct visualization, retrograde pyelography, cystoscopy with intravenous indigo carmine or methylene blue, and intravenous pyelography (IVP). When attempting to identify an area of ureter directly, palpation and recognition of the typical peristalsis may be sufficient. Although palpation is relatively easier in abdominal as compared to vaginal approaches, some have advocated palpation as a reliable technique in vaginal approaches as well,[47,49,64] although this is debated.[35] The ureter is said to be easily palpable transvaginally in the 10 or 2 o'clock position after opening the anterior cul-de-sac during vaginal hysterectomy. Placement of ureteral catheters (usually 5-6 F whistle-tip) has been advocated as a means of facilitating ureteral identification as well as identification of injuries. Patients with conditions tending to distort the trigone, such as large cystoceles or prior anterior colporrhaphy, may benefit from this strategy although stent placement in itself may be challenging. The

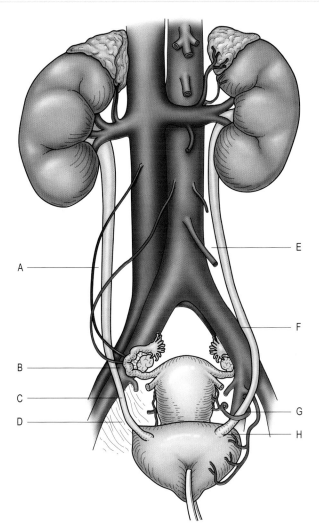

Figure 23.5 Anatomic studies have determined the proximity of the ureter to specific anatomic landmarks and distortion produced by certain surgical procedures. Common site of ureteral injury. **(A)** Division of the gonadal vessels and infundibulopelvic ligament. **(B)** Resection of adnexal masses adherent to the ureter within the broad ligament. **(C)** At the apex of the obturator fossa in pelvic lymphadenectomy. **(D)** Division of the lateral ligaments of the rectum in abdominoperineal resection. **(E)** Division of inferior mesenteric vessels in sigmoid resection. **(F)** At pelvic brim during vascular bypass procedures. **(G)** Division of the uterine artery during hysterectomy. **(H)** At the lateral vaginal fornix, entry into trigone of the bladder during hysterectomy and vaginal procedures.

5- and 15-minute films; however, it should be noted that a "limited" or "one-shot" IVP has poor sensitivity of only 20% whereas that for a complete series is 80–100%.[65] In the operating room, circumstances for obtaining good images are never ideal and this approach may be insufficient to provide a definitive answer in this setting.

Routine intraoperative cystoscopy with intravenous dye to screen for unsuspected ureteric injuries in gynecologic and pelvic reconstructive procedures has been advocated by some as mandatory in all cases,[35,43,66,67] while others have recommended only its selective use.[57,68] Indeed, it has been argued that the rate of preexisting ureteral obstruction or other abnormalities may be more common than intra-operative injury[60] and that very low overall rates of ureteric injury do not justify an additional procedure that will only very rarely change management. At the same time, others argue that cystoscopy adds little time and no morbidity to the procedure and, taking into account the complexity of complications when not recognized and repaired immedi-ately, is likely cost-effective as has been demonstrated in a decision analysis model evaluating the utility of cystoscopy in hysterectomy.[66] The technique involves administration of either indigo carmine or methylene blue intravenously approximately 10–15 minutes prior to cystoscopy. It should be noted that indigo carmine is preferred as it appears in the urinary tract more promptly than methylene blue and does not reduce oxygen saturation, which can occur with methylene blue. Ureteric efflux of blue dye should be brisk in cases of ureteric patency (provided hydration status is adequate); slow or no efflux should prompt further inves-tigation or revision of the repair. Cystoscopy should be performed prior to finalizing any repair (e.g. cutting ties and sutures, closing incisions) rather than as the final step, and may be required multiple times in complex reconstructive procedures, so as to facilitate "taking down" the repair if a ureteric injury is detected. The majority of intraoperative interventions consist of simply removing or replacing sutures, rather than more complex urologic procedures.

The mechanism of injury and location on the ureter will direct intraoperative intervention. In cases of ureteric ligation, removal of the suture may be all that is required. Crush injuries from clamps should usually be stented and drained; rarely, removal of the clamp is all that is required. If viability is in question, then the injured ureter is excised and ureteric reimplantation or end-to-end anastomosis is performed depending on distance of the injury from the ureterovesical junction.

Ureteroneocystostomy is appropriate for distal ureteric defects of up to 5 cm, while a psoas hitch or Boari flap combined with reimplantation will bridge gaps of 5–10 cm and 10–15 cm, respectively.[69,70] As a rule, ureteroureteros-tomy is not recommended below the level of the internal iliac vessels due to concern regarding the distal segment

stent must be removed at the end of the procedure and blue efflux documented as the course of a ureter can be kinked or deviated even with a stent in place. If more extensive dissection is required to identify the ureter abdominally, particularly near the bladder pedicles or paracervical region, attempts should be made to limit dissection to the anterior and medial aspect to minimize potential devascularization. Retrograde pyelography using a cone-tip ureteral catheter via cystotomy or cystoscopy is probably the most accurate method to identify a ureteric injury as the collecting system can be filled and distended reliably. An on-table IVP can be performed using 1–2 cc/kg iodinated contrast and taking

blood supply. Ureteral laceration and excision injuries are repaired based on the level of injury. Usually little or no ischemic injury occurs unless cautery was used. If a ureteric injury consists of a partial laceration, then closure with fine absorbable suture along with ureteric stenting and external drainage may be appropriate; however, in distal injuries of this type, reimplantation with stenting and drainage is usually the simplest, most reliable option. Devascularization injuries can result in delayed necrosis with fistula formation in 10–14 days. If devascularization is a concern, ureteric debridement and repair should be performed, whereas if equivocal, consideration should be given to stenting and coverage with omentum or peritoneum. While the exception, extensive ureteric loss may require more complex urologic reconstruction; options include transuretero-ureterostomy, ileal ureteral substitution/interposition (Fig. 23.6), autotransplantation, and nephrectomy.[70]

URETHRAL INJURY

Urethral injury in pelvic reconstructive procedures is very rare and more likely to occur in transvaginal rather than

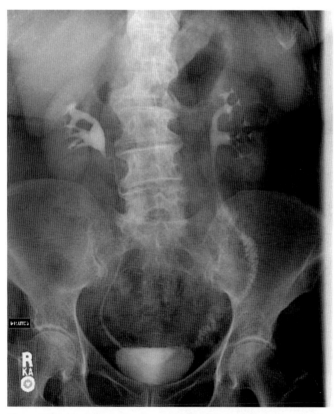

Figure 23.6 Ureteric replacement. Ureteric injury at the level of the infundibulopelvic ligament resulting in a long ureteric stricture. Intraoperatively, dense periureteral scarring extended proximal and distal to the site of injury. Poor anesthetic bladder capacity and extended length of ureteric disease precluded repair using a Boari flap. Thus, an ileal-ureteric interposition was elected. IVP 1 year postoperatively demonstrates the ileal interposition and normal upper tracts bilaterally.

abdominal procedures. In transvaginal procedures, injury most commonly occurs during dissection between the anterior vaginal wall and periurethral fascia. Diverticulectomy occasionally can result in a large urethral defect. Trocar or needle passage during antiincontinence procedures may also injure the urethra.

During anterior vaginal wall dissection, identification of the correct plane between the vaginal wall and periurethral fascia can be facilitated by submucosal infiltration with normal saline, dilute epinephrine or local anesthetic solutions. The periurethral fascia is characterized by subtle white glistening tissue that does not bleed easily, while dissection that penetrates this layer into the spongy periurethral tissue produces bleeding readily. If it is unclear whether an injury has penetrated the full urethral thickness simply by inspecting for the transurethral catheter, either urethroscopy using a ≤30° lens or pericatheter instillation of blue dye through a 5 F feeding tube or small intravenous catheter will facilitate the diagnosis. During abdominal cases in which dissection or suture placement occurs near the urethra (e.g. retropubic bladder neck suspension, urethrolysis), palpating the urethral catheter and balloon facilitates identification of the urethra and bladder neck.

Superficial urethral injuries (i.e. into the spongy periurethral tissue, but not through the mucosa) sustained during transvaginal procedures should be closed immediately using fine absorbable suture to reappose the periurethral fascia. The dissection can then be redirected to avoid reentry into the same space. If injuries are full thickness, they should be repaired in layers over a urethral catheter (14–16 F) or metal sound using running fine (5-0 or 6-0) absorbable suture for the mucosa and periurethral fascia/muscularis. Tensionless, nonoverlapping suture lines are important. Large defects may also require placement of interposition tissue such as fascia and/or Martius labial fat graft.[71] Water-tightness after repair should be confirmed by retrograde pericatheter urethral filling or gentle urethroscopy. Postoperatively, a silastic catheter is left in situ for approximately 3–4 weeks and strong consideration should be given to placement of a suprapubic catheter to optimize diversion of urine away from the site of injury.

BOWEL INJURY

Bowel injury during pelvic reconstructive procedures is extremely rare. Retropubic trocar or needle placement may perforate bowel and result in potentially life-threatening peritonitis if not recognized intraoperatively. This complication has been described in multiple case reports in the midurethral sling literature, in particular the TVT.[31,72-76] It has been suggested that the obturator approach for vaginal tape placement will minimize the risk of visceral perforation. Bowel perforation is also described following suprapubic bladder catheter placement.

To avoid these injuries, it is important to identify patients in whom prior abdominal surgery may have resulted in bowel fixation in the pelvis or adherence to the lower abdominal wall. Selective preoperative cross-sectional imaging might help identify those at risk. For all patients, steep Trendelenburg positioning will help mobilize small bowel cephalad. For retropubic needle or trocar passage, direct fingertip guidance reduces the risk of injury. The entry site for needle and trocar passage should very closely approximate the posterior aspect of the pubis. A suprapubic catheter entry site should be no more than 3 cm proximal to the edge of the symphysis pubis and the catheter should be directed at an angle of approximately 30° from the abdominal wall into a distended bladder. Use of a Lowsley retractor and placement of the catheter under cystoscopic control will also minimize the risk of injury.[42]

Transvaginal procedures in which bowel injury may occur include rectocele and enterocele repair. A rectal injury rate of 0.5% was reported in a series of vaginal hysterectomies, of which 69% included posterior repair.[77] Prior posterior repair was identified as a risk factor for injury, occurring in 25%, compared to 2.5% of those without injury. In all cases, injuries were recognized and repaired immediately intraoperatively using a two-layer closure without drain placement. Prevention of rectal injury is aided by packing the rectum prior to the procedure or using an O'Connor drape, both of which simply allow for more reliable intraoperative identification. If a rectal injury is suspected but not readily visible, examination with one finger in the rectum and one in the vagina should be performed. Alternatively, the vagina can be filled with fluid and air insufflated into the rectum using a catheter or Toomey syringe. All rectal injuries should be repaired at the time of recognition. Any plans for foreign body placement (e.g. mesh) should be deferred. In cases of small bowel injury during enterocele repair, it is important to ensure that all sites of injury are identified. If exposure is inadequate, the injury should be approached transabdominally.

CONCLUSION

Intraoperative injury in pelvic reconstructive surgery occurs infrequently but when it does occur, management can be challenging. Prevention of injuries, as well as efficient and effective intraoperative management, requires a detailed knowledge of the particular case and specific operative anatomy to allow anticipation of potential intraoperative hazards. In this way, the patient can be appropriately counseled preoperatively, particularly in terms of her desires for outcome and willingness to accept the surgeon's estimate for the risk of intraoperative injuries and their sequelae. Preparedness for complications and knowledge of management options will minimize the risk of long-term sequelae.

REFERENCES

1. Mann WJ, Arato M, Patsner B, Stone MC. Ureteral injuries in an obstetrics and gynecology training program: etiology and management. Obstet Gynecol 1988;72:82–85.

2. Miyazawa K. Urological injuries in gynaecological surgery. Hawaii Med J 1980;39:11–12.

3. Carey JM, Leach GE. Transvaginal surgery in the octogenarian using cadaveric fascia for pelvic prolapse and stress incontinence: minimal one-year results compared to younger patients. Urology 2004;63(4):665–670.

4. Ballard RM, Bradley-Watson PJ, Johnstone FD, Kenney A, McCarthy TG. Low doses of subcutaneous heparin in the prevention of deep vein thrombosis after gynecologic surgery. J Obstet Gynaecol Br Commonw 1973;180:469–472.

5. Leach GE, Dmochowski RR, Appell RA, et al. Female stress urinary incontinence clinical guidelines panel report on surgical management of female stress urinary incontinence. The American Urological Association. J Urol 1997;158;875–880.

6. Lambrou NC, Buller MD, Thompson JR, et al. Prevalence of perioperative complications among women undergoing reconstructive pelvic surgery. Am J Obstet Gynecol 2000;183:1355–1360.

7. Kingsnorth AN, Skandalakis PN, Colborn GL, et al. Embryology, anatomy, and surgical applications of the preperitoneal space. Surg Clin North Am 2000;80(1):1–24.

8. Katske FA, Raz S. Use of Foley catheter to obtain transvaginal tamponade. Urol Urotech 1987;8.

9. Aungst M, Wagner M. Foley balloon to tamponade bleeding in the retropubic space. Obstet Gynecol 2003;102(5 Pt 1):1037–1038.

10. Addison WA, Livengood CH, Parker RT. Vaginal vault prolapse with emphasis on management by transabdominal sacral colpopexy. Postgrad Obstet Gynecol 1998;8:1–7.

11. Timmons MC, Kohler MF, Addison WA. Thumb-tack use for control of presacral bleeding with description of an instrument for thumbtack application. Obstet Gynceol 1991;78: 313–315.

12. Barksdale PA, Elkins TE, Sanders CK, et al. An anatomic approach to pelvic haemorrhage during sacrospinous ligament fixation of the vaginal vault. Obstet Gynecol 1998;91(5):715–718.

13. Verdeja AM, Elkins TE, Odoi A, Gasser RF, Lamoutte C. Transvaginal sacrospinous colpopexy: anatomic landmarks to be aware of to minimize complications. Am J Obstet Gynecol 1995;173:1468–1469.

14. Keith LG, Vogelzang RL, Croteau DL. Surgical management of intractable pelvic haemorrhage. In: Sciarra JJ, ed. Gynecology and obstetrics. Philadelphia: Lippincott-Raven; 1996.

15. Kuuva N, Nilsson CG. A nationwide analysis of complications associated with the tension-free vaginal tape (TVT) procedure. Acta Obstet Gynecol Scand 2002;81:72–77.

16. Jarvis G. Surgery for genuine stress incontinence. Br J Obstet Gynaecol 1994;101:371–374.

17. Nygaard IE, Kreder KJ. Complications of incontinence surgery. Int Urogynecol J 1994;5: 353–360.

18. Chaliha C, Stanton SL. Complications of surgery for genuine stress incontinence. Br J Obstet Gynaecol 1999;106:1238–1245.

19. Vierhout MD. Severe haemorrhage complicating tension-free vaginal tape (TVT): a case report. Int Urogynecol J 2001;12:139–140.

20. Primicerio M, De Matteis G, Mantanino OM, et al. Use of the TVT (tension-free-vaginal tape) in the treatment of female urinary stress incontinence [article in Italian]. Minerva Ginecol 1999;51(9):355–358.

21. Zilbert AW, Farrell SA. External iliac artery laceration during tension-free vaginal tape procedure. Int Urogynecol J 2001;12:141–143.

22. Boustead GB. Review: the tension-free vaginal tape for treating female stress urinary incontinence. BJU Int 2002;89:687–692.

23. Mellier G, Benayed B, Bretones S, et al. Suburethral tape via the obturator route: is the TOT a simplification of the TVT? Int Urogynecol J Pelvic Floor Dysfunct 2004;15:227–232.

24. DeTayrac R, Xavier D, Droupy S, et al. A prospective randomized trial comparing tension-free vaginal tape and transobturator suburethral tape for surgical treatment of stress urinary incontinence. Am J Obstet Gynecol 2004;190:602–608.

25. Nicholas C, Lambrou MD, Buller JL, et al. Prevalence of perioperative complications among women undergoing reconstructive pelvic surgery. Am J Obstet Gynecol 2000;183:1355–1360.

26. Leach GE, Raz S. Modified Pereyra bladder neck suspension after previously failed anti-incontinence surgery. Urology 1984;23: 359.

27. Pereyra AJ, Lebherz TB. Combined urethral vesical suspension vaginal urethroplasty for correction of urinary stress incontinence. Obstet Gynecol 1967;30:357.

28. Wang A. The techniques of trocar insertion and intraoperative urethrocystoscopy in tension-free vaginal taping: an experience of 600 cases. Acta Obstet Gynecol Scand 2004;83: 293–298.

29. Niecmczyk P, Klutke JJ, Carlin BI, Klutke CG. United States experience with tension-free vaginal tape procedure for urinary stress incontinence: assessment of safety and tolerability. Tech Urol 2001;7(4):261–265.

30. Lebret T, Lugagne PM, Herve JM, et al. Evaluation of tension-free vaginal tape procedure. Its safety and efficacy in the treatment of female stress urinary incontinence during the learning phase. Eur Urol 2001;40(5):543–547.

31. Kobashi KC, Govier FE. Perioperative complications: the first 140 polypropylene pubovaginal slings. J Urol 2003;170:1918–1921.

32. Croak AJ, Schulte V, Klingele CJ, et al. Needle tip control and its effect in reducing intraoperative complications during tension-free vaginal tape placement. Int Urogynecol J 2004; 15:138–144.

33. Mermieu JF, Messas A, Delmas V, et al. Bladder injury after TVT transobturator [in French]. Prog Urol 2003;13(1):115–117.

34. Stamey TA. Endoscopic suspension of the vesical neck for urinary incontinence in females. Ann Surg 1980;192:465.

35. Harris RL, Cundiff GW, Theofrastous JP, et al. The value of intraoperative cystoscopy in urogynecologic and reconstructive pelvic surgery. Am J Obstet Gynecol 1997;177:1367–1371.

36. Petit PD, Petrou SP. The value of cystoscopy in major vaginal surgery. Obsetet Gynecol 1994;84:318–320.

37. Hadley RH, Myers RC. Complications of vaginal surgery: does unintentional cystotomy result in vesicovaginal fistula? Proceedings of the Western Section, American Urological Association. Scottsdale, 1989, p. 32.

38. But I, Bratu D, Faganelj M. Prolene tape in the bladder wall after TVT procedure: intramural tape placement or secondary tape migration. Int Urogynecol J Pelvic Floor Dysfunct 2005;16:75–76.

39. Wang Y, Hadley HR. The use of rotated vascularized pedicle flaps for complex transvaginal procedures. J Urol 1993;149(3):590–592.

40. Kiricuta I, Goldstein AM. The repair of extensive vesicovaginal fistulas with pedicled omentum: a review of 27 cases. J Urol 1972;108(5):724–727.

41. Hamlin RH, Nicholson EC. Reconstruction of urethra totally destroyed in labour. BMJ 1969;1(650):147–150.

42. Zimmern PE, Hadley HR, Leach GE, et al. Transvaginal closure of the bladder neck and placement of a suprapubic catheter for destroyed urethra after long-term indwelling catheterization. J Urol 1985;134:554–557.

43. Kwon CH, Goldberg RP, Koduri S, et al. The use of intraoperative cystoscopy in major vaginal and urogynecologic surgeries. Am J Obstet Gynecol 2002;187:1466–1472.

44. Harris WJ. Early complications of abdominal and vaginal hysterectomy. Obstet Gynecol Surv 1995;50(11):795–805.

45. Goodno JA Jr, Powers TW, Harris VD. Ureteral injury in gynecologic surgery: a ten-year review in a community hospital. Am J Obstet Gynecol 1995;172:1817–1822.

46. Harkki-Siren P, Sjoberg J, Tiitinen A. Urinary tract injuries after hysterectomy. Obstet Gynecol 1998;92:113–118.

47. Stanhope CR, Wilson TO, Utz WJ, et al. Suture entrapment and secondary ureteral obstruction. Am J Obstet Gynecol 1991;164:1513–1519.

48. Wiskind AK, Thompson JD. Should cystoscopy be done after every gynecologic operation to diagnose unsuspected ureteral injury? J Pelvic Surg 1995;1:134–137.

49. Barber MD, Visco AG, Weidner AC, et al. Bilateral uterosacral ligament vaginal vault suspension with site-specific endopelvic fascia defect repair for treatment of pelvic organ prolapse. Am J Obstet Gynecol 1991;2000:1402–1411.

50. Shull BL, Bachofen C, Boates KC, et al. A transvaginal approach to repair of apical and other associated sites of pelvic organ prolapse with uterosacral ligaments. Am J Obstet Gynecol 2000;183:1365–1374.

51. Tulikangas PK, Weber AM, Larive B, et al. Intraoperative cystoscopy in conjunction with anti-incontinence surgery. Obstet Gynecol 2000;95:794–796.

52. Saidi MH, Sadler RK, Vancaillie TG, et al. Diagnosis and management of serious urinary complications after major operative laparoscopy. Obstet Gynecol 1996;87:272–276.

53. Witters S, Cornelissen M, Vereecken R. Iatrogenic ureteral injury: aggressive or conservative treatment. Am J Obstet Gynecol 1986;155:582–584.

54. Neuman M, Eidelman A, Langer R, et al. Iatrogenic injuries to the ureter during gynecologic and obstetric operations. Surg Gynecol Obstet 1991;173:268–272.

55. Van Nagell Jr, Roddick JW Jr. Vaginal hysterectomy, the ureter and excretory urography. Obsetet Gynecol 1972;39(5):784–786.

56. Higgins CC. Ureteral injuries during surgery. A review of 87 cases. JAMA 1967;199(2): 82–88.

57. Dandolu V, Mathai E, Chatwani A, et al. Accuracy of cystoscopy in the diagnosis of ureteral injury in benign gynecologic surgery. Int Urogyencol J 2003;14:427–431.

58. Piscatelli JR, Simel DL, Addison WA. Who should have intravenous pyelograms before hysterectomy for benign disease? Obstet Gynecol 1987;69:541–545.

59. Larson DM, Malone JM, Copeland LJ, et al. Ureteral assessment after radical hysterectomy. Obstet Gynecol 1987;69(4):612–616.

60. Handa VL, Maddox MD. Diagnosis of ureteral obstruction during complex urogynecologic surgery. Int Urogynecol J 2001,12.345–348.

61. Buller JL, Thompson JR, Cundiff GW, et al. Uterosacral ligament: description of anatomic relationships to optimize surgical safety. Obstet Gynecol 2001;97:873–879.

62. Hurd WW, Chee SS, Gallagher KL, et al. Location of the ureters in relation to the uterine cervix by computed tomography. Am J Obstet Gynecol 2001;184:336–339.

63. American College of Obstetricians and Gynecologists. Lower urinary tract injuries. Educational Bulletin #238. Washington DC: American College of Obstetricians and Gynecologists; 1997.

64. Symmonds RE. Ureteral injuries associated with gynecologic surgery: prevention and management. Clin Obstet Gynecol 1976;19:623–643.

65. Mathews R, Marshall FF. Management of extensive ureteral defects. American Urological Association Update Series 23(XX), 2001.

66. Visco AG, Taber KH, Weidner AC, et al. Cost-effectiveness of universal cystoscopy to identify ureteral injury at hysterectomy. Obstet Gynecol 2001;97:685–692.

67. Jabs CFI, Drutz P. The role of intraoperative cystoscopy in prolapse and incontinence surgery. Am J Obstet Gynecol 2001;185:1368–1373.

SECTION 9 Intraoperative injury

68. Klutke JJ, Klutke CG, Hsieh G. Bladder injury during the Burch retropubic urethropexy: is routine cystoscopy necessary? Tech Urol 1998;4:145–147.

69. Warwick RT, Worth PH. The psoas bladder-hitch procedure for the replacement of the lower third of the ureter. Br J Urol 1969;41(6):701–709.

70. Hinman F Jr. Atlas of urologic surgery. Philadelphia: WB Saunders; 1998: 818–825.

71. Martius H. Diegynakologichen Operationen. Stuttgart: Thieme; 1954.

72. Peyrat L, Boutin JM, Bruyere F, et al. Intestinal perforation as a complication of tension-free vaginal tape procedure for urinary incontinence. Eur Urol 2001;39:603–605.

73. Meschia M, Busacca P, Pifarotti P, et al. Bowel perforation during insertion of tension-free vaginal tape. Int Urogynecol J 2002;13:263–265.

74. Fourie T, Cohen PL. Delayed bowel erosion by tension-free vaginal tape (TVT). Int Urogynecol J 2003;14:352–354.

75. Castillo OA, Bodden E, Olivares RA, et al. Intestinal perforation: an infrequent complication during insertion of tension-free vaginal tape. J Urol 2004;172:1364.

76. Leboeuf L, Mendez LE, Gousse AE. Small bowel obstruction associated with tension-free vaginal tape. Urology 2004;63:1182e11–1182e13.

77. Mathevert P, Valencia P, Cousin C, et al. Operative injuries during vaginal hysterectomy. Eur J Obstet Gynecol Reprod Biol 2001;97:71–75.

SECTION 9 Intraoperative injury

SECTION 10

Congenital abnormalities of the female genital tract

Aspects of the Management of Congenital Abnormalities of the Female Genital Tract

Christopher R Chapple and Richard Turner-Warwick

INTRODUCTION

In this chapter we will discuss vaginal and urethral anomalies and the management of the vesicorectal fistula. Abnormalities of the uterus are a very specialized group of conditions which fall outside the remit of urologic practice.

EMBRYOLOGY

During the fifth week, primordial germ cells migrate from the yolk sac along the dorsal mesentery to populate the mesenchyme of the posterior body wall near the 10th thoracic level. In both sexes, the arrival of primordial germ cells in the area of future gonads serves as the signal for the existing cells of the mesonephros and the adjacent celomic epithelium to proliferate and form a pair of *genital ridges* just medial to the developing mesonephros. During the sixth week, the cells of the genital ridge invade the mesenchyme in the region of future gonads to form aggregates of supporting cells called *primitive sex cords*. The primitive sex cords subsequently invest the germ cells and support their development. The genital ridge mesenchyme containing the primitive sex cords is divided into cortical and medullary regions. Both regions develop in all embryos but after the sixth week they pursue different fates in male and female embryos.

During this time, a new pair of ducts, called the *paramesonephric (müllerian) ducts*, begins to form just lateral to the mesonephric ducts in both male and female embryos. These ducts arise by craniocaudal invagination of thickened celomic epithelium, extending all the way from the third thoracic segment to the posterior wall of the developing urogenital sinus. The caudal tips of the paramesonephric ducts are adherent to each other as they connect with the urogenital sinus between the openings of the right and left mesonephric ducts. The cranial ends of the paramesonephric ducts form funnel-shaped openings into the celomic cavity (the future peritoneum).

In female embryos, the mesonephric (wolffian) ducts degenerate and the paramesonephric (müllerian) ducts give rise to the fallopian tubes, the uterus, and the upper two-thirds of the vagina. The remnants of mesonephric ducts are found in the mesentery of the ovary as the epoöphoron and paroöphoron, and near the vaginal introitus and anterolateral vaginal wall as Gartner's duct cysts. The distal tips of the paramesonephric ducts adhere to each other just before they contact the posterior wall of the urogenital sinus. The wall of the urogenital sinus at this point forms a small thickening called the *sinusal tubercle*. As soon as the fused tips of the paramesonephric ducts connect with the sinusal tubercle, the ducts begin to fuse in a caudal-to-cranial direction, forming a tube with a single lumen. This tube, called the *uterovaginal canal*, becomes the superior portion of the vagina and the uterus. The unfused, superior portions of the paramesonephric ducts become the fallopian tubes (oviducts), and the funnel-shaped superior openings of the paramesonephric ducts become the infundibula.

While the uterovaginal canal is forming during the third month, the endodermal tissue of the sinusal tubercle in the posterior urogenital sinus continues to thicken, forming a pair of swellings called the *sinovaginal bulbs*. These structures give rise to the lower third of the vagina. The most inferior portion of the uterovaginal canal becomes occluded transiently by a block of tissue called the *vaginal plate*. The origin of the vaginal plate is not clear; it may arise from the sinovaginal bulbs, from the walls of the paramesonephric ducts, from the nearby mesonephric ducts or from a combination of these tissues. The vaginal plate elongates between the third and fifth months and subsequently becomes canalized to form the inferior vaginal lumen.

As the vaginal plate forms, the lower end of the vagina lengthens and its junction with the urogenital sinus migrates caudally until it comes to rest on the posterior wall of the definitive urogenital sinus (future vestibule of the vagina) during the fourth month. An endodermal membrane temporarily separates the vaginal lumen from the cavity of the definitive urogenital sinus. This barrier degenerates partially after the fifth month but its remnant persists as the vaginal *hymen*. The mucous membrane that lines the vagina and cervix may also derive from the endodermal epithelium of the definitive urogenital sinus.

The early development of the external genitalia is similar in both sexes. Early in the fifth week, a pair of swellings called *cloacal folds* develops on either side of the cloacal membrane. These folds meet just anterior to the cloacal membrane to form a midline swelling called the *genital tubercle*. During the cloacal division into the anterior urogenital sinus and the posterior anorectal canal, the portion of the cloacal folds flanking the opening of the urogenital sinus becomes the *urogenital folds* and the portion flanking the opening of the anorectal canal becomes the *anal folds*. A new pair of swellings, called the *labioscrotal folds*, then appears on either side of the urogenital folds.

The most popular hypothesis of external genital development is based on work performed in the early part of the 20th century. Inherent to this type of analysis is that many of the conclusions are speculative and unproven in terms of mechanistic validity. The cavity of the urogenital sinus extends onto the surface of the enlarging genital tubercle in the form of an endoderm-lined *urethral groove* during the sixth week. This groove becomes temporarily filled by a solid endodermal structure called the *urethral plate* which disintegrates and recanalizes to form an even deeper secondary groove. In males, this groove is relatively long and broad, whereas in females it is shorter and more sharply tapered. In both sexes, an ectodermal *epithelial tag* is at that time present at the tip of the genital tubercle. The genital tubercle elongates to form the phallus and a primordium of the glans clitoris and glans penis is demarcated from the phallic shaft by a coronary sulcus. The appearance of the external genitalia is similar in male and female embryos up until the 12th week.

VAGINAL ANOMALIES

Varying degrees of maldevelopment of the lower müllerian duct system and others cause a variety of vaginal and paravaginal problems. Naturally, when the uterus is present and there is vaginal occlusion, a hydrocolpos develops in infancy and, if this is not identified, it becomes a hematocolpos at puberty. The cecolovaginoplasty procedure was in fact originally developed for resolution of this particular situation because it obviated not only the undesirable need for regular dilation during adolescence that "split-skin" substitution required, but also the tell-tale donor-site scar that naturally prompted embarrassing questions when wearing a bathing costume.

Maldevelopment of the lower vaginal segment.
Maldevelopment of the lower vaginal segment results in defects that range from an imperforate or abnor-

mally thick hymen to a lower segment agenesis. The upper vagina may or may not be normal. The importance of preserving the hymen is now always taken into account when surgeons are preoccupied with complex paravaginal reconstructions or even minor procedures. Thus, when a young patient has an intact hymen and a vaginal access procedure is required, careful consideration should be given to its preservation. When the periintroital skin is supple, an acceptable reconstructive hymenoplasty may not be a particularly difficult procedure but when there is local scarring, it can become intricate. Fortunately there is usually adequate reasonably thick labial skin that can be redeployed but to achieve a cosmetically acceptable outcome, a two-stage procedure is sometimes required.

Disturbance of an intact hymen can be simply avoided by a bimanual rectal examination of the pelvis. Simple endoscopic vaginoscopy with an irrigating cystourethroscope may provide a better view of the cervix and vaginal epithelium than a speculum. As a result of ultrasound examination, hydrocolpos is more commonly identified in infants than it used to be; previously hematocolpos was only diagnosed at puberty. When this is due to a simple imperforate hymen, since the diaphanous posterior crescenteric sector is the most difficult part of the hymenal narrowing to reconstruct; the situation can be relieved by a limited incision in the anterior 12 o'clock sector that preserves the posterior hymenal fourchette (Fig. 24.1). Similarly, a simple upwards extension of an anterior-sector hymenotomy, into an anterior vaginotomy, provides good access for an intravaginal procedure under direct vision. At the conclusion of the procedure simple anterior suturing closes the vaginotomy and reconstitutes the hymen. The anterior periintroital prevaginal approach to the urethra (Fig. 24.2) leaves both the vagina and the hymen intact. A periintroital prevaginal approach can also be used in association with a high anterior vaginotomy incision to achieve wide access to the vaginal vault without a lower hymenointroital incision.

Labial flap inlay for lower segment vaginal agenesis (Fig. 24.3). A distal agenesis of the vaginal wall segment is often quite short; the upper vaginal segment is commonly quite normal. When the labia minora are of sufficient size they can be mobilized (Fig. 24.3A), flattened by separating their folded layers (Fig. 24.3B), and inlaid to reepithelialize the circumferential defect resulting from excision of the atretic segment (Fig. 24.3C).

Vaginal "pull-down" and "ring" substitution. Alternatively the upper vaginal segment can be mobilized and gently pulled down to a neo-introitus created by simple infolding of the perineal or labial skin. This is often feasible but occasionally, although the caliber of the upper vagina

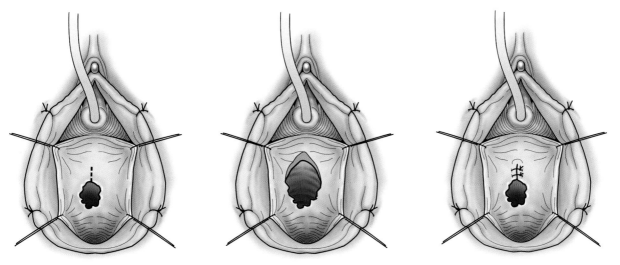

Figure 24.1 Limited incision in the anterior 12 o'clock sector that preserves the posterior hymenal fourchette.

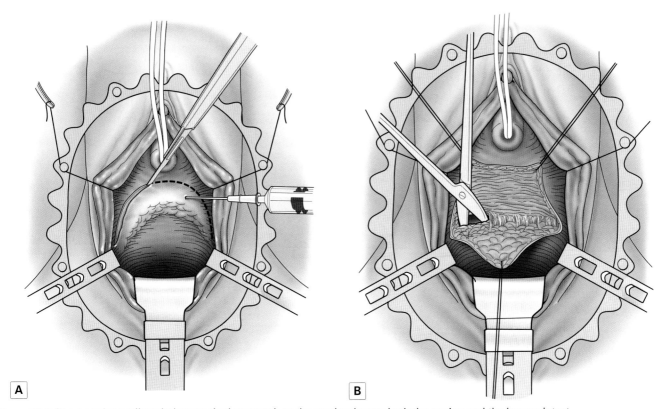

A

B

Figure 24.2 The anterior periintroital prevaginal approach to the urethra leaves both the vagina and the hymen intact

may be normal, its walls may be abnormally thin. When this occurs the urethra may also be underdeveloped with a thin sphincteric mechanism that is easily damaged during the mobilization. This can result in a previously continent patient becoming incontinent.

A partial vaginal "ring" substitution of the lower vagina is occasionally necessary, using either a skin flap from the thigh or a short bowel segment, according to the findings.

A vaginal substitution construction or reconstruction is commonly indicated for congenital vaginal atresia and intersex malformations.

Vaginal substitution: skin and amnion. The normal adult vagina is a cavity some 10–12 cm deep and about three fingerbreadths wide. Its walls are considerably elastic and it is lined with stratified epithelium which, like buccal mucosa

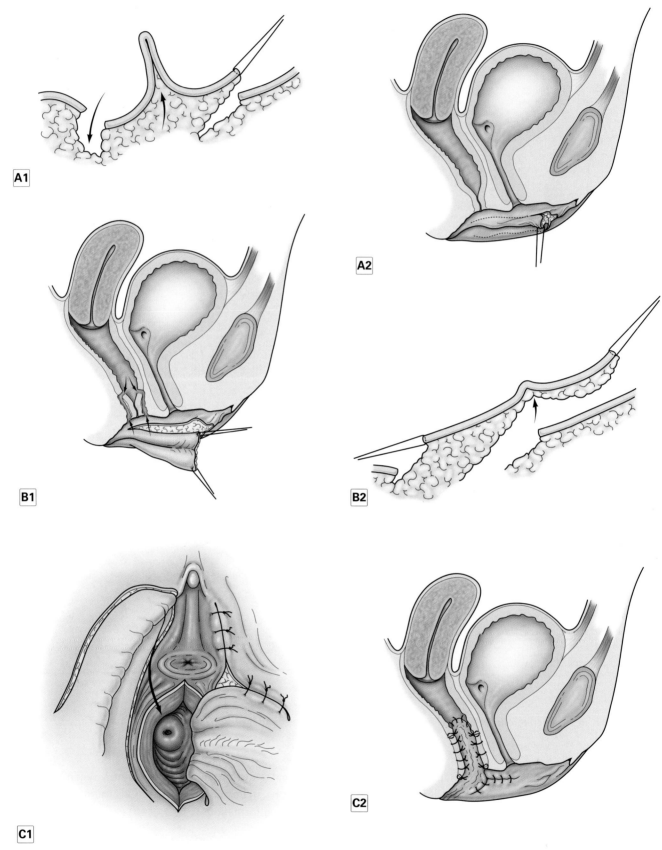

Figure 24.3 When the labia minora are of sufficient size they can be mobilized (**A**), flattened by separating their folded layers (**B**), and inlaid to reepithelialize the circumferential defect resulting from excision of the atretic segment (**C**).

from the mouth, is specially adapted to a "wet" environment. A variety of options have been developed for substitution vaginoplasty; the usual alternatives for its substitution lining are either skin or bowel mucosa.

The earliest vaginal substitution procedures involved the inlay of split-skin grafts mounted on a mold. The success of these depended upon the frequent passage of dilators postoperatively to prevent the natural tendency of such grafts to contract, which is naturally an undesirable focus of attention during early adolescence. Furthermore, the disfiguring donor site of the graft can be a great embarrassment for a girl when she is wearing a bathing costume because

it naturally invites enquiry relating to the reason for the operation.

Amnion was used for a while and this solved the "donor site" problem but not the tendency to contraction. It was also abandoned because of the potential pathogenic implications of utilizing amnion.

A satisfactory and robust neovagina can be constructed from a part of pedicled island skin flaps of suitable dimensions, raised and mobilized from the inner aspect of each thigh and sutured together to create a neovaginal lumen of appropriate caliber (Fig. 24.4). The longitudinal axis of the donor sites of the island skin flaps can be either longitudinal

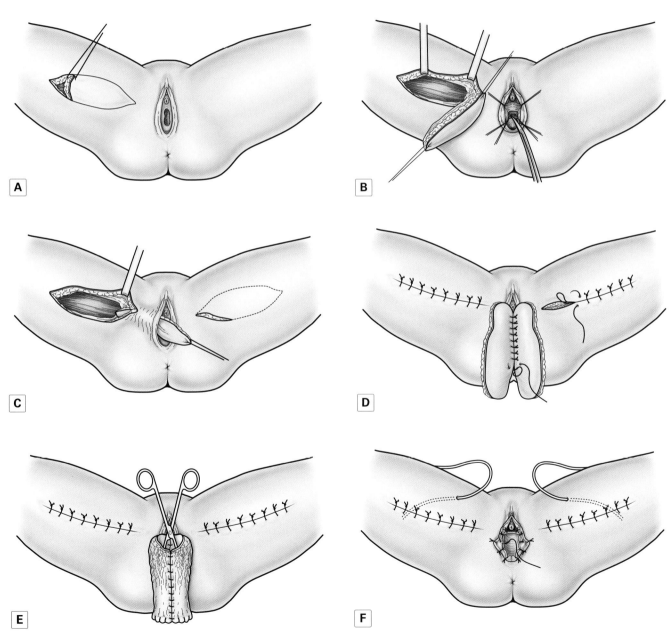

Figure 24.4 A satisfactory and robust neovagina can be constructed from pedicled island skin flaps of suitable dimensions, raised and mobilized from the inner aspect of each thigh and sutured together to create a neovaginal lumen of appropriate caliber.

along the thigh or circumferential, parallel with the skin crease at the junction of the thigh and the pudenda. The longitudinal thigh flaps can be myocutaneous, based on the gracilis muscle, or fasciocutaneous, based on the pedicle vessels coming through it. The inclusion of the gracilis muscle under the island flaps is not necessary to ensure their viability provided these are appropriately raised on the performing vessels; indeed, this tends to make them unnecessarily bulky when they are conjoined at their distal extremity, at the apex of the neovagina. However, foreshortening of the length of the mobilized gracilis, and using it to support just the base of the island flap but not its whole extent, can facilitate and protect the mobilization of the pedicle vessels. Circumferential island skin flaps are then simply fasciocutaneous.

If the thigh skin is tight circumferentially then approximation of the skin margins of a longitudinal island donor site may be somewhat difficult. Skin deficiency can be closed by a skin graft but alternatively, the skin lateral to the donor site can be prestretched by the preliminary insertion of a tissue-expanding balloon. A natural disadvantage of the pedicled island skin vaginoplasty procedures is that the longitudinal donor-site scars on the inner aspect of the thigh are very obvious when wearing a bathing costume. The scar of a circumferential donor site is considerably less obvious.

Bowel segment vaginal substitution: principles and expectations.

There are distinct advantages in using a bowel segment substitution for a neovagina: the natural habitat of its mucosa is wet, its vascularization can be reliable, it is available to reconstruct a capacious vagina, and the reconstruction can be achieved through a cosmetic suprapubic V incision which can be concealed by a modest bikini. The sexual function of a bowel vaginoplasty is remarkably satisfactory. All bowel segments produce some mucus and, when transposed, they continue to do so indefinitely. Naturally, therefore, patients who have a bowel segment vaginoplasty have some discharge but this is clean, clear mucus that is easily controlled by simple vaginal douching which is particularly important when a relatively long bowel segment is used. It is, however, essential that patients are warned of this as a possibility preoperatively with appropriate counseling.

The sigmoid colon was used for the earliest bowel segment vaginoplasty procedures but compared with the right colon, it has disadvantages.

- The musculodynamic activity of the left colon is considerably greater than that of the cecocolon on the right and this tends to result in a lumen that is considerably narrower than that of a normal vagina.
- When a left colonic segment is used for a vaginoplasty it may be advisable to "detubularize" it by a folded

reduplication procedure in order to avoid the regular ongoing neovaginal self-dilation that is necessary to maintain an appropriate caliber unless this is achieved by regular sexual activity.
- The left colon is prone to intrinsic abnormalities, such as diverticulitis, that may preclude its use.
- The restoration of colonic continuity requires careful preoperative bowel preparation and, compared with ileocolic anastomosis, colocolic anastomosis is relatively unreliable and prone to complications.
- Although the pedicle vessels of the sigmoid colon are almost always sufficiently mobilizable to enable one end of the segment to reach the perineal skin, their configuration may prevent both ends of a detubularized segment reaching it with sufficient vascular perfusion to prevent ischemic stenosis of the neo-introital anastomosis.

There are many positive advantages in using the right colon segment of the large bowel for vaginoplasty in preference to the sigmoid colon on the left.

- The relatively large diameter of the cecum approximates to that of the normal vagina and its use for vaginoplasty is rarely compromised by intrinsic inflammatory pathology such as diverticulitis.
- The musculodynamic activity of the cecum is relatively low compared with that of the sigmoid colon, with a minimal intrinsic tendency to become narrow and develop a contracture. Thus neither detubularization nor regular postoperative self-dilation routine is usually required to prevent a cecolovaginoplasty narrowing.
- Because the pattern of the main blood vessels of the cecum and of the right colon is remarkably constant and reliable, their surgical mobilization and transposition is simple and relatively easy.

Thus a particular advantage of a large-caliber cecal bowel segment substitution lying within a large-caliber neovaginal tunnel is that it is generally "stable" and rarely requires routine postoperative dilation. When a cecolovaginoplasty (Fig. 24.5) is used in childhood to resolve a hydrocolpos or hematocolpos, there is a fair expectation that the neovagina will have an acceptable caliber a few years later when the patient becomes adult, without an interim dilation routine.

It is easy to underestimate the length of the ascending colon that is required to enable its upper end to reach the perineum easily, without tension, when the cecolic segment is inverted. The transection of the ascending colon and its ascending vessels (Fig. 24.5A,B) should be high enough to ensure that a small, well-vascularized excess of this hangs out of the perineum (Fig. 24.5C) so that it can be trimmed

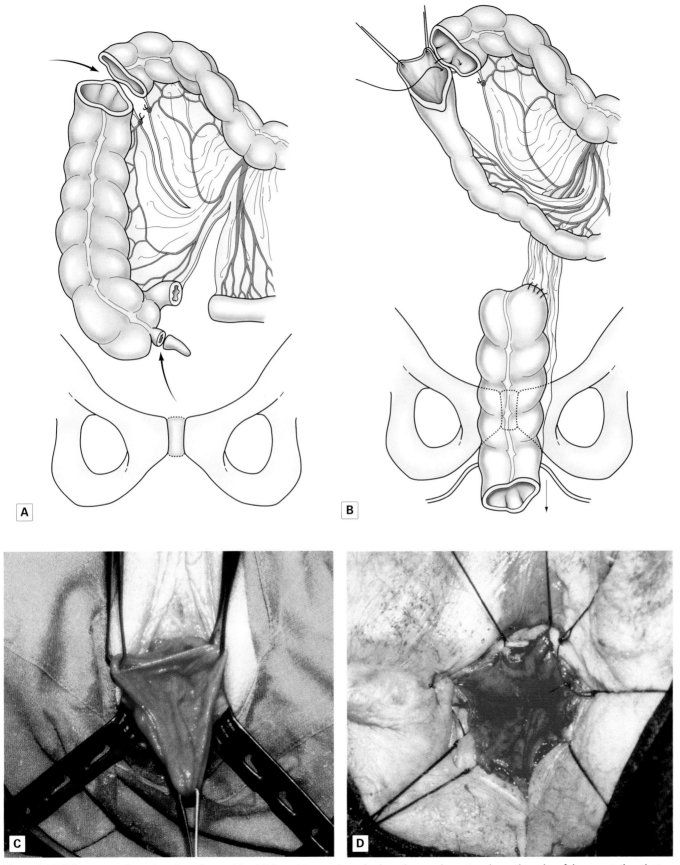

Figure 24.5 When a cecolovaginoplasty is used in childhood to resolve a hydrocolpos or hematocolpos, there is a fair expectation that the neovagina will have an acceptable caliber a few years later when the patient becomes adult, without an interim dilation routine.

Continued

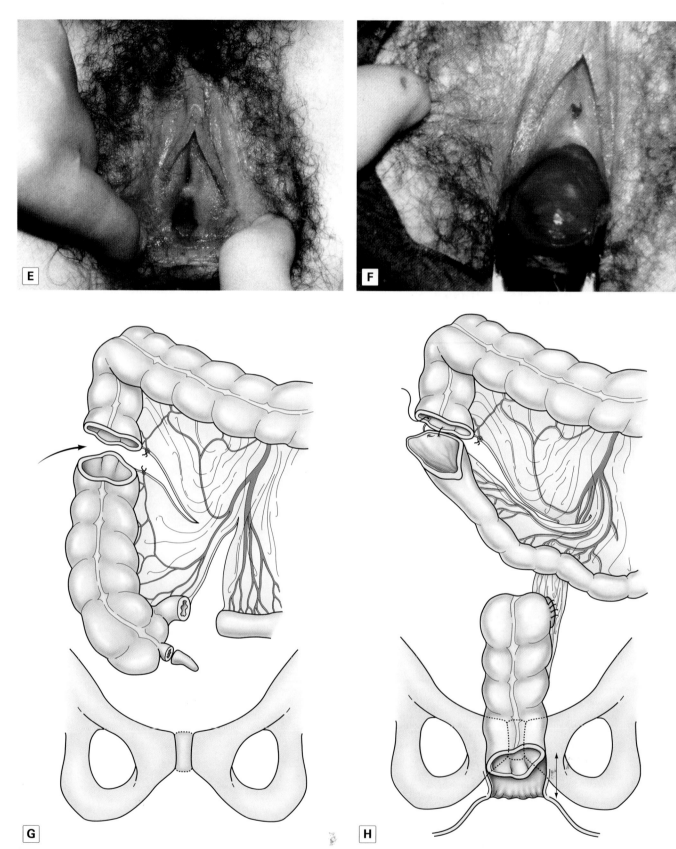

Figure 24.5, cont'd

back to create the neo-introitus (Fig. 24.5D-F). If a segment of insufficient length is taken (Fig. 24.5D), tension and hypovascularization risk the ischemic loss of its subterminal section (Fig. 24.5D) and the development of introital stenosis.

The complications of cecolovaginoplasty tend to be few. As with any bowel segment substitution that reaches the skin surface without tension, it is occasionally necessary to resect a subsequent prolapse of a redundant length by a simple circumcisional procedure with introital reanastomosis.

The rectal segment vaginoplasty has been described with restoration of colonic continuity by anastomosing the sigmoid colon to the lower rectum (Fig. 24.6). The particular advantages of this procedure are that the rectum is relatively capacious so that detubularization is not necessary, and the rectal segment and its inferior hemorrhoidal vascular pedicle require minimal mobilization to achieve the translocation. However, the restorative coloanal anastomosis is relatively difficult compared to ileocolic anastomosis, and particular care is required to avoid suture-line leakage.

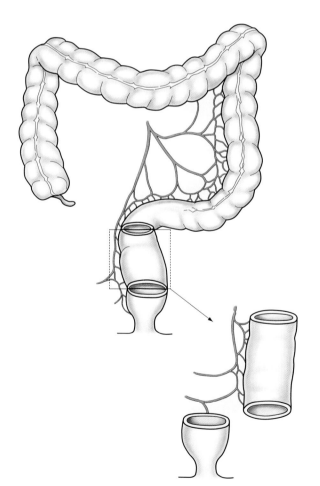

Figure 24.6 The rectal segment vaginoplasty has been described with restoration of colonic continuity by anastomosing the sigmoid colon to the lower rectum.

DEVELOPMENT AND PREVENTION OF NEOVAGINAL INTROITAL NARROWING. Two distinct forms of narrowing can develop at the introitus after a bowel substitution vaginoplasty.

Type 1: junction-ring stenosis (Fig. 24.7A-C). Simple type 1 anastomotic stenosis arises from short mucocutaneous junctional narrowings (Fig. 24.7A). These are generally preventable by avoiding a circumferential ring-form of the anastomosis of the neovaginal bowel to the neo-introitus by a simple V-shaped skin inlay. Because a type 1 stenosis is short, it is usually easy to resolve, either by a series of simple recalibrating dilations (Fig. 24.7B) or by a minimal skin inlay introitoplasty revision (Fig. 24.7C).

Type 2: lining-defect stenoses (Fig. 24.7D-H). A type 2 stenosis is longer and relatively severe (Fig. 24.7D). This type of supraintroital narrowing is generally the result of a continuity defect gap between the distal extremity of the viable length of the neovaginal bowel segment and the neo-introital skin. It is usually due to the ischemic loss of the distal centimeters of the neovaginal bowel segment owing to a terminal vascular deficiency, but it can also result from tension and separation of the introital suture line. The usual situation is that a few centimeters of the lower wall of the neovaginal tunnel has neither a bowel lining nor a skin lining; the natural healing process of this "bare area" results in rapid occlusion of its lumen and the development of a dense fibrotic stenosis, the length of which is that of the distal continuity defect (Fig. 24.7E).

Neither the development nor the process of this type of healing occlusion can be prevented by the repeated passage of recalibrating dilators postoperatively. A type 2 stenosis is preventable by ensuring adequate vascularization of the distal margin of an adequate length of the neovaginal bowel segment. The resolution of a type 2 introital stenosis generally requires remobilization of the distal end of the viable bowel segment (Fig. 24.7F), its "pull-down" (Fig. 24.7G) and its reanastomosis to the neo-introital skin (Fig. 24.7H). The normal elasticity of the bowel wall usually makes this a relatively simple perineal-approach procedure.

A formal vaginal pack is not required to maintain the caliber of a bowel segment neovagina. Indeed, this can be counterproductive if the vascular perfusion of the subterminal bowel wall is marginally precarious because a pack can compress it against the wall of the neovaginal tunnel and this can actually contribute to the failure of the blood supply which is the basic cause of a type 2 supraintroital stenosis. However, a very light pack, for a day or two, may prevent the early accumulation of a venous ooze outside the cecovaginoplasty from the wall of a capacious neovaginal tunnel.

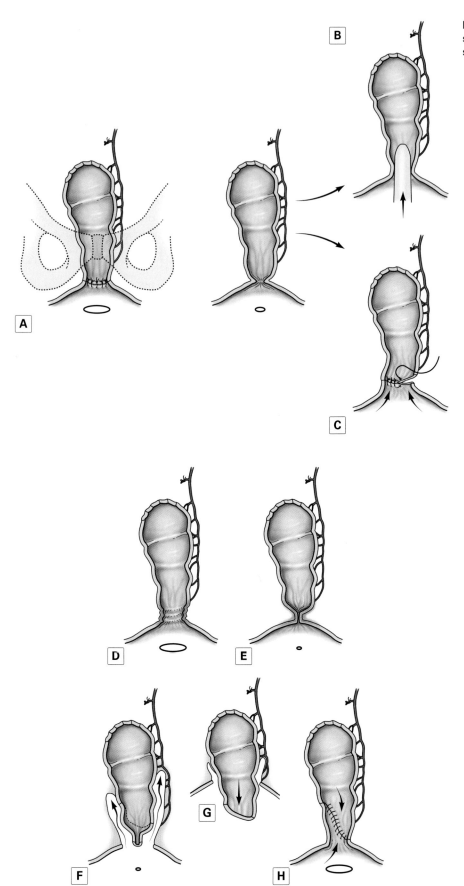

Figure 24.7 **(A-C)** Type 1: junction-ring stenosis. **(D-H)** Type 2: lining-defect stenoses.

Developmental rectovaginal fistulae and anorectal atresia

(Fig. 24.8). Development anorectal atresia results in a deficiency of the anal sphincter mechanism and rectovaginal fistula (Fig. 24.8A). The separation of the fistula (Fig. 24.8B) and the simple rectal pull-through in infancy that used to be the routine procedure for developmental rectovaginal fistula naturally resulted in a simple anterior perineal colostomy (Fig. 24.8C,D); the patient has no sensation of the passage of a motion until this reaches the perineal skin and in this position there is no adjacent functional anal pelvic floor musculature that could possibly control its discharge. Such a perineal colostomy is inevitably incontinent but, understandably, some young women prefer to persist in the endeavor to control and manage a colostomy in this position rather than have it relocated on the abdominal surface.

Pelvic floor stimulation studies often show some contractile activity in the posterolateral margin of the under-

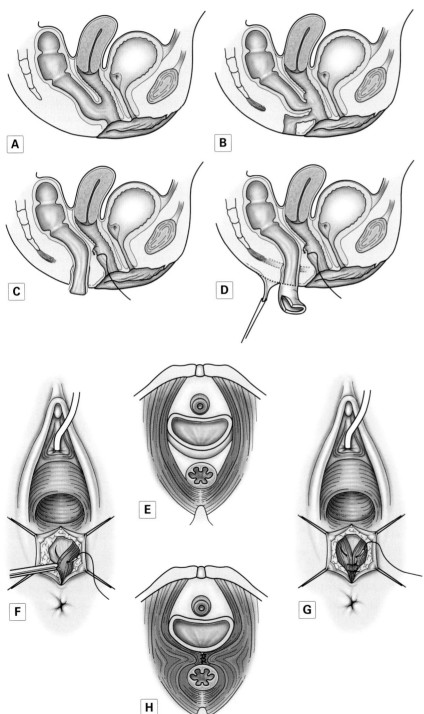

Figure 24.8 Developmental rectovaginal fistulae: anorectal atresia.

SECTION 10 Congenital abnormalities of the female genital tract

Continued

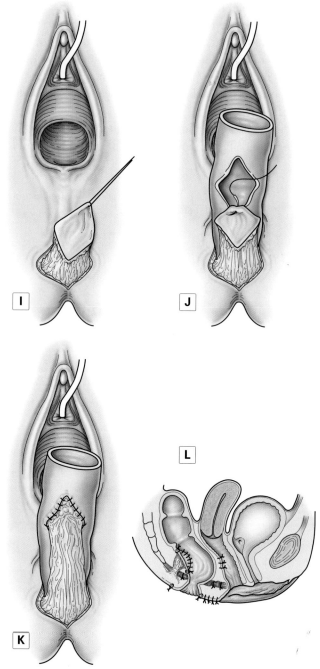

Figure 24.8, cont'd

The mainstay of the practical management of an incontinent colostomy, perineal or abdominal, is the ACE (antegrade colonic evacuation) continent cecostomy procedure which enables a daily "wash-out" of the whole colon to be achieved by a simple antegrade irrigation using a catheterizable leak-proof stoma.

DEVELOPMENTAL ABNORMALITIES OF THE FEMALE URETHRA

Developmental abnormalities of the female urethra naturally compromise its intrinsic sphincteric function to a varying extent and it is this that determines whether the patient is continent or incontinent. The great majority of these abnormalities present in childhood and their treatment is addressed in pediatric urologic texts: however, some may not present until the patient becomes adult and these need appropriate consideration.

Paraurethral "cysts". The surgical excision of paraurethral "cysts" can prove to be a trap for the unwary. Although some sequenced elements of developmental duct systems are indeed localized cysts, others are extensive. Local excision of the lower end of an obstructed duplication of the upper urinary tract is likely to result in a fistulous ureteric drainage. When there is any doubt about the situation, the extent of a paraurethral cystic lesion should be assessed radiographically either by contrast imaging or by MR scanning.

Subsphincteric ectopic ureteric discharge. The great majority of females with incontinence due to a subsphincteric ectopic ureteric orifice present in childhood and are appropriately treated then. It is, however, important to remember that a duplex system can escape identification until the minor leakage becomes troublesome in adolescence. If the possibility of this is overlooked and imaging of the upper tracts is not critically assessed, they are easily missed. However, once identified, they are one of the easiest and most satisfactory causes of incontinence to resolve.

The "short" urethra. A relatively "short" urethra is not an unusual development anomaly but many of these have an adequate functional sphincteric length, at least until this is compromised by the natural hazards of childbirth when the extent of the underlying anatomic anomaly is identified as a result of the leakage.

Atretic vaginourethral fistulae (Fig. 24.9). When the lower segment of the vagina is atretic, the vagina proximal to this may have a developmental fistulous communication with the urethra (Fig. 24.9A). An advantageous clinical side effect of this is that the patient does not develop hemato-

developed puborectal sling element of the levator muscle (Fig. 24.8E). In such cases a marginal degree of muscular control of a perineal colostomy may be potentially achievable by transposing it backwards (Fig. 24.8F), tight onto the sling, and bringing the inner margins of this together in the midline in front of it (Fig. 24.8G,H). The introduction of an innervated pedicled patch of perineal skin into the subterminal segment of a relocated sensory perineal colostomy (Fig. 24.8I-K) has been tried in an endeavor to provide a sensory forewarning of the need for a voluntary pelvic floor contraction (Fig. 24.8L) but this had only limited success.

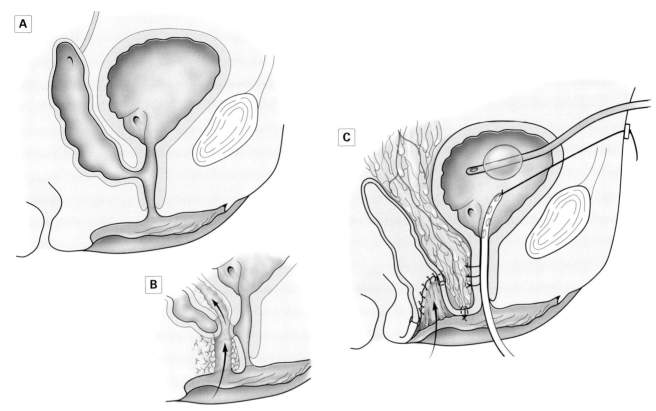

Figure 24.9 Atretic vaginourethral fistulae.

colpos because she menstruates into the urethra. The separation of the vaginourethral communication (Fig. 24.9B) requires great care because both the vaginal wall and the posterior midurethral wall are hypoplastic and thin. In such cases there is usually a sufficiency of proximal vaginal wall to achieve a simple perineal "pull-down" vaginointroitoplasty (Fig. 24.9C) but the urethral closure may be a more delicate procedure. A supporting Martius interposition flap is generally advisable.

When such a developmental fistula is associated with the adrenogenital syndrome, the bladder neck sphincter mechanism is often prominent and somewhat "male" in type. The augmented occlusive function of this may reduce the potential incidence of postoperative incontinence after closure of the fistula.

Intrinsic sphincteric hypoplasia. It is unusual for a patient with an intrinsic sphincteric hypoplasia but with an otherwise intact urethra to present as an adult but it is important to be aware of the possibility of this because it can become unexpectedly troublesome. For instance, an adult patient with the combination of vaginal atresia and a hypoplastic intrinsic sphincter may have been urologically asymptomatic and normally continent on the basis of a precarious balance between a relatively underactive bladder and a competent bladder neck mechanism but she may become unexpectedly and disastrously incontinent after a

vaginal reconstruction as a result of simple separation of a lower segment vaginal atresia from the atretic urethra. A synchronous prophylactic sphincteroplasty may be required.

Urethral fusion defects. The commonest developmental anomalies of the urethra are simple fusion defects which may be either anterior or posterior. In addition to the actual fusion defect, the proximal part of the sphincter mechanism is commonly underdeveloped and this can compromise the result of a functional reconstruction.

Posterior fusion defects: hypospadias, urethro-vaginal, and vesicourethro-vaginal "cloacal" fistulae. Posterior fusion defects range from a minimal hypospadiac urethral meatus upwards to involve the whole length of the urethra or through the bladder neck to form an extensive vesicourethro-vaginal "cloacal" defect, providing a direct view into the bladder, with total incontinence which naturally presents for treatment during childhood. When the fusion defect does not include the bladder neck this may be marginally competent so that, as in the mild degrees of epispadias, the situation may escape identification until adulthood.

The sphincteric deficiency associated with a urethro-vaginal "cloacal" fistula that extends up to the bladder neck is not confined to its posterior aspect; a variable length of the open anterior sphincteric wall is atretic. Thus, although a posterior reconstructive sphincteroplasty for the resolution of this situation naturally involves the whole length of the urethra, the functional efficiency of the result is usually largely confined to the bladder neck area so that an abdominoperineal reconstruction is generally advisable in the endeavor to augment the competence of this by tubularization of the lower trigonal area with omental support.

SHORTCOMINGS OF THE CLOSURE OF URETHROVAGINAL FISTULAE BY SUBSTITUTION URETHROPLASTY. The closure of a fistulous urethrovaginal defect with an inert substitution patch of pedicled vaginal wall or labial skin is functionally misconceived. An inert patch does nothing to augment the circumferential sphincteric closure pressure in its area; indeed, it may actually diminish it. The fundamental principle of functional reconstructions of urethral defects should be to retrieve and to circumferentially redeploy every residual remnant of potentially functional sphincteric muscle in a functional manner, rather than simply "elongate" it with a functionless patch.

A reconstructive sphincteroplasty for a posterior urethrovaginal developmental defect is difficult and often produces a less than adequate result because its muscular component is relatively thin and atretic (this is discussed further in Chapter 22).

Urethral diverticula. Developmental urethral diverticula are outpouchings of the urethral lining through its wall; they are commonly single, the neck of the diverticulum is variable in size, and it is usually located posteriorly in the middle third of the urethra. When their communication with the urethra is relatively large, they empty freely so they are usually impalpable on clinical examination. Occasionally they contain calculi or a tumor and when they drain poorly, they may be mistaken, on clinical examination, for a simple paravaginal cyst. These are discussed further in Chapter 22.

Anterior fusion defects: epispadias and ectopia vesicae. Overt anterior fusion defects of the urethra and bladder, ectopia vesicae, are naturally resolved in infancy. However, minimal defects—the formes frustes of it—are only apparent on close inspection of the genitalia so it is not unusual for them to escape notice until adult life.

The urethral meatus may appear quite normal when the defect is minimal but there is usually an occult defect of the intrinsic sphincter mechanism above this which can compromise its occlusive function and result in varying degrees of incontinence. On examination, the diagnostic feature of this situation is a bifid clitoris and, in the adult, a small central patch of hairless skin above it. Radiograghically the pubic bones may approximate with an underdevelopment of the symphysis.

The patient illustrated in Figure 24.10 was asymptomatic until she developed troublesome incontinence after her first child. Without recognition of the nature of the problem, her incontinence was initially treated by an anterior colporrhaphy and subsequently also by a Burch suspension without significant improvement. In fact, her anterior sphincteric fusion defect extended the whole length of the urethra and a full-length anterior sphincteroplasty was required involving a synchronous perineoretropubic approach, after which the patient was normally continent and had further children without any further incontinence problems. The characteristic hairless area of the forme fruste of the condition was obvious (Fig. 24.10A) and the pubic symphysis defect was minimal (Fig. 24.10B).

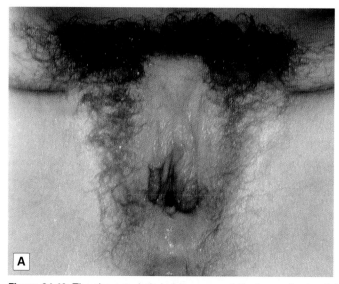
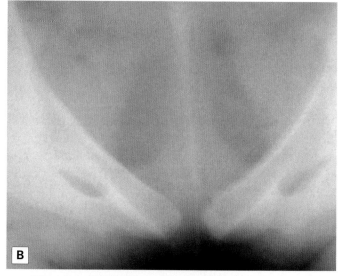

Figure 24.10 The characteristic hairless area of the forme fruste of the condition was obvious (**A**) and the pubic symphysis defect was minimal (**B**).

TECHNIQUE. With the patient in the supine perineo-abdominal position, the initial incision above the urethral meatus is V-shaped with its apex starting at the margin of the meatus and each limb extending up to the inner margin of each half of the bifid clitoris (indicated in Figure 24.11A by the tips of the pick-up blades). The hairless skin is excised in a diamond-shaped configuration.

The anterior aspect of the distal urethra is separated from its adhesion to the back of the attenuated pubis or, if this is deficient, from the fibrous interpubic band between its medial ends.

The retropubic area is exposed using a suprapubic incision via a cosmetic transverse incision to minimize the extent of the skin incision which should be within the pubic hair area; this provides a midline abdominal wall incision underneath it to ensure that this can be upwardly extended if necessary to achieve adequate mobilization of the omental apron to provide appropriate supple "urodynamic" support of the urethral reconstruction.

The bladder is opened by low midline incision so that the patulous bladder neck can be seen (Fig. 24.11B). A finger in the urethra may facilitate its separation from the back of the pubis with preservation of a maximum amount of peri-urethral tissue for the overclosure support of the reconstruction. After the full-length mobilization of the upper urethra from its anterior adhesion, the retropubic abdominoperineal tunnel allows the urethra to drop back to increase the surgical access to it.

The proximal and distal ends of the urethra are longitudinally retracted with stay sutures and the abnormally thin anterior urethral wall of the urethra is opened longitudinally in the midline. The width of the posterior uroepithelial strip is reduced to about 15 mm and it is then a relatively simple matter to overclose the remnants of the sphincter

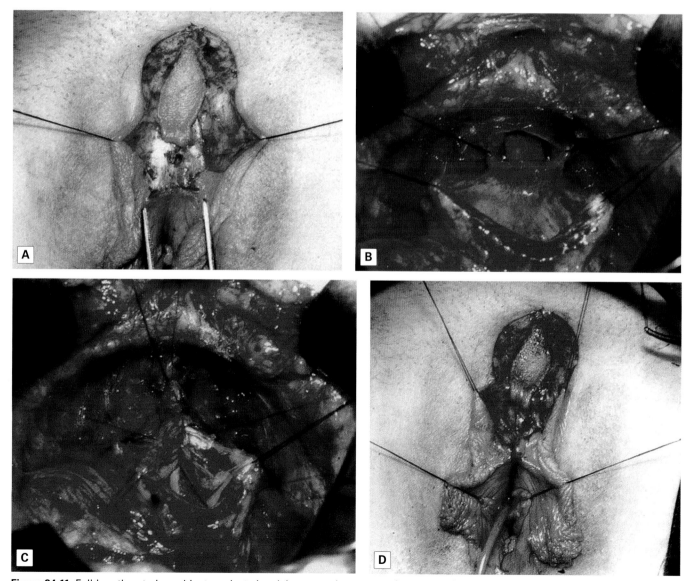

Figure 24.11 Full-length anterior sphincteroplasty involving a synchronous perineoretropubic approach.

Continued

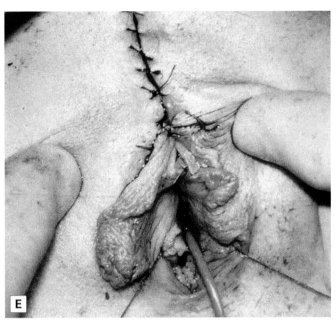

Figure 24.11, cont'd

mechanism in the posterior wall of the urethra around a 12 F stenting urethral catheter that is retained by a sling suture (Fig. 24.11C). A suprapubic catheter is inserted and the bladder and abdomen are closed after prepositioning the mobilized omentum in the retropubic space, the lower extremity of which is included in the sutures closing the anterior perineal incision which approximates the margins of the excised hairless skin area and the two halves of the clitoris (Fig. 24.11D,E).

Vaginorectal fistulae. Vaginorectal fistulae may result from developmental abnormalities and the closure of the rectal defect is generally the more difficult aspect of their resolution, usually requiring a proximal diversion and colorectal expertise. The principles of surgical management are as expounded elsewhere in this textbook (Fig. 24.12) with the creation of an abdominoperineal tunnel, the excision of damaged tissue, and the interposition of omentum. As detailed elsewhere in this chapter, a neovagina can be created as required.

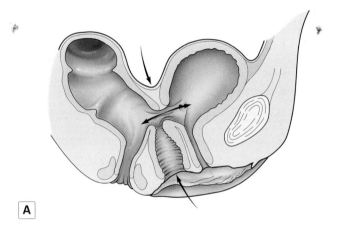

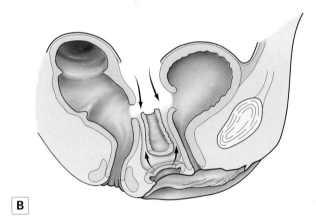

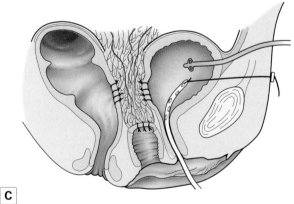

Figure 24.12 The creation of an abdominoperineal tunnel, the excision of damaged tissue, and the interposition of omentum. (Adapted from figures designed and drawn by Richard Turner-Warwick and Paul Richardson.)

SECTION 11

Irritative conditions of the genitourinary tract

Urinary Tract Infections

Naresh V Desireddi and Anthony J Schaeffer

INTRODUCTION

Urinary tract infections (UTIs) represent one of the most common infections in the United States and account for nearly 1.2% of all office visits by women.[1] UTIs are associated with significant morbidity and the financial impact of UTIs is greater than $1 billion in the United States.[2] Recent advances in the pathophysiology of UTIs, including host and bacterial factors, have aided in identifying patients with increased risk of recurrent infections and complications. A systematic approach to diagnosis and treatment results in successful eradication of infection in the majority of patients and identifies high-risk patients at risk for treatment failure. Such patients include elderly women, pregnant women, and patients with chronic indwelling catheters. Shorter treatment regimens and prophylactic therapy have reduced the morbidity of treating infections.

PATHOGENESIS

As with other infections, UTIs represent the interaction between an uropathogen and a host. An infection occurs when a pathogen overcomes a host's natural barriers. Recent advances in the elucidation of these interactions may aid in the management of complicated UTIs.

Uropathogens usually originate from the fecal reservoir and virulent organisms colonize the vagina, with subsequent migration to the urinary tract.[3] The adherence of bacteria to the mucosal surface of the urinary tract represents one of the early initiating events of a UTI. This interaction is mediated by bacterial adhesins located on the tip of filamentous appendages called pili.[4] The pili are subdivided into mannose-sensitive (type 1) and mannose-resistant (P) pili. They are defined by the ability to mediate the hemagglutination of erythrocytes, with type 1 aided by the addition of mannose. The adhesin Fim H on the tip of type 1 pili plays an important role in most uropathogenic *E. coli* adhering to the urothelium.[5] Type 1 pili adhere to bladder surface uroplakins, which are hexagonal arrays of integral membrane glycoproteins.[6] Mannose-resistant (P) pili are found in most pyelonephrogenic strains of *E. coli*.[7] Host cell factors including increased vaginal cell receptivity aid in uropathogen colonization. Initial studies revealed that uropathogenic strains of *E. coli* have increased adherence to vaginal epithelial cells.[8] Subsequent studies have showed an association between vaginal cell receptivity and buccal cell receptivity. These results suggest that a common genotypic trait for epithelial cell receptivity may be an important susceptible factor for UTIs.[9]

Many host defenses prevent UTIs in women, including the flow of urine through the urinary tract, low pH of the urine, neutrophil influx into the bladder, and secretory IgA. Recent work has shown that type 1-piliated uropathogens can invade superficial epithelial cells and set up large foci of intracellular bacteria called factories. Bacteria can form intracellular niches and create a persistent, quiescent reservoir. These reservoirs can persist for months undetected because bacteria are not sloughed into the urine.[10] These reservoirs may be the foci for cystitis or bacteriuria in patients with recurrent UTIs and may be resistant to the usual treatment regimens of acute cystitis.

Hultgren and associates[11] have recently discovered intracellular bacterial biofilm-like pods that protrude from the bacterial surface. These structures are encased in a polysaccharide matrix surrounded by a shell of uroplakin. While encased within these pods, bacteria interact with the host's surrounding matrix but lie hidden from the host's immune system. They are thus resistant to the host's natural defenses and antimicrobial therapy, while making an individual susceptible to recurrent UTIs.

CLINICAL TERMINOLOGY

A urinary tract infection is a clinical entity with various symptoms and characterized by an inflammatory response to the urothelium, often with pyuria and bacteriuria. Bacteriuria is the presence of bacteria in the urine (Fig. 25.1), in what is usually a sterile environment.

Infections of the genitourinary tract are characterized as uncomplicated or complicated. An uncomplicated UTI represents an infection in a healthy patient with an anatomically and functionally normal genitourinary system. A complicated UTI occurs in individuals with structural or functional abnormalities of the urinary tract and in the immunocompromised, which makes them susceptible to infection and poor treatment outcomes.

Urinary tract infections can be classified into four different subcategories:

- isolated infections
- unresolved infections
- recurrent infections secondary to a reinfection
- recurrent infection secondary to bacterial persistence.[12]

Isolated infections are characterized as a first UTI or separated from a previous infection by at least 6 months. An unresolved infection occurs when the initial therapy has been insufficient to eradicate the initial uropathogen. Some of the etiologies for unresolved bacteriuria include bacterial resistance to the initial antimicrobial, development of resistance, infection secondary to two different species, azotemia, and giant staghorn calculi. Recurrent infections are secondary to reinfection from outside the urinary tract or secondary to bacterial persistence within the urinary tract. The majority of recurrent infections in women are reinfections from outside the urinary tract. The recurrence of a UTI with the same organism points to a source within the urinary tract, referred to as bacterial persistence. Common sources of bacterial persistence include infectious stones, unilateral infected atrophic kidneys, ectopic ureters, urethral diverticulum, and foreign bodies.

The elucidation of the infectious cause often requires cystoscopic evaluation and localizing studies of the collecting system. Recurrent UTIs should be documented with cultures. The symptoms associated with recurrent UTIs may be similar to other disease entities like interstitial cystitis and carcinoma in situ. When cultures are negative, these entities should be ruled out during the work-up.

DIAGNOSIS

The urinalysis (U/A) and urine culture remain the key tests during the work-up of a UTI. For the majority of patients with uncomplicated cystitis, urine culture and susceptibilities are often not required. A traditional microscopic examination of a U/A on a wet mount or a urine dipstick for leukocyte esterase and nitrites with clinical symptoms is sufficient.[13] In most other circumstances, a urine culture should be sent.

The accuracy of the U/A and urine culture improves with the collection method. In order of decreasing accuracy, specimens can be obtained via suprapubic aspiration, catheterization, and voided specimens.[14] Catheterized and voided specimens should be obtained from the midstream as this reduces urethral contamination.

The microscopic urinalysis evaluates for bacteriuria, pyuria, and hematuria and the dipstick checks for leukocyte esterase and nitrites, indirect assays for inflammation and bacteria respectively. The presence of bacteriuria can be missed on a urinalysis when bacteria numbers are less than 30,000/ml because of the volume limitations of a slide. A UTI is usually associated with pyuria and the lack of pyuria should make the physician question the diagnosis until culture results are back. The urine dipstick for leukocyte esterase has sensitivities between 75% and 90% for detecting pyuria.[15] Many gram-negative bacteria reduce nitrates to nitrites in the urinary tract so urine nitrites can be used as a surrogate marker for bacteriuria. Urinary nitrites have a low sensitivity since some uropathogens do not reduce nitrates, including enterococci and *S. saphrophyticus*.

Classically, the diagnosis of a UTI required a quantitative urine culture greater than 100,000 colony-forming units (CFU) of bacteria per ml of urine. This convenient number has a few limitations. Twenty to 40% of women with symptomatic UTIs present with bacterial counts between 10^2 and 10^4 CFU/ml of urine. This is likely secondary to frequent urination prompted by irritation and the slow doubling time of some bacterial species. A lower threshold of 100 CFU/ml may be more appropriate for the diagnosis of cystitis in symptomatic women.[16]

Radiologic imaging is usually unnecessary in the majority of patients with a UTI but imaging does aid in the diagnosis and management of complicated UTIs. The presence of

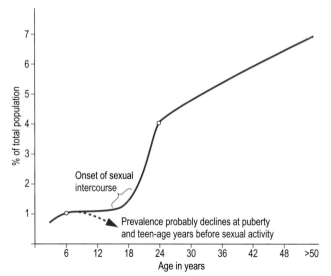

Figure 25.1 Prevalence of bacteriuria with age. (Adapted from Anderson GT, Palermjo JJ, Schilling JD, et al. Science 2003;301:105–7.[11])

risk factors for urinary tract obstruction warrants imaging studies, as antimicrobial therapy alone is insufficient to eradicate the infection in this scenario. Some of these risk factors include a history of kidney stones, ureteral strictures, history of diabetes mellitus, and prior genitourinary surgery (Box 25.1). The lack of a clinical response after 48–72 hours of therapy also warrants imaging. The presence of foci of bacterial persistence may be noted on the imaging study. Renal ultrasound and CT scans are the most common modalities currently utilized. A renal ultrasound can identify hydronephrosis and is advantageous because it is non-invasive and utilizes no radiation or contrast. A CT scan provides better anatomic detail and is more sensitive for identifying renal and perirenal abscesses.[17]

CLINICAL SPECTRUM

Urinary tract infections can range from acute cystitis involving the lower urinary tract to pyelonephritis and frank urosepsis. Acute uncomplicated cystitis is an inflammation of the bladder and characterized by dysuria, suprapubic pain, frequency, and urgency. Cystitis should be differentiated from other conditions in which dysuria is common, including vaginitis and sexually transmitted diseases. Acute pyelonephritis is a clinical syndrome of fevers, chills, and flank pain along with bacteriuria and pyuria. Urine cultures are usually positive but 20% of patients have less than 10^5 CFU/ml.[18] CT imaging is not indicated unless the patient has a poor response to antimicrobial therapy or has risk factors previously mentioned.

Box 25.1 Indications for imaging

- Poor response to antimicrobial therapy after 48–72 hours
- History of nephrolithiasis, especially history of struvite stones
- Predisposition to ureteral obstruction from stone, stricture
- Papillary necrosis
- Neuropathic bladder
- History of urinary tract surgery predisposing to obstruction (e.g. ureteral reimplantation or urethral stricture disease)
- Polycystic kidney disease in hemodialysis patients
- Infection with unusual organisms like tuberculosis, fungi
- Diabetes mellitus

Adapted from Anderson GT, Palermjo JJ, Schilling JD, et al. Science 2003; 301:105–7.[11]

Chronic pyelonephritis is a historical term and is a radiologic and pathologic entity characterized by a contracted, atrophic kidney. Emphysematous pyelonephritis (EP) is a necrotizing infection of the renal parenchyma by gas-forming bacteria. EP is usually seen in diabetic patients or individuals with impairment of renal function and was associated with a mortality of up to 40% in the past. Most patients have the classic triad of fever, vomiting, and flank pain, and often appear acutely ill.[19] The most common organism identified is *E. coli*, with Klebsiella and Proteus also noted.[20] The plain film often shows gas overlying the kidney, but CT remains the diagnostic test of choice (Fig. 25.2).

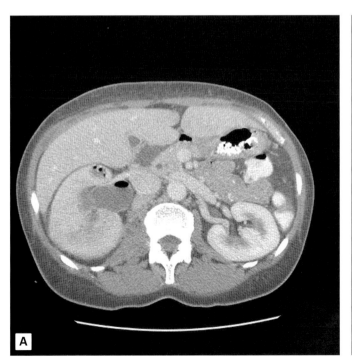
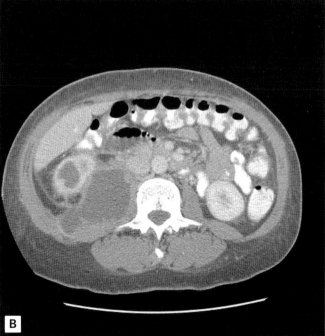

Figure 25.2 CT scan of emphysematous pyelonephritis. Kidney with air in parenchyma and collecting system from a gas-forming bacteria, (**A**) hydronephrosis, and (**B**) psoas abscess.

Renal abscesses are severe complications from a UTI. A carbuncle representing a collection of purulent material in the renal parenchyma can be recognized early in the infection. Usually, they are secondary to ascending infection caused by *E. coli*, Proteus, Klebsiella or Pseudomonas. Occasionally, hematogenous spread from *S. aureus* can be seen in intravenous drug users. The presenting symptoms can be nonspecific and include fevers, night sweats, abdominal or flank pain, malaise, and weight loss. Emphysematous pyelonephritis and abscess should be suspected when there is a minimal response to initial antibiotic therapy.

TREATMENT

The successful treatment of any UTI requires the eradication of the bacteria from the urinary tract. Without the initial elimination of bacteriuria, the etiology of a post-therapy bacteriuria from a reinfection cannot be validated.

UTIs are subdivided into different groups based on clinical syndromes and outcomes. Some of the categories and their treatments that will be discussed include acute uncomplicated cystitis, recurrent cystitis, acute uncomplicated pyelonephritis, complicated pyelonephritis, and complicated infections (Table 25.1). Some of the complicated infections include asymptomatic bacteriuria and infection during pregnancy, asymptomatic bacteriuria in elderly women, and catheter-associated UTIs. The role of prophylaxis and patient-initiated therapy will also be reviewed.

The recommended treatment options for uncomplicated cystitis in women include a short course of empiric antimicrobials and patient-initiated therapy. Since the majority of UTIs in women occur in a normal urinary tract, empiric treatment can be commenced without obtaining a urine culture for outpatients. The culture pattern and sensitivities

Table 25.1	Common treatment regimens for UTIs
Condition	**Treatment regimens**
Acute uncomplicated cystitis— oral therapy	TMP-SMX 160–800 mg b.i.d. × 3 d Ciprofloxacin 500 mg b.i.d. × 3 d Enoxacin 400 mg q.d. × 3d Levofloxacin 500 mg q.d. × 3 d TMP 100 mg b.i.d. × 3 d Nitrofurantoin 100 mg q.i.d. × 3 d Norfloxacin 400 mg b.i.d. × 3 d
Acute uncomplicated cystitis (for symptoms longer than 7 d, recent exposure to antibiotics, history of diabetes, age >65 yrs)—oral therapy	TMP-SMX 160–800 b.i.d. × 7 d Fluoroquinolone × 7 d (as above)
Acute uncomplicated pyelonephritis (outpatient)— oral therapy	TMP-SMX 160–800 mg b.i.d. × 10–14 d Ciprofloxacin 500 mg b.i.d. × 10–14 d Enoxacin 400 mg q.d. × 10–14 d Levofloxacin 500 mg q.d. × 10–14 d Norfloxacin 400 mg b.i.d. × 10–14 d
Acute uncomplicated pyelonephritis (inpatient)— parenteral therapy	Ampicillin 1 g q 6h + gentamicin 1.5 mg/kg q 8h Ciprofloxacin 400 mg q 12h Levofloxacin 500 mg q.d. Ceftriaxone 1 g q.d. Continue regimen until afebrile, then oral TMP-SMX or fluoroquinolone for a total of 14 days
Complicated UTIs (outpatient)— oral therapy	Fluoroquinolone × 10–14 d (see above for doses)
Complicated UTIs (inpatient)— parenteral therapy	Ampicillin 2 g q 6h + gentamicin 1.5 mg/kg q 8h Ciprofloxacin 400 mg 12h Levofloxacin 500 mg q.d. Ceftriaxone 1 g q.d. Ticarcillin-clavulanate 3 g q 8h Imipenem-cilastatin 500 mg q 6–8h Aztreonam 1 g q 8h Continue regimen until afebrile, then oral fluoroquinolone for a total of 14–21 d
Urosepsis—parenteral therapy	Ampicillin 2 g q 6h and gentamicin 1.5 mg/kg q 8h

Adapted from Anderson GT, Palermjo JJ, Schilling JD, et al. Science 2003;301:105–107.[11]

in the outpatient population are predictable and often do not change the treatment plan. This also saves the extra expense of obtaining a urine culture.[21] As *E. coli* remains the most common urinary pathogen, cost-effective treatment requires good efficacy against this organism. Currently, trimethoprim-sulfamethoxazole (TMP-SMX) is the initial recommended therapy in healthy, adult, nonpregnant women in communities with resistance less than 10–20%. Fluoroquinolones are extremely effective and should be utilized in regions where TMP-SMX resistance is greater than 20%. Treatment is recommended for a course of 3 days or less of oral therapy. Longer regimens do not improve efficacy and are associated with higher cost and more side effects.[22] Single-dose therapy has lower cure rates compared to a 3-day course.[23]

Another trend has been the advocation of patient-initiated or "self-start" therapy in individuals with recurrent UTIs. Patients are given a self-culture device and prescription, which is fulfilled upon the start of symptoms. Patient-initiated therapy has been found to be efficacious and represents another alternative to treatment.[24] In individuals with recurrent symptoms of a UTI, symptoms for greater than 7 days, recent antimicrobial therapy or comorbid conditions like diabetes mellitus, urine cultures should be obtained and treatment should be commenced for 7 days.

The treatment of uncomplicated pyelonephritis ranges from outpatient therapy in mild cases to hospitalization with intravenous antibiotics followed by a switch to outpatient therapy in moderate to severe cases. In individuals with no major comorbidities or complicating factors, a mild infection (low-grade fever, mild WBC, no nausea or vomiting) can be treated with an oral antimicrobial as an outpatient for 14 days.[25] Empiric treatment with a fluoroquinolone or TMP-SMX in regions of low resistance to *E. coli* is the recommended first-line treatment option.[26] A urine culture should be obtained and the antimicrobial regimen adjusted as needed after the results are back.

Individuals with moderate to severe pyelonephritis (high fever, high WBC, nausea, vomiting, dehydration, and signs of sepsis) or failure on an outpatient regimen should be admitted for intravenous antibiotics with a fluoroquinolone, aminoglycoside with or without ampicillin, or an extended-spectrum cephalosporin with or without an aminoglycoside.[22] After evidence of clinical improvement for 48 hours (afebrile, decrease in WBC), the patient should be switched to oral antimicrobial therapy tailored to the culture results, with fluoroquinolones, TMP-SMX or amoxicillin (for gram-positive organisms) as recommended treatment options. When no clinical improvement is seen after the initial treatment period, imaging studies should be ordered to evaluate for a possible abscess, infected hydronephrosis or another complicated UTI.

The treatment of emphysematous pyelonephritis classically was open drainage followed by elective nephrectomy at a later date. More recently, percutaneous treatment options and broad-spectrum antibiotic therapy has been an effective treatment option for up to 80% of patients.[27] Using aggressive volume resuscitation, diabetic control, antimicrobials, and percutaneous drainage, the mortality rate was only 8% in the study by Chen and associates.[27] Similarly, renal abscesses were historically treated by open surgical drainage. More recently, small abscesses less than 3 cm in diameter have been treated with antimicrobials only.[28] Percutaneous drainage can be utilized for an abscess between 3 and 5 cm. Larger abscesses greater than 5 cm may require multiple percutaneous drainages or additional surgical drainage.[29]

A complicated UTI occurs in an individual with a structural or functional abnormality of the genitourinary tract. For practical purposes, all men and children should be presumed to have a complicated UTI until proven otherwise. Individuals can present from cystitis to frank urosepsis. The management of these individuals requires a thorough diagnostic evaluation with appropriate imaging and urine culture data. As evidence-based guidelines are lacking, an effective treatment plan relies on clinical judgment and experience. Initial therapy with an oral fluoroquinolone or a parenteral antimicrobial with antipseudomonal activity is recommended with a treatment course of 14 days. After treatment is completed, follow-up urine cultures should be checked.

URINARY TRACT INFECTIONS IN PREGNANCY

UTIs are a common complication of pregnancy. Physiologic changes of pregnancy including decreased ureteral peristalsis, mechanical obstruction of the ureters by the gravid uterus, and displacement of the bladder anteriorly and superiorly all promote urinary stasis. The prevalence of bacteriuria in pregnant females is similar to nonpregnant females, at around 5%.[30] *E. coli*, Klebsiella, and Enterobacter species account for more than 90% of UTIs. All pregnant females should undergo a urinalysis and urine culture in the first trimester. Patients with asymptomatic bacteriuria have a much higher risk of progression to pyelonephritis (between 13.5% and 65%) than individuals without bacteriuria (1.4%).[31] Asymptomatic bacteriuria has also been associated with prematurity, low birthweight, and maternal anemia. Some authors also recommend a repeat urine culture at 16 weeks if the initial culture is negative.

Due to the increased risk of pyelonephritis and other complications, all pregnant women with asymptomatic bacteriuria should be treated with a 3-day course of an antimicrobial. Initial therapeutic options include amoxicillin, ampicillin or a cephalosporin. Nitrofurantoin and TMP-SMX can be utilized in selected trimesters of pregnancy (Table 25.2). Fluoroquinolones, tetracycline, and macrolides should be avoided during pregnancy (see Table

Table 25.2 Antimicrobial options and contraindications in pregnancy

Antimicrobial	Regimen	Comments
Safe in all trimesters		
Amoxicillin	250 mg t.i.d. × 7 d 250 mg t.i.d. × 3 day 3 g dose followed by 3 g dose 12 h later 2 g plus 1 g probenicid	High incidence of *E. coli* resistance
Amoxicillin/clavulanic acid	250 mg/125 mg t.i.d. × 7 d	
Cephalexin	500 mg q.i.d. × 7 d	
Safe in selected trimesters		
Nitrofurantoin	100 mg q.i.d. × 3 or 7 d	Possible hemolytic anemia in patients with G6PD deficiency Contraindicated at term
Sulfisoxazole	1 g then 500 mg q.i.d. × 7 d	Risk of neonatal hyperbilirubinemia Avoid during third TM
TMP-SMX	TMP 320 mg/SMX 1600 mg b.i.d. × 3 d	TMP—may cause megaloblastic anemia because of antifolate properties in first TM SMX—see above
Unsafe during all trimesters		
Fluoroquinolones	Contraindicated	Possible damage to immature cartilage
Tetracyclines	Contraindicated	Inhibits new bone formation in fetus and risk of acute liver decompensation in mother
Erythromycin	Contraindicated	Risk of maternal cholestatic jaundice
Chloramphenicol	Contraindicated	Associated with "gray baby" syndrome

Adapted from Langermann S, Ballou WR Jr. J Infect Dis 2001;183:584–86.[45]

25.2 for specific side effects). A followup urine culture should be checked to ensure eradication after therapy. Due to the high prevalence of recurrent bacteriuria, urine should be screened at each office visit in patients with positive cultures. Patients with follow-up negative cultures do not need additional treatment except for individuals with group B streptococcus infections, who need therapy at labor to prevent GBS sepsis.

Pregnant women with cystitis require the same treatment regimen as patients with asymptomatic bacteriuria. Follow-up urine cultures should be checked 1–2 days after the initiation of treatment to check for resolution of bacteriuria.

If cultures remain positive, antimicrobial suppressive therapy for the remainder of pregnancy may be indicated.[32]

All pregnant women with acute pyelonephritis should be admitted for parenteral microbial therapy. Initial treatment with ampicillin and an aminoglycoside, followed by oral therapy for at least 14 days, is indicated.[33] Due to the increased risk of another episode of pyelonephritis, patients should be monitored for bacteriuria or placed on prophylaxis therapy. Patients who do not respond during the first 48 hours of antimicrobial therapy require imaging evaluation. A renal ultrasound is the initial imaging modality in pregnant women as it evaluates for obstruction without any harmful radiation exposure to the fetus. In patients with obstruction and infection, emergency decompression of the urinary tract is indicated with cystoscopy and retrograde stent placement or a percutaneous nephrostomy tube. Stents should be changed every 6 weeks and patients require continuous antimicrobial prophylaxis until delivery.[34]

ASYMPTOMATIC BACTERIURIA: ELDERLY WOMAN

Urinary infections occur much more frequently in the elderly population. Asymptomatic bacteriuria, defined as greater than 100,000 CFU/ml of voided urine without symptoms of a UTI, is also common in the elderly. Current estimates of asymptomatic bacteriuria in elderly women living in nursing homes range between 25% and 50%.[35] In addition, comorbid conditions that impair elderly individuals increase the risk of asymptomatic bacteriuria.

The assessment of symptoms in elderly individuals with bacteriuria poses a difficult task to the clinician. Elderly patients often present with nonspecific symptoms like confusion, lethargy, dementia, urinary and fecal incontinence.[36] Fever is often not a common presenting symptom in the elderly. In addition, the etiology of fever in patients with bacteriuria and no localizing signs is due to a UTI only 10% of the time.[37] In an elderly febrile patient with a positive culture and no urinary tract symptoms, the diagnosis of a UTI is unlikely. Asymptomatic bacteriuria should not be treated because it does not decrease the risk of a recurrent symptomatic UTI, lower mortality or decrease costs. In addition, treatment of asymptomatic bacteriuria promotes increased drug resistance in a patient population that already has high levels of drug resistance. Some of the few indications to treat asymptomatic bacteriuria are urinary tract obstruction, bacteriuria in renal transplant patients, and prior to urinary tract surgical procedures.

CATHETER-ASSOCIATED URINARY TRACT INFECTIONS

The most common hospital-acquired infections are UTIs, with urethral instrumentation the main risk factor. Catheter-associated UTIs account for 40% of nosocomial infections and the most common source of gram-negative sepsis. Around 10–15% of hospitalized patients receive an indwelling catheter[38] and the risk of acquiring bacteriuria is about 5–10% per day. Most patients will inevitably become bacteriuric if the catheter remains. The use of a closed catheter drainage system has reduced the risk of catheter-associated bacteriuria from around 90% at 4 days to around 30%.[39]

A count of 100 CFU/ml or more represents significant bacteriuria. The diagnosis of infection requires symptoms localizing to the urinary tract as cultures and pyuria have a low positive predictive value. Asymptomatic bacteriuria should not be treated because it may lead to increased resistance and the bacteriuria eventually returns. Symptomatic bladder infections should be treated for 10–14 days with an oral fluoroquinolone. Patients with fever and flank pain should be treated for acute pyelonephritis with parenteral antibiotics, followed by oral agents for 14–21 days. The urinary tract should also be imaged to rule out obstruction.

In cases of symptomatic infections, the urinary catheter should be changed or removed if feasible. Patients with long-term catheters have an increased risk of bladder cancer and nephrolithiasis and should be monitored periodically. In patients with struvite stones from Proteus infection, removal of the stone and antimicrobial treatment are indicated.

PROPHYLAXIS

Current strategies to prevent UTIs include antimicrobial prophylaxis, postcoital therapy, and estrogen replacement therapy in postmenopausal women. The use of natural compounds to prevent UTIs is also being investigated. Cranberry juice has been used for many years to prevent UTIs. It contains the compound hippuric acid, which may reduce adherence of bacteria in vitro. It has been shown to reduce bacteriuria but not the incidence of symptomatic UTIs.[40] Some other studies have shown a decreased risk of symptomatic UTIs with cranberry juice, but long-term clinical outcomes still need to be measured.[41]

Successful prophylactic therapy requires elimination of pathogenic strains from the introital flora without causing bacterial resistance. Prophylactic therapy decreases the incidence of recurrent UTIs by as much as 95%.[42] The use of prophylaxis has reduced the reinfection rate from 2.0–3.0 per patient-year to 0.1–0.4 per patient-year. Common antimicrobials utilized for prophylaxis are single-day, low-dose TMP-SMX, TMP, nitrofurantoin, and cephalexin. Fluoroquinolones should be utilized only in nonpregnant women or when resistance to the other antimicrobials is present.

In individuals with recurrent UTIs associated with intercourse, postcoital therapy with a single-dose antimicrobial reduces the incidence of reinfection.[43] In addition, spermicidal agents should be avoided in women with recurrent UTIs. Estrogen replacement therapy in postmenopausal women restores the normal vaginal flora, including lactobacillus, and reduces E. coli colonization. The use of vaginal estrogen has been shown to reduce the incidence of symptomatic UTIs.[44]

RESEARCH STRATEGIES

Active exciting research is currently being done to elucidate the basic pathogenesis of UTIs and efforts to prevent UTIs. Future research strategies to prevent colonization of bacteria and progression to UTIs will need to be investigated. Immunization techniques are currently being investigated to prevent UTIs. The Fim H subunit of *E. coli* has been the focus of a vaccine to prevent bacterial attachment.[45] Other avenues to prevent colonization, including the blockage of adherence and immunomodulation, will need to be researched. Recently, there has been increasing resistance to the fluoroquinolones in Europe. New methodology and treatment strategies to deal with changing resistance patterns will also be a focus in the future.

REFERENCES

1. Schappert SM. Ambulatory care visits to physician offices, hospital outpatient departments, and emergency departments: United States, 1997. Vital Health Stat 1999;13(143): i–iv, 1–39.
2. Rosenberg M. Pharmacoeconomics of treating uncomplicated urinary tract infections. Int J Antimicrob Agents;1999;11(3-4):247–251.
3. Schaeffer AJ, Jones JM, Dunn JK. Association of in vitro E. coli adherence to vaginal and buccal epithelial cells with susceptibility of women to recurrent urinary tract infections. N Engl J Med 304(18):1062–1066.
4. Klemm P. Fimbrial adhesins of Escherichia coli. Rev Infect Dis 7(3):321–340.
5. Connell H, Agace W, Klemm P, et al. Type 1 fimbrial expression enhances Escherichia coli virulence for the urinary tract. Proc Natl Acad Sci USA 1996;93(18): 9827–9832.
6. Mulvey MA, Lopez-Boado YS, Wilson CL, et al. Induction and evasion of host defenses by type 1-piliated uropathogenic Escherichia coli. Science 1999;282(5393):1494–1497.
7. Kallenius G, Mollby R, Svenson SB, et al. Occurrence of P-fimbriated Escherichia coli in urinary tract infections. Lancet 1981;2(8260-61):1369–1372.
8. Fowler JE Jr, Stamey TA. Studies of introital colonization in women with recurrent urinary infections. VIII: The role of bacterial adherence. J Urol 1977;118(2):296–298.
9. Schaeffer AJ, Navas EL, Venegas MF, et al. Variation of blood group antigen expression on vaginal cells and mucus of secretor and nonsecretor women. J Urol 1994;152(3):859–864.
10. Mulvey MA, Schilling JD, Hultgren SJ. Establishment of a persistent Escherichia coli reservoir during the acute phase of a bladder infection. Infect Immun 69(7):4572–4579.
11. Anderson GT, Palermjo JJ, Schilling JD, et al. Intracellular bacterial biofilm-like pods in urinary tract infections. Science 2003;301(5629):105–7.
12. Schaeffer AJ. Infections of the urinary tract. In: Walsh PC, Wein AJ, Vaughan ED Jr, Retik AB, eds. Campbell's urology, 8th edn. Philadelphia: WB Saunders; 2002
13. Stamm WE, Hooton TM. Management of urinary tract infections in adults. N Engl J Med 329(18):1328–1334.
14. Stamey TA, Govan DE, Palmer JM. The localization and treatment of urinary tract infections: the role of bactericidal urine levels as opposed to serum level. Medicine 1965;44:1–36.
15. Kunin CM. Urinary tract infections in females. Clin Infect Dis 1994;18(1):1–10.
16. Kunin CM, White LV, Hua TH. A reassessment of the importance of "low-count" bacteriuria in young women with acute urinary symptoms. Ann Intern Med 1993;119(6):454–460.
17. Soulen MC, Fishman EK, Goldman SM, et al. Bacterial renal infection: role of CT. Radiology 1989;171(3):703–707.
18. Rubin RH, Beam TR, Stamm WE. An approach to evaluating antibacterial agents in the treatment of urinary tract infections. Clin Infect Dis 1992;14(Suppl 2):S246–251.
19. Schainuck LI, Fouty R, Cutler RE. Emphysematous pyelonephritis, a new case and review of previous observations. Am J Med 1968;44(1):134–139.
20. Ahlering TE, Boyd SD, Hamilton CL. Emphysematous pyelonephritis. J Urol 1985;134(6):1086–1088.
21. Andriole VT. When to do culture in urinary tract infections. Int J Antimicrob Agents 1999;11(3-4):253–255.
22. Warren JW, Abrutyn E, Hebel JR, et al. Guidelines for antimicrobial treatment of uncomplicated acute bacterial cystitis and acute pyelonephritis in women. IDSA. Clin Infect Dis 1999;29(4):745–758.
23. Goto T, Kitagawa T, Kawahara M, et al. Comparative study of single-dose and three-day therapy for acute uncomplicated cystitis. Hinyokika Kiyo 1999;45(2):85–89.
24. Schaeffer AJ, Stuppy BA. Efficacy and safety of self-start therapy in women with recurrent urinary tract infections. J Urol 1999;161(1):207–211.
25. Mombelli G, Pezzoli R, Pinoja-Lutz G, et al. Oral vs intravenous ciprofloxacin in the initial empirical management of severe pyelonephritis or complicated urinary tract infections: a prospective randomized clinical trial. Arch Intern Med 1999;159(1):53–58.
26. Naber KG. Which fluoroquinolones are suitable for the treatment of urinary tract infections? Int J Antimicrob Agents 2001;17(4):331–341.
27. Chen MT, Huang CN, Chou YH, et al. Percutaneous drainage in the treatment of emphysematous pyelonephritis: 10-year experience. J Urol 1997;157(5):1569–1573.
28. Levin R, Burbige KA, Abramson S, et al. The diagnosis and management of renal inflammatory processes in children. J Urol 1984;132(4):718–721.
29. Siegel JF, Smith A, Moldwin R. Minimally invasive treatment of renal abscess. J Urol 1996;155(1):52–55.
30. Ovalle A, Levancini M. Urinary tract infections in pregnancy. Curr Opin Urol 2001;11(1):55–59.
31. Sweet RL. Bacteriuria and pyelonephritis during pregnancy. Semin Perinatol 1977;1(1):25–40.
32. Pfau A, Sacks TG. Effective prophylaxis for recurrent urinary tract infections during pregnancy. Clin Infect Dis 1992;14(4):810–814.
33. Sanchez-Ramos L, McAlpine KJ, Adair CD, et al. Pyelonephritis in pregnancy: once-a-day ceftriaxone versus multiple doses of cefazolin. Am J Obstet Gynecol 1995;172(1 Pt 1):129–133.
34. Pearle MS, Taxer OA. Renal urolithiasis: therapy for special circumstances. Part I. American Urological Association update series, vol. XX, lesson 39, 2001
35. Nicolle LE. Urinary tract infections in long-term-care facilities. Infect Control Hosp Epidemiol 2001;22(3):167–175.
36. Stark RP, Maki DG. Bacteriuria in the catheterized patient: what quantitative level of bacteriuria is relevant? N Engl J Med 1984;311(9):560–564.
37. Nicolle LE. Urinary tract infection in long-term-care facility residents. Clin Infect Dis 2000;31(3):757–761.
38. Stamm WE. Guidelines for prevention of catheter-associated urinary tract infections. Ann Intern Med 1975;82(3):386–390.
39. Pearman JW. Prevention of urinary tract infection following spinal cord injury. Paraplegia 1971;9(2):95–104.
40. Avorn J, Monane M, Gurwitz JH, et al. Reduction of bacteriuria and pyuria after ingestion of cranberry juice. JAMA 1994;271(10):751–754.
41. Kontiokari T, Sundqvist K, Nuutinen M, et al. Randomised trial of cranberry-lingonberry juice and Lactobacillus GG drink for the prevention of urinary tract infections in women. BMJ 2001;322(7302):1571.

42. Nicolle LE, Ronald AR. Recurrent urinary tract infection in adult women: diagnosis and treatment. Infect Dis Clin North Am 1987;1(4):793–806.

43. Stapleton A, Latham RH, Johnson C, et al. Postcoital antimicrobial prophylaxis for recurrent urinary tract infection. A randomized, double-blind, placebo-controlled trial. JAMA 1990;264(6):703–706.

44. Raz R, Stamm WE. A controlled trial of intravaginal estriol in postmenopausal women with recurrent urinary tract infection. N Engl J Med 1993;1329(11):753–756.

45. Langermann S, Ballou WR Jr. Vaccination utilizing the FimCH complex as a strategy to prevent Escherichia coli urinary tract infections. J Infect Dis 2001;183 Suppl 1:S84–86.

46. Weiser AC, Schaeffer AJ. The use and misuse of antimicrobial agents in urology. American Urological Association Update Series 2002: Vol XXI, Lesson 37

SECTION 11 Irritative conditions of the genitourinary tract

Interstitial Cystitis: An Overview

C Sage Claydon and Kristene E Whitmore

INTRODUCTION

Interstitial cystitis (IC) presents as chronic debilitating pelvic/bladder/urethral pain, urinary frequency, and urgency. It is a diagnosis of exclusion made in the absence of other identifiable causes. This condition was first described in 1836 by Parrish, who called it "tic douloureux of the bladder." The term interstitial cystitis was later coined by Skene in 1887. In 1915, Hunner described five patients with contracted fibrotic bladders, hyperemic bladder mucosa with adjacent ulcers, and mucosal hemorrhage following hydrodistension.[1,2]

Although the medical field has been aware of IC for over 100 years, both the natural history and pathophysiologic mechanisms of IC remain elusive. In 1987, the National Institutes of Health-National Institute of Diabetes and Digestive and Kidney Disorders (NIH-NIDDK) established a set of standardized criteria for inclusion in research studies[3] in an effort to perform meaningful and reproducible research in the field of IC. These criteria were revised in 1988[3] (Box 26.1). Between 1993 and 1997, in an effort to better understand the natural history of IC, the NIH initiated a multicenter longitudinal observational study group: the Interstitial Cystitis Data Base (ICDB).[4] Enrollment criteria varied from the NIH-NIDDK, with the main difference being that IC diagnosis was symptom driven and cystoscopy was optional (Box 26.2).[4] During the study 637 patients were enrolled.[5]

EPIDEMIOLOGY

The reported prevalence of IC varies. The largest published study to date, the Nurse's Health Study data (NHS), reported in 1999, estimated the prevalence of IC in women in the United States to be 52–67/100,000.[6] The study was based on self-report of IC by participants. Participants' medical records demonstrating cystoscopic findings and symptoms consistent with IC were then used to confirm the

---

> **Box 26.1 NIH-NIDDK criteria for inclusion in interstitial cystitis research trials (revised November 1988)[3]**
>
> **Inclusion criteria**
>
> Must meet criteria for both A and B.
>
> (A) Glomerulations on cystoscopic exam under anesthesia (at least 10/quadrant and in at least three quadrants) **or** Hunner's ulcers on cystoscopic exam under anesthesia
>
> (B) Pain associated with the bladder **or** urinary urgency
>
> **Exclusion criteria**
>
> ■ Bladder capacity >350 ml on waking cystometrogram (either gas or liquid)
>
> ■ No intense urge to void when the bladder is filled to 150 ml (or 100 ml of gas) while awake
>
> ■ Involuntary bladder contractions on cystometrogram at a medium filling rate
>
> ■ Duration of symptoms <9 months
>
> ■ Absence of nocturnal frequency
>
> ■ Symptoms relieved by antimicrobials, antiseptics, anticholinergics or antispasmodics
>
> ■ Waking urinary frequency <8
>
> ■ Diagnosis of bacterial cystitis or prostatitis within 3 months. Must be abacteriuric for 3 months
>
> **Other exclusion criteria include the presence of:**
>
> ■ Bladder or lower ureteral calculi
>
> ■ Active genital herpes
>
> ■ Uterine, cervical, vaginal or urethral cancer
>
> ■ Urethral diverticulum
>
> ■ Cyclophosphamide cystitis
>
> ■ Vaginitis
>
> ■ Tuberculosis cystitis
>
> ■ Radiation cystitis
>
> ■ Benign or malignant bladder tumors
>
> ■ Age <18 years

Box 26.2   Interstitial Cystitis Data Base criteria[4]

Inclusion criteria

- Willing to provide informed consent
- Willing to undergo cystoscopy under anesthesia
- Symptoms of urinary urgency, frequency or pain for more than 6 months
- Daytime frequency of ≥7 or urgency or pain measured on a linear analog scale

Exclusion criteria

- History of genitourinary tuberculosis
- History of urethral cancer
- History of bladder malignancy, high-grade dysplasia or carcinoma in situ
- History of prostate cancer
- Ovarian, vaginal or cervical cancer within the last 3 years
- Current vaginitis
- Bacterial cystitis within the past 3 months
- History of cyclophosphamide treatment
- Radiation cystitis
- Neurogenic bladder
- Bladder outlet obstruction (determined by urodynamic testing)
- Bacterial prostaties within the past 6 months
- Urethritis for the previous 3 months
- Urethral dilation, cystometrogram, cystoscopy under anesthesia or bladder biopsy in the past 3 months
- History of augmentation cystoplasty, cystectomy, cystolysis or neurectomy
- Urethral stricture of <12 F

---

diagnosis. However, these figures are limited since all the participants were women and 90% were Caucasian. Therefore the actual prevalence may be greater.

DEMOGRAPHICS

Data collected from the ICDB study demonstrated a male/female ratio of 1/10.8 in IC. The report noted that more than 93% of the subjects were Caucasian but the authors point out this may reflect referral patterns rather than racial selectivity of the disease. Although IC can occur at any age, most studies demonstrate a mean symptom onset between 30 and 50 years old.[4-6]

PATHOPHYSIOLOGY

To date, the pathogenesis of IC remains unclear. Recently biopsies from 206 patients from the ICDB were evaluated. Using multivariate analysis, the authors demonstrated that

increased nighttime frequency was associated with four biopsy features: complete loss of urothelium, granulation tissue in the lamina propria, increased vascular density in lamina propria (using factor VIII stain), and increased tryptase staining mast cell count in the lamina propria. Pain was highly associated with the percentage of submucosal hemorrhage and denuded urothelium.[7]

Given these findings, several theories examining the etiology of IC are currently under investigation. They include increased bladder permeability, ultrastructural derangements of the lamina propria, increased mast cells, neurogenic inflammation, autoimmune disorders, and infectious agents. The true etiology is most likely multifactorial, involving one or more steps in a pathway which results in the clinical syndrome of IC (Fig. 26.1).

Increased bladder permeability. One of the leading theories for IC pathogenesis is that a defect in the glycosaminoglycan (GAG) layer of the urothelium allows noxious solutes to cross into the bladder interstitium, damaging the bladder and stimulating pain neurons (C fibers). There are several ultrastructural, animal, and clinical studies supporting this theory.[8-10] In a recent study evaluating molecular markers for cell permeability, Slobodov et al compared bladder biopsies from 27 IC patients with seven controls.[11] In addition to decreased cell thickness of the urothelium, from five cells to 1–2 cells, they found significant differences in the distribution of chondroitin sulfate proteoglycan (a GAG protein), ZO-1 (cell junction protein), uroplakin (urothelial protein), and E-cadherin (urothelial differentiation). According to the authors, these findings are consistent with abnormal cell differentiation, which in turn could lead to increased urothelial permeability.

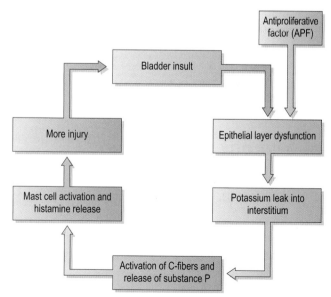

Figure 26.1 Pathogenesis of interstitial cystitis.

In 1998, Parsons et al reported urgency in 79% (15/19) and pain in 37% (7/19) of normal volunteers in response to intravesical instillation of protamine sulfate, a substance known to disrupt the GAG layer, followed by potassium chloride (KCl). Intravesical heparin was then administered followed by KCl, and a reversal of urgency and pain was noted in 47% (7/15) and 87% (13/15) respectively.[12] This theory is the basis of several current therapeutic interventions including intravesical heparin cocktails and pentosan polysulfate.

Mast cells. Elevated mast cell counts in the bladder muscularis and lamina propria have been well described in the literature.[7,8,13,14] Increased mucosal mast cells were seen in nonulcerative IC; however, detrusor mastocytosis was seen in both ulcerative (classic) as well as nonulcerative IC.[13] In a case–control study, Peeker et al found a 6–8-fold increase in detrusor mast cells in patients with ulcerative IC and a 2–3-fold increase in the nonulcerative IC group.[14] Studies have also demonstrated increased mast cell granulation products methylhistamine and tryptase in IC urine.[7] Although there are conflicting reports on the diagnostic utility of mastocytosis in IC,[7] these findings suggest that mast cells occupy an intermediary role in the pathogenesis of IC. Mast cell release can be triggered by either allergic/immune response (type 1 hypersensitivity) or other non-immune sources including, but not limited to, neuropeptides (substance P), cytokines, leukotrienes (IL-2, IL-6), and neurotransmitters.[13]

Neurogenic inflammation. Ultrastructural studies of the IC bladder demonstrate an increased number of C fibers (unmyelinated sensory afferents) in close proximity to mast cells.[13,15] When stimulated, these fibers release substance P, calcitonin gene-related peptide, and acetylcholine. This promotes mast cell degranulation and the release of inflammatory mediators such as histamine, tryptase, bradykinin, vasoactive intestinal peptide, cytokines, prostaglandins, and nitric oxide. Subsequently additional C fibers are activated, resulting in an increase in substance P, vasodilation, increased vascular permeability, mast cell migration, and degranulation with propagation of the pain and inflammation cycle.[2] Initiation of this cycle may be triggered by a number of events (see Fig. 26.1).

Antiproliferative factor (APF). Antiproliferative factor (APF) has been isolated from the urine of both women and men with IC.[16,17] In an elegant study, Keay et al extracted APF from IC urine and added it to tissue cultures of age-matched normal urothelium. They demonstrated a decreased rate of epithelial cell proliferation (increased APF), with a decreased rate of heparin binding–epidermal growth factor (HB-EGF) production. When APF was removed from the culture medium, both HB-EGF and cell proliferation were noted to normalize, thus demonstrating that these changes were reversible.[17] APF may likely serve as a diagnostic marker for IC.

Autoimmune/genetic. IC is often associated with systemic autoimmune diseases such as Sjögren's syndrome, inflammatory bowel disease, and systemic lupus erythematosus as well as irritable bowel syndrome, fibromyalgia, and atopic conditions. In addition to mast cells, T lymphocytes are also noted to occupy the bladder wall. Some studies demonstrate an increased expression of growth factors similar to those in rheumatoid arthritis. It is hypothesized that these growth factors may accumulate in the GAG layer and promote inflammation.[18]

Central sensitization/chronic pain. One of the hallmark symptoms of IC is chronic pain. Integral in the pathogenesis of all chronic pain syndromes is the concept of central sensitization. Normally, a certain threshold of input has to be received by the dorsal horn cells of the spinal cord before the pain signal is transmitted to the brain. With central sensitization, the transmission threshold is reset at a lower level.[9] Specifically, in IC increased and/or uninterrupted transmission of pain signals from the bladder to the spinal cord (as seen in neurogenic inflammation) eventually allows the dorsal horn cells in the spinal cord to fire with less peripheral input, thereby increasing pain perception with less stimulation (neural plasticity).[9,15]

Clinical presentation. IC is classically characterized as chronic pain in the form of suprapubic pressure, which is exacerbated by bladder filling and relieved by voiding, in combination with increased daytime and nighttime frequency in the absence of a proven urinary tract infection or other obvious pathology. Until further work-up is done to rule out such conditions as endometriosis, carcinoma and prostatitis, the International Continence Society (ICS)[19] dictates this condition be termed painful bladder syndrome.

IC is a progressive disorder resulting in a range of presentations. The severity of symptoms ranges from mild to debilitating. Pain may be experienced in the urethra, bladder, lower abdomen, lower back, perineum, medial thighs or inguinal area. Dyspareunia is often present.[8] Typically, patients experience episodic exacerbations of symptoms called "flares." Physical or emotional stress is the most common precipitating event for IC flares,[20] along with physical activity.[8,21] In 60% of cases consumption of acidic beverages or foods has been demonstrated to exacerbate symptoms.[22] In addition, many women report flares during the luteal phase of the menstrual cycle.

Symptoms start an average of 5–7 years before the diagnosis of IC is made.[6] Therefore patients frequently present

SECTION 11 Irritative conditions of the genitourinary tract

frustrated and/or angry after extensive evaluations and treatments for endometriosis, dysmenorrhea, dyspareunia, gastrointestinal dysfunction, and recurrent urinary tract infection (UTI) have failed to provide symptom relief. In addition, patients are often sleep deprived (due to pain and nighttime frequency) and clinically depressed. Many experience disruption in interpersonal relationships and activities of daily living due to symptoms.[8,20,21]

DIAGNOSTIC WORK-UP

IC is a diagnosis of exclusion. Therefore, the history and physical examination are symptom driven. The history begins with a query about lower urinary tract symptoms (LUTS) and includes an account of the onset of symptoms, all prior treatments for LUTS, culture results from prior "UTIs," gastrointestinal symptoms, obstetric and gynecologic history, as well as prior history of: pelvic surgeries, pelvic radiation, chemotherapy, tuberculosis, and spinal trauma. The severity and duration of symptom flares should be recorded. The presence of conditions associated with IC should also be noted. These include the diagnosis or suspected diagnosis of: fibromyalgia, endometriosis, migraines, SICCA syndrome (dry eyes and mouth), Sjögren's syndrome, drug hypersensitivity, sinusitis, vulvodynia, urethral syndrome, and irritable bowel syndrome. At the initial visit patients may be asked to complete a validated quality of life questionnaire such as the Interstitial Cystitis Symptom/Problem Indices[23] or the Pelvic Pain and Urgency/Frequency Scale (PUF).[24] Although not diagnostic, these allow objective quantification of symptom severity and bother as well as facilitating accurate assessment of treatment outcomes.[25] A voiding diary is beneficial, both for initial evaluation as well as for following treatment outcomes.

Physical examination should include evaluation for vaginitis (atrophic or infective), urethral diverticulum, active herpes, and pelvic organ prolapse. Patients with IC often experience suprapubic and anterior vaginal wall tenderness to palpation. High tone pelvic floor muscle dysfunction (HT-PFD) (aka short pelvic floor) should be noted as IC treatments are less likely to be effective unless HT-PFD is also treated.

The pelvic floor muscles (PFMs) are evaluated with the patient in lithotomy position; with one or two fingers inserted into the vagina, a reflex contraction of the PFM should be palpable as the patient coughs. Strength on digital palpation is assessed using a scale from no contraction to unmistakably strong (0–5).[26] The quality of the PFM can be assessed by either transvaginal or transrectal palpation of the obturator internus, coccygeus, iliococcygeus, and pubococcygeus muscles. As the PFMs are contracted and relaxed, each muscle is examined for tenderness, resting tone, and contractile tone. They should feel supple and be minimally

tender to palpation. The degree of individual muscle spasm can also be subjectively rated on a scale of 0–5.[26,27]

A urinalysis and postvoid residual are routinely performed. Although the presence of leukocytes and microscopic hematuria is common among patients with IC, if they are noted a urine culture and sensitivities should be performed. In addition, the presence of hematuria mandates evaluation for nephrolithiasis, upper tract disease, and bladder carcinoma. Urine cytology, renal ultrasound, and cystoscopy should be performed in all patients with persistent urgency and hematuria; this enables detection of both carcinoma and foreign bodies in the bladder.

Traditionally, the diagnosis of IC required cystoscopy with bladder hydrodistension under anesthesia (BOD): general, regional or conscious sedation with local. The bladder is distended to its maximum capacity at a pressure of 70–90 cmH$_2$O held for 2–8 min, drained and the contents measured. The average maximum capacity under anesthesia (MCUA) for patients with IC is 575 ml and 1115 ml for patients without IC.[2,28] The bladder is refilled and evaluated for petechial hemorrhages called glomerulations (Fig. 26.2) and Hunner's ulcers (Fig. 26.3). The presence of a Hunner's ulcer remains pathognomonic for IC. A 1 mm cup biopsy of the bladder is obtained to rule out carcinoma in situ, eosinophilic cystitis or infection as well as to evaluate for the presence of mast cells in the lamina propria and detrusor muscle.[2,8] Patients are divided into two categories of IC based on findings noted at BOD: *classic* (ulcerative, late stage), and *"nonulcerative"* (early stage) with findings of restricted bladder capacity <350 ml and Hunner's ulcers, or glomerulations, submucosal hemorrhages, and a bladder capacity >350 ml.[2,28]

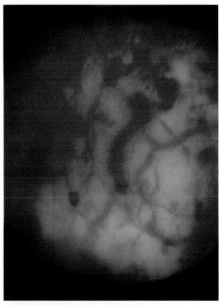

Figure 26.2 Glomerulations.

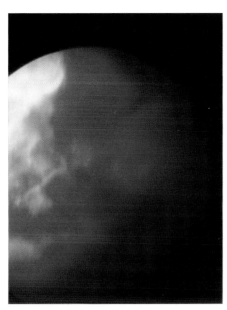

Figure 26.3 Hunner's ulcers.

At present there is debate regarding the utility of cystoscopy with BOD. The advent of the NIH-NIDDK research criteria (see Box 26.1) resulted in an increased awareness of IC as well as increased disease recognition in clinical practice. However, data from the ICDB demonstrated that up to 60% of patients with clinical symptoms consistent with IC would be misdiagnosed if strict NIH-NIDDK enrollment criteria were adhered to.[4] Recently, an analysis of 204 patients from the ICDB demonstrated that glomerulations were not predictive of IC symptoms.[7] In addition, there are reports of glomerulations noted on cystoscopy with BOD of "normal controls." These findings have led some IC practitioners to question the clinical utility of bladder hydrodistension in the diagnosis of IC, and to recommend a symptom-based approach to diagnosis.[29]

In March 2003, IC researchers from around the world met in Kyoto, Japan, to discuss the diagnosis and treatment of IC. Although many representatives from North America questioned the diagnostic utility of cystoscopy with BOD, most felt it is clinically useful and admitted to continuing BOD in their routine practice.[30] The main reasons given were:

- it allows inclusion in research protocols
- it enables maximum capacity under anesthesia to be determined
- it facilitates bladder biopsy which may help guide treatment and may advance knowledge of the pathophysiology of IC
- it helps distinguish ulcerative from nonulcerative types
- approximately 30% of patients experience symptom relief after BOD.[31]

Bladder permeability testing. Theoretically, IC symptoms may result from increased bladder permeability. Parsons proposed a diagnostic office procedure for confirming IC: the potassium sensitivity test (PST). Forty milliliters of normal saline are instilled into the bladder, the bladder is drained, and 40 ml of 0.4 M KCl solution is instilled. The patient is asked to rate pain and urgency from each instillation on a 0–5 scale. An increase in pain or urgency scale response of 2 or more to KCl is considered positive for increased permeability. Although positive results were noted in patients with other conditions that increase bladder permeability, such as bacterial and radiation cystitis, the authors believed a positive PST in combination with symptoms of frequency, urgency, and pain in the absence of other disease was adequate to confirm an IC diagnosis. However, a negative PST does not exclude IC as not all patients with cystoscopic evidence of IC will exhibit a positive PST.[17] Controversy exists about the diagnostic certainty of the PST. Kuo, in a study of 196 women with urgency-frequency syndrome, found that only 34% of those with a positive PST had cystoscopic findings consistent with IC.[32] Overall, the false-positive rate for the diagnosis of IC by PST is reported to be less than 2% while the false-negative rate remains unknown.[33]

Finally, lactulose and rhamnose are being tested as a "nonpainful" measure of bladder permeability.[34] These and other reports suggest that a positive permeability test, though not pathognomonic for IC, may help support the diagnosis.

Urodynamic testing (UDT). To meet the current NIH-NIDDK research criteria, a patient must undergo UDT.[3] However, during the Kyoto meeting in 2003 many investigators questioned the utility of UDT in IC diagnosis.[35] No specific urodynamic values define IC. Patients with IC routinely experience early first sensation on filling, early first desire to void and/or strong desire to void at low bladder volumes. In addition, they exhibit a low cystometric capacity associated with pain on filling. Results from the ICDB demonstrate that volume at first sensation to void is inversely proportional to daytime frequency. Those with daytime frequency greater than 15 exhibited first sensation to void at 74 ± 61 ml and maximum cystometric capacity 184 ± 114 ml compared to 114 ± 81 ml and 244 ± 149 ml in those voiding more than five times while awake.[36] Similar trends were seen for 24-h frequency. The volume at first sensation to void is markedly reduced in the presence of Hunner's ulcers: 34.7 ± 20.5.[28] Finally, although listed as an NIH-NIDDK exclusion criterion, the ICDB study demonstrated that 14% of IC patients have detrusor overactivity.

Diagnostic markers. Currently there is no diagnostic marker for IC. Symptom criteria supported by cystoscopic findings and/or permeability testing remain the primary

SECTION 11 Irritative conditions of the genitourinary tract

diagnostic means. Research to examine potential markers for IC in urine, serum, and/or bladder biopsy specimens is ongoing. These include but are not limited to urinary APF, noradrenalin, IGF binding protein-3, EGF, HB-EGF, CGMP, IL-6, and glycoprotein 51 (GP51). Urinary leukotriene E4, eosinophil protein X, IL-6, and CD45R0 positive leukocytes may be useful as markers for disease progression. Serum markers currently under investigation include HB-EGF and EGF. Finally, bladder cell fraction of stretch-activated ATP release, IL-4 gene variants, nitric oxide synthase, and mast cell activation are also being evaluated. Currently the most promising marker is urine APF level and as research develops, this may serve as a pathognomonic marker for IC.[37,38]

TREATMENT

At present there is no cure for IC. Treatment goals are directed toward managing symptoms and/or inducing remission by healing the urothelium. To date, only two medications have FDA approval for the treatment of IC: oral pentosan polysulfate (PPS) and intravesical dimethyl sulfoxide (DMSO). However, these medications are not effective in all IC patients. Therefore most practitioners use a multimodal approach to treatment which includes behavioral, pharmacologic, and surgical modes of therapy. It is our experience that a team approach is often needed to fully address the complex issues associated with IC. This may include supplemental stress management, sex counseling, nutritional counseling, physical therapy, and pain management.

Behavioral treatment.
Initial management of IC includes behavioral measures such as bladder retraining, dietary modification, and treatment of high tone pelvic floor muscle dysfunction.

Bladder retraining includes increasing the voiding interval with timed toileting.[39] Initially a 24-hour voiding diary is recorded. Patients are then asked to add an additional 15–30 minutes to their voiding interval every 3–4 weeks, until a 3–4-hour period between voids is achieved. In a study of 42 IC patients, Chaiken et al employed timed toileting with pelvic floor muscle exercises and audio relaxation tapes. After 3 months of treatment, voiding diary data revealed that 98% had a significant decrease in the number of voids per day while 71% had a significant increase in their functional bladder capacity.[40]

Approximately 51–60% of IC patients can identify foods or beverages that exacerbate their IC symptoms within 4 hours of ingestion.[22] These are listed in Box 26.3. Although the mechanism of symptom exacerbation is unknown, studies have shown a relationship between substances that produce acidic urine and exacerbation of IC symptoms.[22] Many clinicians recommend elimination of these substances

---

Box 26.3   Consumables associated with lower urinary tract symptoms

Foods to avoid

- Alcoholic beverages
- Aspartame
- Carbonated beverages
- Cheese
- Chili
- Chocolate
- Coffee
- Citrus fruit
- Spicy foods
- Tomato
- Tea
- Vinegar/condiments containing vinegar

Foods to limit

- Apples/apple juice
- Avocados
- Bananas
- Beans
- Cantaloupe melon
- Corned beef
- Cranberries
- Grapes
- Nuts (except almonds and cashews)
- Peaches
- Pineapple
- Plums
- Prunes/raisins
- Sour cream
- Rye bread
- Yogurt

---

from the diet.[41] Patients are able to identify specific food sensitivities by adding them back to their diet one at a time. In a prospective open label trial of 203 IC patients with food-related flares, Bologna et al reported a significant reduction in urgency and pain when these substances were consumed with 1.32 g calcium glycerophosphate (Prelief™).[22]

Treatment of HT-PFD.
The role of musculoskeletal involvement in chronic pelvic pain syndromes is just starting to be investigated. Normally, a reflex increase in pelvic floor muscle tone occurs during bladder filling as a result of stimulation of sensory afferents for stretch, which contributes to urinary continence; this is called the guarding

reflex. In IC, HT-PFD is theorized to result from a sustained guarding reflex, caused by increased C-fiber afferent activity leading to a tonic somatic efferent response.[27] HT-PFD in turn contributes to urgency/frequency and possibly pain.

In a pilot study of 16 IC patients with HT-PFD and sacroiliac malalignment, 94% exhibited improvement in irritative voiding symptoms and dyspareunia after treatment for HT-PFD.[42] Therapy included myofascial release, joint mobilization, muscle energy techniques, strengthening, stretching, neuromuscular reeducation, and home exercises. Thiele massage is initiated after realignment of the sacrum and ileum to restore normal tension to the pelvic floor musculature.[42] This technique involves myofascial release of trigger points through either a transvaginal or a transanal approach. A study of 21 IC patients with HT-PFD employing Thiele massage twice a week for 5 weeks noted a significant improvement in QOL scales that was maintained for at least 4.5 months following treatment.[43] Patients with persistent HT-PFD are prescribed biofeedback with functional electrical stimulation (FES). The goal of biofeedback is to break the cycle of muscle spasm by facilitating conscious control of pelvic floor muscle contraction and relaxation. The addition of FES has been demonstrated to significantly reduce detrusor overactivity in studies of patients with urge or mixed incontinence.[44,45] Although no studies are published to date, there is an ongoing randomized controlled trial addressing the role of FES in IC management. Trigger point injections of 1% lidocaine and/or corticosteroid into contracted pelvic floor muscles may be useful prior to internal massage in the recalcitrant patient.

Pharmacologic therapy (Table 26.1)
Oral agents
PENTOSAN POLYSULFATE. Pentosan polysulfate (PPS) is a heparin-like compound which is similar to the GAGs in the urothelium. It is hypothesized to replace the defective GAG layer of the urothelium, thus decreasing bladder permeability. Recent work by Chiang et al demonstrated that PPS also functions as a mast cell stabilizer,[46] potentially decreasing neurogenic inflammation. PPS is the only FDA-approved oral medication for the relief of bladder pain associated with IC. It is dosed 100 mg t.i.d. or 200 mg b.i.d. It takes 6–8 weeks for initial symptom relief and 6 months may be required for clinical improvement.

In an open label trial of 2809 IC patients, Hanno demonstrated a 42–62% improvement in pain and urgency after 3 months of treatment. He also reported continued benefit and a low occurrence of side effects (alopecia, headache, GI distress) with 3 years of continued treatment.[47] Placebo-controlled trials of PPS in the United States have demonstrated mixed results. In a study of 62 patients with

IC, Parsons et al reported a statistically significant improvement in subjective frequency, urgency, nocturia, and pain as well as an increase in voided volume when compared to controls.[48] In a subsequent study of 148 IC patients, 38% noted a >50% reduction in pain after 3 months on PPS compared to 18% receiving placebo.[49] However, a recent placebo-controlled study of 121 patients from the IC Clinical Trials Group (ICCTG) demonstrated only a slight improvement with PPS compared to placebo; these numbers failed to reach clinical significance.[50] This may have been due to the "cross-over" study design. The authors allowed patients taking hydroxyzine (a mast cell stabilizer) into the placebo group, assuming that the two drugs had different mechanisms of action. However, recent studies suggest PPS may also play a role in mast cell stabilization,[46] thereby possibly confounding the findings.

ANTIHISTAMINES Hydroxyzine is thought to provide symptom relief by mast cell stabilization, anticholinergic effects, and sedation. To date, there are limited reports on the efficacy of hydroxyzine in IC symptom relief. In an open label study of 90 IC patients given 25–75 mg of hydroxyzine daily, an average of 40% reduction in symptom score was noted over 3 months.[51] In a recent placebo-controlled trial of 121 patients, no statistically significant difference was found between placebo and 50 mg/day hydroxyzine after 24 weeks of treatment.[50] Again, these data may be affected by the inclusion of patients taking PPS in the control group.

ANTIDEPRESSANTS. Tricyclic antidepressants provide central and peripheral anticholinergic effects, block the reuptake of serotonin and norepinepherine, and provide H1-receptor blocking activity. Recent placebo-controlled trials as well as long term open label studies of the effect of Amitriptyline in IC, show it effective per urgency/frequency and pain.[52,53] Dosing should start at 10 mg and may be increased up to 100 mg HS at 2–3 week intervals. Selective serotonin reuptake inhibitors may also be used.

OTHER ORAL AGENTS. Gabapentin is an anticonvulsant proven effective in mediating neuropathic pain syndromes, including those from genitourinary origin. Muscle relaxants like hyoscyamine and tizanidine may be beneficial in relief of pain due to bladder spasm and HT-PFD; these may also provide anticholinergic effects which may decrease urgency/frequency. Detrusor-selective anticholinergics such as oxybutinin and tolteridine may provide symptom relief when combined with other treatments. Narcotics may be added to the treatment regimen. The amount and frequency of narcotic medication can be coordinated with a pain specialist. Finally dietary supplements such as L-arginine may be beneficial.[39] Table 26.1 provides dosing information as well as common side effects of these medications.

SECTION 11 Irritative conditions of the genitourinary tract

Table 26.1 Common medications used to treat interstitial cystitis

Medication	Symptom	Dose***	Mode of action	Common side effects	Other
Oral					
Pentosan polysulfate*	P	100 mg t.i.d. or 200 mg b.i.d.	Repair GAG layer Possible mast cell stabilization	GI distress (4%), hair loss (1–4%), elevated LFTs (1%)	Minimum 6 months for symptom relief
Hydroxyzine	U,F,P	10–75 mg daily	Inhibits mast cell release (H1-receptor blocker) Anticholinergic effects	Sedation	Often used if mast cells present on biopsy
Amitriptyline	P,U,F	10–100 mg HS	Inhibits NE and 5-HT reuptake Anticholinergic effects	Sedation Dry mouth	Tricyclic antidepressant
Nortriptyline	P,U,F	10–25 mg HS	Inhibits NE and 5-HT reuptake Anticholinergic effects	Sedation Dry mouth	Tricyclic antidepressant often better tolerated than amitriptyline
Gabapentin	P	100 mg HS: titrate to 300 mg t.i.d.	Unknown	Sedation, fatigue, dizziness	Anticonvulsant May titrate to max dose of 3600 mg daily
Oxybutinin extended release (XR)	U,F	5–30 mg q.d.	Anticholinergic	Dry mouth, constipation, headache	Contraindicated for narrow-angle glaucoma and renal or hepatic insufficiency
Tolteridine extended release (LA)	U,F	4 mg q.d.	Anticholinergic	Dry mouth, constipation, headache	Contraindicated for narrow-angle glaucoma and renal or hepatic insufficiency
Tizanidine	P	2 mg HS; may titrate to 8 mg t.i.d. as needed	α_2-adrenergic receptor agonist Smooth muscle relaxant	Sedation Dry mouth Hepatic dysfunction (3%) Visual hallucination Prolonged Q-T interval	Check LFTs for first 6 months of use Dose affected by renal insufficiency
Hyoscyamine	U,F	0.125–0.3 mg up to q.i.d.	Anticholinergic Smooth muscle relaxant	Sedation Constipation Dry mouth Blurred vision	Can have additive effects with other anti-cholinergic
Narcotics	P	Varied	Central analgesia	Sedation Constipation	
Nutraceuticals					
L-Arginine	P	1.5 g/day	Nitric oxide synthetase inhibitor		6 months for effect
Intravesical					
DMSO *	P,U,F	50 ml for 15 min weekly for 6 weeks	Unknown: possible antiinflammatory or disruption of pain pathway	Lens changes in animal studies PDR: recommends q 6 mo, CBC,Cr, LFTs	May taste/smell garlic for 72 h Instillation is painful Effects noted 3–4 weeks after 6th instillation Contraindicated for bladder Ca

P, pain; U, urgency; F, frequency; CBI, continuous bladder instillation; LFTs, liver function tests; NE, norepinephrine; 5-HT, serotonin
*FDA approved for the treatment of IC
** Our center's formula
***Additional information obtained from PDR Electronic Library 2004.1 S,Thompson-micromedex, 2004

Table 26.1 Common medications used to treat interstitial cystitis—cont'd

Medication	Symptom	Dose***	Mode of action	Common side effects	Other
Heparin cocktail	P,U,F	**10,000u heparin, 50 cc of 0.5% bupivacaine, 100 mg hydrocortisone, 80 mg gentamicin, 50 cc of 8.4% NaHCO₃ weekly for 6 weeks	Repair of GAG layer, anti-inflammatory, local analgesia	NaHCO₃ will precipitate if mixed with other ingredients before instillation	May be mixed with 1LNS and used as CBI (omit NaHCO₃ and gentamicin) for flare rescue
BCG	P,U,F	50 mg in 60 ml sterile saline	Unknown: live attenuated mycobacterium Possible local immunomodulation		Limited long-term effect in preliminary studies
Botox	U,F	300 u in 3 ml sterile saline	Blocks acetylcholine release, paralytic	Transient hematuria	Effects up to 6 months

P, pain; U, urgency; F, frequency; CBI, continuous bladder instillation; LFTs, liver function tests; NE, norepinephrine; 5-HT, serotonin
*FDA approved for the treatment of IC
** Our center's formula
***Additional information obtained from PDR Electronic Library 2004.1 S,Thompson-micromedex, 2004

Intravesical agents. DMSO is the only intravesical medication with FDA approval for IC treatment. It is administered 50 ml weekly for 6 weeks. Clinical trials demonstrate a 53–93% initial response rate after four treatments but the relapse rate is reported at between 40% and 59%, with 50–60% of relapsers responding to repeat treatment.[54] The mechanism of action is unknown; theories include interruption of the pain pathway and decreased inflammation. Intravesical heparin has also been shown beneficial in treating IC, either alone or as part of a cocktail.[54,55] Heparin is thought to help heal the defective GAG layer. The addition of a corticosteroid, bupivacaine, and gentamicin may decrease inflammation, provide local analgesia, and prevent infection, respectively.

Preliminary studies of intravesical bacillus Calmette-Guerin (BCG)[56] and resiniferotoxin (RTX) demonstrated short-term benefit in IC patients however recent multi center randomized controlled trials failed to demonstrate significant improvement over placebo.[57,58] Similarly, initial open label studies found hyaluronic acid beneficial to IC patients, however more recent placebo-controlled trials in the United States failed to show a significant difference over controls (personal communication, publication pending).

Surgical treatment. BOD was demonstrated to provide symptom relief in 30–54% of patients for up to 6 months, when the bladder was distended at 80 cmH₂O for 8 minutes.[31] The mechanism of benefit is unknown. Some theories include ischemic or mechanical damage to the bladder's submucosal nerve plexus, exhaustion of C-fiber neurotransmitters (substance P), and widespread mast cell degranulation with exhaustion of inflammatory mediators.[55]

Sacral neuromodulation has been shown to decrease LUTS in patients recalcitrant to anticholinergic therapy. A recent open label study of 21 refractory IC patients demonstrated a 60–70% reduction in subjective pain, frequency, and urgency as well as a 50–60% objective improvement in frequency based on voiding diary data.[59] Other studies have demonstrated similar results.[60,61] The exact mechanism of action is unknown but it is thought to cause a disruption of sensory afferent input to the pontine micturition center. The technique involves transcutaneous placement of an electrode into the S3 foramen, either unilaterally or bilaterally. The electrode is then tested for efficacy by an external impulse generator. If patients experience a >50% objective symptom improvement by voiding diary and questionnaire data, an internal pulse generator is placed. Reported complications are small but include lead migration, local wound complication, implant site pain, and change in pain location.[61]

Botulinum neurotoxin type A (BTX) has demonstrated recent success in treatment of refractory urgency/frequency.[62] The technique involves transurethral intramural injection of the trigone. Symptom relief is reported for up to 6 months. Continued research will determine the exact extent of the benefit that BTX may offer.

Lumbar sympathetic epidural nerve blocks may assist in managing chronic pain.[63] In addition, a differential epidural nerve block may help distinguish somatic and psychogenic pain.[2] A pain management specialist should be skilled in both of these techniques.

Major surgical intervention is reserved for intractable cases after all other therapeutic modalities have been exhausted and a psychologic evaluation as well as a differential epidural block to rule out psychogenic pain has been performed. Interventions include urinary diversion and partial cystectomy with augmentation enterocystoplasty. Given the risk of recurrent pain, augmentation enterocystoplasty should be reserved for patients with classic/ulcerative IC.[64,65]

Success rates of up to 70% are reported for urinary diversion.[2,54] Surgical approaches include continent (pouch) or incontinent (ileal loop) diversion either with or without cystourethrectomy. There are reports of recurrent symptoms as well as pouch spasm in continent diversions which have led some surgeons to recommend incontinent loops. The etiology of symptom recurrence is unknown. Reported complications from the in situ bladder post diversion include pyocystitis, hemorrhage, severe pain, and bladder spasm.[66] Persistent pain from urethral remnants has been reported.[65]

Finally, alternative therapies such as nutraceuticals, Chinese herbs, and acupuncture may provide additional symptom relief in the recalcitrant patient.[39]

CONCLUSION

In spite of recent interest in the natural progression and etiology of IC, relatively little is known. The criteria established by the NIH-NIDDK in 1988 to standardize research protocols are now being questioned. There is consensus that future IC research should focus on validating the diagnostic criteria of IC as well as the criteria used for research protocols. It has been suggested that since pain is the hallmark of IC, control groups in future IC studies might be limited to those with urgency-frequency syndrome.[67] This debate may be settled if a biologic marker is validated for IC diagnosis, the most promising of which is APF. Future DNA studies of bladder biopsies may also provide the key to both the etiology and natural progression of IC. Until then, thoughtful examination of the clinical criteria we currently use to define IC should be undertaken.

REFERENCES

1. Parsons JK, Parsons CL. The historical origins of interstitial cystitis. J Urol 2004;17(1):20–22.
2. Bologna RA, Tu LM, Whitmore KE. Hypersensitivity disorders of the lower urinary tract. In: Walters MD, Karram MM, eds. Urogynecology and reconstructive pelvic surgery. St Louis: Mosby; 1999.
3. Striker GE. Division of Kidney, Urologic, and Hematologic Diseases (DKUHD) of the National Institute of Diabetes and Digestive and Kidney Diseases (NIDDK): diagnostic criteria for research studies (interstitial cystitis). Am J Kidney Dis 1989;13:353–354.
4. Hanno PM, Landis JR, Matthews-Cooke Y, et al. The diagnosis of interstitial cystitis revisited: lessons learned from the National Institute of Health Interstitial Cystitis Database Study. J Urol 1999;161:553–557.
5. Profert KJ, Schaeffer AJ, Bresnsinger CM, et al. A prospective study of interstitial cystitis: results of a longitudinal follow up of the interstitial cystitis data base cohort. J Urol 2000;163: 1434–1439.
6. Curhan GC, Speizer FE, Hunter DJ, et al. Epidemiology of interstitial cystitis: a population based study. J Urol 1999;161:549–552.
7. Tomaszewski JE, Landis R, Russack V, et al. Biopsy features are associated with primary symptoms in interstitial cystitis: results from the interstitial cystitis data base study. Urology 2001;57(Suppl 6A):67–81.
8. Roseamilia A, Igawa Y, Higashi S. Pathology of interstitial cystitis. Int J Urol 2003;10:S11–S15.
9. Lukban JC, Parkin JV, Holzberg AS, et al. Interstitial cystitis and pelvic floor dysfunction: a comprehensive review. Pain Med 2001;2(1):60–71.
10. Westropp JL, Buffington CA. In vivo models of interstitial cystitis. J Urol 2002;167:694–702.
11. Slobodov G, Feloney M, Gran C, et al. Abnormal expression of molecular markers for bladder impermeability and differentiation in the urothelium of patients with interstitial cystitis. J Urol 2004;171:1554–1558.
12. Parsons CL, Greenberger M, Gabal L, et al. The role of urinary potassium in the pathogenesis and diagnosis of interstitial cystitis. J Urol 1998;159:1862–1867.
13. Theoharides TC, Kempuraj D, Sant GR. Mast cell involvement in interstitial cystitis: a review of human and experimental evidence. Urology 2001;57(Suppl 6A):47–55.
14. Peeker R, Enerback L, Fall M, et al. Recruitment, distribution and phenotypes of mast cells in interstitial cystitis. J Urol 2000;163:1009–1015.
15. Pang X, Marchand J, Sant GR, et al. Increased number of substance P positive nerve fibers in interstitial cystitis. Br J Urol 1995;75:744–750.
16. Keay S, Zhang CO, Chai T, et al. Antiproliferative factor, heparin-binding epidermal growth factor-like growth factor and epidermal growth factor in men and women with interstitial cystitis verses chronic pelvic pain syndrome. Urology 2004;63:22–26.
17. Keay S, Zhang CO, Shoenfelt JO, et al. Decreased in vitro proliferation of bladder epithelial cells from patients with interstitial cystitis. Urology 2003;61:1278–1284.
18. Van De Merwe JP, Yamada T, Sakamoto Y. Systemic aspects of interstitial cystitis, immunology and linkage with autoimmune disorders. Int J Urol 2003;10:S35–S38.
19. Abrams P, Cardozo L, Fall M, et al. The standardization of terminology in lower urinary tract function: report from the standardization sub-committee of the International Continence Society. Urology 2003;61:37–49.
20. Lutgendorf SK, Kreder KJ, Rothrock NE, et al. Stress and symptomatology in patients with interstitial cystitis: a laboratory stress model. J Urol 2000;164:1265–1269.
21. Koizol JA, Clark DC, Gittes R, et al. The natural history of interstitial cystitis: a survey of 374 patients. J Urol 1993;149:465–469.
22. Bologna RA, Gomelsky A, Lukban JC, et al. The efficacy of calcium glycerophosphate in the prevention of food related flares in interstitial cystitis. NIDDK Interstitial Cystitis and Bladder Research Symposium, 2000, Minneapolis.

23. O'Leary MP, Sant GR, Fowler FJ, et al. The interstitial cystitis symptom index and problem index. Urology 1997;49(Suppl 5A):58–63.

24. Parsons CL, Dell J, Stanford EJ, et al. Increased prevalence of interstitial cystitis: previously unrecognized urologic and gynecologic cases using a new symptom questionnaire and intravesical potassium sensitivity. Urology 2002;60:573–578.

25. Bade J, Ishizula O, Yoshida M. Future research needs for the definition/diagnosis of interstitial cystitis. Int J Urol 2003;10:S31–S34.

26. Claydon CS. The evaluation of pelvic organ prolapse. J Pelvic Med Surg 2004;10(4):173–192.

27. Lukban JC, Whitmore KE. Pelvic floor muscle re-education. Treatment of the overactive and painful bladder syndrome. Clin Obstet Gynecol 2002;45(1):273–285.

28. Nigro DA, Wein AJ, Foy M, et al. Associations among cystoscopic and urodynamic findings from women enrolled in the interstitial cystitis data base (ICDB) study. Urology 1997;49(Suppl 5A):86–92.

29. Payne CK, Terai A, Komatsu K. Research criteria verses clinical criteria for interstitial cystitis. Int J Urol 2003;10:S7–S10.

30. Rabe HH, Gotoh M, Momose H. The place of cystoscopy and hydrodistension in the diagnosis of interstitial cystitis: a potpourri of opinions emanating from an international consultation on IC in Kyoto, Japan, March 28–30, 2003. Int J Urol 2003;10:S16–S18.

31. Hanno PM, Wein AJ. Conservative therapy of interstitial cystitis. Semin Urol 1991;9:143–147.

32. Kuo HC. Urodynamic study and potassium sensitivity test for women with frequency-urgency syndrome and interstitial cystitis. Urol Int 2003;71:61–65.

33. Parsons CL, Forrest J, Nickel JC, et al. Effect of pentosan polysulfate therapy on intravesical potassium sensitivity. Urology 2002;59:329–333.

34. Erikson DR, Herb N, Ordille S. et al. A new direct test of bladder permeability. J Urol 2000;164:419–422.

35. Irwin PP, Takei M, Sugino Y. Summary of the Urodynamics workshop on IC, Kyoto, Japan. Int J Urol 2003;10:S19–S23.

36. Kirkemo A, Peabody M, Diokno AC, et al. Associations among urodynamic findings and symptoms in women enrolled in the interstitial cystitis data base (ICDB) study. Urology 1997;49(Suppl 5A):76–80.

37. Erikson DR, Xie SX, Bhavaadan VP, et al. A comparison of multiple urine markers for interstitial cystitis. J Urol 2002;167:2461–2469.

38. Keay S, Takeda M, Tamaki M, et al. Current and future directions on diagnostic markers in interstitial cystitis. Int J Urol 2003;10:S27–S30.

39. Whitmore KE. Complementary and alternative therapies as treatment approaches for interstitial cystitis. Rev Urol 2002;4(Suppl 1):S28–S35.

40. Chaiken DC, Blavis JG. Behavioral therapy for the treatment of refractory interstitial cystitis. J Urol 1993;149:1445–1448.

41. Rovner E, Propert KJ, Brensinger C, et al. Treatments used in women with interstitial cystitis: the interstitial cystitis data base (ICDB) study experience. Urology 2000;56:940–945.

42. Lukban JC, Whitmore KE, Kellogg-Spadt S, et al. The effect of manual physical therapy in patients with interstitial cystitis, high tone pelvic floor dysfunction, and sacroiliac joint dysfunction. NIDDK Interstitial Cystitis and Bladder Research Symposium, 2000, Minneapolis.

43. Oyama IA, Rejba A, Fletcher E, et al. Modified Thiele massage as a therapeutic intervention for female interstitial cystitis patients with high-tone pelvic floor dysfunction. Urol, 2004;64(5):862–865.

44. Brubaker L, Benson JT, Clark A, et al. Transvaginal electrical stimulation for female urinary incontinence. Am J Gynecol 1997;177:536–540.

45. Yamanishi T, Yasuda K, Sakakibara R, et al. Randomized double-blind study of electrical stimulation for urinary incontinence due to detrusor overactivity. Urology 2000;55:353–357.

46. Chiang G, Patra P, Letourneau R, et al. Pentosan polysulfate inhibits mast cell histamine secretion and intracellular calcium ion levels: an alternative explanation of its beneficial effects in interstitial cystitis. J Urol 2000;164:2119–2125.

47. Hanno PM. Analysis of long-term elmiron therapy for interstitial cystitis. Urology 1997;49 (Suppl):93–99.

48. Parsons CL, Mulholland SG. Successful therapy of interstitial cystitis with pentosan polysulfate. J Urol 1987;138:513–516.

49. Parsons CL, Benson G, Childs SJ, et al. A quantitatively controlled method to study prospectively interstitial cystitis and demonstrate the efficacy of pentosan polysulfate. J Urol 1993;150:845–848.

50. Sant GR, Popert KJ, Hanno PM, et al. A pilot clinical trial of oral pentosan polysulfate and oral hydroxyzine in patients with interstitial cystitis. J Urol 2003;170:810–815.

51. Theoharides TC, Sant GR. Hydroxyzine therapy for interstitial cystitis. Urology 1997;49(Suppl 5A):108–110.

52. VanOphoven A, Pokupic S, Heinecke A, et al. A prospective randomized, placebo controlled, double-blind study of amytriptyline for the treatment of interstitial cystitis. J Urol 2004;172(2):533–536.

53. VanOphoven A, Hertle L. Long-term results of amytriptyline treatment for interstitial cystitis. J Urol 2005;174(5):1837–1840.

54. Parkin J, Shea C, Sant GR. Intravesical dimethyl sulfoxide (DMSO) for interstitial cystitis: a practical approach. Urology 1997;49(Suppl 5A):105–107.

55. Lukban JC, Whitmore KE, Sant GR. Current management of interstitial cystitis. Urol Clin North Am 2002;29:649–660.

56. Peters KM, Doikno AC, Steinert BW, et al. The efficacy of intravesical bacillus calmette guerin in the treatment of interstitial cystitis: long-term follow-up. J Urol 1998;159(5):1483–1486.

57. Mayer R, Propert KJ, Peters KM, et al. A randomized controlled trial of intravesical bacillus calmette-guerin for treatment refractory interstitial cystitis. J Urol 2005;173(4):1186–1191.

58. Peters KM, Carey JM, Konstandt DB. Sacral neuromodulation for the treatment of refractory interstitial cystitis: outcomes based on technique. Int Urogynecol J 2003;14:223–228.

59. Payne CK, Mosbaugh PG, Forrest JB, et al. Intravesical resiniferatoxin for the treatment of interstitial cystitis: a randomized, double blind, placebo controlled trial. J Urol 2005;173(5):1590–1594.

60. Whitmore KE, Payne CK, Diokno AC, et al. Sacral neuromodulation in patients with interstitial cystitis; a multicentered trial. Int Urogynecol J 2003;14:305–309.

61. Seigel S, Paszkiewicz E, Kirkpatrick C, et al. Sacral nerve modulation in patients with chronic intractable pelvic pain. J Urol 2001;166:1742–1745.

62. Rapp DE, Lucioni A, Katz EE, et al. Use of botulinum-A toxin for the treatment of refractory overactive bladder symptoms: an initial experience. Urology 2004;63:1071–1075.

63. Irwin PP, Hammond WD, Galloway NT. Lumbar epidural blockade for management of pain in interstitial cystisis. Br J Urol 1993;71(4):413–416.

64. Peeker R, Aldenborg F, Fall M. The treatment of interstitial cystitis with supratrigonal cystectomy and ileocystoplasty: difference in outcome between classic and non-ulcer disease. J Urol 1998;159(5):1479–1482.

65. Chakravarti A, Ganta S, Somani B, et al. Caecocystoplasty for intractable interstitial cystitis: long term results. Eur Urol 2004;46:114–117.

66. Adeyoju AB, Thornhill J, Lynch T, et al. The fate of the defunctioned bladder following supravesical urinary diversion. Br J Urol 1996;78(1):80–83.

67. Bade J, Ishizuka O, Yoshida M. Future research needs for the definition/diagnosis of interstitial cystitis. Int J Urol 2003;10:S31–S34.

Chronic Pelvic Pain: Diagnosis and Management

Malcolm Lucas, Andrew Pickersgill and Anthony R B Smith

INTRODUCTION

Chronic pelvic pain is a clinical enigma that, whilst often leading to utter despair on the part of the sufferer, regrettably often engenders responses in clinicians varying from bored lack of interest to avoidance and denial. This probably reflects the frustration felt by clinicians who usually prefer the reassurance of dealing with recognizable pathology and conventional medical models of care. Such frustration is not surprising as many cases of pelvic pain are difficult to explain and extremely difficult to treat effectively. This chapter will present a conceptual framework for some of the mechanisms involved together with a pragmatic guide to management based, as far as is possible, on evidence.

A CONCEPTUAL FRAMEWORK

Pain models. Much has been written about chronic pain and numerous models have been proposed for defining and categorizing the condition. The traditional biomedical model holds that pain is a physiologic response of the body to tissue damage or a pathologic process and that any psychologic response is secondary. The corollary of this would be that if no pathology can be found, the pain would be said to be psychologic in origin—or psychosomatic. This is an outmoded, often stigmatizing concept that is of little help to many patients except those with readily identifiable causes. Most workers would now prefer the biopsychosocial model which recognizes that pain is a complex subjective, sensory and emotional experience which can be affected by many factors including physiologic, social and cultural conditions.[1] This is a more useful concept, the acceptance of which implies the need for multidisciplinary skills in the provision of care.

The traditional biomedical model, however, still forms the basis of a great deal of our structured thinking about chronic pain and has to be understood by medical practitioners in detail. Within this model we recognize the existence of *somatic* pain, which is mediated by sensory fibers, is well localized and in which referred pain is rare. An example would be pain from a hernia, an injury or fracture. Visceral pain, on the other hand, is typically poorly localized, mediated by autonomic nerves and referred pain is common. The pain associated with constipation is typical of this route of pain mediation.

Any pain which is chronic (defined by the pain societies as lasting more than 6 months) may in addition become "centralized." This phenomenon, presumably caused by the "overuse" of certain pain pathways, becomes upregulated and no longer requires the same intensity of stimulus, or indeed any stimulus at all, to generate the pain. This is known as "wind-up" or centralization of pain and has two recognized stages.

- *Hyperalgesia*: the pain response is more intense and prolonged than would be expected from the type of stimulus.
- *Allodynia*: the pain response occurs spontaneously from nonnoxious stimuli such as the touch of clothing or a cotton wool ball. This type of centralization is extremely common in chronic pelvic pain.

Pelvic and genitourinary pain terminology. The plethora of terms used to describe subtle clinical variations of genitourinary pain has led to much confusion and obscurity. The term "urethral syndrome," for instance, though widely used, may mean quite a different thing to a gynecologist than to a urologist and may be little different in meaning from, say, "urethrotrigonitis." Neither term conveys meaning to fellow clinicians or to patients. Academics will argue about the relative features of "vaginismus" versus "dyspareunia",[2] a semantic debate which most sufferers would regard as esoteric and unhelpful. Such expressions have sometimes evolved with the aim of offering precision in diagnosis, sometimes completely the opposite, and occasionally deliberately to obfuscate with jargon. Other examples are shown in Box 27.1.

The International Continence Society has tried to address this issue and introduced a new system of terminology

Box 27.1 Obsolete terminology

Urethral syndrome

Trigonitis

Urethrotrigonitis

Strangury

Dysuria

Bladder spasm

Interstitial cystitis

Vulvodynia

Vaginismus

Vestibulitis

Vestibulodynia

Dysesthesia

Hunner's ulcer

Frequency-urgency dysuria syndrome

Urethritis

Detrusor mastocytosis

Cystitis parenchymatosa

Other related terms

Pelvic fibromyalgia

Pelvic congestion syndrome

Proctalgia fugax

Levator ani syndrome

Pudendal neuralgia

Coccygodynia

which, though simplistic in concept, helps to clarify meaning. The full detail can be found at the website *www.icsoffice.org* but in summary the principles (relating to women only) are as follows.

The symptom of pain should be defined in relation to its anatomic site such that:

- *bladder pain* is felt suprapubically or retropubically, and usually increases with bladder filling and may persist after voiding
- *urethral pain* is felt in the urethra and the woman indicates the urethra as the site
- *vulval pain* is felt in and around the external genitalia
- *vaginal pain* is felt internally, above the introitus
- *perineal pain* is felt between the posterior fourchette (posterior lip of the introitus) and the anus
- *pelvic pain* is less well defined than, for example, bladder, urethral or perineal pain and is less clearly related to the micturition cycle or to bowel function and is not localized to any single pelvic organ
- *anal pain* is felt in or around the anal canal.

There are some problems with this. Not all pain is so readily localizable in site though the factors that trigger it may be organ specific. Nor does this scheme allow for pain felt in the pelvic ring or in the suprapubic region. Pain may occur in numerous sites which together make up a pattern for that individual. It would be useful to describe the triggers of pain separately from the site. For instance, bladder filling or vaginal penetration may induce spastic and painful contraction of the pelvic floor. How would this pain be classified?

Pain syndromes. The ICS has tried to identify pain syndromes which describe functional abnormalities where a precise cause has not been defined. "Syndromes describe constellations, or varying combinations of symptoms, but cannot be used for precise diagnosis. The use of the word syndrome can only be justified if there is at least one other symptom in addition to the symptom used to describe the syndrome." It is presumed therefore that a diagnostic process has taken place that excludes other recognized causes of pain, a process of exclusion (see Table 27.1). Each of the "syndromes" described requires, within its definition, that all other identifiable pathology and signs of infection have been eliminated.

Most women experience some *uterine pain* in association with menstruation. The severity ranges from mild and transient at the onset of menstruation to severe and debilitating pain predating menstruation and continuing until the loss has ceased. The pain is typically a cramp-like spasmodic pain. Terms such as primary and secondary dysmenorrhea are generally unhelpful and the focus in managing such pain should be on defining whether there is evidence of uterine or other pelvic pathology. Fibroids and intramural endometriosis are the most common uterine pathologies seen, the former being relatively obvious on ultrasound imaging. Menstrual loss is often increased in association with more painful menstruation. A woman presenting with increased menstrual loss should have the cause of the heavy loss determined (pathologic, hematologic, and endocrine).

Painful bladder syndrome is the complaint of suprapubic pain related to bladder filling, accompanied by other symptoms such as increased daytime and nighttime frequency, in the absence of proven urinary infection or other obvious pathology. The ICS believes this to be a preferable term to "interstitial cystitis" which is a very specific diagnosis (see Chapter 26) with which many patients with a painful bladder syndrome will not conform.[3] The traditional definition of interstitial cystitis by the National Institute of Diabetes, Digestive and Kidney Diseases (NIDDK)[4] was established to help researchers standardize the patient group that they were researching. Whilst this helped with the science, it effectively disenfranchised many patients who shared the syndrome but failed to meet all diagnostic criteria. We now recognize that few patients actually have a true ulcer[3] and

Table 27.1 Diagnostic measures for the identification of underlying causes of pelvic pain syndrome

Condition	History	Examination	Cultures	Imaging	Endoscopy	Urodynamics	PST	Histology	Special tests
Bladder									
Bacterial UTI	y		y						Special cultures
Fistula	y	y		Contrast study	Cyst				
Stone	y			Plain film or US	Cyst				
CIS					Cyst			y	
"IC"	y		y		Cyst		y	y	
Radiation cystitis	y				Cyst				
Bladder endometriosis	y				Cyst		y		
TB	Y		y		Cyst				
Diverticulum				Contrast study or US	Cyst				
Cyclophosphamide	y								
Tiaprofenic acid	y								
Urethral caruncle		Y							
Detrusor overactivity						y			
Genital/vaginal/pelvic									
Endometriosis				US	Lap			y	
Fibroids				US	Lap				
Pelvic inflammatory disease	Y		y		Lap				
Tubovarian abscess		y		US					
Salpingitis		y							
Malignancy		y		US				y	
Pelvic adhesions					Lap				
Pelvic congestion/pelvic varices				US/MR/Doppler	Lap				
Ovarian cyst		y		US					
Ectopic pregnancy	y			US					
Anatomic abnormalities, e.g. non-communicating rudimentary horn vaginal atresia				y					
Other peritoneal causes, e.g. chronic inflammation								y	
Iatrogenic, e.g. IUCD Vulvodynia									

Table 27.1 Diagnostic measures for the identification of underlying causes of pelvic pain syndrome—cont'd

Condition	History	Examination	Cultures	Imaging	Endoscopy	Urodynamics	PST	Histology	Special tests
Anorectal									
Constipation	y	y		Plain film					
Fissure	y	y			Sig				
Anal or rectal carcinoma	y	y			Sig			y	
Inflammatory bowel disease	y			Contrast studies	Sig			y	
Irritable bowel syndrome	y								
Appendicitis	y	y			Lap				
Hernia	y	y		US/CT					
Neurologic									
Conus or root lesion	y	y		MRI					
Nerve entrapment	y	y							
Psychosocial problems									
Depression	y								
Sexual abuse	y								
Substance abuse	y								
Eating disorder	y								
Need for contraception	y								
School avoidance	y								
General medical									
Vascular, e.g. Raynaud's	y	y							y
Sjögren's	y	y							y
SLE	y	y							y
RA	y	y							y
Cutaneous disease	y	y						y	

that glomerulations may be seen in asymptomatic women. Classic histologic features, such as mast cell infiltration, are often absent in women who otherwise share the same clinical syndrome. The ICS and other recent publications have recommended abandoning the term interstitial cystitis or at least relaxing the criteria for diagnosis.[5,6] There have been three consensus meetings on the diagnosis of painful bladder syndrome recently which have brought some agreement to the process of diagnosis.[7-9]

Urethral pain syndrome describes the combination of pain felt in the urethra associated with other lower urinary tract symptoms or sexual symptoms, in the absence of known pathology or proven urinary tract infection. The term "urethral syndrome" has been used for years by some to represent the same thing but there is confusion because others would use this term to describe early symptoms of interstitial cystitis. Difficulty arises from the inadequacy of definition of urine infection and there is recognition that insistence on 10^5 organisms per HPF is too dogmatic for asymptomatic women.[10]

Vulval pain syndrome, vaginal, perineal, perianal and pelvic pain syndrome all describe the combination of pain at the anatomic site associated either with the micturition cycle or with symptoms suggestive of urinary tract or sexual dysfunction in the absence of proven infection or other obvious pathology. Vulval pain may be generalized or specific, characterized by the degree to which a point of tenderness can be defined.

CAUSES OF CHRONIC PELVIC PAIN

Conventionally, an understanding of etiology is important because it directs treatment strategy. There are, of course, important recognized causes of pelvic pain which are summarized in Table 27.1. The pelvic pain syndromes remain more of an enigma, however, with numerous putative mechanisms involved.

Much has been written about the etiology of "interstitial cystitis" and rather less about the pain syndromes described above. It is helpful to the clinician to think in terms of interrelationships of causation rather than attempting always to categorize. This helps to provide a framework for diagnosis, just as the use of a urodynamic mindset for describing bladder and urethral dysfunction helped the management of incontinence.

Potential etiologic causes for any pelvic pain syndrome include infection and inflammation, physical trauma, the effects of local hypoxia, autoimmune abnormalities, and neurogenic dystrophy. The possible mechanisms involved in the genesis of interstitial cystitis have been discussed in Chapter 26.

Pelvic floor dysfunction. The pelvic floor muscle complex is essential for the support of the pelvic organs and the prevention of incontinence. These muscles may become underactive, as seen in incontinence and prolapse, but may also become overactive. Overactive pelvic floor muscles will cause difficulty with voiding (urine or stool) and an increasing problem with constipation and urinary retention. This is a vicious cycle which may exacerbate the underlying pelvic floor "spasm."[11] It may result from habitual avoidance of voiding or defecation, for instance in jobs which do not permit ready access to a toilet, and may be related to psychosocial problems, including anxieties about sex. There is a recognized association with a history of sexual abuse in earlier life, though this association must never be assumed.[12,13] An overactive pelvic floor will result in aching and pain.[14-16]

There will often be triggers for the pain which bear no direct relationship to the etiology; for instance, sexual

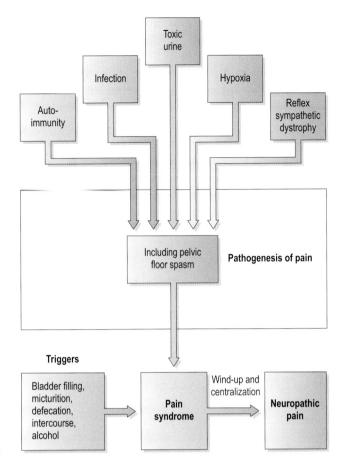

Figure 27.1 A conceptual model of the relationship between underlying etiologies, triggering mechanisms and clinical syndromes.

intercourse or simple bladder distension may be powerful triggers for a painful bladder syndrome which might have its underlying cause in an autoimmune phenomenon (Fig. 27.1). Consequently treatment remains empirical in most cases where a precise cause for pain has not been identified.

Some of the concepts discussed in the above section are summarized in Figure 27.1.

A PRAGMATIC APPROACH TO MANAGEMENT

Whilst our first step in management must be the exclusion of serious conditions, patients usually want help and not just a diagnosis. We should therefore try to provide support and practical help from the start and this is best done with the help of specialist nurses who will see the patient too. Patients should be warned at the outset that it is possible, even likely, that no organic cause for pain will be found. This encourages the subsequent acceptance of this fact, after numerous tests have been carried out, and it is less likely to result in them simply seeking help from another doctor.

Diagnosis

History and examination. A detailed history is essential to characterize the symptoms. It is absolutely critical to establish a relationship with the patient based on trust, and spending time with them trying to understand the detail of their particular pain experience is a vital part of this process. In particular, one must know the precise site of each component of the pain, the system to which it relates (is it related to micturition, defecation or intercourse?), its temporal relationships, its intensity, and what triggers and relieves it.

A symptom index and problem index was developed by O'Leary[17] to help with this, and other generic quality of life scoring systems, such as the SF-36, SF-12, and King's Health Questionnaire,[18] may be of value particularly in monitoring the response to treatment.[19]

Quantification of pain is routine in pain practice using standardized pain scoring tools. A pain diary is useful for demonstrating the relationships of pain to micturition, defecation, and sex.

Table 27.1 shows how important the general medical, surgical, obstetric, and psychosocial history may be in determining a diagnosis of generalized medical disease. A general and localized clinical examination (which must include careful vaginal examination) is also important in exclusion of conditions such as genital malignancy, cutaneous disease, and hernia. Pelvic examination must be extremely careful and aimed at identifying areas of tenderness and pelvic floor spasm as well as obvious pelvic pathology.

Initial investigations

URINE CULTURES. Urinalysis is important to exclude diabetes as well as identifying pyuria and hematuria which mandate further investigation. Many patients will already have had multiple midstream urine cultures performed with little or no abnormality detected. It is always worth repeating these but consider taking urethral swabs and suprapubic punctures of bladder urine.

Current standard definitions of UTI allow for a state where a painful bladder syndrome may exist in which no bacterial infection can be identified on standard culture criteria. However, infection, particularly with fastidious organisms such as gardnerella, *Mycoplasma hominis*, *Chlamydia trachomatis* or *Ureaplasma urealyticum* has long been suggested as a cause of painful bladder syndrome. Special culture techniques (including early morning specimens for TB) ought to be used to try to identify any low-grade chronic infection. It is worth discussing these protocols with your local microbiologist who should understand the difficult group of patients to whom these tests refer. Studies on bladder biopsies with DNA probes for specific bacteria have so far failed to identify a common infective pathogen.[20]

VAGINAL TESTS. High vaginal swabs are mandatory to exclude chlamydia, gonorrhea and other vaginal pathogens.[21] Screening for chlamydia with serology is also important in sexually active young women to reduce the risk of chronic PID and infertility.

A cervical smear is advisable to exclude cervical cancer or CIN disease. Vaginal pH should be checked (5–6.5 suggests infection).

IMAGING. A transabdominal scan may identify ovarian cysts and other adnexal pathology (e.g. hydrosalpinx). It also allows assessment of the kidneys and extrapelvic manifestations of malignancy, e.g. ascites, and permits visualization of the uterus (e.g. for fibroids), the endometrial cavity, and the bladder before and after menstruation. The investigation will only identify endometriosis if there are endometriomas present.

Transvaginal scanning (TVS) is much more sensitive when looking at the pelvis, especially the endometrial cavity. It will provide better images of endometriotic cysts or adenomyosis, though MR scanning may be even more reliable for the latter. Pelvic varices can be identified by using transvaginal US with color Doppler and Doppler spectral analysis.[22]

Hydrosonography can also be employed to delineate polyps and intracavity fibroids. It may identify adenomyosis and provide clearer images of the ovaries.

A plain abdominal x-ray will exclude urinary calculus.

MRI is as sensitive as scanning to detect endometriomas. Spinal MRI may be necessary to exclude conus or root pathology, particularly if there were any identifiable neurologic signs.

Barium enema can be used to detect sigmoid/rectal disease in severe endometriosis.

ENDOSCOPY. Cystoscopy is essential to exclude bladder pathology as the cause of pain. Flexible cystoscopy is a useful investigation for testing the patient's tolerance of urethral instrumentation and for conscious pain mapping.[9,23,24]

Cystoscopy and examination under anesthetic, however, are more widely used as they allow for an objective assessment of both the pain reaction to bladder filling (patients with an inflammatory bladder syndrome will often hyperventilate when the bladder is distended, even under deep anesthesia) and also of any ulceration, the presence of release bleeding or petechiae and an opportunity to both biopsy and hyperdistend the bladder (see below). It has been shown, however, that some of these abnormalities are no more common in patients with painful bladders than in patients being cystoscoped for other reasons.[5]

For any patient in whom pain is perianal, a full examination of the rectum is essential. This can only be carried out using the sigmoidoscope and a proctoscope is inadequate for this purpose, giving views only of the anal canal. Flexible sigmoidoscopy and colonoscopy should be considered to exclude colonic pathology in anyone who has associated alteration in bowel habit.

Laparoscopy may be particularly valuable to exclude conditions such as hydrosalpinges, ovarian disease, endometriosis, and pelvic adhesions, and for identifying pelvic vascular congestion.[25-28]

Hysteroscopy is useful if polyps or submucosal fibroids are suspected.

BIOPSIES. Bladder biopsy is useful to confirm the presence of inflammatory changes in a painful bladder and occasionally to identify the presence of carcinoma in situ.[29] It may also be useful to diagnose endometriosis and other painful conditions of the peritoneum.

URODYNAMICS. The role of urodynamics has been debated and accepted as a recommendation in the diagnosis of bladder pain. Its main value in diagnosis is the exclusion of detrusor overactivity but it also provides a further form of conscious pain mapping with quantification of response to measured bladder volumes. This is essential for the NIDDK definition of interstitial cystitis and, of course, is a condition that can be treated specifically.[9]

The potassium sensitivity test (PST) identifies patients with increased epithelial permeability.[30-32] Most patients with severe painful bladder syndrome went through an initial phase of more limited symptoms, perhaps with frequency and nocturia alone or with recurrent limited episodes of abacterial cystitis. The PST may have a role in identifying these patients at an early stage before they have developed serious pathologic changes in the bladder wall or begun to convert somatic inflammatory pain into neuropathic pain.. There is a window of opportunity here to treat patients at an early stage of their disease if the possibility of the diagnosis is kept in mind.

The maximum tolerated bladder volume with and without potassium chloride is recorded, a positive result being a smaller value for KCl. This correlates well with the presence of a diagnosis of IC.[33] However, there are also false positives in other inflammatory conditions so the consensus is that the test has poor discriminating power.

Pain related to the menstrual cycle. Pain which follows a cyclical pattern with the menstrual cycle raises the suspicion of a gynecologic etiology although women will often report that conditions such as irritable bowel syndrome are worse at different times of the menstrual cycle.

Box 27.2   Gynecologic causes of chronic pain

Uterus
- Period pains (primary dysmenorrhea)
- Intramural endometriosis (adenomyosis)
- Fibroids

Fallopian tube
- Chronic salpingitis
- Hydrosalpinx

Ovary
- Benign/malignant ovarian cysts
- Endometriotic cysts
- Ovarian entrapment by adhesions

General
- Endometriosis
- Peritoneal changes leading to chronic inflammation
- Fibrosis
- Venous congestion
- Adhesions secondary to infection/endometriosis
- Congenital anomalies

INVESTIGATION. Chronic infective conditions such as salpingitis, in addition to endometriosis and fibroids, are often associated with heavy and painful periods. Pelvic ultrasound can identify many gynecologic pathologies and many women are sufficiently reassured by negative ultrasound to decline further investigation. Diagnostic laparoscopy is clearly more invasive but may be necessary to determine whether endometriosis is present and whether there are adhesions within the pelvis. Since there is evidence that early endometriosis, superficial or mild, has a better prognosis if treated, laparoscopy may be justified in the investigation of women with chronic pelvic pain. If ultrasound demonstrates increased endometrial thickness in the presence of pain and menstrual abnormality, hysteroscopy may be appropriate since an intrauterine fibroid/polyp may require removal.

If ultrasound and laparoscopy are negative in the presence of cyclical pain, suppression of ovulation may be indicated. The combined oral contraceptive pill is the simplest method but GnRH analogs may be required.

Treatment Strategies
Basic principles. Because of the perceived rarity of each of these clinical syndromes, there are few data available from randomized controlled trials and our knowledge of efficacy is based on sporadic reports, largely of longitudinal series. It is also important to remember that for most functional disease, there is a high placebo effect and measurable

rate of spontaneous resolution. All other treatments should be compared against this baseline but rarely are. If ever there was a type of suffering ripe for exploitation by unproven treatments and unscrupulous practitioners, then this would be it. A quick review of internet sites relating to this topic rapidly reveals this to be the case.

Most of these patients are likely to go through a period of protracted investigation and repeated treatments. It is important to provide some structure to this process both to ensure the completeness of investigative pathways and for the patient to understand that there is a rationale to their treatment. The use of symptom scores, structured pro-formas, and a dedicated multidisciplinary clinic all help to provide this framework.

Avoidance of triggers. All patients with painful bladder or urethra syndromes find there are triggers to their pain. Identifying these is a process of careful detective work that some will take to with compulsion. Drugs, allergens or dietary components, bubble baths, tampons, and deodorant soaps are common noxious agents but others are extensively described within the support literature from the help organizations. Avoidance often involves significant and unwelcome changes in lifestyle. Treatment of associated constipation may require the use of laxatives or fecal softeners but suppositories should be avoided.

Patients will usually have tried some form of self-help, ranging from the use of hot baths and heating pads to rest and inactivity, but usually with little reward.[34]

Support. Psychologic support and practical advice are essential for these patients and only rarely is this best provided by the doctor. The Interstitial Cystitis Support Group, Interstitial Cystitis Network, and the Interstitial Cystitis Association are all very professional organizations who provide a wealth of information for sufferers, much of it web based. The only disadvantage is their use of the name interstitial cystitis, which implies to all patients that they have a precise diagnosis, with associated expectations, when often they do not.

The National Endometriosis Society and Simply Holistic Endometriosis may be helpful for endometriosis sufferers.

Generic treatments

TREATMENTS FOR PAIN AND SPASM. All patients want pain relief and whilst it is appealing to try to address the underlying cause primarily, the reality is that this is rarely known and takes a long time to determine. A pragmatic guide to pain relief is therefore a vital part of this treatment schedule. The input of a chronic pain specialist is a highly desirable addition to a specialist pelvic pain clinic.

Primarily inflammatory pain (somatic or visceral) may respond to nonsteroidal antiinflammatory drugs (NSAIDs) such as ibuprofen or maproxen. Most of the evidence available for their use in pelvic pain relates to dysmenorrhea in which they are shown to be more effective than paracetamol.[35,36] Beware triaprofenic acid (Surgam) which has been shown to cause an inflammatory cystitis.[37] The COX-2 inhibitors such as celecoxib also have a role as alternative antiinflammatory approaches but should be reserved for those patients who are unable to tolerate NSAIDS because of gastric or other GI complications.

The use of regular opioids for chronic pelvic pain causes anxiety for both clinician and patient. They should only be used once the antiinflammatory options have been fully tried but remember that NSAIDS may also have a synergistic effect when used in tandem with opioids. Chronic opioid use must be carefully controlled, preferably by a single consistent source such as the pain clinic or the GP. Longer acting opioids (e.g. MST, oxycodone) are better than short-acting drugs, and fentanyl patches are well tolerated.

Remember that what starts as somatic pain may often become centralized neuropathic pain. Characteristically this type of pain is out of all proportion to the apparent somatic cause and tends to be triggered at increasingly lower thresholds. It is also not relieved by local therapies. Opiates are not effective for this type of pain. Tricyclic antidepressants are commonly used for neuropathic pain but also have anticholinergic and antihistaminic effects. There is no controlled study of their use but they may improve symptoms, particularly when taken at night. Indeed, the use of amitriptyline has been given a grade B recommendation by the consensus meetings on bladder pain.[9] Serotonin reuptake inhibitors such as fluoxetine enhance the adrenergic regulation of pain pathways in the spinal cord and may also be useful but have not been investigated. Anticonvulsants will reduce the excitability of afferent pain pathways. Though carbamazapine has been used, gabapentin is rapidly becoming the first-line treatment for neuropathic pain and can be safely prescribed in gradually increasing doses up to 900 mg three times per day, and is well tolerated. The data regarding its use in pelvic pain syndromes are, as yet, thin on the ground.

It is possible that painful bladder syndrome sometimes results from a state of painful pelvic floor spasm which is triggered by bladder filling or emptying. This theory has led some workers to try pelvic floor relaxation techniques in the treatment protocols for these patients. Diazepam or baclofen may be useful in this respect but physiotherapy (pelvic muscle training aimed at teaching relaxation) may be more effective. Extracorporeal magnetic stimulation is a technique in which a powerful electromagnet resides beneath a chair and delivers pulsatile magnetic field that induces pelvic muscle contraction. The technique has been used in 21 patients with chronic pelvic pain syndrome in our unit but was found to be ineffective.

TENS. Transcutaneous electrical nerve stimulation is commonly used for relief of chronic pain syndromes. Whilst this is a self-administered treatment, best results probably occur when a trained therapist can spend time explaining the technique to the patient. The effect is cumulative over time and may operate through the gate control mechanism or by modulating pain pathways or autonomic reflexes.[38]

The results of treatment are difficult to assess in a randomized controlled trial because of the high intensity of stimulation. Twenty-one of 33 patients with ulcerative interstitial cystitis were effectively relieved of pain though this required continued use of the stimulator.[39] However, the results were less good with nonulcerative, painful bladder syndrome. It is possible that electrode positioning will affect the results of treatment. Suprapubic,[40] vaginal-anal,[41,42] and tibial nerve sites[43,44] have been tested, all with some success.

Acupuncture has also been used and anecdotally clinicians will usually be aware of patients who appear to have benefited from this treatment. Chang[45] showed an 85% improvement in symptoms after acupuncture but that the improvement wore off with time. A randomized trial of acupuncture and moxibustion therapy (n=128) versus "western medicine" (n=52) in women with "urethral syndrome" showed short-term response in 91% versus 21% and prolonged improvement in 80%.[46] However, the definitions of both the traditional Chinese techniques used and the western medicine employed were not clear.

NERVE BLOCK TECHNIQUES. Nerve blockade may be used temporarily as a diagnostic or therapeutic trial (usually using bupivacaine) or permanently, by using a neurolytic agent such as phenol. Pudendal nerve section has already been discussed. The caudal epidural space, the sacral roots as they pass through the sacral foramina, and the presacral plexus in the presacral space can all be injected under imaging control. The lumbar sympathetic plexus can also be injected if pain is thought largely to be visceral in origin.

These are techniques for the anesthetist who has specialized in pain management and is another area in which the need for multidisciplinary care of these patients is paramount.

Treatments specific to the painful bladder or urethra

BLADDER DISTENSION. Hydrodistension has been popular for treating bladder pain since the 1930s. Sensory nerve sprouting is often seen histologically in painful bladders and there is an increase in neuropeptides in muscle samples. Release of these substances and others may induce an inflammatory reaction. We also know that patients with chronic pelvic pain syndrome have altered sensation of pain generated by heat, indicating an abnormality of small-diameter unmyelinated C fibers.[47] Whatever the cause of this neuropathy might be, it is the rationale behind the use of hydrodistension as a treatment option, because the effect of hydrodistension is to create a state of submucosal ischemia which renders the sensory nerves inactive. The effect may increase with duration of distension but tends to be short-lived. Thus, a classic Helmstein distension under epidural anesthesia for 2 hours works better than a short hydrostatic distension with the cystoscope.[48] Glemain, however, showed that only 43% of 63 patients remained in remission at 1 year.[49]

The evidence on hydrodistension amounts to level 2– at best and whilst it is widely practiced, there is little scientific justification for its use as a routine intervention.

ANTIINFECTIVE TREATMENTS. Any routinely proven bacterial urine infection should be treated in the conventional way with appropriate antibiotics.

There are few data about the routine use of antibiotics in the absence of proven infection. Warren carried out a RCT in 50 patients and clinical improvement occurred in 12/25 on antibiotics compared to 6/25 on placebo;[50] 10/25 compared to 5/25 became pain free. One school of thought proposes that most chronic pelvic pain is infection related and that it is the inadequacy of diagnostic techniques that leads to a failure to identify the cause. However, much of this work is based on nonpeer-reviewed data and must be viewed with some caution.

In a study of antibiotic therapy for urethral pain syndrome, 58 patients versus 51 with proven UTI were treated with antibiotics. There was no difference in recovery time for urgency or dysuria, suggesting that positive culture may be irrelevant to clinical practice.[51] However, this study did not examine the longer term outcomes of antibiotic therapy in these groups.

Sexually transmitted infections may also be important in causation and require urethral and opportunistic organism culture techniques and serology for identification.

ANTIINFLAMMATORY TREATMENTS/ORAL THERAPY. Many patients with a painful bladder syndrome will have chronic inflammatory changes in bladder histology. Mast cell granules are known to release vasoactive and nociceptive substances, including histamine, that attract inflammatory cells and may be a stimulus to increased nerve density, in turn responsible for the sensory phenomena and further stimulation of the inflammatory response. Mast cells are not always visible but the presence of inflammatory changes would support the use of antihistamines in treatment. Other antiinflammatory treatments are more nonspecific but equally justified.

Antihistamines alone have been ineffective in the management of painful bladder though they are often included in bladder instillations. Hydroxyzine has been evaluated in a case series of 150 patients in which there was a 40% reduction in symptoms score.[52] Cimetidine has a known immunosuppressive effect and offers symptomatic improvement to some patients though its mechanism of action remains unclear.[53] Steroids might be expected to have some value, particularly in the light of the good association with other autoimmune conditions such as SLE and IBD. They have been reported to show 70% initial response but there is a high relapse rate.[54] Further evidence of their value is pretty sparse though they are often included in intravesical cocktails.

INTRAVESICAL TREATMENTS. Dimethyl sulfoxide (DMSO) is an industrial solvent akin to bleach which has been found to have powerful antiinflammatory properties and used as a bladder instillation in a course of weekly 1-hour instillations for 6 or 8 weeks. Response rates vary from 50% to 80%. In a 33-patient crossover trial comparing DMSO with placebo, there was a 53% vs 18% symptomatic improvement.[55] This is probably the commonest form of intravesical therapy used in the UK and is often made up as a cocktail by local pharmacies along with steroids and antihistamine.

It is proposed that the protective glycoprotein layer of the urothelium is defective in patients with painful bladder syndrome, resulting in leakage of urinary constituents into the detrusor muscle. This causes a widespread inflammatory response. On this basis, pentosan polysulfate (Elmiron), heparin, and hyaluronic acid have all been used as intravesical therapies with varying success. In some series patients have been taught to give themselves intravesical heparin washouts.

Pentosan polysulfate (Elmiron). Of forty-eight patients in a randomized trial, 32% improved on Elmiron versus 16% of the placebo group. There was a decrease in pain and increase in voided volumes.[56] A metaanalysis of four randomized studies (n=398) where pain was the main outcome variable showed a 16% difference overall between the two groups. The number needed to treat (NNT) was 7.[57]

Heparin. Heparin has some antiinflammatory action and also helps to simulate the GaG layer of the urothelium. Because of the cheapness of this drug, it can be instilled by the patient regularly (10,000 IU in 10 ml) several times per week[58] and may reduce the need for more intensive courses of DMSO.

Hyaluronic acid. Hyaluronic acid (30–40 mg in weekly instillations) is now also available for this use, but is much more expensive. Small case series have reported up to 70% response rates.[59]

URETHRAL DILATION. This time-honored technique beloved of gynecologists but scorned by some urologists may have some justification for use in patients with pain that is indisputably of urethral origin. A randomized trial with subjective outcome evaluation in 60 women showed 75% improvement in the dilation group compared to 50% with tetracycline or 20% on placebo.[60] Uroflowmetry only improved in the dilation group. Unfortunately, we do not have evidence on which women are likely to benefit from this technique.

Endometriosis. Endometriosis and its treatment are a major challenge for patients and clinicians. Extrauterine endometriosis may be classified into peritoneal, ovarian, and rectovaginal disease. Whilst localized disease in an ovary or the rectovaginal septum may produce symptoms confined to the relevant area, the pain is often more widespread and may be limited to the time of menstruation or may be continuous with exacerbations during a period.

Diagnosis of endometriosis may require a combination of ultrasound, laparoscopy, and histology in addition to clinical examination, during which rectovaginal deposits are often missed. Pelvic examination has 79% sensitivity and 32% specificity to establish endometriosis.

Management of endometriosis can be divided into nonsurgical and surgical modalities. Nonsurgical treatments are designed to inhibit the estrogenic driver for endometrial growth through suppression of ovarian activity. Medical treatments are all equally effective in ameliorating the symptoms of dysmenorrhea, dyspareunia, and chronic pelvic pain for as long as they are taken and a few months afterwards. Simplistically, they act by creating a pseudopregnancy, peudomenopause or a male-type hormonal environment. The continuous use of the combined oral contraceptive pill is the simplest choice, and progestagens may also be used to mimic a pseudopregnancy. A pseudomenopause can be created by using GnRH analogs, particularly when other treatments have failed, but they do also have unwanted side effects like hot flushes. Add-back estrogen therapy is advised simultaneously to prevent osteoporosis and the other associated hypoestrogenic side effects.[61]

Danazol is less popular with patients on account of the androgenic side effects of hair growth, voice deepening, and weight gain. There are also some concerns that it may be associated with ovarian cancer and insulin resistance. Gestrinone is an alternative androgenic drug.[62]

Surgical treatment of endometriosis can be very challenging, particularly when the disease is widespread and deeply infiltrating, involving structures such as the ureter and rectum. There is no place for a hysterectomy and castration (bilateral salpingo-oophorectomy) to treat this disease. The aim of surgery should be to remove or destroy all of the endometriotic tissue, with adjoining fibrosis and angiogenesis. The laparoscopic approach is increasingly being employed by surgeons who have developed high levels of skill; results are at least equivalent to laparotomy with less morbidity.[63] For deeply infiltrating endometriosis, a multidisciplinary team approach is essential and this has led to the evolution of centers of excellence for such surgery.[64] Excisional surgery is associated with statistically significant reduction in pelvic pain; the more severe the disease, the better the results. Over 50% will experience long-term relief.

All forms of treatment of endometriosis are associated with recurrence although there is a lack of clarity about how much is recurrence and how much is new disease. Whilst the etiology is so poorly understood, treatment will remain an ongoing challenge.

Pelvic cancer. Occasionally pelvic pain will be the presenting feature of a pelvic malignancy. This is one reason why thorough investigation at the beginning of a management encounter is so important. Most pelvic malignancy should now be managed by multidisciplinary teams including oncologists and surgeons who have both the training and experience to deal with cancers that may involve more than one organ system.

Pudendal nerve entrapment. Compression of the pudendal nerve as it passes through the ischiorectal fossa can cause chronic pain in the perineum, between the posterior fourchette and anal canal. External clinical examination is usually normal but palpation of the ischial spine on rectal examination will usually exacerbate the pain. The diagnosis might be confirmed by performing pudendal nerve terminal motor latencies using the "Kiff" glove, a test which is still used in some colorectal research departments but rarely employed in routine clinical practice.[65,66] The proof of the pudding in this diagnosis is whether surgical release of the nerve in Alcock's canal actually relieves the pain.

The sciatic and obstetric nerves have previously been found to be involved in some cases of endometriosis ensheathing and compressing the nerves.

Perianal pain syndrome. Chronic perianal pain may be related to underlying cancer, fissure, fistula, inflammatory bowel disease or hemorrhoids. A confident diagnosis to exclude these conditions is therefore essential. However, in the absence of a clear pathologic cause, the pain is assumed to be related to levator spasm and often associated with anismus or inappropriate sphincter activity during attempted defecation.

Treatment may then be directed at assisting the easy passage of stool by use of bulking laxatives and fecal softeners, and techniques to reduce levator spasm. Muscle relaxation techniques as described above may be useful and biofeedback has also been used with some success.

Nonsurgical therapies. Genitourinary pain in the postmenopausal woman with hypoestrogenic state may be helped by estrogen.[67]

Recent studies have also utilized a programme of BCG (Tice) bladder instillation with some success.[68,69] Thirty patients were treated with a 6-week course and followed up for a minimum of 6 months. There was a 60% response rate versus 27% placebo response. However, a further crossover study comparing BCG with DMSO in 21 patients showed no benefit to BCG.[70]

Capsaicin and resiniferatoxin (RTX) are members of the vanilloid family, a group of powerful neurotoxins that prevent the upregulation of VR1 receptors in the primary afferent C fibers which are important in mediating chronic bladder pain.[71] Both drugs are effective though capsaicin is very toxic and unfortunately RTX, whilst being more effective and less toxic, adheres to the plastic surface of bottles and syringes so that it is difficult to control the dosing adequately.

Recent interest in botulinum toxin for the treatment of overactive detrusor has spread to the painful bladder and some groups are experimenting with this novel therapy though the mechanism of action is mysterious. Whilst the mechanism of action on depletion of presynaptic vesicles of acetylcholine is known, there is emerging evidence that sensory neurotransmitters may also be inactivated by this toxin.[71,72]

Surgery. Surgery has traditionally been regarded as a treatment of last resort in these patients but some new developments merit a reexamination of this philosophy. In gynecology, removal of damaged tubes and ovarian cysts may help to relieve pain. The risks of surgical exploration may be considerable and preoperative counseling must include a full risk appraisal.

If chronic pelvic pain is indeed manifest though pelvic muscle spasm then chronic neuromodulation, such as may be achieved with the implantable Interstim device, may be helpful in providing permanent relief up to 14 months follow-up (Stone AR, personal communication). Whether this is appropriate in patients who have a demonstrable inflammatory change in the bladder is doubtful.

Sacral neuromodulation is known to help patients with detrusor overactivity[73,74] and urinary retention and has also been applied to chronic pelvic pain.[75] Electrical stimulation of sacral sensory fibers appears to modulate transmission of pain through ascending pathways or activation of inhibitory pathways.[76,77]

The technique has been used in a number of small series of pain patients and improvements have been shown in frequency, pain, and urgency towards normal values, while urinary markers for IC were normalized.[78] Reduction of narcotic requirement and improvement in symptom scores were also recorded in similar studies.[79-81]

Patients with refractory pelvic floor dysfunction and pelvic pain have also been treated with sacral neuromodulation, and benefit has been reported.[82]

So far, no data are available from any large-scale or randomized studies of this technique. The implants are expensive and have a significant technical failure rate which poses problems for healthcare systems with limited resources.

Transurethral resection of the bladder ulcer in ulcerative interstitial cystitis has been shown to be effective, with 92/103 patients initially relieved, but only 40% remained symptom free at 4 years.[23] Treatment of the ulcer with ND YAG laser showed a response in 21/27 ulcers but this compared to less than 40% response in nonulcerative disease.[83]

Cystectomy (partial or total) has been employed with varying success.[84,85] It is disappointing that removal of the (apparently) painful organ can fail to relieve pain. This may be because there is an underlying abnormality of visceral sensation which is just as bad for an intestinal bladder as for a natural one or that it is possible to experience "phantom bladder pain" even after removal of the organ. Alternatively, this failure may imply that the original cause lies within the urine such that the augmented bladder suffers just as much. Van Ophoven et al[86] reviewed 10 series of surgical cases with more than 10 patients in each series (n=14) who underwent cystectomy with supratrigonal substitution. Success ranged from 55% to 83%. Patients with trigonal disease, urethral pain, large bladder capacities, and neuropathic conversion faired poorly. Patient selection for some of these series may not have been very tightly defined, however.

If there is no clinical doubt that the pain is of bladder origin and not urethral then cystectomy and bladder substitution still offers a chance of improvement, albeit with all the short-and long-term sequelae of this type of surgery. If the urethra seems to be the site of pain, then cystourethrectomy and urinary diversion is still an option but there are no data on this.

UTERINE NERVE TRANSECTION AND PRESACRAL NEURECTOMY. Many patients with apparent resolution of disease have problems with chronic pelvic pain. Uterine nerve resection and presacral neurectomy may have a role in their management although the literature provides conflicting evidence for the value of both procedures.

Uterine nerve transaction was first described over 40 years ago and its use has been reviewed.[87] Laproscopic uterine nerve ablation (LUNA) has been evaluated in the treatment of dysmenorrhea with no obvious pathology in a prospective randomized study.[88] Complete pain relief in 81% was reported at 3 months in the LUNA group, although this reduced to 45% at 12 months. The control group derived no benefit. Women with endometriosis and dysmenorrhea have also been shown to gain relief from dysmenorrhea with LUNA.

Presacral neurectomy (PSN) has been reviewed and reveals conflicting evidence of its value.[88] There is some evidence that it is of most value in midline pain.[89]

Both LUNA and PSN are procedures which carry a significant risk of hemorrhage and should not be performed by inexperienced surgeons.

MICROLAPAROSCOPY. Microlaparoscopy under local anesthesia has been used for conscious pain mapping of chronic pelvic pain. Adhesiolysis has similarly been employed at the same time if adhesions are identified which are demonstrably associated with pain.[90] Surgery has traditionally been regarded as a treatment of last resort in these patients but some new developments merit a reexamination of this philosophy.

REFERENCES

1. Weisberg MB, Clavel AL Jr. Why is chronic pain so difficult to treat? Psychological considerations from simple to complex care. Postgrad Med 1999;106(6):141–164.

2. de Kruiff ME, ter Kuile MM, Weijenborg PT, van Lankveld JJ. Vaginismus and dyspareunia: is there a difference in clinical presentation? J Psychosom Obstet Gynecol 2000;21(3):149–155.

3. Hanno PM, Landis JR, Matthews-Cook Y, Kusek J, Nyberg L and the Interstitial Cystitis Database Study Group. The diagnosis of interstitial cystitis revisited: lessons learned from the National Institute of Health Interstitial Database Study. J Urol 1999:161:553–557.

4. Gillenwater JY, Wein AJ. Summary of the National Institutes of Arthritis, Diabetes, Digestive and Kidney diseases workshop on interstitial cystitis. National Institutes of Health, Bethesda. J Urol 1988;140:203–206.

5. Waxman JA, Sulek PJ, Kuehi TJ. Cystoscopic findings consistent with interstitial cystitis in normal women undergoing tubal ligation. J Urol 1998;160:1663–1667.

6. Agarwal M, O'Reilly PH, Dixon RA. Interstitial cystitis—a time for revision of name and diagnostic criteria in the new millennium? BJU Int 2001;87:348–350.

7. Payne CK, Terai A, Komatsu K. Research criteria versus clinical criteria for interstitial cystitis. Int J Urol 2003;10(Suppl):S7–S10.

8. Nordling J. Interstitial cystitis: how should we diagnose it and treat it in 2004? Curr Opin Urol 2004;14(6):323–327.

9. Fall M, Baranowski AP, Fowler CJ, et al. EAU guidelines on chronic pelvic pain. Eur Urol 2004;46(6):681–689.

10. Pappas PG. Laboratory in the diagnosis and management of urinary tract infections. Med Clin North Am 1991;75:313–325.

11. Messelink EJ. The overactive bladder and the role of the pelvic floor muscles. BJU Int 1999;83(Suppl 2):31–35.

12. Howard FM. Pelvic floor pain syndrome. In: Howard FM, ed. Pelvic pain. Diagnosis and management. Philadelphia: Lippincott Williams and Wilkins; 2000: pp 429–432.

13. Rapkin AJ, Kames LD, Darke LL, Stampler FM, Naliboff BD. History of physical and sexual abuse in women with chronic pelvic pain. Obstet Gynecol 1990;76:92–96.

14. Walling MK, Reiter RC, O'Hara MW, Milburn AK, Lilly G, Vincent SD. Abuse history and chronic pain in women: I. Prevalences of sexual abuse and physical abuse. Obstet Gynecol 1994;84:193–199.

15. Raphael KG, Widom CS, Lange G. Childhood victimization and pain in adulthood: a prospective investigation. Pain 2001;92:283–293.

16. Walling MK, O'Hara MW, Reiter RC, Milburn AK, Lilly G, Vincent SD. Abuse history and chronic pain in women: II. A multivariate analysis of abuse and psychological morbidity. Obstet Gynecol 1994;84:200–206.

17. O'Leary MP, Sant GR, Fowler FJ, White KE, Spolarich-Kroll J. The interstitial cystitis symptom index and problem index. Urology 1997;49(Suppl. 5A):58–63.

18. Kelleher C, Cardozo LD, Khullar V, Salvatore S. A new questionnaire to assesss the quality of life of urinary incontinent women. Br J Obstet Gynaecol 1997;104:1374–1379.

19. Lubeck DP, Whitmore K, Sant GR, Alvarez-Horine S, Lai C. Psychometric validation of the O'Leary–Sant interstitial cystitis symptom index in a clinical trial of pentosan polysulfate sodium. Urology 2001;57:62–66.

20. Duncan JL, Schaeffer AJ. Do infectious agents cause interstitial cystitis? Urology 1997; 49: 48–51.

21. Ness RB, Soper DE, Holley RL, et al. Effectiveness of inpatient and outpatient strategies for women with pelvic inflammatory disease. Am J Obstet Gynecol 2002;186(5):929–937.

22. Kuligowska E, Deeds L 3rd, Lu K 3rd. Pelvic pain: overlooked and underdiagnosed gynecologic conditions. Radiographics 2005;25(1):3–20.

23. Peeker R, Aldenborg F, Fall M. Complete transurethral resection of ulcers in classic interstitial cystitis. Int Urogynecol J Pelvic Floor Dysfunct 2000;11(5):290–295.

24. Messing E, Pauk D, Schaeffer A, et al. Associations among cystoscopic findings and symptoms and physical examination findings in women enrolled in the Interstitial Cystitis Data Base (ICDB) Study. Urology 1997;49:81–85.

25. Howard FM. The role of laparoscopy as a diagnostic tool in chronic pelvic pain. Baillière's Best Pract Res Clin Obstet Gynaecol 2000;14(3):467–494.

26. Porpora MG, Gomel V. The role of laparoscopy in the management of pelvic pain in women of reproductive age. Fertil Steril 1997;68(5):765–779.

27. Fauconnier A, Chapron C, Dubuisson JB, Viera M, Doussett B, Breart G. Relation between pain symptoms and the anatomic location of deep infiltrating endometriosis. Fertil Steril 2002;78(4):719–726.

28. Goldstein DP, De Cholnoky C, Emans SJ. Adolescent endometriosis. J Adolesc Health Care 1980;1(1):37–41.

29. Johansson SL, Fall M. Pathology of interstitial cystitis. Urol Clin North Am 1994;21:55–62.

30. Parsons CL, Zupkas P, Parsons JK. Intravesical potassium sensitivity in patients with interstitial cystitis and urethral syndrome. Urology 2001;57(3):428–432.

31. Chambers GK, Fenster HN, Cripps S, Jens M, Taylor D. An assessment of the use of intravesical potassium in the diagnosis of interstitial cystitis. J Urol 1999;162:699–701.

32. Gregoire M, Liandier F, Naud A, Lacombe L, Fradet Y. Does the potassium stimulation test predict cystometric, cystoscopic outcome in interstitial cystitis? J Urol 2002;168:556–557.

33. Parsons CL, Greenberger M, Gabal L, Bidair M, Barme G. The role of urinary potassium in the pathogenesis and diagnosis of interstitial cystitis. J Urology 1998;159(6):1862–1866.

34. Koziol JA. Epidemiology of interstitial cystitis. Urol Clin North Am 1994;21(1):7–20.

35. Zhang WY, Li Wan Po A. Efficacy of minor analgesics in primary dysmenorrhoea: a systematic review. Br J Obstet Gynaecol 1998;105:780–789.

36. Furniss LD. Nonsteroidal anti-inflammatory agents in the treatment of primary dysmenorrhea. Clin Pharm 1982;1:327–333.

37. Buchbinder R, Forbes A, Kobben F, Boyd I, Snow RM, McNeil JJ. Clinical features of tiaprofenic acid (surgam) associated cystitis and a study of risk factors for its development. J Clin Epidemiol. 2000;53(10):1013–1019.

38. Melzack R, Wall PD. Pain mechanisms: a new theory. Science 1965;150:971–979.

39. Fall M, Lindström S. Electrical stimulation. A physiologic approach to the treatment of urinary incontinence. Urol Clin North Am 1991;18:393–407.

40. Fall M. Conservative management of chronic interstitial cystitis: transcutaneous electrical nerve stimulation and transurethral resection. J Urol 1985;133:774–778.

41. Fall M, Carlsson CA, Erlandson BE. Electrical stimulation in interstitial cystitis. J Urol 1980;123:192–195.

42. Eriksen BC. Painful bladder disease in women: effect of maximal electric pelvic floor stimulation. Neurourol Urodynam 1989;8:362–363.

43. Geirsson G, Wang YH, Lindström S, Fall M. Traditional acupuncture and electrical stimulation of the posterior tibial nerve. A trial in chronic interstitial cystitis. Scand J Urol Nephrol 1993;27:67–70.

44. McGuire EJ, Zhang SC, Horwinski ER, Lytton B. Treatment of motor and sensory detrusor instability by electrical stimulation. J Urol 1983;129:78–79.

45. Chang PL. Urodynamic studies in acupuncture for women with frequency, urgency and dysuria. J Urol 1988;140(3):563–566.

46. Zheng H, Wang S, Shang J, et al. Study on acupuncture and moxibustion therapy for female urethral syndrome. J Trad Chinese Med 1998;18(2):122–127.

47. Lee JC, Wyang CC, Kromm BG, Berger RE. Neurophysiologic testing in chronic pelvic pain syndrome: a pilot study. Urology 2001;58:246–250.

48. Dunn M. Interstitial cystitis: treated by prolonged bladder distension. J Urol 1977;49:641–645.

49. Glemain P, Riviere C, Lenormand L, Karam G, Bouchot O, Buzelin JM. Prolonged hydrodistention of the bladder for symptomatic treatment of interstitial cystitis: efficacy at 6 months and 1 year. Eur Urol 2002;41(1):79–84.

50. Warren JW, Horne LM, Hebel JR, Marvel RP, Keay SK, Chai TC. Pilot study of sequential oral antibiotics for the treatment of interstitial cystitis. J Urol 2000;163(6):1685–1688.

51. Baerheim A, Digranes A, Hunskaar S. Equal symptomatic outcome after antibacterial treatment of acute lower urinary tract infection and the acute urethral syndrome in adult women. Scand J Primary Health Care 1999;17(3):170–173.

52. Theoharides TC, Sant GR. Hydroxyzine therapy for interstitial cystitis. Urology 1997;49(5A Suppl):108–110.

53. Dasgupta P, Sharma SD, Womack C, Blackford HN, Dennis P. Cimetidine in painful bladder syndrome: a histopathological study. BJU Int 2001;88(3):183–186.

54. Badenoch AW. Chronic interstitial cystitis. BMJ 1971;43:718–721.

55. Perez-Marrero R, Emerson LE, Feltis JT. A controlled study of dimethyl sulfoxide in interstitial cystitis. J Urol 1988;140:36–39.

56. Parsons CL, Mulholland SG. Successful therapy of interstitial cystitis with pentanopolysulfate. J Urol 1987;138:513–516.

57. Hwang P, Auclair B, Beechinor D, et al. Efficacy of pentosanpolysulfate in the treatment of interstitial cystitis: a meta-analysis. Urology 1997;50:39–43.

58. Parsons CL, Benson G, Childs SJ. A quantitatively controlled method to study prospectively interstitial cystitis and demonstrate the efficacy of pentanopolysulfate. J Urol 1993; 159: 845–848.

59. Morales A, Emerson L, Nickel JC. Intravesical hyaluronic acid in the treatment of refractory interstitial cystitis. Urology 1997;49(5A Suppl):111–113.

60. Bergman A, Karram M, Bhattia N. Urethral syndrome. A comparison of different treatment modalities. J Reprod Med 1989;34:157–162.

61. Pickersgill A. Review: GnRH analogues and add-back therapy. Is there a perfect combination? Br J Obstet Gynaecol 1998;105:475–485.

62. Teirney R, Prentice A. The medical management of endometriosis. Rev Gynecol Pract 2002;6:91–98.

63. Gambone JC, Mittman BS, Munro MG, et al, for the Chronic Pelvic Pain/Endometriosis Working Group. Consensus statement for the management of chronic pelvic pain and endometriosis: proceedings of an expert-panel consensus process. Fertil Steril 2002;78:961–972.

64. Koh CH, Janik GM. The surgical management of deep rectovaginal endometriosis. Curr Opin Obstet Gynecol 2002;14:357–364.

65. Amarenco G, Kerdraon J. Pudendal nerve terminal sensitive latency: technique and normal values. J Urol 1999;161:103–106.

66. Robert R, Prat-Pradal D, Labat JJ, et al. Anatomic basis of chronic perineal pain: role of the pudendal nerve. Surg Radiol Anat 1998;20:93–98.

67. Youngblood VH, Tomlin EM, Davis JB, Senile urethritis in women. J Urol 1957;78:150–153.

68. Peters K, Diokno A, Steinert B, et al. The efficacy of Tice strain bacillus Calmette-Guerin in the treatment of interstitial cystitis; a double-blind, prospective, placebo controlled trial. J Urol 1997;157:2090–2094.

69. Peters KM, Diokno AC, Steinert BW, Gonzalez JA. The efficacy of intravesical bacillus Calmette-Guerin in the treatment of interstitial cystitis; long-term follow up. J Urol 1998;159:1483–1486.

70. Peeker R, Haghsheno MA, Holmang S, Fall M. Intravesical bacillus Calmette-Guerin and dimethyl sulfoxide for treatment of classic and nonulcer interstitial cystitis: a prospective, randomized double-blind study. J Urol 2000;164(6):1912–1915.

71. Cruz F. Mechanisms involved in new therapies for overactive bladder. Urology 2004;63(3 Suppl 1):65–73.

72. Sahai A, Khan M, Fowler CJ, Dasgupta P. Botulinum toxin for the treatment of lower urinary tract symptoms: a review. Neurourol Urodynam 2005;24(1):2–12.

73. Ruud Bosch JL, Groen J. Sacral nerve neuromodulation in the treatment of refractory motor urge incontinence. Curr Opin Urol 2001;11:399–403.

74. Schmidt RA. Applications of neuromodulation. Urol Neurourol Urodynam 1988;7:585.

75. Paszkiewicz EJ, Siegel SW, Kirkpatrick C, Hinkel B, Keeisha J, Kirkemo A. Sacral nerve stimulation in patients with chronic, intractable pelvic pain. Urology 2001;57:124.

76. Schmidt RA, Senn E, Tanagho EA. Functional evaluation of sacral nerve root integrity. Report of a technique. Urology 1990;35:388–392.

77. Kemler MA, Barendse GA, van Kleef M, Egbrink MG. Pain relief in complex regional pain syndrome due to spinal cord stimulation does not depend on vasodilation. Anesthesiology 2000;92:1653–1660.

78. Maher CF, Carey MP, Dwyer PL, Schluter PL. Percutaneous sacral nerve root neuromodulation for intractable interstitial cystitis. J Urol 2001;165:884–886.

79. Whitmore KE, Payne CK, Diokno AC, Lukban JC. Sacral neuromodulation in patients with interstitial cystitis: a multicenter clinical trial. Int Urogynecol J Pelvic Floor Dysfunct 2003;14(5):305–308.

80. Peters KM, Konstandt D. Sacral neuromodulation decreases narcotic requirements in refractory interstitial cystitis. BJU Int 2004;93(6):777–779.

81. Comiter CV. Sacral neuromodulation for the symptomatic treatment of refractory interstitial cystitis: a prospective study. J Urol 2003;169(4):1369–1373.

82. Aboseif S, Tamaddon K, Chalfin S, Freedman S, Kaptein J. Sacral neuromodulation as an effective treatment for refractory pelvic floor dysfunction. Urology 2002;60:52–56.

83. Malloy TR, Shanberg AM. Laser therapy for interstitial cystitis. Urol Clin North Am 1994;21(1):141–144.

84. Linn JF, Hohenfellner M, Roth S et al. Treatment of interstitial cystitis: comparison of subtrigonal and supratrigonal cystectomy combined with orthotopic bladder substitution. J Urol 1998;159:774–778.

85. Hughes OD, Kynaston HG, Jenkins BJ, Stephenson TP, Vaughton KC. Substitution cystoplasty for intractable interstitial cystitis. Br J Urol 1995;76(2):172–174.

86. Van Ophoven A, Oberpenning F, Hertle L. Long-term results of trigone-preserving orthotopic substitution enterocystoplasty for interstitial cystitis. J Urol 2002;167(2 Pt 1):603–607.

87. Daniell JF, Lalonde CJ. Advanced laparoscopic procedures for pelvic pain and dysmenorrhoea. In: Sutton C, ed. Advanced laparoscopic surgery. London: Baillière Tindall; 1995.

88. Biggerstaff ED, Foster SN. Laparoscopic surgery for dysmenorrhoea: uterine nerve ablation and presacral neurectomy. In: Sutton C, ed. Gynecological endoscopic surgery. London: Chapman and Hall; 1997.

89. Sutton CJ, Ewen SP, Whitelaw N, Haines P. Prospective, randomized, double-blind, controlled trial of laser laparoscopy in the treatment of pelvic pain associated with minimal, mild, and moderate endometriosis. Fertil Steril 1994;62(4):696–700.

90. Dover RW, Sutton CJG. Laparoscopic treatment of pelvic pain. In: Cardozo L, Staskin D, Kirby A eds. Textbook of female urology and urogynaecology. London: Isis Medical Media; 2001.

SECTION 12

Neurogenic bladder

Neurogenic Bladder: Pathophysiology

Timothy B Boone

INTRODUCTION

Our understanding of storage and micturition is rapidly changing as advances in the science are occurring at a quickening pace. Likewise, our knowledge of the pathophysiology of vesicourethral neurogenic disorders will follow, to include molecular changes in both the target organs and the neural circuitry devoted to micturition. The physiology of voiding function is highly regulated by the central and peripheral nervous systems.[1] Injury, disease, and metabolic disorders of the nervous system can have profound effects on vesicourethral function. The purpose of this chapter is to review the pathophysiology of some of the more common neurogenic bladder disorders, realizing that our knowledge will advance in this area as molecular tools are applied to neuropathic detrusor muscle, interstitium, and urothelium.

Many of the normal neural-controlled mechanisms which maintain urinary continence and provide "pressure-safe" storage of urine are bypassed in neurogenic vesicourethral dysfunction. The accommodation of urine by the bladder during filling has both passive and active properties. The elastic and viscoelastic components of the bladder wall allow tremendous stretch to accommodate increasing volumes while maintaining low-pressure storage. At the same time the lack of excitatory parasympathetic input along with active urothelial release of nitric oxide (NO) provide a local neural mechanism to reinforce stretch-induced relaxation and send forward the sensation of filling.[2] These active and passive processes determine detrusor compliance, the most important physiologic parameter in neurogenic vesicourethral dysfunction. Neural injury and disease have a strong influence on bladder storage and compliance due to changes induced in the smooth muscle, interstitium, and urothelium. Neurogenic models of disease are beginning to demonstrate profound changes in the detrusor muscle.[3] The absence of involuntary bladder contractions while maintaining outlet closure at rest, even with increases in abdominal pressure, are important features to normal vesicourethral physiology,

and these functions are often lost when neurologic injury impacts the micturition cycle.

An overview of the neural regulation of micturition and storage is illustrated in Figure 28.1A. Multiple reflex pathways organized in the brain and spinal cord coordinate the bladder and urethra during storage and urethra during storage and voiding. The "on/off" switch in the pontine reticular formation controls the storage of urine, followed by effective voiding to completion. Ascending and descending neural pathways converge in this brainstem area to regulate the voiding cycle. A coordinated and sustained contraction of the detrusor smooth muscle in concert with lowered urethral resistance at the internal (smooth) and external (striated) sphincter is often disrupted in neurologic disease. A state of dyssynergia or discoordination between the bladder and sphincter exists.

Figure 28.1B illustrates some of the functional changes that can occur after neurologic injury. Normally, sensory pathways conveying filling sensation and volume to the nervous system are mediated by thinly myelinated Aδ fibers. Numerous animal studies and indirect human data demonstrate a change to C fiber-mediated sensory input following neural injury to the spinal cord.[1] A change in the afferent pathway from the bladder along with damage to the spinal cord pathways ascending to and descending from the pontine micturition center results in a loss of bladder and sphincter coordination. Detrusor–sphincter dyssynergia (DSD) is a functional type of outlet obstruction, as opposed to the classic anatomic obstruction the prostate can induce to obstruct urine flow and elevate voiding pressures. Involuntary bladder contractions (detrusor overactivity) from the loss of central inhibition along with discoordination between the bladder and urethral sphincter(s) are a common manifestation of neurogenic vesicourethral dysfunction (Fig. 28.2).

Reflexic contraction of the bladder against a closed urethra generates elevated intravesical pressure, which over time can induce vesicoureteral reflux or loss of detrusor compliance. Left untreated, more than 50% of patients

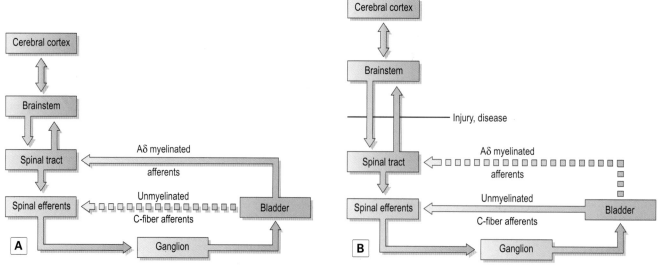

Figure 28.1 (**A**) Normal micturition with Ad afferent-mediated sensation. (**B**) Neurogenic dysfunction with C fiber afferent-mediated sensation.

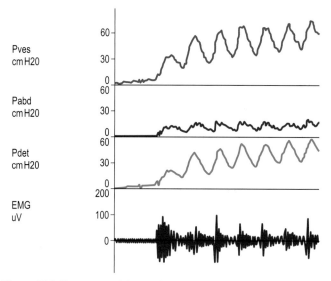

Figure 28.2 Detrusor–sphincter dyssynergia.

Box 28.1   Neurogenic functional classification

Failure to store
Due to the bladder

- Detrusor overactivity
  Suprasacral neurologic disease
  Suprapontine neurologic disease

- Loss of compliance
  Increased muscle tone
  Fibrosis

- Detrusor hypersensitivity
  Urothelial changes
  Local afferent neural changes

Due to the outlet

- Neurogenic sphincter dysfunction

- Fixed outlet (fibrosis)

Failure to empty
Due to the bladder

- Detrusor underactivity
  Sacral neurologic disease
  Peripheral nerve disease

Due to the outlet

- Internal (smooth) sphincter dyssynergia

- External (striated) sphincter dyssynergia

with DSD will develop urologic complications in less than 5 years.[4]

The pathophysiology of neurogenic vesicourethral dysfunction can be simplified by considering failure of storage or emptying of the bladder.[5] Box 28.1 illustrates the popular Wein classification scheme modified to focus on neurogenic vesicourethral dysfunction. Overall, some general statements can be made about discrete neurologic lesions. Focal infarcts, spinal cord lesions or tumors, and focal plaques are usually associated with predictable vesicourethral dysfunction. Neurologic disease or lesions above the pontine micturition center (PMC) in the brainstem usually result in detrusor overactivity (loss of inhibition) with sphincter synergy at both the internal and external urethral sphincters always being the result from suprapontine neural insults. Injury or disease below the PMC and above the sacral nuclei (S2–4) subserving bladder and urethral function results in detrusor overactivity and a substantial risk for sphincter dyssynergia. Some common clinical neurologic disorders that can affect vesicourethral function will be discussed, based on the location of the neurologic impairment.

CEREBROVASCULAR ACCIDENT

Ischemia or infarction of the brain is caused by arterial occlusion, thrombosis or hemorrhage. Cerebrovascular accident (CVA) or stroke is a major cause of morbidity and mortality with a prevalence of 60 per 1000 patients over 65 years of age. For those over 75 years, the prevalence increases to 95 per 1000.[6] Two studies have emphasized the prognostic relationship between CVA and urinary incontinence. Taub and associates found initial incontinence after CVA to be the strongest indicator of long-term disability.[7] Wade and Hewer studied over 500 patients after CVA and reported a high mortality rate in those with early incontinence.[8] Furthermore, reduced mobility in the long term was associated with early urinary incontinence.

A range of vesicourethral dysfunction can occur following a CVA. Initial urinary retention is very common, and it resembles the areflexic shock phase after a spinal cord injury. The mechanism of "cerebral shock" is unknown, with 20% of unilateral stroke patients showing frank hyporeflexia with early urodynamic testing.[9] Soon after the shock phase resolves, detrusor overactivity with intact sensation becomes the major neurogenic bladder dysfunction. Urinary frequency and urgency, with or without urge incontinence, is common with bladder overactivity, and sphincter synergy is the most frequent urodynamic finding.[10,11]

Other patterns of neurogenic voiding dysfunction are seen, including detrusor underactivity and pseudodyssynergia. Suprapontine input can also help facilitate complete bladder emptying. The exact CNS sites for this input are not currently known but noninvasive imaging with PET scanning and functional MRI will define this in the future. True DSD does not occur following a CVA, although the sensation of urgent voiding leads many patients to try and avoid incontinence with a sudden external sphincter contraction noted with the onset of detrusor overactivity (pseudodyssynergia). Lower urinary tract symptoms alone in patients with some impaired cognition can be difficult to manage, especially when potential impaired contractility can complicate the clinical history. Therefore, urodynamic testing, especially in men with potential prostate-mediated obstruction, is advisable when early conservative management is not working.

BRAIN TUMOR

One of the earliest references to the influence of the cerebral cortex over vesicourethral function came from Drs Andrew and Nathan, two neurosurgeons operating on frontal lobe lesions.[12] The association of intracranial tumors in the superomedial part of the frontal lobes and urinary incontinence, frequency, and urgency has been substantial in a larger series by Maurice-Williams.[13] He found the overactive neurogenic symptoms only in patients with frontal lobe lesions. Other small case reports describe suprapontine tumors with impaired contractility and retention.[14]

CEREBRAL PALSY

Cerebral dysfunction secondary to prenatal or perinatal infection or hypoxia causes cerebral palsy, usually characterized by neuromuscular disability. Up to one-third of children with cerebral palsy will have lower urinary tract symptoms.[15] The most common symptom is incontinence, which is diurnal and associated with uninhibited detrusor contractions on urodynamic testing.[16]

SHY–DRAGER SYNDROME

A clinical triad consisting of orthostatic syncope, impotence, and bladder dysfunction was described in patients by Shy and Drager in 1960.[17] Parkinsonian features accompany this syndrome, including tremor, gait disturbance, bradykinesia, anhidrosis, and rigidity. Urinary symptoms usually occur earlier than problems with orthostatic hypotension. Detrusor areflexia with sphincteric bradykinesia or pseudodyssynergia is the most common voiding pattern seen on urodynamic testing.[18] Loss of detrusor compliance is a common finding as global autonomic failure progresses for 8–10 years, which is the usual time to death following the diagnosis of Shy–Drager syndrome.

PARKINSON'S DISEASE

A deficit of dopamine in the substantia nigra region in the brain leads to Parkinson's disease, characterized by tremor, bradykinesia, and muscular rigidity. Men and women are usually equally afflicted by this leading neurologic disease, which affects 100–150 per 100,000 people in the United States.[19] Voiding dysfunction is reported in 40–70% of patients with Parkinson's disease.[20,21] Loss of suprapontine inhibition leading to detrusor overactivity with urgency, frequency, and urge incontinence is the most common vesicourethral abnormality seen.[22] Obstructive symptoms secondary to two common manifestations of external urethral sphincter dysfunction characterize the remaining patients with lower urinary tract symptoms. Since the neurologic deficit is above the pons, true DSD is not possible. However, pseudodyssynergia may be seen as the urge to void which accompanies detrusor overactivity, and the patient attempts to abort the bladder contraction with a voluntary increase in sphincter activity.

The second external sphincter abnormality is bradykinesia of the rhabdosphincter and pelvic floor, wherein urinary flow is slow due to poor relaxation of the muscle with the onset of a detrusor contraction. The combination of detrusor overactivity with sphincter abnormalities in an elderly male at risk for prostate-mediated obstruction makes careful urodynamic evaluation mandatory before any surgical intervention to the lower urinary tract. Furthermore, impaired detrusor contractility can be seen in up to 16% of men and women, emphasizing the need for urodynamic testing to formulate management decisions.[23]

MULTIPLE SCLEROSIS

Focal neural demyelination causing impairment of nerve conduction is the central pathologic lesion in multiple sclerosis (MS). Focal demyelinating plaques with associated edema lead to multiple exacerbations and remissions with a variety of neurologic abnormalities. Affecting one in 1000 Americans, MS is twice as common in women as men and is the number one neurologic disorder seen in 20–45 year olds.[24] Up to 80% of MS patients will have lower urinary tract symptoms, and 10% will present with voiding complaints as the initial manifestation of this neurologic disease.[19] Detrusor overactivity with symptoms of frequency, urgency, and urge incontinence is the most common urodynamic abnormality seen, occurring in 62% of patients, followed by DSD in 25%, and detrusor hypocontractility in 20%.[25]

Unlike some neurologic lesions, the effect of MS on the central nervous system can change urodynamic patterns and symptoms in up to 55% of patients.[26,27] The prevalence of voiding dysfunction in MS patients, along with the likelihood of urodynamic pattern changes with symptomatic deterioration, demands that urodynamic testing play a central role in the diagnosis and management of MS patients. Watanabe and associates noted three urodynamic patterns that predispose the MS patient to grave urologic complications.[18] The presence of DSD in men, loss of detrusor compliance, and the use of an indwelling catheter to manage bladder dysfunction all create a significant risk for damage to the lower urinary tract.

SPINAL CORD INJURY

With an estimated annual incidence of 8000–10,000 new spinal cord injuries a year in the United States, neurogenic bladder dysfunction in this population is common.[28] A period of decreased spinal cord activity below the injury, referred to as spinal shock, usually follows any significant spinal cord injury (SCI). Somatic and autonomic reflex activity is absent, and the bladder is areflexic with a closed bladder neck. Urethral sphincter tone is maintained, so incontinence is generally not a problem, except with overflow from bladder overdistension. After a period of weeks to months, somatic and autonomic reflex activity will resume.

When the distal spinal cord is intact but is isolated from higher control, the reflex behavior starts out with poorly sustained detrusor contractions under no voluntary control. The final pattern of vesicourethral dysfunction will be determined by the completeness of the SCI, level of the SCI, and the state of coordination between the bladder and urethral sphincter mechanisms.

Suprasacral SCI. Lesions between the sacral spinal cord and the pontine micturition center are characterized by detrusor overactivity (hyperreflexia) with or without sphincter synergy. In general, DSD is more common in complete suprasacral SCI. For injuries at T6 or higher, both the internal smooth sphincter and the external striated sphincter can exhibit DSD. As the bladder contracts reflexively against a closed urethra, elevated pressures are generated which, over time, will damage both the lower and upper urinary tracts. Urodynamic testing is required to diagnose the pattern of dysfunction, make proper management decisions, and follow storage pressures with compliance measurement to assure safe storage of urine. The often-quoted study by McGuire and associates established 40 cmH_2O as the pressure limit beyond which one would see significant upper tract damage if left untreated in children with myelodysplasia and neurogenic bladder dysfunction.[29] The same risk applies to SCI patients, where detrusor compliance during storage is the most important urodynamic parameter to be determined and followed over time. Along with a comprehensive initial evaluation, periodic follow-up evaluation is required to detect and manage high-pressure storage, high detrusor leak point pressure, bladder overdistension, vesicoureteral reflux, urolithiasis, and recurrent infection. Guidelines for the urologic evaluation of patients with SCI have been published by the American Paraplegia Society.[30]

The classic urodynamic survey of 489 neurogenic bladder patients by Kaplan et al reported a general correlation between the neurologic lesion level and the predicted pattern of vesicourethral dysfunction.[31] However, up to 15% of patients would be misclassified and poorly managed if the sole diagnostic tool was a neurologic examination. At either SCI extreme, opposite results with urodynamic testing (i.e. areflexia with cervical lesions and DSD with sacral cord lesions) were seen, as has also been reported by Weld and Dmochowski.[32]

Spinal cord injury is classified as complete or incomplete, using a grading classification based on somatic neurologic findings. Complete SCI in the somatic domain does not assure the same damage to autonomic pathways. In addition, multiple injuries may exist, although what is detected clinically may reflect only as single-level SCI. For these reasons, urodynamic testing should guide management. The reverse argument also can be made. Neurologic diagnoses should not be made solely on the findings of urodynamic testing.

Sacral SCI. SCI involving the conus medullaris and cauda equina presents with lower motor neuron dysfunction. Both afferent and efferent pathways are present in the local reflex arc to the S2–4 spinal cord. These are damaged, resulting in detrusor underactivity (areflexia), saddle anesthesia, loss of voluntary sphincter control, absence of the bulbocavernosus reflex, and reduced anal sphincter tone. Initial detrusor underactivity with normal or elevated compliance is common. However, over time, storage pressures can increase with an insidious loss of compliance secondary to the loss of normal innervation.

Autonomic hyperreflexia. SCI patients with autonomic hyperreflexia (AH) have injuries above the T6 vertebral level, which is superior to the sympathetic outflow exiting the spinal cord to innervate visceral and somatic organs. AH is a syndrome of exaggerated sympathetic activity triggered by sensory stimulation entering the nervous system below the lesion level. The sensory stimulation elicits sympathetic outflow, causing arteriolar and pilomotor spasm, leading to hypertension and a reduction in skin temperature. Above the lesion level, compensatory vasodilation results in flushing and sweating in the face and neck, a pounding headache, and reflex bradycardia. AH-induced hypertension can be severe, leading to seizure or cerebral hemorrhage. Bladder and rectal obstruction are common precipitating factors. Simple urodynamic testing can elicit AH, where immediate decompression of the bladder should be undertaken. Other inciting factors include bone fractures, appendicitis, decubitus ulcers, fecal impaction, instrumentation, clot retention, and catheter-related obstruction.

DIABETES MELLITUS

Diabetes mellitus is the most common metabolic disorder in the United States, with neuropathy being the presenting complication seen with most patients. Segmental demyelinization and neural vasculopathy are thought to damage nerve conduction. When innervation of the bladder is affected, the term diabetic cystopathy is used, coined by Frimodt-Moller in 1976.[33] Over 5 million people in the United States are diabetic and 20–40% show autonomic dysfunction.[34] The insidious onset of bladder sensation loss describes the classic description of diabetic cystopathy. A gradual increase in voiding intervals leads to detrusor distension and chronic decompensation. Loss of contractility results and patients may void once or twice daily with ever-increasing postvoid residual urine volumes. Diabetic cystopathy has been described in 26–87% of diabetics without symptoms of

bladder dysfunction,[19] and the cystopathy seems to occur about 10 years after the diagnosis of diabetes.

More recently, Kaplan studied 182 consecutive diabetics with voiding symptoms.[35] Both motor and sensory neuropathy was detected in men and women with a mixture of irritative and obstructive voiding symptoms. Nocturia, frequency, and hesitancy were the top three voiding complaints. Urodynamic testing revealed delayed sensation with over half the patients showing uninhibited contractions on filling cystometry. Frank areflexia was found in 10%, and 23% of the patients demonstrated impaired detrusor contractility. Urodynamic testing in 173 diabetics by Kitami[36] showed fewer patients with uninhibited contractions (14%), and 67% had a reduction in maximum detrusor pressure. DSD was reported in one-third, although the spinal cord pathogenesis of this finding is unclear to this author.

Based on more contemporary studies, it is clear that diabetic patients with voiding symptoms require urodynamic testing to guide proper diagnosis and management.

MYELODYSPLASIA

Myelodysplasia, or spina bifida, is the most common cause for neurogenic bladder dysfunction in children, with an incidence of one in 1000 births in the United States. Multidisciplinary centers manage the spectrum of serious malformations of the spine, nervous system, and somatovisceral targets of faulty innervation. Spina bifida cystica (meningocele), myelomeningocele (sac and neural elements), lipomeningocele (sac, neural elements, and fatty tissue), and myeloschisis (spinal cord open without covering) all represent spina bifida variants. This variability accounts for the variety of neurologic deficits seen in children with myelodysplasia. Maldevelopment and fibrosis of the lumbosacral spinal cord can lead to neurogenic bowel and bladder dysfunction along with lower extremity weakness or paralysis.

Neurologic examination is insufficient to predict the type of vesicourethral dysfunction secondary to spina bifida.[37] Over half of the children studied will have bladder contractions, with 48% of newborns exhibiting an intact sacral reflex arc, 23% with partial external sphincter denervation, and 29% showing complete loss of sacral cord function.[38] The typical patient with myelodysplasia and a neurogenic bladder shows an areflexic bladder with an open bladder neck and potential loss of detrusor compliance. Managing the neurogenic bladder in children is based on five findings gathered over the years from the clinical literature.[39]

1. Lower urinary tract dysfunction is common in children with myelodysplasia. This dysfunction results in urinary incontinence, urinary tract infection, and renal damage.

2. Bladder leak point pressure greater than 40 cmH$_2$O places the upper urinary tract at risk along with detrusor–sphincter dyssynergia, loss of bladder compliance, detrusor overactivity, recurrent bladder infections, and significant residual urine volumes.

3. Upper urinary tract damage is not always reversible. The chance of bladder augmentation is doubled in children with neurogenic bladder storage disorders, where intermittent catheterization is utilized for bladder management.

4. Maintenance of normal renal and bladder function requires regular examination to detect early upper tract deterioration.

5. The combination of intermittent catheterization and anticholinergic medication is very effective. Using this combination, 60–70% of vesicoureteral reflux disappears, 70–75% of hydronephrosis improves, and 55–84% of urinary incontinence is cured.

DISK DISEASE

Intervertebral disk prolapse with posterolateral protrusion causes direct neurologic damage by nerve root or spinal cord compression. Disk prolapse or herniation occurs frequently at the L4–5 and L5–S1 levels. More centrally based disk prolapse seems to affect the nerves to the bladder, pelvic floor, and penis. A large prospective study of 114 patients with lumbar disk herniation requiring surgical treatment revealed 27% with detrusor areflexia.[40] All the areflexic patients had to strain to void. Urodynamic testing was performed before and after surgery in 86% of the patients. Of note, only 22% of the patients with preoperative areflexia regained normal function following disk surgery. O'Flynn and associates reported similar results following disk surgery.[41] Areflexia with straining to void was detected postoperatively in 37% of the patients. Only one patient regained normal bladder function.

Cauda equina syndrome is a severe form of disk herniation with lower extremity weakness, bilateral sciatica, saddle-type hypesthesia, and bowel and bladder dysfunction. Often patients lose voluntary control of both the anal and urethral sphincters. Since most disk herniation occurs at the L4–5 or L5–S1 level, when it is central in distribution, the S2–4 roots can be affected. Shin et al reported on 50 patients with cauda equina injuries. Loss of detrusor compliance was detected in 28%, and almost half of the patients had temporary hyperreflexia as well, until compliance and capacity normalized.[42]

RADICAL PELVIC SURGERY

Two common causes of neurogenic vesicourethral dysfunction are abdominoperineal resection (APR) for rectal carcinoma and radical hysterectomy with pelvic lymphadenectomy for cervical carcinoma. Both procedures can damage or injure the peripheral innervation of the bladder, including the pelvic plexus.

Voiding dysfunction following conventional or wide APR was reported on by Michelassi and Block.[43] Wide APR caused 18% of the patients to need self-catheterization postoperatively. Within 8 months, all of the patients were able to stop catheterization and void normally. By contrast, low anterior resection is associated with a lower rate of vesicourethral dysfunction. Hojo et al showed that preservation of the autonomic nerves resulted in spontaneous voiding in 88% versus 78% of patients undergoing complete resection of the pelvic nerves, resulting in urinary retention and chronic catheterization.[44]

Voiding dysfunction following radical hysterectomy is usually secondary to parasympathetic denervation of the bladder, with up to 50% of patients showing additional sympathetic denervation.[45] Iio and associates found urodynamic evidence of detrusor compliance loss and sphincteric denervation in 24 patients undergoing radical hysterectomy.[46]

Overall, neurogenic bladder dysfunction is seen in 10–60% of patients. Voiding dysfunction is permanent in 15–20%. Often voiding dysfunction is transient, and nondestructive methods of management are mandatory. As a rule of thumb, it is wise to wait a year following surgery before more permanent treatment options are performed to give the bladder and urethra time to reinnervate.

REFERENCES

1. Yoshimura N, Satoshi S, Chancellor MB. Integrated physiology of the lower urinary tract. In: Corcos J, Schick E, eds. Textbook of the neurogenic bladder. London: Martin Dunitz; 2004.
2. de Groat WC. The urothelium in overactive bladder: passive bystander or active participant? Urology 2004;64(Suppl 6A):7–11.
3. Nagatomi J, Gloeckner DC, Chancellor MB, et al. Changes in the biaxial viscoelastic response of the urinary bladder following spinal cord injury. Ann Biomed Eng 2004;32(10):1409–1419.
4. Rivas DA, Abdill CK, Chancellor MB. Current management of detrusor sphincter dyssynergia. Topic Spinal Cord Injury Rehabil 1996;1:1–17.
5. Wein AJ. Pathophysiology and categorization of voiding dysfunction. In: Retik AB, Vaughn ED, Wein AJ, eds. Campbell's urology. Philadelphia: WB Saunders; 2002.
6. Nitti VW, Adler H, Combs AJ. The role of urodynamics in the evaluation of voiding dysfunction in men after cerebrovascular accident. J Urol 1996;155:263–266.
7. Taub NA, Wolfe CD, Richardson E, et al. Predicting the disability of

first-time stroke suffers at 1 year. 12-month follow-up of a population-based cohort in Southeast England. Stroke 1994;25:352–357.

8. Wade DT, Hewer RL. Outlook after an acute stroke: urinary incontinence and loss of consciousness compared in 532 patients. Q J Med 1985;56:601–608.

9. Gelber DA, Good DC, Laven LJ, et al. Causes of urinary incontinence after acute hemispheric stroke. Stroke 1993;24:378–382.

10. Marinkovic SP, Badlani G. Voiding and sexual dysfunction after cerebrovascular accidents. J Urol 2001;165:359–370.

11. Tsuchida S, Noto H, Yamaguchi O, et al. Urodynamic studies in hemiplegic patients after cerbrovascular accidents. Urology 1983;21:315–318.

12. Andrew J, Nathan PW. Lesions of the anterior frontal lobes and disturbances of micturition and defaecation. Brain 1964;87:233–262.

13. Maurice-Williams RS. Micturition symptoms in frontal tumors. J Neurol Neurosurg Psychiatr 1974;37:431–436.

14. Lang EW, Chestnut RM, Hennerici M. Urinary retention and space occupying lesions of the frontal cortex. Eur Neurol 1996;36:43–47.

15. McNeal DM, Hawtrey CE, Wolraich ML, et al. Symptomatic neurogenic bladder in a cerebral-palsied population. Dev Med Child Neurol 1983;25:612–616.

16. Decter RM, Bauer SB, Khoshbin S, et al. Urodynamic assessment of children with cerebral palsy. J Urol 1987;138:1110–1112.

17. Shy GM, Drager GA. A neurological syndrome associated with orthostatic hypotension: a clinico-pathologic study. Arch Neurol 1960;2:511–527.

18. Salinas JM, Berger Y, De La Roacha RE, et al. Urological evaluation in the Shy–Drager syndrome. J Urol 1986;135:741–743.

19. Leu PB, Diokno AC. Epidemiology of the neurogenic bladder. In: Corcos J, Schick E, eds. Textbook of the neurogenic bladder. London: Martin Dunitz; 2004.

20. Langworthy OR, Lewis LG, Dees JE, Hesser FH. Clinical study of control of bladder by central nervous system. Bull Johns Hopkins Hosp 1936;58:89.

21. Murnaghan GF. Neurogenic disorders of the bladder in parkinsonism. Br J Urol 1961;33:403–409.

22. Pavlakis AJ, Siroky MB, Goldstein I, Krane RJ. Neurourologic findings in parkinson's disease. J Urol 1983;129:80–83.

23. Araki I, Kitahara M, Oida T, Kuno S. Voiding dysfunction and parkinson's disease: urodynamic abnormalities and urinary symptoms. J Urol 2000;164:1640–1643.

24. Fingerman JS, Finkelstein LH. The overactive bladder in multiple sclerosis. J Am Osteopath Assoc 2000;100:S9–S12.

25. Litwiller SE, Frohman EM, Zimmern PE. Multiple sclerosis and the urologist. J Urol 1999;161:743–757.

26. Wheeler JS Jr, Siroky MB, Pavlakis AJ, et al. The changing neurourologic pattern of multiple sclerosis. J Urol 1983;130:1123–1126.

27. Ciancio SJ, Mutchnik SE, Rivera VM, Boone TB. Urodynamic pattern changes in multiple sclerosis. Urology 2001;57:239–245.

28. Waites KB, Canupp WC, DeVivo MJ, et al. Compliance with annual urologic evaluations and preservation of renal function in persons with spinal cord injury. J Spinal Cord Med 1995;18:251–254.

29. McGuire EJ, Woodside JR, Borden TA, Weiss RM. Prognostic value of urodynamic testing in myelodysplastic patients. J Urol 1981;126:205–209.

30. Linsenmeyer TA, Culkin D. APS recommendations for the urological evaluation of patients with spinal cord injury. J Spinal Cord Med 1999;22:139–142.

31. Kaplan SA, Chancellor MB, Blaivas JG. Bladder and sphincter behavior in patients with spinal cord lesions. J Urol 1991;146:113–117.

32. Weld KJ, Dmochowski RR. Association of level of injury and bladder behavior in patients with post-traumatic spinal cord injury. Urology 2000;55:490–494.

33. Frimodt-Moller C. Diabetic cystopathy: a clinical study of the frequency of bladder dysfunction in diabetics. Dan Med Bull 1976;23:267–278.

34. Ross MA. Neuropathies associated with diabetes. Med Clin North Am 1993;77:111–124.

35. Kaplan SA, Te AE, Blaivas JG. Urodynamic findings in patients with diabetic cystopathy. J Urol 1995;153:342–344.

36. Kitami K. Vesicourethral dysfunction of diabetic patients. Nippon Hinyokika Gakkai Zasshi 1991 Jul; 82(7):1074–1083.

37. Bauer SB, Hallett M, Khoshbin S, et al. Predictive value of urodynamic evaluation in newborns with myelodysplasia. JAMA 1984;252:650–652.

38. Spindel MR, Bauer SB, Dyro FM, et al. The changing neurourologic lesion in myelodysplasia. JAMA 1987;258:1630–1633.

39. Kondo A, Gotoh M, Kamihira O. Spina bifida in infancy and childhood. In: Corcos J, Schick E, eds. Textbook of the neurogenic bladder. London: Martin Dunitz; 2004.

40. Bartolin Z, Vilendecic M, Derezic D. Bladder function after surgery for lumbar intervertebral disk protrusion. J Urol 1999;161:1885–1887.

41. O'Flynn KJ, Murphy R, Thomas DG. Neurogenic bladder dysfunction in lumbar intervertebral disc prolapse. Br J Urol 1992;69:38–40.

42. Shin JC, Park CI, Kim HJ, Lee IY. Significance of low compliance bladder in cauda equina injury. Spinal Cord 2002;40:650–655.

43. Michelassi F, Block GE. Morbidity and mortality of wide pelvic lymphadenectomy for rectal adenocarcinoma. Dis Colon Rectum 1992;35:1143–1147.

44. Hojo K, Vernava AM, Sugihara K, Katumata K. Preservation of urine voiding and sexual function after rectal cancer surgery. Dis Colon Rectum 1991;34:532–539.

45. Kershen RT, Boone TB. Peripheral neuropathies of the lower urinary tract, following pelvic surgery and radiation therapy. In: Corcos J, Schick E, eds. Textbook of the neurogenic bladder. London: Martin Dunitz; 2004.

46. Iio S, Yoshioka S, Nishio S, et al. Urodynamic evaluation for bladder dysfunction after radical hysterectomy. Jpn J Urol 1993;84:535–540.

Neurogenic Bladder: Evaluation and Management

Gary E Lemack

INTRODUCTION

Patients with neurologic conditions frequently develop significant lower urinary tract dysfunction during the course of their disease. Since in many of these conditions, normal sensation is altered, one often cannot rely on the typical signs and symptoms to aid in diagnosing the type of bladder dysfunction present. It is also clear that certain specific patterns of bladder dysfunction may be associated with greater, and potentially life-threatening, morbidity. As such, accurately diagnosing patients with neurogenic bladder conditions is imperative to both improving quality of life and minimizing the risk of complications, by implementing condition-specific therapy.

NEUROLOGIC HISTORY

In patients with progressive neurologic conditions, it is useful to establish the onset of symptoms (often not the same as the timing of diagnosis) as well as recent changes in symptom severity, as this information may clearly influence treatment recommendations. In addition, disease duration has been correlated with the development of urinary symptoms, particularly in multiple sclerosis (MS) and Parkinson's disease (PD).[1] Even patients with presumably fixed neurologic conditions (ie. spinal cord injury, myelomeningocele) may have symptomatic deterioration (ie. due to development of a syrinx or tethered cord), and therefore any recent changes in sensory or motor function should be directly assessed.

Patients with movement disorders should be carefully questioned as to the onset of their neurologic symptoms in comparison to their urinary symptoms, since those with more progressive syndromes, such as multiple systems atrophy (MSA), often develop autonomic disturbances (such as bladder and erectile dysfunction) early during the course of their illness. Patients with Parkinson's disease should be assessed for their Hoehn and Yahr stage, which can be useful in predicting the severity of bladder dysfunction and prospects for further deterioration.[2]

Patients with multiple sclerosis should be queried as to the timing of the onset of their symptoms, and for recent exacerbations, as frequently such exacerbations can be initiated by urologic events.[3] In addition, inquiring about the status of their condition (relapsing, remitting, primary progressive, secondary progressive) may be quite important in planning therapy, particularly when considering surgical options which might require considerable dexterity.

In patients with more recent acute events, such as cerebrovascular accident (CVA), information about the stroke location and recovery since the event can be useful, since stroke location can impact on prognosis.[4] Patients with history of back surgery (often several procedures) should be questioned about the vertebral level of the surgery and the presence of ongoing sensory deficit.

Current treatments should also be documented, with particular attention paid to medications. Medications with properties that can affect the bladder outlet (typically with either α-agonist or antagonist properties) or detrusor contractility (typically those with anticholinergic properties) should be recorded, along with narcotic and skeletal muscle relaxant use.

PHYSICAL EXAMINATION

General observations. Mode of ambulation and recent progression of ambulatory disturbances should be assessed at the initial visit. Clearly, the degree of physical independence of the patient, particularly as it relates to the ability to get to the toilet, often affects the degree of urge-related leakage episodes. Additionally, some patients who are non-ambulatory may have great difficulty with self-urethral catheterization. If so, an abdominal catheterizable stoma may be a more reasonable option in the appropriately selected patient who is considering surgical intervention.

Hand function in patients with cervical spinal cord injury (SCI), and particularly the ability to grasp firmly between the thumb and index or middle finger, must be carefully judged in those who may require intermittent catheterization following treatment. However, it is no longer mandatory that patients have use of both hands prior to such an intervention, as single-unit catheter/collection systems are commercially available.

An evaluation of the skin, particularly in the gluteal region, should be carried out, as localized skin and subcutaneous infections as well as more severe skin breakdown are not uncommon among patients with restricted mobility. Such issues will need to be addressed before major reconstructive procedures are considered. Some patients may also have intrathecal pumps in place and their location, as well as that of their tubing, should be assessed prior to surgical endeavors.

Neurologic examination.

A brief neurologic examination is essential when first evaluating patients with presumed neurovesical dysfunction. Mental status should be assessed, as significant cognitive dysfunction and memory disturbances have been independently associated with abnormal voiding function. An appreciation of past and present intellectual capacity may also provide insight into the progression of lower urinary tract disorders, as well as guiding the degree of complexity of treatment strategies. Both motor strength and sensory level should be determined, as distribution of motor and sensory disturbances can often predict lower urinary tract dysfunction, particularly in multiple sclerosis.[5]

There should also be a thorough evaluation of both cutaneous and motor reflexes at the time of the initial encounter. The bulbocavernosus reflex, elicited by gently squeezing the glans penis in men or gentle compression of the clitoris against the pubis in women and simultaneously feeling for an anal sphincter contraction (by placing a finger in the rectum), assesses the integrity of the S2–4 reflex arc. The anal reflex, which assesses integrity of S2–5, can be checked by applying a pinprick to the mucocutaneous junction of the anus and evaluating for anal sphincter contraction. The cremasteric reflex may be somewhat less reliable but assesses sensory dermatomes supplied by L1–2.

Muscle motor reflexes should also be routinely evaluated. The most common of these are the biceps reflex (assesses C5–6), patellar reflex (L2–4), and Achilles (ankle) reflex (L5–S2). Evidence of an upper motor neurologic injury would include spasticity of the involved skeletal muscle, heightened response to reflex testing, and an upgoing toe on gentle stroking of the plantar surface of the foot (positive Babinski).

Genitourinary examination.

Pelvic examination should be carried out to assess for vaginal estrogenization (noting a loss of lubrication, rugation, and blanching of the mucosal surface) and pelvic prolapse. One should also observe for urine loss (either spontaneous or induced by Valsalva or cough). An assessment of the urethra is essential in both men and women, particularly those with chronic indwelling catheters, as traumatic hypospadias in men and bladder neck erosion in women may require surgical repair. A careful examination of sensation of the genitalia may provide insight into the nature of sexual dysfunction, if present, as both hypo- and hyperesthesia have been described among patients with neurologic conditions. A rectal examination should assess for sphincter tone and for stool impaction, as chronic constipation may aggravate voiding dysfunction.

In men, the prostate should be examined for areas of tenderness or fluctuance since prostatitis and prostatic abscesses are not uncommon among men with severe neurovesical dysfunction, particularly those with chronic indwelling catheters.

ROLE OF URODYNAMICS AND NEUROPHYSIOLOGIC TESTING

Attempting to manage patients with neurourologic conditions without urodynamic assessment can lead to inappropriate treatment and significant morbidity. The use of urodynamics has been, in part, responsible for the improved care and longer life expectancy of many patients with neurologic conditions, such as spinal cord injury. In its simplest form, urodynamics can consist of an evaluation of urine flow and postvoid residual. In its most complex form, it involves a multisystem test of vesical and extravesical pressures during filling and voiding, coupled with fluoroscopic evaluation of the bladder and simultaneous neurophysiologic testing of pelvic floor function.

Since most patients with trauma-related SCI will suffer neurovesical dysfunction, it is generally agreed that all should undergo baseline urodynamic assessment, though the frequency at which that should occur is somewhat controversial.[6] Because these patients have also been traditionally at risk for upper tract deterioration, monitoring of the kidneys at periodic intervals is also recommended, particularly in those with fairly severe bladder dysfunction.[7] The timing of the initial evaluation generally can be delayed until the spinal shock phase of the initial injury dissipates. During this phase, spinal reflex activity below the level of the injury ceases, resulting in skeletal muscle flaccidity and a depression of smooth muscle activity, which generally results in urinary retention due to detrusor areflexia. Patients can either be managed with indwelling catheters or be taught clean intermittent catheterization (CIC) during this time. With the emergence from spinal shock, bladder reflex activity returns (often in the form of leakage) in patients on CIC, along with skeletal muscle spasticity, to a varying degree depending on the location of the lesion. It is at this time that urodynamic assessment is warranted.

While fairly predictable patterns of neurovesical dysfunction follow spinal cord injury, depending on the level and completeness of the injury, the same cannot be said of other neurologic disorders. Patients who may be at the greatest risk of significant morbidity are those found to have evidence of detrusor–external sphincter dyssynergia (DESD), which is true of most patients with thoracic and cervical SCI, as well as up to 70% of patients with primary progressive MS (Fig. 29.1), and a minority of patients with other common disorders.[8] Simultaneous fluoroscopic evaluation of the bladder outlet will demonstrate ballooning of the proximal urethra and impaired emptying (Fig. 29.2). Interestingly, lesion site in MS may correlate with bladder dysfunction, as the presence of cervical lesions has been associated with the urodynamic diagnosis of DESD.[9] Given that most of these patients have sustained pathologic overactive detrusor contractions, intravesical pressures are frequently raised, a finding which has been shown to be associated with long-term renal dysfunction in patients with myelomeningocele.[10] Therapeutic efforts therefore concentrate on reducing intravesical pressures.

The majority of patients with other common neurologic conditions (including most with MS, PD, and CVA) will be found to have neurogenic detrusor overactivity (DO) on urodynamic studies (UDS) (Fig. 29.3). While symptoms will vary, typically sensate patients will note urgency, frequency,

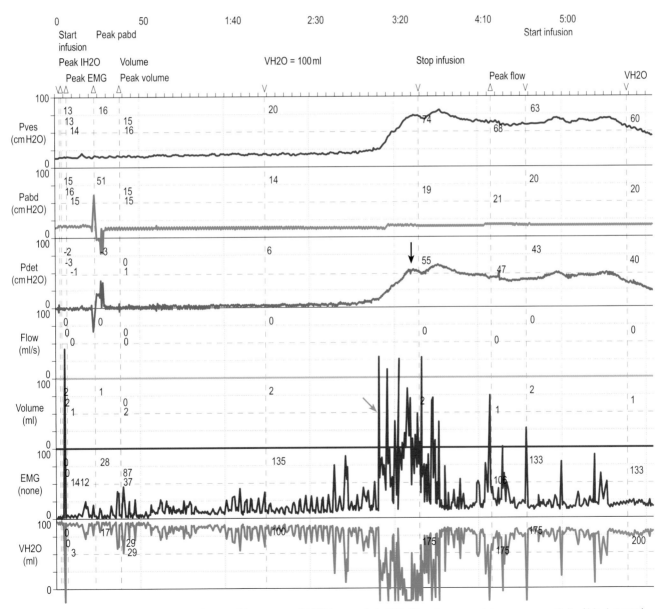

Figure 29.1 Urodynamic tracing from a 26-year-old woman with T5 incomplete SCI. Simultaneous detrusor overactivity (*black arrow*) with dyssynergic sphincteric activity noted on EMG tracing (*gray arrow*) leads to sustained elevated intravesical pressures and poor emptying.

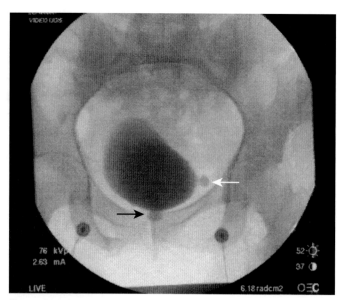

Figure 29.2 Voiding cystogram performed at time of urodynamics reveals ballooning of the proximal urethra secondary to external sphincter dyssynergia (*black arrow*). Also noted is a left-sided bladder diverticulum (*white arrow*).

urge incontinence, and nocturia that typically are progressive. Though there are no clear criteria to distinguish neurogenic DO from idiopathic DO (Fig. 29.4), there are emerging data that suggest the former is more likely to be associated with urge incontinence during UDS and the emergence of DO earlier during filling in patients with PD than those with bladder outlet obstruction (BOO)-induced DO.[11] These types of findings may have practical uses for predicting the likelihood of resolution of DO following treatment for BOO due to prostatic disease in patients with PD.

Urodynamic assessment of bladder compliance is also essential. Patients with chronic neurogenic bladder (NGB) conditions (such as SCI), particularly those who have been treated with indwelling catheters for prolonged periods of time, may develop poorly compliant bladders, which can place the upper tract at substantial risk if left untreated. Detrusor leak point pressure, the detrusor pressure at which leakage is noted urodynamically, should be determined and if elevated (typically above 40 cmH_2O) must be appropriately treated.

The emergence of the specific complaint of voiding dysfunction in patients with MS and movement disorders should also prompt urodynamic examination. In the case of MS, this may indicate the progression from the typical finding of neurogenic DO to DESD or detrusor failure, which will clearly alter therapy. For many men with PD, it is often impossible to sort out the contribution of typical processes associated with this age group (such as BOO secondary to benign prostatic growth) to neurogenically mediated events. Since surgical endeavors used to treat men with BOO may have an unacceptable rate of incontinence in patients with PD (up to 20%), it is imperative to study these patients urodynamically.

Specific evaluation of the pelvic floor in patients with movement disorders may be the best example of how neurophysiologic testing can be useful clinically. Patients with movement disorders, particularly those with MSA and to a lesser extent those with PD, have significant external sphincter dysfunction. In the case of MSA, denervation motor unit potentials (MUPs) have been demonstrated in the majority, indicating a very specific loss of sphincteric activity due to involvement of anterior horn cells in Onuf's nucleus.[12] Electromyographic (EMG) assessment of MUPs utilizing concentric needle electrodes allows one to differentiate normal from denervated and reinnervated muscle. These findings may help in distinguishing neurologic conditions affecting the pelvic floor, and may have distinct prognostic implications.[13]

In many urodynamic laboratories, a more simple kinesiologic assessment of overall pelvic floor muscle activity utilizes a surface electrode placed perineally adjacent to the anus or needle electrodes in a similar location. In general, while surface electrodes are more easily tolerated by sensate patients, they are prone to artefacts and can become easily dislodged during testing. Regardless, when used for a kinesiologic assessment, recording of EMG allows a determination of pelvic floor (and, by inference, external sphincter) activity during storage (continuous low-frequency tonic activity) and during voiding (loss of activity immediately prior to detrusor contraction). Abnormal activity during voiding indicates a dyssynergic pattern, which may indicate a cervical or upper thoracic cord lesion, though dyssynergia from other nonneurologic sources such as dysfunctional voiding (Hinman syndrome) is not uncommon.

NONSURGICAL THERAPY
Oral medications for the overactive bladder (detrusor overactivity). The mainstay of therapy in neurogenic bladder conditions resulting in detrusor overactivity remains anticholinergic medications. The goal of this therapy is to decrease intravesical pressures, increase bladder capacity, and reduce incontinence episodes. Given the dense innervation of the detrusor smooth muscle by muscarinic-type cholinergic nerves, the main mechanism by which overactive contractions are muted is by blocking synaptic excitation at the level of the muscarinic receptor. While many medications have anticholinergic properties, relatively few have traditionally been used specifically for the purpose of detrusor relaxation, and those include propantheline, hyoscyamine, and oxybutynin. Since some of these molecules have other properties, including direct antispasmodic and anesthetic properties, it is possible that part of their effect is not related to muscarinic blockade.

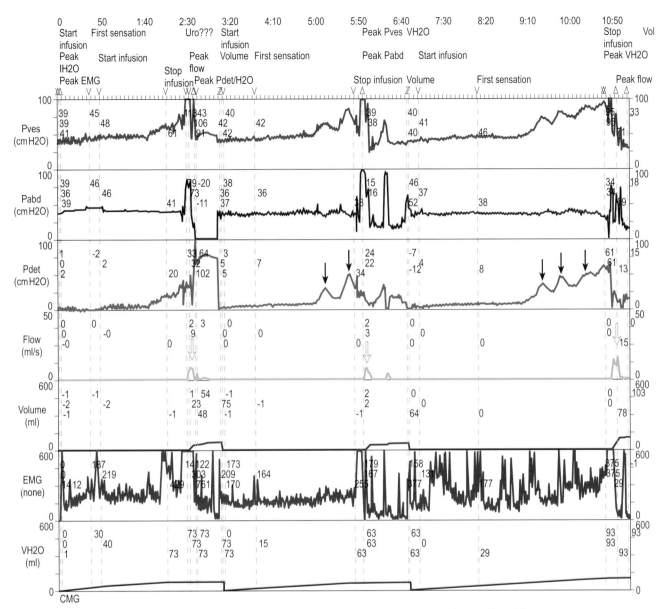

Figure 29.3 Severe neurogenic (phasic) detrusor overactivity (*black arrows*). Leakage event denoted by white arrows.

In addition to the oral use of oxybutynin, intravesical[14] and combined intravesical and oral uses[15] have been recommended for treatment of patients with SCI, even those with indwelling catheters.[16]

The last few years have witnessed the development of alternative anticholinergic medications with lower side-effect profiles, such as tolterodine (with extended-release formulation), extended-release oxybutynin, transdermal oxybutynin, and trospium. While none has shown superior efficacy to oxybutynin, each has shown improved tolerability. There does not appear to be compelling evidence that one is superior to any of the others, particularly with regard to treating patients with NGB conditions. Data are now emerging that tolterodine, extended-release oxybutynin and trospium, a quaternary amine antimuscarinic, are effective in treating NGB conditions and that higher doses

may be tolerated using some of these medications.[17-19] The efficacy of the new M3 muscarinic receptor-specific anticholinergic agent darifenacin, as well as solifenacin (YM905) which is believed to have greater bladder selectivity, has not yet been directly assessed in NGB populations. There are data to suggest that the M2 receptor may be responsible for overactive contractions in patients with NGB, allowing the possibility that M3-specific agents will not be as effective in these populations.[20]

In most patients with thoracic and cervical SCI who have sufficient manual dexterity, anticholinergic therapy will be coupled with CIC, since the vast majority will have DESD. Patients with sacral cord lesions or cauda equina syndrome typically will not require anticholinergic therapy in the presence of low filling pressures though they will rely on CIC. While many patients with distal cord lesions will be

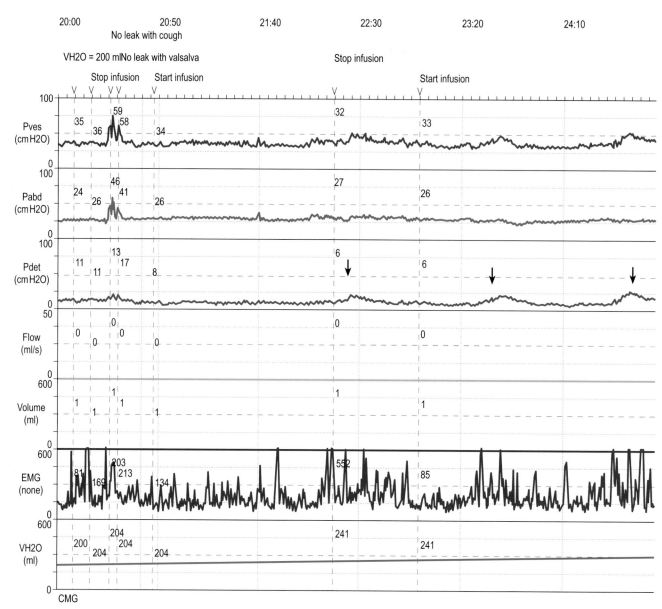

Figure 29.4 Idiopathic detrusor overactivity (*black arrows*).

continent due to the absence of DO, some may have inadequate sphincteric function, resulting in troublesome leakage between catheterizations with minor degrees of bladder fullness.

Intravesically delivered agents. Patients with refractory neurogenic bladder conditions resulting in upper tract damage, repeated infections or intractable incontinence traditionally have been treated surgically. The emergence of new treatment options, while still not approved and/or commercially available, has allowed some patients to avoid surgery. The recognition of the importance of the unmyelinated afferent C fiber as an important mediator of pain reflexes from the bladder in pathologic conditions, and a fiber which plays more of a dominant role in the micturition reflex following SCI,[21] raised the possibility of desensitizing

these nerves as a means of treating refractory conditions of overactive bladder. By binding at the (vanilloid-sensitive) afferent nerve fiber, capsaicin was the first agent noted to initially excite and ultimately desensitize the nerve, and prevent the development of neurogenic inflammation and the release of inflammatory mediators and substance P.[22,23] Several clinical trials of capsaicin for patients with neurogenic DO have been conducted, with an average response rate of 84%, including improvements in frequency, incontinence, and urodynamic bladder capacity with a durable response noted for 2–6 months.[24] Resiniferatoxin, a more potent vanilloid derived from a cactus-like plant, has also been studied for the treatment of neurogenic DO, since it does not seem to initially excite but rather exclusively desensitizes the afferent fiber, and therefore potentially results in minimal pain with instillation. Randomized trials have been conducted and demonstrate fairly dramatic improvements in bladder capacity and reductions in incontinence episodes, with minimal discomfort, superior to capsaicin.[25,26]

Recent studies have focused on the use of botulinum toxin, delivered by cystoscopic injection into the detrusor wall, for the treatment of neurogenic detrusor overactivity.[27,28] Impressive increases in cystometric capacity and reduction in voiding pressures were noted after injection of a total of 300 U of botulinum toxin into the detrusor wall in 30 different sites, sparing the trigone, an effect which seems to persist for 6–9 months. Many patients were able to discontinue anticholinergic agents altogether, and complete continence was restored in 73% of patients. No adverse sequelae were reported in the largest experience reported to date, though case reports of adverse reactions have been noted.[29] Botulinum toxin has also been injected into the urethral sphincter for the treatment of DESD, with varying degrees of success.[30]

SURGICAL THERAPY

Suprapubic catheters. Patients with debilitating incontinence unresponsive to medical therapy and those with recurrent urinary infections secondary to indwelling urethral catheter use may require further intervention to improve their quality of life and/or stabilize their disease. As a first step in the treatment of refractory neurogenic DO, patients frequently inquire about catheter use. While urethral catheter use is the simplest option, its association with bladder neck erosion in women, traumatic hypospadias in men, recurrent urinary infections and bacteriuria, as well as the impact on sexual function, make long-term urethral catheter use less desirable.[31] Suprapubic catheters (SPC), while still associated with higher rates of recurrent infections, bladder stone formation,[32] and bladder cancer[33] than CIC, are generally easier to care for and associated with fewer urethral and prostate-related complications. One needs to be sure to assess for intrinsic sphincteric deficiency (ISD), particularly in patients with a history of long-term urethral catheter use, since ongoing urethral leakage can continue despite placement of an SPC.

Treatment of sphincteric insufficiency.

In patients with incompetent outlets, treatment aimed at ISD may be necessary at the time of SPC placement. Typically in women, this involves either therapy aimed at increasing outlet resistance, such as pubovaginal sling,[34] or bladder neck closure, which may be most useful in patients with severe ISD secondary to bladder neck erosion and long-term catheter use (Fig. 29.5). Artificial urinary sphincter placement has been advocated in both men and women with urethral incompetence, though complications such as urethral ero-

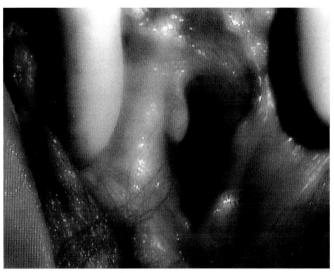

Figure 29.5 Bladder neck erosion secondary to long-term catheter use.

sion have been associated with its use in this population due to repeated catheterization. In males, bladder neck closure, as well as bladder neck tapering with suburethral sling placement, has been advocated for patients with minimal outlet resistance.[35]

Augmentation cystoplasty and urinary diversion.

Patients who seek to remain catheter free, as well as those who develop repeated infections despite placement of an SPC, might be candidates for continent or incontinent urinary diversion, and/or augmentation cystoplasty alone. Since any form of augmentation carries the risk of impaired emptying, all patients considered for such an approach should be carefully evaluated for their manual dexterity, ability, and commitment to perform intermittent catheterization. Patients unable to catheterize via their native urethra may be candidates for continent diversion to the abdominal wall, though they still must demonstrate the ability to catheterize independently. For those unable to do so, and for those in whom the risk of disease progression might readily affect their ability to catheterize, incontinent diversion is often the best selection.

Incontinent diversion to the abdominal wall may involve construction of either an ileovesicostomy, leaving the ureterovesical junction intact, or an ileal conduit, with or without concomitant cystectomy. Ileovesicostomy has been advocated by several authors for its relative ease of reconstruction and versatility, though complications such as impaired bladder drainage and recurrent infections have been reported (Fig. 29.6).[36,37] Ileal conduit diversion eliminates the risk of impaired drainage, though it is associated with other perioperative complications, including recurrent pyocystitis in roughly 25% of patients who do not undergo simultaneous cystectomy,[38] as well as long-term renal damage.[39]

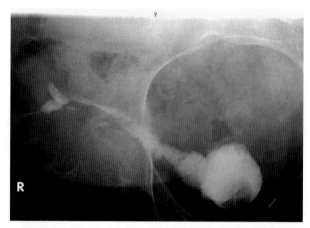

Figure 29.6 Cystogram image of ileovesicostomy.

Augmentation cystosplasty, with or without creation of a catheterizable stoma to the skin, can reliably increase bladder capacity, reduce intravesical pressures, and decrease incontinence rates in NGB patients with refractory neurogenic DO (Table 29.1). The portion of bowel used for augmentation and the method of creating the catheterizable channel have varied. In general, ileal segments appear to be favored for augmentation when available, due to the relative abundance of ileum and the relatively lower rate of metabolic disturbances and long-term mucus production. Catheterizable channels utilizing appendix (Mitrofanoff), tapered ileum (Indiana), reconfigured ileum (Monti and extended Monti), and retubularized native bladder, as well as several other modifications, have all met with considerable success. Still, complication rates in this patient population are considerable, including the potential risk of bladder rupture in patients with augmentation, which may present a surgical emergency, as well as a described tumor risk in augmented bladders,[40] stone formation, recurrent bladder infections, and bowel dysfunction depending upon the segment used.

Other methods of augmentation have also been attempted given the complications associated with bowel use. Auto-augmentation has been attempted, in which the muscular wall of the bladder is incised and often removed (detrusor myectomy), allowing the mucosa to balloon out. This method has not met with good long-term success in terms of durable increases in bladder capacity,[41] though it may have application in patients with idiopathic detrusor overactivity.[42] Ureterocystoplasty may be an appropriate option to consider when dilated upper tracts are present in order to utilize urothelial tissue rather than bowel.[43] Augmentation using allograft small intestinal submucosa, either alone[44] and more recently as a scaffolding for the growth of smooth muscle cells and urothelial cells,[45] has also been described in animal models. Finally, recent investigations have evaluated the use of cultured urothelial cells for use in bladder augmentation.[46]

Treatment of sphincter dyssynergia. Male patients with DESD incapable of performing CIC may desire continuous urethral drainage of urine rather than incontinent diversion or indwelling catheterization. Sphincterotomy, which results in ongoing urinary drainage by reducing outlet resistance, can be accomplished cystoscopically by incising the sphincter with the cold knife, cautery or laser,[47] or chemically by injecting the sphincter with botulinum toxin.[30,48] In both cases, repeat treatments are often required over time. Different types of urethral stents have also been advocated for this purpose, including the Memokath[49] and Urolume,[50,51] though complications of the stent, including migration and difficulty with removal, if required, have been reported, particularly with the Urolume.[52]

NEURAL STIMULATION

Emerging data suggest that direct CNS stimulation may effectively treat symptoms of urinary urgency, frequency, and incontinence with certain neurologic disorders. Patients with SCI classically have been treated with posterior rhizotomy, in order to abolish reflex detrusor contractions, along with implantation of a device for periodic voluntary anterior root stimulation (Finetech–Brindley stimulator).[53] Traditionally, the difficulty has been with selective activation of a detrusor contraction without simultaneous pelvic floor/sphincteric contraction, inducing a DESD type of response and impaired bladder drainage. Newer systems have sought to address that challenge, though at this point implantation is still not widely recommended or available.[54,55]

Bladder dysfunction in the setting of other neurologic conditions has also been treated by neuromodulation. Sacral cord stimulation has been used to treat urge incontinence in patients with MS, with modest success.[56,57] Deep brain stimulation has been used to attempt to control tremors in various neurologic conditions, particularly Parkinson's disease. Patients undergoing subthalamic nucleus stimulation were noted to have a significant increase in both overall bladder capacity as well as threshold for the development of detrusor overactivity, and a reduction in voiding pressures compared to before stimulation, indicating a secondary benefit of this treatment modality.[58]

CONCLUSION

The majority of patients with the most common neurologic disorders, including multiple sclerosis, Parkinson's disease, stroke, and spinal cord injury, will be found to have neurovesical dysfunction on thorough evaluation. However, since urinary symptoms are not always a reliable indicator of whether bladder dysfunction exists and since the spectrum of bladder disorders seems to change over time with progression of disease in many instances, careful and ongoing

Table 29.1 Representative series of augmentation cystoplasty for neurogenic and nonneurogenic bladder dysfunction

Lead author	Year	# pts	Patient diagnosis	Bowel used	Follow-up (mos)	Preop capacity (ml)	Postop capacity (ml)	% complete continence	% requ. CIC
Kockelbergh[i]	1991	45	Mixed	Ileum*	20	404	471	69%	33%
Radomski[ii]	1995	14	Neuro	Ileum	18	177	441	100%	NR
		12	Neuro	Sigmoid	37	170	538	42%	NR
Flood[iii]	1995	102	Mixed	Ileum*	37	108	438	78%	88%
Hasan[iv]	1995	48	Mixed	Ileum*	38	307	588	NR	85%
Greenwell[v]	2001	267	Mixed	Ileum	60–204	NR	NR	87%–neuro. 93%–idiop.	60%– neuro. 6%–idiop.
Khastgir[vi]	2003	32	Neuro	Ileum	72	143	589	100%	100%
Quek[vii]	2003	26	Neuro	Ileum	96	201	615	69%	100%

NR, not reported; neuro, neurogenic bladder disorders; idiop., idiopathic detrusor overactivity; *, primarily ileum used, with a small fraction requiring augmentation using colon segments.
[i] Kockelbergh RC, Tan JBL, Bates CP, et al. Clam enterocystoplasty in general urological practice. Br J Urol 1991;68:38–41.
[ii] Radomski SB, Herschorn S, Stone AR. Urodynamic comparison of ileum vs. sigmoid in augmentation cystoplasty for neurogenic bladder dysfunction. Neuro Urodynam 1995;14:231–237.
[iii] Flood HD, Malhotra SJ, O'Connell HE, et al. Long-term results and complications using augmentation in reconstructive urology. Neuro Urol 1995;14:297–309.
[iv] Hasan ST, Marshall C, Robson W, et al. Clinical outcome and quality of life following enterocystoplasty for idiopathic detrusor instability and neurogenic bladder dysfunction. Br J Urol 1995; 76:551–557.
[v] Greenwell TJ, Venn SN, Mundy AR. Augmentation cystoplasty. BJU Int 2001;88:511–525.
[vi] Khastgir J, Hamid R, Arya M, et al. Surgical and patient reported outcomes of clam augmentation ileocystoplasty in spinal cord injured patients. Eur Urol 2003;43:263–269.
[vii] Quek ML, Ginsberg DA. Long-term urodynamics follow-up of bladder augmentation for neurogenic bladder. J Urol 2003;169: 95–198.

evaluation of these patients is the most accurate means of assuring appropriate care for their urologic issues. Future research efforts should focus on more promptly recognizing vesical dysfunction, as well as developing minimally invasive end-organ (bladder) treatments for patients with symptoms refractory to conventionally available medications.

REFERENCES

1. Koldewijn EL, Hommes OR, Lemmens WAJG, et al. Relationship between lower urinary tract abnormalities and disease related parameters in multiple sclerosis. J Urol 1995;154:169–173.

2. Lemack GE, Dewey RB, Roehrborn CG, et al. Questionnaire-based assessment of bladder dysfunction in patients with mild to moderate Parkinson's disease. Urology 2000;56:250–254.

3. Rapp NS, Gilroy J, Lerner AM. Role of bacterial infection in exacerbation of multiple sclerosis. Am J Phys Med Rehab 1995;74:415–418.

4. Khan Z, Starer P, Yang YC, Bhola A. Analysis of voiding disorders in patients with cerebrovascular accidents, Urology 1990;32:265–270.

5. Betts CD, D'Mellow MT, Fowler CJ. Urinary symptoms and the neurologic features of bladder dysfunction in multiple sclerosis. J Neurol Neurosurg Psychiatr 1993;56(3):245–250.

6. Razdan S, Leboeuf L, Meinbach DS, et al. Current practice patterns in the urologic surveillance and management of patients with spinal cord injury. Urology 2003;61:893–896.

7. Bodley R. Imaging in chronic spinal cord injury—indications and benefits. Eur J Radiol 2002;42:135–153.

8. Ukkonen M, Elovaara I, Dastidar P, et al. Urodynamic findings in primary progressive multiple sclerosis are associated with increased volumes of plaques and atrophy in the central nervous system. Acta Neurol Scand 2004;109:100–105.

9. Araki I, Matsui M, Ozawa K, et al. Relationship of bladder dysfunction to lesion site in multiple sclerosis. J Urol 2003;169:1384–1387.

10. Ghoniem GM, Bloom DA, McGuire EJ, et al. Bladder compliance in meningomyelocele children. J Urol 1989;141:1404–1406.

11. Defreitas GA, Lemack GE, Zimmern PE, et al. Distinguishing neurogenic from non-neurogenic detrusor overactivity: a urodynamic assessment of lower urinary tract symptoms in patients with and without Parkinson's disease. Urology 2003;62:651–655.

12. Kirby RS, Fowler CJ, Gosling J, et al. Urethro-vesical dysfunction in progressive autonomic failure in multiple systems atrophy. J Neurol Neurosurg Psychiatr 1986;49:554–562.

13. Vodusek DB, Fowler CJ. Clinical neurophysiology. In: Fowler CJ, ed. Blue books of practical neurology: neurology of bowel, bladder and sexual dysfunction. Boston: Butterworth Heinemann; 1999: 109–143.

14. Haferkamp A, Staehler G, Garner HJ, et al. Dosage escalation of intravesical oxybutynin in the treatment of neurogenic bladder patients. Spinal Cord 2000;38:250–254.

15. Pannek J, Sommerfield HJ, Botel U, et al. Combined intravesical and oral oxybutynin chloride in adult patients with spinal cord injury. Urology 2000;55:358–362.

16. Kim YH, Bird ET, Priebe M, et al. The role of oxybutynin in spinal cord injury patients with indwelling catheters. J Urol 1997;158:2083–2086.

17. Raes A, Hoebeke P, Segaert I, et al. Retrospective analysis of efficacy and tolerability of tolterodine in children with overactive bladder. Eur Urol 2004;45:240–244.

18. Bennett N, O'Leary M, Patel AS, et al. Can higher doses of oxybutynin improve efficacy in neurogenic bladder? J Urol 2004;171:749–751.

19. Stohrer M, Bauer P, Giannetti BM, et al. Effect of trospium chloride on urodynamic parameters in patients with detrusor hyperreflexia due to spinal cord injuries. A multicentre placebo-controlled, double blind trial. Urol Int 1991;47:138–143.

20. Pontari MA, Braverman AS, Ruggieri MR Sr. The M2 muscarinic receptor mediates in vitro bladder contractions from patients with neurogenic bladder dysfunction. Am J Physiol Regul Integr Comp Physiol 2004;286:R874–880.

21. de Groat WC, Kawatani M, Hisamitsu T, et al. Mechanisms underlying the recovery of urinary bladder function following spinal cord injury. J Auton Nerv Syst 1990;30:S71–S77.

22. Szallasi A, Blumberg PM. Vanilloid (capsaicin) receptors and mechanisms. Pharmacol Rev 1999;51:159–212.

23. Dasgupta P, Chandiramani VA, Beckett A, et al. The effect of intravesical capsaicin on the suburothelial innervation in patients with detrusor hyperreflexia. BJU Int 2000;85:238–245.

24. de Seze M, Wiart L, Ferriere JM, et al. Intravesical instillation of capsaicin in urology: a review of the literature. Eur Urol 1999;36:267–277.

25. Giannantoni A, Di Stast SM, Stephen RL, et al. Intravesical capsaicin versus resiniferatoxin in patients with detrusor hyperreflexia: a prospective randomized study. J Urol 2002;167:1710–1714.

26. Kim JH, Rivas DA, Shenot PJ, et al. Intravesical resiniferatoxin for refractory detrusor hyperreflexia: a multicenter, randomized, placebo-controlled trial. J Spinal Cord Med 2003;26:358–363.

27. Schurch B, Stohrer M, Kramer G, et al. Botulinum-A toxin for treating detrusor hyperreflexia in spinal cord injured patients: a new alternative to anticholinergic drugs? Preliminary results. J Urol 2000;164:692–697.

28. Reitz A, Stohrer M, Kramer G, et al. European experience of 200 cases treated with botulinum-A toxin injections into the detrusor muscle for urinary incontinence due to neurogenic detrusor overactivity. Eur Urol 2004;45:510–515.

29. Wyndaele JJ, Van Dromme SA. Muscular weakness as side effect of botulinum toxin for neurogenic detrusor overactivity. Spinal Cord 2002;40:599–600.

30. de Seze M, Petit H, Gallien P, et al. Botulinum a toxin and detrusor sphincter dyssynergia: a double-blind lidocaine-controlled study in 13 patients with spinal cord disease. Eur Urol 2002; 42:56–62.

31. Weld KJ, Dmochowski RR. Effect of bladder management on urologic complications in spinal cord injured patients. J Urol 2000;163:768–772.

32. Ord J, Lunn D, Reynard J. Bladder management and risk of bladder stone formation in spinal cord injured patients. J Urol 2003;170:1734–1777.

33. West DA, Cummings JM, Longo WE, et al. Role of chronic catheterization in the development of bladder cancer in patients with spinal cord injury. Urology 1999;53:292–297.

34. Fontaine E, Bendaya S, Desert JF, et al. Combined modified rectus fascial sling and augmentation ileocystoplasty for neurogenic incontinence in women. J Urol 1997;157:109–112.

35. Dik P, Van Gool JD, De Jong TP. Urinary continence and erectile function after bladder neck sling suspension in male patients with spinal dysraphism. BJU Int 1999;83:971–975.

36. Atan A, Konety BR, Nangia A, et al. Advantages and risks of ileovesicostomy for the management of neuropathic bladder. Urology 1999;54:636–640.

37. Leng WW, Faerber G, Del Torzo M, et al, Long-term outcome of incontinent ileovesicostomy management of severe lower urinary tract dysfunction. J Urol 1999;161:1803–1806.

38. Chartier-Kastler EJ, Mozer P, Denys P, et al. Neurogenic bladder management and cutaneous non-continent ileal conduit. Spinal Cord 2002;40:443–448.

39. Pitts WR, Muecke EC. A 20 year experience with ileal conduits. The fate of the kidneys. J Urol 1979;122:154–161.

40. Barrington JW, Fulford S, Griffiths D, et al. Tumors in bladder remnant after augmentation cystoplasty. J Urol 1997;157:482–486.

41. MacNeily AE, Afshar K, Coleman GU, et al. Autoaugmentation by detrusor myototomy: its lack of effectiveness in the management of congenital neuropathic bladder. J Urol 2003;170:1643–1646.

42. Leng WW, Blalock HJ, Frdericksson WH, et al Enterocystoplasty or detrusor myectomy? Comparison of indications and outcomes of bladder augmentation. J Urol 1999;161:758–763.

43. Husmann DA, Snodgrass WT, Koyle MA, et al. Ureterocystoplasty: indications for a successful augmentation. J Urol 2004;171:376–380.

44. Patterson RF, Lifshitz DA, Beck SD, et al. Multilayered small intestinal submucosa is inferior to autologous bowel for laparoscopic bladder augmentation. J Urol 2002;168:2253–2257.

45. Zhang Y, Kropp BP, Lin HK, et al. Bladder regeneration with cell seeded small intestinal submucosa. Tissue Eng 2004;10:181–187.

46. Atala A. Future trends in bladder reconstructive surgery. Semin Ped Surg 2002;11:134–142.

47. Reynard JM, Vass J, Sullivan ME, et al. Sphincterotomy and the treatment of detrusor sphincter dyssynergia: current status, future, and prospects. Spinal Cord 2003;41:1–11.

48. Schurch B, Hauri D, Rodic B, et al. Botulinum-A toxin as a treatment of detrusor sphincter dyssynergia: a prospective study in 24 spinal cord injury patients. J Urol 1997;155:1023–1029.

49. Hamid R, Arya M, Wood S, et al. The use of the Memokath stent in the treatment of detrusor sphincter dyssynergia in spinal cord injury patients: a single-centre seven-year experience. Eur Urol 2003;43:539–543.

50. Chartier-Kastler EJ, Thomas L, Bussel B, et al. A urethral stent for the treatment of detrusor striated-sphincter dyssynergia. BJU Int 2000;86:52–57.

51. Juan Garcia FJ, Salvador S, Montoto A, et al. Intraurethral stent prosthesis in spinal cord injured patients with sphincter dyssynergia. Spinal Cord 1999;37:54–57.

52. Wilson, TS, Lemack GE, Dmochowski RR. Urolume stents: lessons learned. J Urol 2002;167:2477–2480.

53. Brindley GS. The first 500 patients with sacral anterior root stimulation: general description. Paraplegia 1994;32:795–805.

54. Rijkhoff NJ, Wijkstra H, van Kerrebroeck PE, et al. Selective detrusor activation by sacral ventral nerve-root stimulation: results of intraoperative testing in humans during implantation of a Finetech-Brindley system. World J Urol 1998;16:337–341.

55. Kirkham AP, Knight SL, Craggs MD, et al Neuromodulation through sacral nerve roots 2 to 4 with a Finetech-Brindley sacral posterior and anterior root stimulator. Spinal Cord 2002;40:272–281.

56. Ruud Bosch JL, Groen J. Treatment of refractory urge urinary incontinence with sacral spinal nerve stimulation in multiple sclerosis patients. Lancet 1996;348:717–719.

57. Chartier-Kasler EJ, Ruud Bosch JLH, Perrigot M, Chancellor MB, Richard F, Denys P. Long-term results of sacral nerve stimulation (S3) for the treatment of neurogenic refractory urge incontinence related to detrusor hyperreflexia. J Urol 2000;164:1476.

58. Finazzi-Agro E, Peppe A, D'Amico A, et al. Effects of subthalamic nucleus stimulation on urodynamic findings in patients with Parkinson's disease. J Urol 2003;169:1388–1391.

SECTION 12 Neurogenic bladder

SECTION 13

Statistics

Statistical Concepts for Pelvic Floor Clinicians

Linda Brubaker

INTRODUCTION

This chapter highlights statistical issues relevant to researchers in female pelvic floor disorders. The reader should be aware that no single chapter could replace broad-based texts or coursework in statistics. Since most clinicians have limited training in trial design and statistical analysis, it is critical to identify a collegial statistician for assistance in these areas.

How does a researcher find a "good" statistician? There are a variety of individuals who call themselves "statisticians." Expertise may range from a PhD degree in biostatistics all the way to a heightened interest, backed up with as little as a medical school course. It is not unreasonable to review a CV and ask other research colleagues about their experiences with the potential statistician, especially to determine compatibility with clinician researchers.

Once the initial project meeting has been planned, a collaborative relationship has begun. Both the researcher and the statistician have special obligations to ensure effective communication because neither individual completely speaks the other's professional language. The researcher should be able to clearly present the project, patiently answer questions while avoiding excessive "doctor" jargon, clarify issues that are unclear, and carefully consider all statistical recommendations. The statistician should be able to clearly reiterate the primary aims of the study and the broad medical issues under study, assist the researcher with appropriate forms of data collection, generate sample sizes, and present a brief overview of the analytic plan. If each individual persists with his or her own language (clinicians in "doc-speak" and statisticians in "stat-speak") it is unlikely that clear communication will be established, creating a barrier to high-quality research.

In many ways, statistics is like surgery. It is imperative to know *when* to use a procedure and *which* procedure is most appropriate. Box 30.1 lists some "golden rules" for pelvic floor researchers to consider.

Box 30.1 Golden rules for clinical researchers

- Consult a statistician during the design phase of the research project (be sure to have data collection techniques approved by the statistician).

- Plan and revise the project aims very carefully.

- Select the optimal study design (usually in concert with other research colleagues and statisticians).

- Develop the study protocol (even for retrospective chart reviews).

- Maintain ethical research practices at all times (including compliance with all human subjects research regulations).

- Conduct the study in compliance with the study protocol.

- Complete the analysis according to the a priori analytic plan.

- Disseminate the results in a scientifically appropriate manner.

- Plan the follow-up study.

CONSULT A STATISTICIAN DURING THE DESIGN PHASE OF THE RESEARCH PROJECT

Clinical researchers are strongly encouraged to discuss all research plans with their statistician *while the project is in the planning phase*. Regrettably, the common scenario is that a researcher plans and executes a research protocol and approaches a statistician only after the data have been collected. Often such "statistical emergencies" occur immediately prior to meeting abstract submission deadlines. This is a dreadful time to discover that the study design is hopelessly flawed, the data are not amenable to formal statistical analyses or a data file is seriously corrupted.

The researcher should plan a presentation of the project for the statistician. It is often helpful to provide written materials to aid the statistician, especially if this is the first collaborative project. The presentation should include the purpose of the project, the stage of planning (hopefully early planning!), the proposed methods of the conduct of the study, the proposed outcome measures (how and when these will be collected), and the proposed timeline (e.g. before you graduate from residency, fellowship or before a certain abstract deadline date). It is important to confirm that both parties are at ease working together and have sufficient interest to complete tasks according to the proposed timeline.

PLAN AND REVISE THE PROJECT AIMS VERY CAREFULLY

Following the first meeting, the project aims are likely to be clarified. Most researchers underestimate the yield from reconsidering and redefining project aims. An initial idea may be simply stated as "determine which procedure is better." An improved revision may be stated in the standard null hypothesis format: "procedure A is the same as procedure B." Most clinical researchers actually believe that one procedure is better and that is why they are conducting the trial. This belief is phrased as the alternative hypothesis and the wording of this must be carefully considered. If the researcher believes that procedure A is better than procedure B, a one-sided alternative hypothesis is appropriate (A is better than B). If the researcher decides that this is the only clinically relevant situation, the statistician will be unable to test that procedure B is better than procedure A. Therefore, unless there are compelling circumstances for use of one-sided testing, two-sided alternative hypotheses are recommended by most statisticians.

Further revision of this hypothetic project may be stated as "there is no difference in the stress continence rates as measured by standardized cough stress test 3 months after procedure A or B." Compared to the first statement of the research purpose, this revised version allows the statistician to begin framing the analytic plan. Moreover, the research task is further clarified in the researcher's mind.

Clear concise statement of the research project aims is an important habit for researchers to develop. One technique for enhancing skills in this area is to write the first half of your paper prior to even meeting with the statistician. This assures that a proper literature review has occurred and will help the researcher answer the statistician's questions about rates of clinical events necessary for trial planning (e.g. how many people are incontinent following this procedure?). In addition, the proposed methodology is written out, forcing the researcher to carefully define the manner and method of data collection. Another major benefit is that the researcher has completed half of their final manuscript already, facilitating the final dissemination of the research work.

SELECT THE OPTIMAL STUDY DESIGN

Once the researcher has determined the research aims, the most appropriate study design should be selected. The statistician and other research colleagues can be extremely helpful participants in this process. If, for example, the researcher wishes to determine "which procedure was better," there are several study designs that could be used. The final design may depend on pragmatic issues, such as timing and funding. Another important pragmatic issue is determining the individual(s) who will actually do the research consent process, collect and analyze the data, and prepare the final study findings.

Conceptually, there are two main forms of studies: observational and experimental. Observational studies are generally less expensive and quicker to perform but limited by several forms of bias. Experimental studies tend to be more expensive and require more time but bias may be reduced if techniques such as randomization are used.

A common form of resident and fellow research is the retrospective chart review. It should be obvious that no form of retrospective chart review can be a randomized trial. Chart reviews should be conducted carefully because this type of research may provide important information for planning a prospective clinical trial. There are significant limitations to using data collected from chart reviews. These limitations can be minimized by carefully writing the protocol to ensure the highest data quality.

DEVELOP THE STUDY PROTOCOL (EVEN FOR RETROSPECTIVE CHART REVIEWS)

The study protocol is essentially a detailed explanation of your materials and methods. When the intelligent researcher puts their thoughts on paper giving clear guidelines for study completion, it is easier for others (coinvestigators, study nurses, other researchers) to understand the research plan. This is not as difficult as many novice researchers fear. It is essentially the "how to" manual for the study.

Creating a study protocol is essential for ethical human subjects research and obtaining high-quality data. Novice researchers may find it helpful to follow the format of a research colleague's study protocol, using the main topic headings and subheadings to individualize items to your specific project. Typical headings include background, hypothesis, aims, study population including recruitment, data-related issues (including the type of data that you plan to collect), an analytic plan (what you will do with the data), IRB and ethical issues (have you looked after patient privacy, are all risks to subjects disclosed, including possible breach of confidentiality?), and references. The protocol should allow an intelligent colleague to do your study if you were unable to complete it.

While you are developing the study protocol, maintain close communication with your statistician regarding data collection, data entry, and the analytic plan. Common mistakes made by novice researchers are virtually all preventable with a bit of advice from experienced colleagues. Data integrity depends on following the study protocol and safeguarding your data. This includes regular back-up of data files in a HIPAA-compliant manner. An early decision is whether you will enter data directly into the computer or instead use a paper form. Although we all like to think we enter data without errors, there is abundant research to demonstrate that there is an inherent error rate for all data entry procedures. Techniques such as double-data entry, read aloud and central data checking can minimize this error rate. Novice researchers who are doing their own data entry often enter too much data at one sitting, causing the error rate to rise.

MAINTAIN ETHICAL RESEARCH PRACTICES AT ALL TIMES

When you seek IRB approval, even for a retrospective chart review, you agree to an important role as a researcher. You agree to comply with institutional, federal, and even international regulations regarding human subjects research. These issues are not to be taken lightly. Learn to think of unconsented research like unconsented surgery. Most surgical researchers would never consider doing surgery without informed consent and research should occur in the same stringent settings—always voluntary, always with consent, and always with oversight.

CONDUCT THE STUDY IN COMPLIANCE WITH THE STUDY PROTOCOL

Once the appropriate plans and approvals are in place, the study should be completed according to the study protocol. Occasionally, the researcher must revise the protocol after beginning the study, but this should occur very rarely. The data collected must be entered and checked regularly. The data entry file should be backed up regularly to a separate server or disk drive. Paper forms should be duplicated and kept separate from other data. Although this may seem cumbersome, it is essentially the equivalent of keeping your money in a few different places when you travel internationally. If someone steals your wallet, you still have the stash from your suitcase or passport case! If your data forms get lost, you should have a duplicate in another place or have the data at least partially entered.

There are several simple methods of data entry, including Excel and SPSS. Learn to use one well. Once the data are correctly entered, check the data file for correctness. For example, you do not want to do an analysis of demographic characteristics of adult women who had continence surgery only to find that you have four study participants who are under the age of 10. Clearly, this is a data entry error and it must be corrected before you bring that file to your statistician.

COMPLETE THE ANALYSIS ACCORDING TO THE A PRIORI ANALYTIC PLAN

Once you have completed your study and have entered and cleaned your data, the fun really starts! It is time to test the hypothesis that you described in your study protocol. Work closely with your statistician so that you can learn at least a little bit about statistics with each study you do.

Typically the decisions regarding formal statistical analysis follow a series of steps. The first question is whether the data warrant statistical inference. When statistician testing is not warranted, the analysis is called "descriptive"; that is, no statistical inference is made. Many chart reviews should be used only for descriptive statistics because of the severe limitations and biases in these data sets.

Let's use an example. You have collected data on a new procedure that your group has started doing in the last year and finds very impressive (procedure WOW). You would like to review charts to see if the old procedure (procedure Pre-WOW) was really worse. After receiving IRB approval, you abstract all charts from women who had either Pre-WOW or WOW during the time-period specified in your study protocol. Demographics and clinical measures are carefully abstracted onto paper forms then double-data entered into your HIPAA-approved database. The data file is carefully cleaned and you are ready to do the analysis with your statistician.

Typically the statistician will first simply "get to know" the data file. What are the variables (data points), what is the range of these (for example, age range), and how are the data points distributed?

Frequency testing usually includes an assessment of the measures of central tendency. The spread of the data can be easily and quickly determined with these simple analyses. The most familiar test of central tendency is the *mean* which is simply the arithmetic average of a variable. Although this is commonly reported, it is often more appropriate to report the *median* which is simply the middle measurement. Let's assume for a moment that the following data set represents the number of incontinence episodes reported by seven different patients at the beginning of your study: 2, 3, 5, 6, 8, 27, 58. The mean of this data set is 17 whereas the median is 6. You can see that this data set contains two relatively large numbers. What if the data set were revised to "throw out" the subjects who had 27 and 58 baseline incontinence episodes? Now the mean is 6 and the median is 5. You can see from this simple example that the mean is very sensitive to "outliers" whereas the median is a more reliable report of the central measure. You can try this again by using seven subjects and changing two high numbers to numbers that are closer to the others.

There are other reasons to use the median instead of mean. One excellent example is when you are describing a woman's parity. It is clinically impossible to have a portion of a birth—a .2 parity. When you use the mean to describe parity, you often report a result such as 2.2 children. However, when you use the median, you report a clinically appropriate whole number. Many researchers are using this measure of central tendency for reporting incontinence episodes because, like parity, these occur in whole numbers and the median is less altered by extreme values.

Let's consider this concept further. Imaging your data set of baseline incontinence episodes again, let's assume your treatment improved only one patient—the one who had 58 incontinence episodes at baseline. She now has only 30 incontinence episodes (still by anyone's clinical judgment quite incontinent). You have the option of reporting the mean improvement of four incontinence episodes (data set of improvement = 0,0,0,0,0,0,28) or the median improvement of zero. Clearly the median is the most honest assessment of this data set. Small decisions like these are important to reporting the study findings in a scientifically rigorous fashion.

Researchers often include a measure of the spread of the data set. These measures include the range (from smallest to largest value) and the interquartile range (25th quartile to 75th quartile). These can be efficiently displayed using a box plot (Fig. 30.1). Be sure to indicate what is being displayed in the legend accompanying the box plot.

Other plots are also helpful during the initial phase of data exploration; the distribution of data points is typically explored with a scatter plot (Fig. 30.2). Scatter plots and histograms are helpful to determine preliminary relationships, prior to determining whether the data set is appropriate for formal statistical inference testing.

Following data exploration, it may be appropriate to perform a test of statistical inference. Just like a clinical diagnosis, one can never definitely *prove* something. As clinicians, we can only determine the probability of that diagnosis. Doctors typically think (even subconsciously) about the chance that this set of observations or findings could occur with or without that diagnosis. Similarly, the statistician is testing the data set to determine the chance of that diagnosis (the test statistic) given this set of observations and findings. The statistician and researcher predetermine the threshold for this at the start of the study. In clinical medicine, the threshold is typically set at 5% (more commonly seen as $P<.05$). This means that there is a 5% chance (1 in 20) that the test statistic could occur even if the hypothesis is truly incorrect. (That is, we say it is significant, we now believe and accept those clinical data, but there is always a chance that we are still wrong.) Most clinical researchers do not appreciate the simple fact that even the most optimally conducted research with highly statistically significant results could still cause incorrect conclusions.

Let's go back to the concept of a test statistic. This is "stat-speak." Every statistical test (t-test, chi-square, McNemar) is a mathematical equation that results in a test statistic (a number). These test statistics have difference letters—a t statistic, a z statistic, etc. After generating the test statistic, the statistician determines the probability of finding that

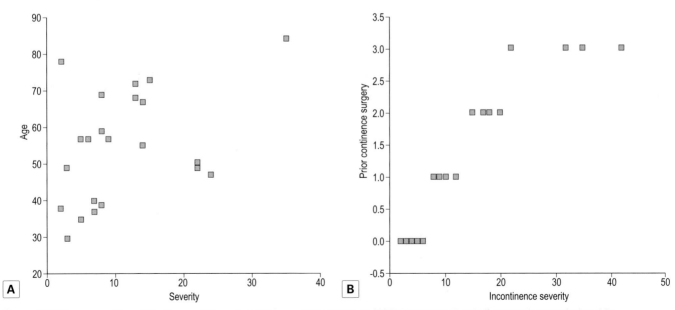

Figure 30.1 Several scatter plots (from artificial datasets) are demonstrated. (**A**) This scatter plot demonstrates no relationship whatsoever between the two variables that are explored together (age and continence severity). (**B**) This scatter plot demonstrates that as the number of prior continence surgeries increases, the continence severity worsens in incontinent women.

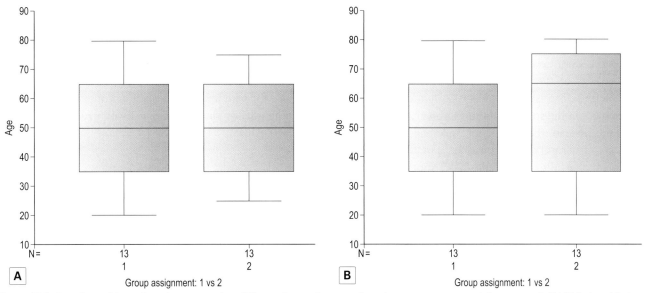

Figure 30.2 A variety of box plots demonstrating different issues in central tendency measures and data spread. **(A)** Side-by-side box plots demonstrating identical medians and means but different ranges. **(B)** Side-by-side box plots demonstrating identical ranges but different medians.

particular test statistic if the null hypothesis is true. If the probability of finding that exact test statistic for your data set is very unlikely, the statistician will recommend that you "reject" the null hypothesis. Unfortunately, that does not "prove" your alternative hypothesis.

Think about this in clinical medicine. You may get an imaging study and see a finding that really makes you think about a certain diagnosis. You therefore "reject" the null (there is no problem here—the patient is normal) and you begin to favor the alternative hypothesis ("there is an abnormality here—or even a particular diagnosis"). But you cannot *prove* that diagnosis (of course, you bright people are thinking of exceptions but try to stay with the analogy).

It is important to test the hypothesis that you stated at the beginning of your study prior to beginning other data analyses (also known as data dredging). Although there is a role for further analyses, there are also mathematical risks to this, including a problem statisticians call "multiple comparisons." Simply stated, this means that by doing so many tests, eventually one is bound to be positive. This also has a corollary in clinical medicine. Occasionally, you may see someone who is really a "worried-well" patient who requests excessive testing. The clinician's reluctance to perform so much testing is similar to the statistician's reluctance to perform so much testing; however, the statisticians have an advantage because they can mathematically adjust for multiple testing—clinicians are just left with a positive test in an otherwise healthy patient!

The statistician will generally recommend (and perform) a certain type of statistical test depending on the data set. The distinct types of data are important for the researcher to understand. Continuous data are something that can be measured continuously—imagine that you could measure to

an infinite number of decimal points. Age and weight are common examples of continuous data. Ordinal data are "ordered"—that is, there is a logical sequence. The stages of pelvic organ prolapse are ordinal: I is the lowest, followed by II, III, and finally IV. Why are these not continuous? There is clearly no stage of 2.2 or 3.7. Another important type of data are nominal. This is particularly important when performing the retrospective chart review. The name of the prior surgery (hysterectomy) or the name of the surgeon (perhaps you!) is nominal—"named." Most researchers convert nominal data to numeric data during data entry. But it is important not to use this type of data as continuous or ordinal. For example, imagine that you have coded race as 0=African-American, 1=Hispanic, 2=Caucasian, 3=Asian, 4=Mixed, 5=Other. Now the data set for your seven patients looks like this {3, 4, 2, 0, 0, 1, 2}. It clearly does not make any sense to report a "mean race." Likewise, these data points are not continuous; there is no such thing as a race value of 1.7. Neither are these data ordinal as there is no logical sequence for the order. So, although you have converted these nominal data to numeric data, be careful to always treat them as nominal data.

Researchers often wish to compare two (or more) groups. The means (or, better yet, the median) of two groups are often compared. For example, the mean blood loss between two surgical groups could be compared. There are certain criteria that the data set must meet prior to making these comparisons. The list of all statistical assumptions is beyond the scope of this small chapter but there are several important concepts that all clinical researchers must understand.

The concept of *independence* is critical. Many biomedical research articles have published analyses with obvious violations of this assumption. Fortunately, pelvic floor researchers have not significantly contributed to this problem. Imagine, however, a clinical researcher who works with eyes. He wishes to compare pretreatment with posttreatment eyesight. Both eyes are treated in seven patients. The research reports on 14 eyes (two from each subject). But subject 1's left eye is related to subject 1's right eye! Likewise for each subject in the study so these 14 observations are not independent. Instead, the researcher must use only left eye observations, only right eye observations, a randomly chosen eye, or a test that allows "paired" data. Another common example of paired data is when the patient is used as their own control—multiple observations

The concept of *normality* is also important. This is not the same as normal from a clinical standpoint, although there are some similarities. In statistical normality, two broad groups of tests are often used. The tests that require the normal (or near-normal) distribution of data include familiar tests such as the t-test. Another group of tests, "nonparametric," should be used when the data are not normally (or near-normally) distributed. *Almost always, nonparametric tests are more appropriate for pelvic floor researchers.* The inappropriate use of a statistical test that requires normally distributed data is just as incorrect as performing the wrong surgery (for example, putting in a sling for urge incontinence!).

DISSEMINATE THE RESULTS IN A SCIENTIFICALLY APPROPRIATE MANNER

Hopefully your manuscript was started (Introduction, Materials and Methods) prior to your data analysis. Now that you have completed your data analysis, you are ready to disseminate the results of your study. It is important to provide sufficient statistical details so that the audience can determine whether 1) the data set was appropriate for the statistical procedures that were performed and 2) the conclusions are supported based on the analysis. The statistical methods should always state which statistical tests were used for which variables. (Just as you wouldn't think of publishing a study that talked about surgery without saying which procedure!)

PLAN THE FOLLOW-UP STUDY

At the conclusion of the study, you have much more information than when you started. Now is the time to consider further studies. Is it important to plan a randomized clinical trial? You should be able to estimate effect sizes much better after your first study. Do you have an idea of how often complications or side effects occur? Do you know how often patients are followed up or drop out? What did you learn from performing this study? What would you do differently next time?

CONCLUSION

Statistics is an important topic for clinical researchers. Some individuals choose to remain completely reliant on their statistician. We know from clinical care, however, that the best communication is when each individual understands the main concepts but doesn't try to replace the other. Statistical collaboration is similar. Rather than trying to become a statistician yourself, it is preferable to start by learning how to communicate effectively, improve your skills, and be able to participate in the conversation.

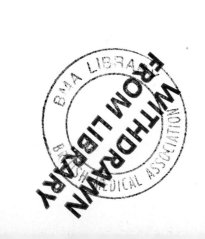